Hematology: Clinical Research and Advances

Hematology: Clinical Research and Advances

Edited by Cyril Goode

hayle
medical

New York

Hayle Medical,
750 Third Avenue, 9th Floor,
New York, NY 10017, USA

Visit us on the World Wide Web at:
www.haylemedical.com

ISBN: 978-1-63241-440-3

Cataloging-in-Publication Data

Hematology : clinical research and advances / edited by Cyril Goode.
   p. cm.
Includes bibliographical references and index.
ISBN 978-1-63241-440-3
1. Hematology. 2. Blood--Diseases. 3. Hematology--Research. 4. Blood--Diseases--Diagnosis.
5. Clinical medicine. I. Goode, Cyril.
RC633 .H46 2017
616.15--dc23

Table of Contents

Permissions

List of Contributors

Index

Preface

I am honored to present to you this unique book which encompasses the most up-to-date data in the field. I was extremely pleased to get this opportunity of editing the work of experts from across the globe. I have also written papers in this field and researched the various aspects revolving around the progress of the discipline. I have tried to unify my knowledge along with that of stalwarts from every corner of the world, to produce a text which not only benefits the readers but also facilitates the growth of the field.

This book provides significant information about hematology to help develop a good understanding of this subject and related fields. Blood cells are the cells found in blood and are produced by hematopoiesis. They are essential for the survival of all the living organisms. The three main types of blood cells are white blood cells, red blood cells and platelets. This text includes some of the vital pieces of work being conducted across the world, on various topics related to blood cells. This book elucidates the concepts and innovative models around prospective developments with respect to hematology. It will provide comprehensive knowledge to the readers. Students, researchers, doctors and all associated with this subject will benefit alike from this book.

Finally, I would like to thank all the contributing authors for their valuable time and contributions. This book would not have been possible without their efforts. I would also like to thank my friends and family for their constant support.

Editor

TCR Triggering by pMHC Ligands Tethered on Surfaces via Poly(Ethylene Glycol) Depends on Polymer Length

Zhengyu Ma[1]*, David N. LeBard[2,9], Sharon M. Loverde[3,9], Kim A. Sharp[4], Michael L. Klein[5], Dennis E. Discher[6], Terri H. Finkel[7,8]

1 Department of Biomedical Research, Nemours/A.I. duPont Hospital for Children, Wilmington, Delaware, United States of America, 2 Department of Chemistry, Yeshiva University, New York, New York, United States of America, 3 Department of Chemistry, College of Staten Island, City University of New York, Staten Island, New York, United States of America, 4 Department of Biochemistry and Biophysics, University of Pennsylvania, Philadelphia, Pennsylvania, United States of America, 5 Institute for Computational Molecular Science and Department of Chemistry, Temple University, Philadelphia, Pennsylvania, United States of America, 6 Department of Chemical and Biomolecular Engineering, University of Pennsylvania, Philadelphia, Pennsylvania, United States of America, 7 Department of Pediatrics, Nemours Children's Hospital, Orlando, Florida, United States of America, 8 Department of Biomedical Sciences, University of Central Florida College of Medicine, Orlando, Florida, United States of America

Abstract

Antigen recognition by T cells relies on the interaction between T cell receptor (TCR) and peptide-major histocompatibility complex (pMHC) at the interface between the T cell and the antigen presenting cell (APC). The pMHC-TCR interaction is two-dimensional (2D), in that both the ligand and receptor are membrane-anchored and their movement is limited to 2D diffusion. The 2D nature of the interaction is critical for the ability of pMHC ligands to trigger TCR. The exact properties of the 2D pMHC-TCR interaction that enable TCR triggering, however, are not fully understood. Here, we altered the 2D pMHC-TCR interaction by tethering pMHC ligands to a rigid plastic surface with flexible poly(ethylene glycol) (PEG) polymers of different lengths, thereby gradually increasing the ligands' range of motion in the third dimension. We found that pMHC ligands tethered by PEG linkers with long contour length were capable of activating T cells. Shorter PEG linkers, however, triggered TCR more efficiently. Molecular dynamics simulation suggested that shorter PEGs exhibit faster TCR binding on-rates and off-rates. Our findings indicate that TCR signaling can be triggered by surface-tethered pMHC ligands within a defined 3D range of motion, and that fast binding rates lead to higher TCR triggering efficiency. These observations are consistent with a model of TCR triggering that incorporates the dynamic interaction between T cell and antigen-presenting cell.

Editor: Marek Cebecauer, J. Heyrovsky Institute of Physical Chemistry, Czech Republic

Funding: This work was supported by NIH 1R21 AI087516, NIH 1R21 AI078387, NIH P20GM103464, the University of Pennsylvania Center for AIDS Research pilot grant (2-P30-AI-045008-11), the Children's Hospital of Philadelphia (CHOP) and the CHOP Research Institute, and the Nemours Foundation and Nemours Children's Hospital. The funders had no role in study design, data collection and analysis, decision to publish, or preparation of the manuscript.

Competing Interests: The authors have declared that no competing interests exist.

* Email: zma@nemours.org

⑨ These authors contributed equally to this work.

Introduction

T cells recognize antigens through the binding between T cell receptors (TCRs) and peptide-major histocompatibility complexes (pMHCs) at the interface between T cell and antigen presenting cells (APCs). pMHC-TCR binding triggers TCR signaling that activates T cells. T cell activation initiates T cell-mediated adaptive immune responses, which are responsible for pathogen clearance or autoimmune disease, depending on the source of peptide antigen. Despite its critical importance, it remains unclear how specific pMHC-TCR binding initiates, or triggers, a signal from the TCR in the first place. The mechanism of TCR signal initiation, also called "the TCR triggering puzzle", cannot be explained by classical models such as receptor conformational change or crosslinking [1,2].

A key feature of TCR triggering is the two dimensional (2D) nature of pMHC-TCR interaction. pMHC and TCR are anchored on plasma membranes and their movement is limited to 2D diffusion. The binding between pMHC and TCR, therefore, can only occur when the two plasma membranes are brought together through cell-cell contact and are closely aligned by adhesion molecules. The membrane-membrane contact, however, is not static. The T cell-APC interaction is dynamic and their relative motion inevitably applies mechanical stress to the interacting membranes and pMHC-TCR binding. Several models of TCR triggering have been proposed by taking into consideration certain features of the complex 2D pMHC-TCR interaction. The kinetic segregation model of TCR triggering, for example, proposes that the closely aligned membranes create steric barriers that segregate surface molecules based on their size [3]. The exclusion of large molecules such as tyrosine phosphatase CD45 from the vicinity of bound pMHC and TCR, which are both relatively small, initiates TCR signaling by creating tyrosine kinase-rich zones around the TCR. The receptor deformation model, on the other hand, postulates that the binding between membrane-anchored pMHC and TCR transfers mechanical forces associated with cell locomotion to the TCR/CD3 complex.

The mechanical forces deform the TCR/CD3 into a conformation or configuration that favors signal initiation [4,5].

The binding properties that determine the efficiency of TCR triggering should also be considered in a 2D context. The kinetics of 3D binding is largely determined by the overall binding activation energy and bond formation detail at the binding interface. 2D binding kinetics, on the other hand, is additionally influenced by factors such as ligand and receptor size, lateral diffusion rate, pre-aligned binding interface [6,7], and mechanical stress associated with membrane dynamics [8]. Studies on the relationship between the 2D kinetics of pMHC-TCR binding (on-rate, off-rate and affinity) and its signaling potential have started to emerge recently [9,10,11]. The results, however, have been highly inconsistent.

To delineate how the 2D nature of pMHC-TCR interaction contributes to TCR triggering, here we altered the 2D pMHC-TCR interaction by tethering pMHC on surfaces with flexible poly(ethylene glycol) (PEG) polymer linkers of varying lengths, and compared their effects on T cell activation. With increase in polymer length, tethered pMHC ligands have an increased range of motion in the third dimension. Thus, the pMHC-TCR interaction becomes more 3D-like. We found that pMHC ligands tethered with PEG polymers of up to 380 nm were capable of triggering TCR. The efficiency of triggering, however, gradually decreased with increase in linker length. Molecular dynamics simulation suggested that pMHC tethered with longer polymers binds its receptors with slower on-rates and off-rates. These observations are consistent with the receptor deformation model of TCR triggering.

Results

Tethering pMHC Ligands to a Surface with PEG Polymer Linkers

To tether pMHC ligands to a surface using PEG linkers, we first conjugated pMHC with a PEG polymer, then tethered the pMHC-PEG conjugates onto a plastic surface through biotin-streptavidin interactions (Fig. 1). To this end, mouse MHC class II molecule IEk with covalently linked moth cytochrome c (MCC) peptide (aa88-103) was engineered to have a free cysteine at the C-terminal end of the IEk β chain. The protein was expressed in a baculovirus insect expression system in secreted form and purified with affinity chromatography (Fig. S1A) [12,13]. The purified protein eluted as 50 kDa monomers in gel filtration chromatography (Fig. S1B). The protein was then conjugated with hetero-bifunctional polymer linker Maleimide-PEG-Biotin (Mal-PEG-Bio) through the reaction between the maleimide group of the PEG linker and the sulfhydryl group (−SH) of the protein C-terminal cysteine. Nine PEG linkers of different lengths with molecular weights ranging from 88 to 60000 Da were used (Table 1). In gel filtration, these polymers were eluted in the expected volumes and order (Fig. 2A). After the reaction, the mixture containing IEkMCC-PEG conjugates, unreacted IEkMCC, and unreacted PEG polymers was subjected to chromatography for separation (Fig. 2B). The three products of the reaction with mid-length polymers (PEG 3500, PEG 5000, and PEG 7500) were separated by a single round of gel filtration chromatography and the conjugate peaks were collected. For reactions with large polymers (PEG 15000, PEG 30000, and PEG 60000), the conjugates and the polymers could not be separated by gel filtration. The polymers were therefore first eliminated with an IEk-specific antibody 14-4-4s affinity column. The remaining IEkMCC-PEG conjugates and free IEkMCC were then separated using gel filtration. For reactions with small polymers (PEG 88,

PEG 484 and PEG 2000), gel filtration could not separate IEkMCC and conjugates, but polymers could be eliminated. In this case, the peaks containing both IEkMCC and conjugates were collected. The concentrations of those conjugates were calculated based on measured biotin concentration and the knowledge that each IEkMCC molecule can have at most one biotin. Any free IEkMCC in the mixture has no affect on the subsequent tethering step since it cannot bind streptavidin.

As shown with the gel filtration analyses (Fig. 2A), the hydrodynamic sizes of the polymers are much larger than those of globular proteins of similar molecular weights, indicating a relatively extended conformation of the PEG polymers in aqueous solution. For example, PEG 7500 was eluted with a similar volume to a protein with molecular weight of 44000 Da. Conjugation of PEG polymers significantly increased the hydrodynamic size of IEkMCC protein (Fig. 2B). Addition of a PEG 7500 polymer to IEkMCC almost doubled its apparent molecular weight, leading to baseline separation of the conjugates and unreacted IEkMCC. Consistent with their monomeric nature, the conjugates did not activate T cells when used in solution even at high concentrations (data not shown).

FRET Characterization of Surface-tethered pMHCs

IEkMCC-PEG conjugates, each with a biotin at the free end of the PEG polymer, were tethered on plastic surfaces covalently coated with streptavidin (Fig. 1). To analyze the average distance of IEkMCC protein to the surface, the efficiency of fluorescence resonance energy transfer (FRET) between DyLight 549-labeled IEkMCC and DyLight 649-labeled streptavidin was measured (Fig. S2). As shown in Fig. 3A, high FRET efficiency was observed between IEkMCC and streptavidin linked with the shortest linker PEG 88. FRET efficiency gradually decreased with increasing length of the PEG linker. FRET efficiency was no longer measurable when linkers longer than PEG 7500 were used.

The acceptor photobleaching-based FRET assay used here compares the fluorescence intensity of FRET donor (DyLight 549) before and after the photobleaching of the FRET acceptor (DyLight 649). The photobleaching step takes many minutes. Therefore, the FRET efficiency indicates an average distance between IEkMCC and streptavidin, rather than an instantaneous distance. The FRET results are consistent with the average shape of the PEG polymer as a sphere of Flory radius in an aqueous medium. Indeed, after normalization against the FRET efficiency of PEG 88, the measured FRET efficiencies of PEG polymers matched closely with the ones calculated based on the Flory radii of the polymers (Fig. 3B). It should be noted, however, that IEkMCC proteins are not fixed at a particular distance from the surface for each surface-tethered pMHC. Behaving similarly to an ideal chain [14], a PEG polymer is highly dynamic in solution. The IEkMCC protein can therefore be positioned at any distance within the contour length (fully extended length) of the polymer at any given moment. Taken together, the FRET data indicate that IEkMCC ligands tethered on the surface via PEG polymers behaved as predicted based on known PEG behavior.

T Cell Activation by pMHC Ligands Tethered to a Surface

To determine how T cell activation is affected by ligand-surface tethering by PEG polymers, IEkMCC ligands tethered to a surface with nine different PEG polymers were used to stimulate IEkMCC-specific 5C.C7 T cells. The surface densities of ligands tethered with different polymers were comparable when detected using the IEk-specific antibody 14-4-4s (Fig. S3). T cells were stimulated in ligand-coated wells for 6 hours, and IL2 production was measured by intracellular staining and flow cytometry. Dose-

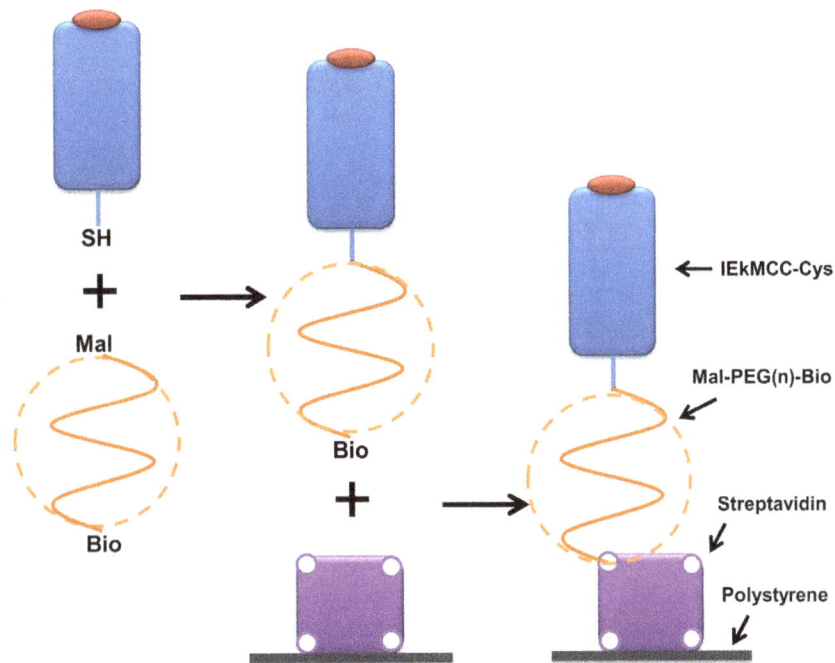

Figure 1. Schematic illustration of IEkMCC ligands tethered onto a plastic surface with PEG polymer linkers. IEkMCC proteins with free c-terminal cysteines were first conjugated with heterobifunctional PEG linkers Mal-PEG-Bio through interactions between the sulfhydryl group and the maleimide group. Conjugates with biotin at the free ends of the polymer were then tethered to a plastic surface coated with streptavidin.

dependent responses were observed for all linkers, as well as an inverse correlation between the percentage of IL2 producing cells and linker length above a critical size (Fig. 4A). IEkMCC tethered with PEG 88, PEG 484, PEG 2000, and PEG 3500 appeared to stimulate IL2 production with similar and high efficiency. Linkers larger than PEG 3500 showed a gradually decreasing ability to stimulate IL2 production, although IEkMCC tethered with the longest linker, PEG 60000 (contour length = 380 nm), was still capable of inducing low levels of IL2 production at high coating concentrations (>100 pM).

IEkMCC with the shortest linker, PEG 88, had the same efficiency as IEkMCC without a PEG linker but biotinylated at the lysine residue of a c-terminal AviTag sequence (IEkMCC-bio) [15] (Fig. S4A). This was expected, since PEG 88 has a contour length

of only 0.6 nm, or the length of about 5 peptide bonds (0.13 nm). Consistent with the dispensable role of costimulatory molecules in activating pre-activated T cells [16,17], addition of costimulatory molecule B7.1 to the surface did not enhance the ability of IEkMCC-PEG 88 to induce cytokine production (Fig. S4A). Addition of free polymers did not affect T cell activation by pMHC-bio (Fig. S4B). The maleimide group at one end of the free polymer was hydrolyzed to abolish its reactivity. The biotin group on the other end allows binding to streptavidin on the plate. T cells adhered well to plate surfaces coated with all IEkMCC-PEGs regardless of PEG length (Fig. S5). T cell adhesion may have been facilitated by binding to RYD sequences in streptavidin, which mimic the integrin-binding RGD sequence [18].

Table 1. PEG linkers and properties.

Linkers	MW (Dalton)	Number of PEO units	Contour length (nm)[1]	Flory radius (nm)[2]	FRET efficiency (%)
PEG 88	88	2	0.6	0.5	58
PEG 484	484	11	3.1	1.2	53
PEG 2000	2000	45	12.7	2.8	34
PEG 3500	3500	80	22.3	3.9	20
PEG 5000	5000	114	31.8	4.8	14
PEG 7500	7500	170	47.7	6.1	2
PEG 15000	15000	341	95.5	9.3	–
PEG 30000	30000	682	190.9	14.0	–
PEG 60000	60000	1364	381.8	21.3	–

[1]PEG contour length is calculated based on the PEO unit length of 0.28 nm in water [32].
[2]The Flory radius (R_F) of the PEG polymer of N subunits and unit length a was calculated using $R_F = a \cdot N^{3/5}$, where a is 0.28 nm.

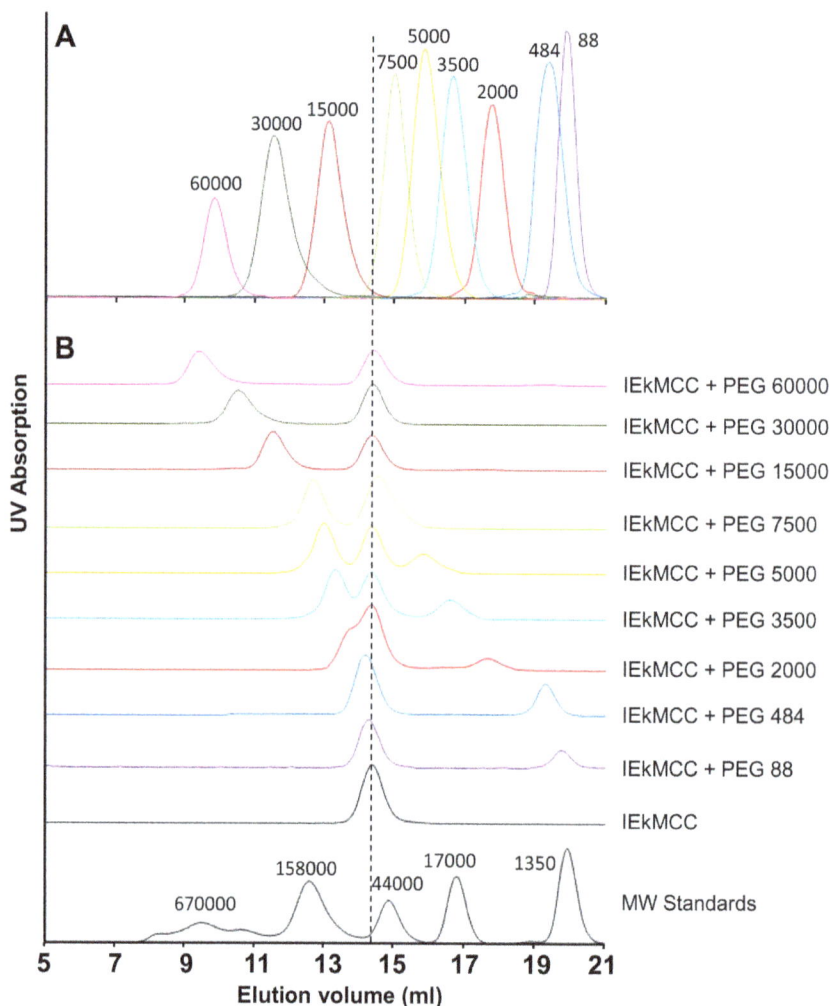

Figure 2. Characterization and separation of PEG polymer linkers and IEkMCC-PEG conjugates. (A) Compiled elution curves of nine PEG polymer linkers from a Superdex 200 10/300 GL gel filtration column. The polymers were detected through the weak UV absorption of the biotin group using a 245 nm UV detector. (B) Separation of the IEkMCC and PEG polymer reaction products. The reaction products were loaded on a Superdex 200 10/300 GL gel filtration column to separate IEkMCC-PEG conjugates, unreacted IEkMCC, and unreacted PEG polymers. The reaction products of PEG 15000, PEG 30000 and PEG 60000 were first purified with an IEk-binding affinity column to eliminate unreacted PEG polymers. The dotted vertical line indicates the elution volume of IEkMCC protein. The late elution peaks of unreacted polymers can be seen for PEGs ranging from PEG 88 to PEG 5000. In reaction with PEG 7500, unreacted IEkMCC and unreacted polymer formed a single peak that was eluted at a position between unconjugated IEkMCC and pure PEG 7500.

T cell responses to different concentrations of ligands at a given time point may not accurately reflect the relationship between T cell response and PEG linker length. It is possible, for example, that similar responses to the shorter polymers are due to saturation of the response at the time of stimulation termination. In other words, these polymers may have stimulated T cells to similar levels of response at a particular end point, but with a different rate. To explore this, T cells were stimulated with a fixed concentration of pMHC ligand and IL2 production assayed at different time points. As shown in Fig. 4B and 4C, the rate of T cells committing to IL2 production depended on the PEG linker length in a manner similar to that observed for dose response. Taken together, these results demonstrate that T cell responses inversely correlate with PEG polymer length, with the exception of PEGs smaller than PEG 5000.

Kinetics of TCR Interaction with pMHC Tethered on a Surface by Molecular Dynamics Simulation

To explore how PEG length influences the kinetics of pMHC-TCR binding, we carried out coarse-grained Molecular Dynamics (CG-MD) simulations to examine the binding *in silico*. As shown in Fig. S6, the interaction between PEG-tethered pMHC ligand and TCR on a cell surface was represented by the interaction between the free end of a fully flexible PEG polymer (with another end fixed in position) and a patch of DMPC lipid bilayer [19,20]. A weak binding potential mimicking the affinity of pMHC-TCR binding ($\sim$10 μM) was added between the free end of the PEG polymer and the lipid bilayer. Binding was defined as an event in which the mobile tail bead of the polymer moves within a 1 nm cutoff distance from any portion of the lipid bilayer. The PEG-bilayer system was simulated as a function of PEG length to examine how polymer length (chain entropy) affects rate of binding. PEG 4000, PEG 10000 and PEG 20000 were chosen

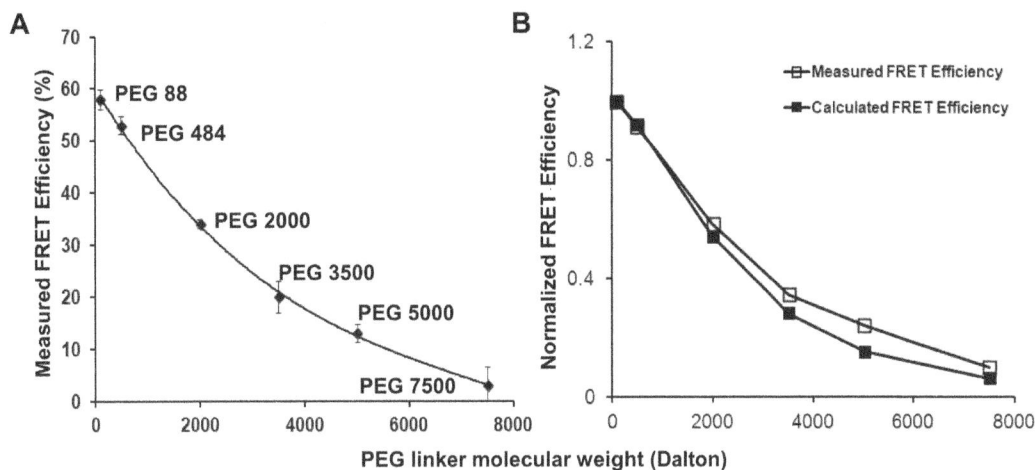

Figure 3. FRET between streptavidin on plastic plates and IEkMCC tethered with PEG polymers. (A) Measured FRET efficiencies of IEkMCC tethered with six different PEG polymers. The intensity of DyLight 549 was captured before and after DyLight 649 was photobleached. The measured FRET efficiency (E_m) was calculated using the intensity of DyLight 549 before (Ib) and after (Ia) DyLight 649 photobleaching ($E_m = \frac{Ia - Ib}{Ia}$). The averaged values of two measurements were plotted with standard deviations. (B) After normalization, the measured FRET efficiencies match those calculated based on the Flory radius (R_F) of the PEG polymers. The R_F of the PEG polymer of N subunits and unit length a was calculated using $R_F = a \cdot N^{3/5}$, where a is 0.28 nm [32]. Theoretical FRET efficiency (E_t) was calculated using the equation $E_t = \frac{1}{1 + (r/R_0)^6}$, where the Förster distance (R_0) of the DyLight 549-DyLight 649 donor-acceptor pair is 5 nm and the distance between the pMHC ligand and streptavidin r is R_F of the PEG polymer plus the pMHC radius of 2 nm. The FRET efficiencies were normalized by dividing the FRET efficiencies by the FRET efficiency of PEG 88.

mainly because of the clear PEG length effect on T cell activation in this MW range. Also, MD simulations of longer PEG lengths are unrealistic due to their long relaxation times (≥ 200 ns). Consideration of protein geometry was omitted to make the simulation feasible with available computational resources. While this simplification hinders derivation of absolute values for binding kinetics, the relative impact of polymer length on binding kinetics may be assessed. Details of the multiple-replica CG-MD [21,22] simulations accelerated by graphics processing units (GPU's) [23] are fully described in Text S1.

To assess the relative impact of polymer length on binding kinetics, we scaled the binding rates of PEG 10000 and PEG 20000 against the rates of PEG 4000. As shown in Figure 5, both the on-rate and off-rate of the binding decreased with linker length. The decrease of the on-rate is possibly due to steric effects of long polymers limiting access to binding sites, as shown in Text S1. The decrease of the off-rate with polymer length may be explained by the lower entropic force applied to the binding by longer polymers, since the entropic force of the polymer is inversely proportional to the length of the polymer chain. The decrease of overall binding rate with polymer length can also be justified in a conceptual context by considering the longer relaxation time of the longer polymers (Text S1). We also estimated the effective force applied to the pMHC-TCR binding from the CG-MD simulations using the potential of mean force acting at the most probable binding distance. Around 40 pN of force was applied by PEG 4000 and the force decreased slightly for longer polymers. It has been shown that 40 pN is large enough to initiate protein conformational changes [24,25]. Together, our CG-MD results suggest that the ability of tethered pMHC to activate T cells correlates with the rates of TCR binding. In addition, pMHC-TCR may sustain a significant amount of mechanical force derived from polymer entropic energy.

Discussion

To investigate how 2D pMHC-TCR interaction contributes to TCR triggering, we gradually increased the range of motion of pMHC ligands in the third dimension using flexible PEG polymers. Our approach differs from previous studies where pMHC or scFv of anti-CD3 antibody were fused on top of CD4 and other transmembrane proteins [26,27]. The TCR binding sites of these molecules are elevated from the cell surface at a fixed distance by the added protein domains. Their movement in the third dimension, however, still fully depends on the movement of the cell membrane. Therefore, these molecules still interact with TCR in a strictly 2D fashion. In contrast, pMHC ligands in our system are tethered to a surface through flexible PEG linkers. Although these polymers take on a spherical equilibrium configuration in an aqueous environment, their chain units move much more freely than the amino acid residues in a folded protein molecule. For instance, PEG 7500 and pMHC were eluted at similar volumes from gel filtration columns, indicating their similar hydrodynamic radii. When attached to a surface on one end, however, the free end of PEG 7500 polymer could be at any position within the contour length of the polymer ($\sim$48 nm) at a given moment, whereas the distal end of pMHC would stay 5 nm above the surface. On the other hand, it should be noted that the "free" end of the polymer does not diffuse freely like an untethered molecule. Its positional dynamics is determined by thermal motion, which will be affected by the chain entropy of the polymer.

The interaction between TCR and pMHC tethered to a surface with PEG polymers therefore must have characteristics of both 2D and 3D interactions. Ideally, their binding kinetics should be determined experimentally. This, however, is technically highly challenging and is beyond the scope of this paper. Unlike 3D interaction kinetics that can be routinely characterized with the mature surface plasmon resonance technology using commercially

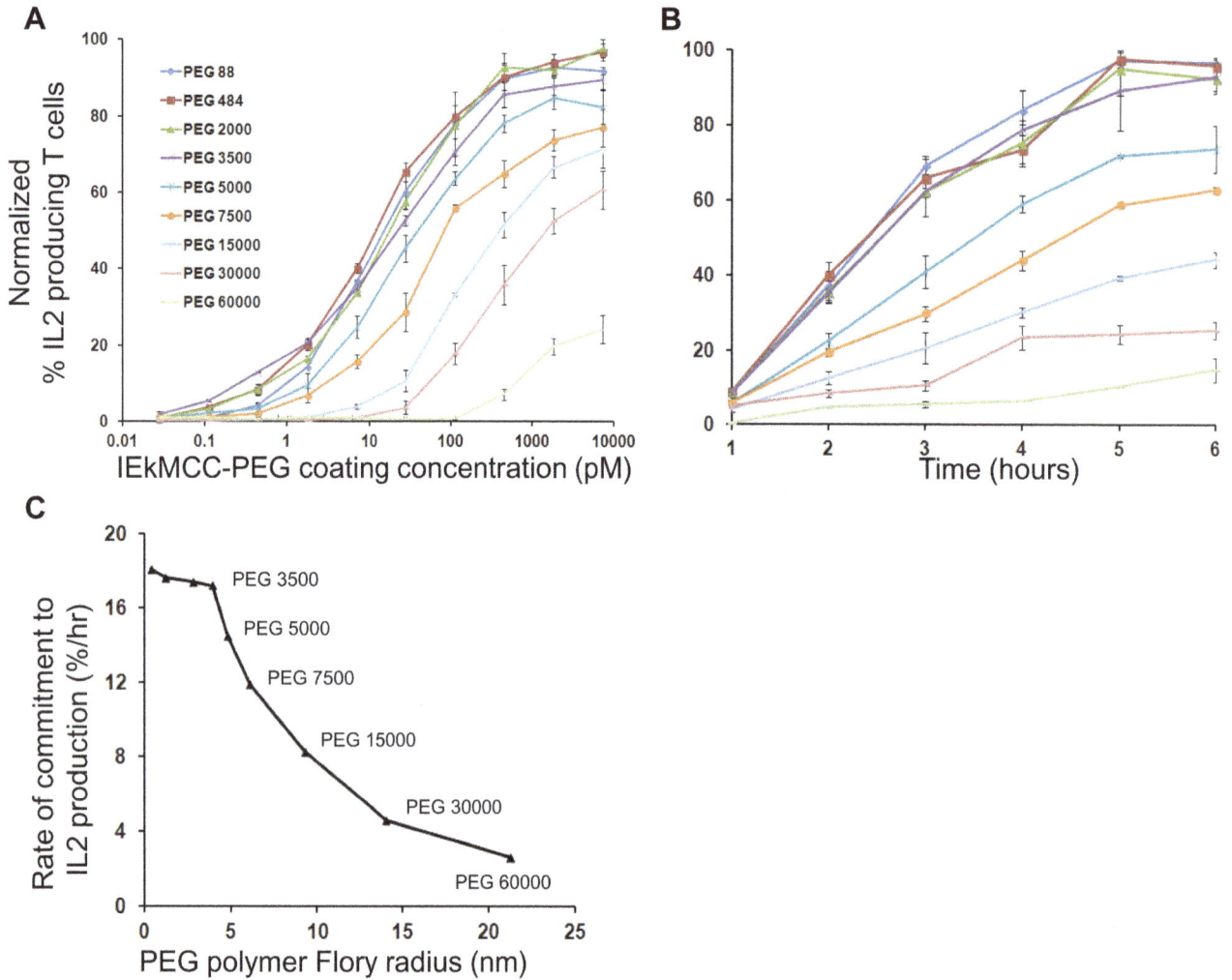

Figure 4. T cell activation by IEkMCC tethered with PEG polymers of different lengths. (A) T cell IL2 production in response to IEkMCC-PEG ligands of varying coating densities after 6 hours of stimulation. Data are representative of three independent experiments. The percent of T cells producing IL2 was determined by intracellular staining and flow cytometry. Three experiments using T cells from three different mice were performed (see Fig. S8 for flow cytometry plots). The percent of T cells producing IL2 was normalized to the highest value in each experiment. The data points are averages of the normalized values with standard errors of the means. (B) The rate of T cell response to IEkMCC ligands tethered with PEG polymers of different lengths. T cell IL2 production in response to stimulation on 96 well plates coated with 110 pM IEkMC-PEG ligands. T cells were harvested every hour for 6 hours and levels of IL2 expression were assayed by flow cytometry. Three experiments using T cells from three different mice were performed (see Fig. S9 for flow cytometry plots). The percent of T cells producing IL2 was normalized to the highest value in each experiment. The data points are averages of the normalized values with standard errors of the means. (C) The rates of T cell IL2 responses to IEkMCC ligands tethered with PEG polymers were extracted from the slope of linear fitting curves in Fig. 4B and plotted against the Flory radius of the polymers. The linear regressions and equations for deriving the rates are shown in Fig. S7.

available systems, such as Biacore, 2D kinetics characterization is still a developing field of research. Different methodologies often give dramatically different results for similar ligand-receptor interactions. For example, 2D pMHC-TCR interactions have been characterized using laminar flow chamber [9], fluorescence microscopy imaging [10], and micropipette and biomembrane force probes [11]. The 2D off-rates obtained varied from being similar to the 3D off-rate [9], to about ten-fold higher than the 3D off-rate [10], to a thousand fold higher than the 3D off-rate [11]. To the best of our knowledge, no attempt has been made to date to experimentally measure protein binding behavior in a system that tethers ligands on a 2D surface using flexible polymer linkers to better understand the parameters governing 2D interactions in T cell activation.

CG-MD simulation offered an alternative approach for assessing the influence of PEG polymers on pMHC-TCR binding at the T cell-surface interface. CG-MD simulations have proven useful for understanding complex molecular level phenomena including pMHC-TCR interactions [28,29,30]. The combination of state-of-the-art GPU computing and a CG-MD approach in our study enabled us to simulate nearly the entire range of PEG lengths to characterize the kinetics of pMHC-TCR binding. Our simulation setup is based on a robust model for the interaction between a free end of PEG polymer and the lipid bilayer, with a binding potential added to match the affinity of pMHC-TCR interaction. It should be noted, however, that certain assumptions and simplifications were required to make the approach computationally feasible. First, the physical dimension and geometry of the pMHC and TCR proteins were not considered. Second, a

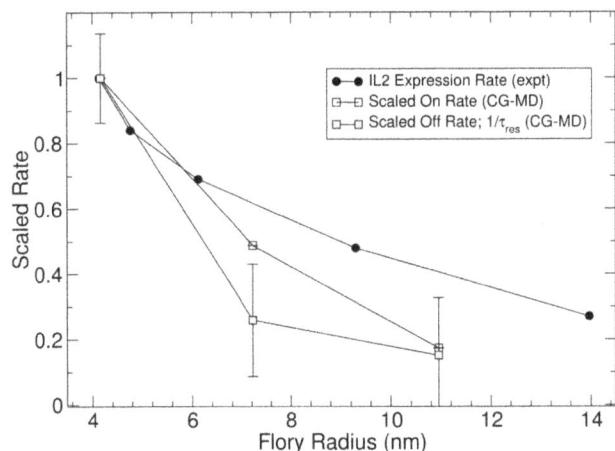

Figure 5. The impact of polymer length on pMHC-TCR binding kinetics based on CG-MD simulation. The on-rates and off-rates derived from the simulation for the PEG 4000, PEG 10000 and PEG 20000 were scaled against the data for the PEG 4000 and plotted as a function of the polymer Flory radius. To display the relationship between binding rates and TCR triggering efficiency, the experimentally determined IL2 expression rates for PEG 3500, PEG 5000, PEG 7500, PEG 150000 and PEG 30000 shown in Fig. 4A were scaled against PEG 3500 and plotted as a function of the polymer Flory radius.

binding event is arbitrarily defined as when the binding partners are within 1 nm of distance. And third, the distance between the two surfaces were fixed. With these simplifications, it is difficult to reliably derive realistic absolute values for kinetics parameters. The qualitative influence of PEG length on binding rates, however, may be reasonably assessed. The simulation showed that the on-rate and off-rate of pMHC-TCR binding decreases with the length of the linker. Also, the PEG polymer entropy applies a significant amount of force to the pMHC-TCR binding to better understand the parameters governing 2D interactions in T cell activation.

Our T cell activation experiments show that T cell responses to PEG-tethered ligands in terms of IL2 production displayed two distinct phases (Fig. 4C). pMHCs tethered by the four smallest PEGs, PEG 88, 484, 2000, and 3500, stimulated T cells similarly and with high efficiency. At this small MW range, the effect of PEG polymer dynamics is relatively small, and the kinetics of pMHC-TCR interaction is dominated by factors associated with intrinsic cell membrane dynamics. The relatively fixed "upright" orientation of pMHC ligands tethered with these short linkers may also play a dominant role in the kinetics of pMHC-TCR binding. In addition, we cannot exclude the possibility of TCR crosslinking for these short polymers, especially at high ligand density. Starting with PEG 5000, T cell responses gradually deceased with increasing PEG linker length. T cells responded to the largest PEG 60000 polymer, although only at high coating concentrations. In addition to IL2 production, we attempted to assay tyrosine phosphorylation using anti-phosphotyrosine antibodies and flow cytometry. The differences between ligands with different polymer lengths, however, could not be clearly resolved due to weak staining.

The results of our study are not consistent with the receptor crosslinking model or the kinetic segregation model. pMHCs tethered with PEG 2000 (contour length = 12.7 nm) or longer were able to trigger TCR. It is unlikely that TCR was triggered through TCR crosslinking by dimeric pMHCs. It has been shown that for activation through pMHC dimerized with linkers, the contour length of the linkers must be less than 10 nm [31].

Moreover, T cells were activated by low densities of pMHCs on a surface that would have only a small probability of forming dimers (Text S2). Our results do not support or disprove the co-receptor crosslinking model. Longer polymers might reduce pMHC potency by interfering with binding between pMHC and co-receptor. We think it is more likely, however, that the polymers interfere with the pMHC-TCR-CD4 three-party binding as a whole, given the closeness of the binding sites. The kinetic segregation model of TCR triggering relies on pMHC-TCR interaction at a tight space between two closely aligned membranes for the exclusion of large tyrosine phosphatase molecules such as CD45. In our study, pMHC ligands tethered through flexible PEG polymers such as PEG 5000 and longer should be able to interact with TCRs on relatively distant T cell plasma membranes. The gap between two membranes in this case should be able to accommodate CD45 and not cause its segregation with TCRs. Moreover, our CG-MD simulation results suggest that ligands with longer polymers bind TCRs more stably but trigger TCR less efficiently. This contradicts the kinetic segregation model, where TCR triggering depends on stable pMHC-TCR interaction [3].

Our results are consistent with the receptor deformation model of TCR triggering. In this model, pMHC-TCR bindings are pulled apart, or ruptured, by mechanical forces associated with the dynamic T cell-APC interaction. Before each rupture, signaling is triggered via the TCR through receptor deformation [5]. The overall triggering efficiency is determined by the frequency of rupture events, which is in turn determined by the on-rate and off-rate of binding. Higher rupture frequency facilitated by faster on-rate and off-rate translates to better integration of signals from multiple rupture events, thus, higher TCR triggering efficiency. While our work does not provide direct evidence for TCR triggering by receptor deformation, our simulation suggests that TCRs are subjected to mechanical forces derived from PEG polymer entropy. In addition, the experimental and simulation data show that pMHC ligands tethered with shorter polymers have higher on-rates and off-rates and trigger TCR more efficiently (Fig. 5). The correlation between binding rates and TCR triggering efficiency in our study is supported by a recent study that experimentally measured the 2D on-rates and off-rates of different pMHC-TCR binding pairs using micropipette and biomembrane force probes [11]. Furthermore, this study showed that 2D off-rates of pMHC-TCR binding were 30 to 8300-fold faster than the 3D off-rate [11], strongly suggesting that pMHC-TCR binding is under mechanical stress at the T cell-APC interface.

In summary, using pMHC ligands tethered to a surface with flexible PEG polymers, our study sheds light on the mechanism of the TCR triggering from a unique perspective. This approach of altering the 2D pMHC-TCR interaction should continue to offer valuable insights, in conjunction with methods to experimentally determine the kinetics of TCR binding to surface-tethered pMHC ligands.

Materials and Methods

Mice, cells and reagents

B10.BR H-2k mice and 5C.C7 TCR transgenic mice were purchased from Jackson Laboratories and Taconic, respectively. To generate T cell blasts, splenocytes from 5C.C7 TCR transgenic mice and irradiated splenocytes from B10.BR mice were mixed in complete Click's medium (Irvine Scientific, Santa Ana, CA) supplemented with 50 U/ml IL2 and 50 µM moth cytochrome c peptide. T cell blasts were used on day 7 to day 10 post stimulation. All animal experiments were approved by the Institutional Animal Care and Use Committee (IACUC) of Nemours/A.I. duPont Hospital for Children. All efforts were made to minimize the number of animals used and their suffering. Heterobiofunctional PEG 88 and PEG 484 linkers with a maleimide group at one end and a biotin group at the other end were from Pierce (Rockford, IL). All other heterobiofunctional linkers with longer PEG linkers were purchased from Jenkem Technology USA (Allen, TX). EDC (1-Ethyl-3-[3-dimethylami-nopropyl] carbodiimide Hydrochloride), Sulfo-NHS, TCEP (Tris(2-Carboxyethyl) phosphine Hydrochloride), streptavidin-Dy-Light 649, DyLight 549, and PBS (0.1 M phosphate and 0.15 M NaCl) were from Pierce (Rockford, IL). Brefeldin A, streptavidin, BSA (bovine serum albumin), MES (2-(N-morpholino)ethanesul-fonic acid), and APTES (3-Aminopropyltriethoxysilane) were from Sigma-Aldrich (St. Louis, MO). DPBS (Dulbecco's PBS) was from Invitrogen (Carlsbad, CA). 14-4-4s mAb was generated from a hybridoma kindly provided by John Kappler (National Jewish Health).

Protein Preparation

Plasmid construct for expressing the extracellular domain of IEk with covalently linked MCC peptide was a gift from John Kappler (National Jewish Health). For conjugation with polymers, the construct was modified by PCR to add a cysteine at the C-terminus of the β chain. Baculoviruses were generated with the construct and BaculoGold Linearized baculovirus DNA (BD Biosciences, San Diego, CA) in Sf9 insect cells (Invitrogen, Calsbad, CA). High titer stocks of cloned recombinant baculovirus were used to infect Hi5 insect cells (Invitrogen, Calsbad, CA) cultured in spinner flasks. IEkMCC protein was purified from the supernatant of infected Hi5 cell cultures using an affinity chromatography column conjugated with 14-4-4s antibody. The protein was further purified using a Superdex 200 10/300 GL gel filtration column (GE Healthcare, Piscataway, NJ) before conju-gating with PEG linkers. The design and production of IEkMCC with a C-terminal AviTag was described previously [15]. The protein was biotinylated at the lysine residue of the AviTag using BirA enzyme as described previously [15].

Conjugate Formation and Purification

IEkMCC-Cys protein was first treated with 0.1 mM TCEP for 1 hour at room temperature to reduce the sulfhydryl group of the c-terminal free cysteine. The protein was then reacted with PEG polymer at 1:20 molar ratio in PBS buffer pH 7.4 for 4 hours. For reactions with PEG 88, PEG 484 and PEG 2000, unreacted PEG linkers were separated from the conjugates and unreacted IEkMCC by gel filtration using a Superdex 200 10/300 GL gel filtration column, and the mixture of conjugates and unreacted IEkMCC protein was collected. The molar ratio of biotin to IEkMCC of the mixture was determined using a HABA (4'-hydroxyazobenzene-2-carboxylic acid)-based assay (Pierce, Rock-ford, IL). For reactions with PEG 3500, PEG 5000, and PEG 7500, IEkMCC-PEG conjugates were separated from unreacted IEkMCC and PEG linkers in one step using a Superdex 200 10/300 GL column. For reactions with PEG 15000, PEG 30000, and PEG 60000, unreacted PEG linkers were first eliminated using an affinity column conjugated with IEk specific antibody 14-4-4s. IEkMCC-PEG conjugates were then separated from unreacted IEkMCC by gel filtration using Superdex 200 10/300 GL.

Covalent Coating of Streptavidin to Polystyrene Surfaces

96-well strip well tissue culture treated polystyrene plates (Corning, Lowell, MA) were treated with 5 mM EDC and 5 mM Sulfo-NHS in MES buffer (0.1 M MES, 0.15 M NaCl, pH 6.0) for 40 minutes to add NHS ester to the carboxyl groups on the polystyrene surface. After washing, 100 µg/ml streptavidin in PBS pH 7.4 was added and incubated overnight at room temperature. The plate was then blocked with DPBS with 1% BSA. The amount of bound streptavidin was determined as 40 ng per well using an assay based on the quenching of biotin-FITC (Invitrogen, Calsbad, CA) fluorescence by streptavidin binding.

FRET Imaging and Analyses

For FRET imaging, DyLight 649-labeled streptavidin was coated on biotinylated plates (Pierce, Rockford, IL). IEkMCC-PEG(n)-Bio conjugates were labeled with DyLight 549 and coated on the plates via biotin-streptavidin binding. The bottom of the wells was imaged under a 60× water immersion objective on a Zeiss Axioplan 2 upright microscope. Using a 300 W xenon light source, we were able to achieve 95% photobleaching of DyLight 649 in about 5 minutes, and no photoconversion from DyLight 649 to DyLight 549 was observed (Fig. S2C). The intensity of DyLight 549 was recorded before and after DyLight 649 was photobleached. All images were analyzed with SlideBook software (Intelligent Imaging Innovations, Denver, CO).

T Cell Stimulation and Flow Cytometry

IEkMCC-PEG conjugates in DPBS with 1 mg/ml BSA were incubated in streptavidin-coated wells overnight at 4°C. Plates were washed, and 2.5×10^5 T cells in complete Click's medium were added. For IL2 production, 20 µg/ml brefeldin A was added to the medium. After stimulation, T cells were harvested, fixed with 3% formaldehyde in DPBS, permeabilized with DPBS buffer containing 1% BSA and 0.1% saponin, and stained with APC-labeled anti-mouse IL2 antibody JES6-5H4 (Biolegend, San Diego, CA).

Coarse-grained Molecular Dynamics Simulation

MD simulations were performed on the sticky membrane PEG systems, in which polymer length was varied from 4000 to 20000 Da. Multiple replica random-walker MD simulations were employed and run in the NPT ensemble using a GPU-accelerated CG model at a temperature of 300 K and pressure of 1 atm. Individual simulations were run for 500 ns each, and a total of 20 replicas were used per system, producing 10 microseconds of aggregate trajectory data per polymer. Details of these simulations and the resulting theoretical calculations can be found in Text S1.

Supporting Information

Figure S1 Characterization of IEkMCC proteins. (A) Purified IEkMCC protein with a free c-terminal cysteine was analyzed by SDS-PAGE and Coomassie Blue staining. The denatured protein migrated as two distinct bands with molecular weights consistent with the α and β chains. (B) Purified protein was analyzed by gel filtration chromatography using a Superdex 200 10/300 GL column. The protein was eluted as a single peak with a molecular weight of ~55 KDa.

Figure S2 Measurement of FRET between surface-tethered IEkMCC ligands and streptavidin on a plastic surface. (A) Schematic of FRET setup. The IEkMCC protein was labeled with DyLIght 549 (red star). The streptavidin on a plastic surface was labeled with DyLight 649. (B) Acceptor photobleaching FRET for linkers PEG 88 and PEG 7500. For the short PEG 88 linker, a significant increase in DyLight 549 intensity was seen after

DyLight 649 was photobleached. For the long PEG 7500 linker, only a slight increase in DyLight 549 intensity was observed after DyLight 649 photobleaching. (C) Photobleaching of DyLight 649 does not lead to photoconversion to DyLight 549. Streptavidin labeled with DyLight 649 (Cy5-like dye) was continuously imaged at both DyLight 549 and DyLight 649 channels with 1 s exposure time and 0 second intervals.

Figure S3 Similar densities of IEk-MCC tethered on plastic through PEG linkers of different lengths. IEkMCC-PEG conjugates at the indicated concentrations were incubated overnight at 4°C on streptavidin-coated 96-well plates. After washing, IEkMCC was detected using the IEk-specific antibody 14-4-4s and goat anti-mouse HRP.

Figure S4 T cell activation by IEkMCC-PEG 88 is independent of PEG tether, constimulatory molecules, or free PEG linkers. Streptavidin plates were coated with IEkMCC-PEG 88 or IEkMCC-bio (IEkMCC without a PEG linker but biotinylated at the lysine residue of a c-terminal AviTag sequence) at indicated concentrations. To test the effect of costimulatory molecules, plates coated with IEkMCC-PEG 88 were washed and further coated with B7.1-Fc fusion protein (1 nM; R&D Systems, biotinylated at 2.3 biotins per molecule). T cell IL2 production was measured by intracellular staining and flow cytometry after 6 hrs of stimulation. (B) IEkMCC-bio without PEG linker (7.2 nM) was anchored on streptavidin coated plates by incubating overnight at 4°C. Polymers (200 pM) were then added for 1 hr at room temperature. The PEG polymers were pre-incubated in PBS overnight at room temperature to hydrolyze the maleimide group. T cells were added to the washed plates and incubated for 6 hrs. Percent of IL2 producing cells was determined using intracellular cytokine staining and flow cytometry. The data points are averages of the values from replicate samples with standard deviations.

Figure S5 T cell adhesion to plates with tethered ligands is independent of linker length. T cells were added to plates coated with IEkMCC-PEG88, IEkMCC-PEG 5000, or IEkMCC-PEG

60000 at 7.2 nM. Cells were imaged 1 hr later using Evos microscope (Life Technologies) with a 20× objective.

Figure S6 Snapshot of the molecular dynamics simulation. The PEG-bilayer system was simulated as a function of PEG length (from 4000 to 20000 Dalton as shown in red) with a distance of 9 nm between the fixed end of the polymer and the center of the bilayer to examine how polymer length (chain entropy) affects both the rate and affinity of binding.

Figure S7 Linear regression trend lines and equations are displayed for Fig. 4B to show the rate of T cell commitment to IL2 production.

Figure S8 Flow cytometry plots for the three experiments done for Fig. 4A. At least 5000 live cells were collected for each sample. Note that in Experiment #1, IEkMCC-PEG 88 was not assayed.

Figure S9 Flow cytometry plots for the three experiments done for Fig. 4B. At least 5000 live cells were collected for each sample. Note that only three time points were assayed in Experiment #1.

Text S1 CG-MD Simulation.

Text S2 Calculation of the number of pMHC-PEG-bio bound to each streptavidin on a plastic surface.

Acknowledgments

We thank D. Shivers, Huihui Han and X. Zhang and for technical assistance and J. Kappler of National Jewish Health for DNA constructs encoding IEkMCC.

Author Contributions

Conceived and designed the experiments: ZM. Performed the experiments: ZM DNL SML. Analyzed the data: ZM DNL SML KAP MLK DED THF. Wrote the paper: ZM DNL SML KAP THF.

References

1. van der Merwe PA (2001) The TCR triggering puzzle. Immunity 14: 665–668.
2. van der Merwe PA, Dushek O (2011) Mechanisms for T cell receptor triggering. Nat Rev Immunol 11: 47–55.
3. Davis SJ, van der Merwe PA (2006) The kinetic-segregation model: TCR triggering and beyond. Nat Immunol 7: 803–809.
4. Ma Z, Discher DE, Finkel TH (2012) Mechanical Force in T Cell Receptor Signal Initiation. Front Immunol 3: 217.
5. Ma Z, Janmey PA, Finkel TH (2008) The receptor deformation model of TCR triggering. Faseb J 22: 1002–1008.
6. Dustin ML, Bromley SK, Davis MM, Zhu C (2001) Identification of self through two-dimensional chemistry and synapses. Annu Rev Cell Dev Biol 17: 133–157.
7. Shaw AS, Dustin ML (1997) Making the T cell receptor go the distance: a topological view of T cell activation. Immunity 6: 361–369.
8. Mempel TR, Henrickson SE, Von Andrian UH (2004) T-cell priming by dendritic cells in lymph nodes occurs in three distinct phases. Nature 427: 154–159.
9. Robert P, Aleksic M, Dushek O, Cerundolo V, Bongrand P, et al. (2012) Kinetics and mechanics of two-dimensional interactions between T cell receptors and different activating ligands. Biophys J 102: 248–257.
10. Huppa JB, Axmann M, Mortelmaier MA, Lillemeier BF, Newell EW, et al. (2010) TCR-peptide-MHC interactions in situ show accelerated kinetics and increased affinity. Nature 463: 963–967.
11. Huang J, Zarnitsyna VI, Liu BY, Edwards LJ, Jiang N, et al. (2010) The kinetics of two-dimensional TCR and pMHC interactions determine T-cell responsiveness. Nature 464: 932–U156.
12. Crawford F, Kozono H, White J, Marrack P, Kappler J (1998) Detection of antigen-specific T cells with multivalent soluble class II MHC covalent peptide complexes. Immunity 8: 675–682.
13. Kozono H, White J, Clements J, Marrack P, Kappler J (1994) Production of soluble MHC class II proteins with covalently bound single peptides. Nature 369: 151–154.
14. Rubenstein M, Colby RH (2003) Polymer Physics: Oxford University Press.
15. Ma Z, Sharp KA, Janmey PA, Finkel TH (2008) Surface-anchored monomeric agonist pMHCs alone trigger TCR with high sensitivity. PLoS Biol 6: e43.
16. London CA, Lodge MP, Abbas AK (2000) Functional responses and costimulator dependence of memory CD4+ T cells. J Immunol 164: 265–272.
17. Pardigon N, Bercovici N, Calbo S, Santos-Lima EC, Liblau R, et al. (1998) Role of co-stimulation in CD8+ T cell activation. Int Immunol 10: 619–630.
18. Alon R, Bayer EA, Wilchek M (1990) Streptavidin Contains an Ryd Sequence Which Mimics the Rgd Receptor Domain of Fibronectin. Biochemical and Biophysical Research Communications 170: 1236–1241.
19. Shinoda W, DeVane R, Klein ML (2007) Multi-property fitting and parameterization of a coarse grained model for aqueous surfactants. Molecular Simulation 33: 27–36.
20. Shinoda W, DeVane R, Klein ML (2010) Zwitterionic lipid assemblies: molecular dynamics studies of monolayers, bilayers, and vesicles using a new coarse grain force field. J Phys Chem B 114: 6836–6849.
21. LeBard DN, Levine BG, Mertmann P, Barr SA, Jusufi A, et al. (2012) Self-assembly of coarse-grained ionic surfactants accelerated by graphics processing units. Soft Matter 8: 2385–2397.
22. Levine BG, LeBard DN, DeVane R, Shinoda W, Kohlmeyer A, et al. (2011) Micellization Studied by GPU-Accelerated Coarse-Grained Molecular Dynamics. Journal of Chemical Theory and Computation 7: 4135–4145.
23. Anderson JA, Lorenz CD, Travesset A (2008) General purpose molecular dynamics simulations fully implemented on graphics processing units. J Comput Phys 227: 5342–5359.

24. Johnson CP, Tang HY, Carag C, Speicher DW, Discher DE (2007) Forced unfolding of proteins within cells. Science 317: 663–666.

25. del Rio A, Perez-Jimenez R, Liu R, Roca-Cusachs P, Fernandez JM, et al. (2009) Stretching single talin rod molecules activates vinculin binding. Science 323: 638–641.

26. Choudhuri K, van der Merwe PA (2007) Molecular mechanisms involved in T cell receptor triggering. Semin Immunol 19: 255–261.

27. Li YC, Chen BM, Wu PC, Cheng TL, Kao LS, et al. (2010) Cutting Edge: mechanical forces acting on T cells immobilized via the TCR complex can trigger TCR signaling. J Immunol 184: 5959–5963.

28. Cuendet MA, Michielin O (2008) Protein-protein interaction investigated by steered molecular dynamics: The TCR-pMHC complex. Biophysical Journal 95: 3575–3590.

29. Cuendet MA, Zoete V, Michielin O (2011) How T cell receptors interact with peptide-MHCs: A multiple steered molecular dynamics study. Proteins-Structure Function and Bioinformatics 79: 3007–3024.

30. Knapp B, Omasits U, Schreiner W, Epstein MM (2010) A Comparative Approach Linking Molecular Dynamics of Altered Peptide Ligands and MHC with In Vivo Immune Responses. PLoS One 5.

31. Cochran JR, Cameron TO, Stern LJ (2000) The relationship of MHC-peptide binding and T cell activation probed using chemically defined MHC class II oligomers. Immunity 12: 241–250.

32. Oesterhelt F, Rief M, Gaub HE (1999) Single molecule force spectroscopy by AFM indicates helical structure of poly(ethylene-glycol) in water. New J Phys 1: 6.1–6.11.

2

Lymphotoxin-LIGHT Pathway Regulates the Interferon Signature in Rheumatoid Arthritis

Jadwiga Bienkowska[1], Norm Allaire[1], Alice Thai[1], Jaya Goyal[1], Tatiana Plavina[1], Ajay Nirula[2], Megan Weaver[3], Charlotte Newman[3], Michelle Petri[4], Evan Beckman[2], Jeffrey L. Browning[2*¤]

1 Translational Medicine, Biogen Idec, Cambridge, Massachusetts, United States of America, 2 Immunobiology, Biogen Idec, Cambridge, Massachusetts, United States of America, 3 Global Clinical Operations, Biogen Idec, Cambridge, Massachusetts, United States of America, 4 Johns Hopkins University School of Medicine, Baltimore, Maryland, United States of America

Abstract

A subset of patients with autoimmune diseases including rheumatoid arthritis (RA) and lupus appear to be exposed continually to interferon (IFN) as evidenced by elevated expression of IFN induced genes in blood cells. In lupus, detection of endogenous chromatin complexes by the innate sensing machinery is the suspected driver for the IFN, but the actual mechanisms remain unknown in all of these diseases. We investigated in two randomized clinical trials the effects on RA patients of baminercept, a lymphotoxin-beta receptor-immunoglobulin fusion protein that blocks the lymphotoxin-$\alpha\beta$/LIGHT axis. Administration of baminercept led to a reduced RNA IFN signature in the blood of patients with elevated baseline signatures. Both RA and SLE patients with a high IFN signature were lymphopenic and lymphocyte counts increased following baminercept treatment of RA patients. These data demonstrate a coupling between the lymphotoxin-LIGHT system and IFN production in rheumatoid arthritis. IFN induced retention of lymphocytes within lymphoid tissues is a likely component of the lymphopenia observed in many autoimmune diseases.

ClinicalTrials.gov NCT00664716.

Editor: Sylvie Bisser, INSERM U1094, University of Limoges School of Medicine, France

Funding: Biogen Idec conducted, funded and provided infrastructure for these studies and had a role in study design, data collection and analysis, decision to publish, or preparation of the manuscript. The specific roles of the authors are listed in the authors contributions section.

Competing Interests: All authors except MP were salaried employees of Biogen Idec during the conduct of these trials. JB, NA, AT, JG, TP, JO, MW and CN report being current employees of Biogen Idec with an equity interest in the company. AN, EB and JLB are former Biogen Idec employees without equity stakes. MP has received consulting fees from Biogen Idec. There are no patents or marketed products to declare and the drug remains in use in a NIH sponsored clinical study in Sjogren's disease.

* Email: browninj@bu.edu

¤ Current address: Department of Microbiology and Section of Rheumatology, Boston University School of Medicine, Boston, Massachusetts, United States of America

Introduction

Systemic lupus erythematosus (SLE), rheumatoid arthritis (RA), Sjogren's syndrome, systemic sclerosis, myositis and multiple sclerosis patients have circulating blood cells with elevated levels of RNA from IFN-induced genes, i.e. an 'IFN signature' [1–3]. A number of observations point towards a role for IFN in some autoimmune diseases. Notably, risk alleles for SLE include several genes involved in IFN responses. Multiple immunological activities are enhanced by IFN and rodent models of lupus can be accelerated by exogenous IFN. Several rare diseases with lupus-like aspects have mutations in components of the IFN response and are termed 'interferonopathies' [4]. Thus, there is very active interest in whether inhibition of IFN signaling has therapeutic benefit [5]. However, the questions of whether the IFN signature is tightly coupled to the pathology in human disease, which immunological detection systems are engaged and what are the actual cellular sources of the IFN, remain unanswered. Moreover, type I (IFN-α, β, ϵ, τ and ω), type II (IFN-γ) and type III (IFN-λ) IFNs can induce similar patterns of gene expression despite being

produced by different spectra of cell types and being under fundamentally different regulation. The varying distribution of receptors for each IFN type also dictates responsive populations and these aspects further confound the problem.

We have investigated the effects of inhibition of the lymphotoxin-LIGHT system in RA using a soluble lymphotoxin-beta receptor (LTBR, TNFRSF3) immunoglobulin fusion protein called baminercept. LTBR is a central component of a signaling system whereby lymphocytes instruct stromal cells to differentiate into specialized vasculature and certain reticular networks [6–9]. These components form the gateways for lymphocyte entry into organized lymphoid tissues and the reticular scaffolds that guide and position cells for optimal encounters with antigen. As such, adaptive immune responses within the lymphoid organs are impaired to varying degrees in the absence of LTBR signaling. Additionally, the differentiation of critical sentinel macrophages in the subcapsular sinus of the lymph node (LN) and the splenic marginal zone depend on LTBR signaling [10]. More recently, it has become clear that LTBR signaling is interwoven with aspects of myeloid cell homeostasis as well as more innate elements of the immune system such as communication between dendritic cells, innate lymphoid cells and epithelial surfaces especially in mucosal environments [11–15]. Baminercept binds to both LTBR ligands, namely, a membrane bound heterotrimeric lymphotoxin (LT) form LTα1β2 and the ligand called LIGHT (TNFSF14). LIGHT interacts with both LTBR and an additional receptor called HVEM (TNFRSF14) and it has pro-inflammatory roles as well being implicated in aspects of T cell survival [16]. Therefore, baminercept is a dual pathway inhibitor blocking signaling triggered by both membrane LT and LIGHT ligands.

Unexpectedly, we found that baminercept reduced the IFN signature in RA patients. The reduced IFN signature in RA patients following baminercept treatment is the first time outside of high dose steroid therapy that an IFN signature was decreased by a pharmacological treatment not targeting IFN itself. Taken together with the known effects of LTBR inhibition, these studies not only link the LTBR axis to IFN production in man, but also provide potential insight into the nature of the IFN signature.

Results

Baminercept reduces the IFN signature in RA patients

Two randomized phase IIb controlled studies of the effects of baminercept in rheumatoid arthritis were conducted. One study enrolled patients with an inadequate response to disease-modifying antirheumatic drug therapy (DMARD-IR) and the other involved patients with an inadequate response to tumor necrosis factor inhibition (TNF-IR) (flow diagrams Figure 1, patient demographics defined in Supplemental Table 1 in File S1). To examine whether baminercept treatment had an impact on the immune system, the transcriptional profiles of whole blood RNA from all RA patients at 0 and 14 weeks were assessed using Affymetrix microarrays. An unsupervised analysis revealed multiple drug-induced changes that fell into three major clusters. First baminercept treatment led to an increased B cell signature. Second, patients with elevated expression at baseline of a collection of IFN response genes had the signature decreased by baminercept treatment and, third, expression of some genes associated with NK cells were decreased following treatment.

At baseline, roughly 25% of the RA patients in both the DMARD-IR and TNF-IR groups had a high IFN signature (Figure 2) and a 15-gene IFN score was calculated from the genes shown in Figure 2 (Supplemental Table 2 in File S1). Many IFN response gene sets and scores have been utilized in the literature including other sets reported by our group [17]. In general, we found similar results regardless of the selected genes. The IFN signature has been best characterized in SLE and for comparison a control cohort of 292 SLE patients from the Johns Hopkins clinic was analyzed using an identical platform. As expected about 50% of the SLE patients had an elevated IFN signature and the IFN signature in RA patients was slightly weaker than in SLE consistent with a previous study (Supplemental Figure 1 in File S1) [1,3]. Therefore, in terms of the IFN signature, the RA patients in these studies compare favorably to previous analyses.

We divided the patients from the TNF-IR study into four groups- placebo and baminercept treated with baseline low or high IFN signature scores. Figure 3 shows a heat map of the expression changes after 14 weeks for all the genes identified in the unsupervised analysis. There was a general increase in a wide range of B cell associated genes, yet interestingly, IgA1 and IgG3 expression decreased. Baminercept can disrupt follicular dendritic cell networks and germinal center reactions and perhaps this decrease reflects impaired class switching and reduced numbers of

circulating B cells or plasma cells expressing these immunoglobulins. The second cluster of genes is comprised of genes induced by IFN. Patients with a baseline high IFN score displayed substantial decreases in the IFN score following treatment. The third cluster contains multiple NK related genes and these often decreased following baminercept treatment.

To further document the IFN signature, the expression of three IFN stimulated genes, Ly6E, ISG15 and OAS1 was determined by quantitative PCR (qPCR) and an IFN score calculated (Supplemental Table 2 in File S1). The qPCR and microarray scores correlated well (Figure 4a). Figure 4b shows the change in the TNF-IR study following 14 weeks of placebo or baminercept treatment in the 3-gene PCR based IFN score as a function of the pre-treatment IFN score. This analysis revealed a significant interaction between the pre-treatment IFN and treatment, interaction p value $= 2 \times 10^{-7}$. A substantial reduction in the IFN signature was also observed at 6 weeks. To extend this observation, the 3-gene qPCR IFN signature was determined for patients in DMARD-IR study. Patients were binned into baseline IFN^{high} and IFN^{low} groups based on the 3-gene qPCR IFN score of greater or less than one. The DMARD-IR study had 6 treatment cohorts and only the 70 and 200 mg q2w cohorts were analyzed by qPCR. Baminercept treatment led to a trend towards a reduced IFN signature in both cohorts and combining the two cohorts showed significant reduction (Figure 4c). The biomarker data indicated approximate saturation of the pharmacodynamic response in both these cohorts justifying combining the data (see below and serum LIGHT measurements Supplemental Figure 2 in File S1). We questioned whether the incidence of infectious events could impact the observation and there was little indication that infection rates were substantially increased or decreased following baminercept treatment (Supplemental Table 3 in File S1). Since baminercept potentially dampens the immune system, an increased rate of infection was possible and therefore treatment could have increased the IFN signature. As an increased IFN signature was not observed, infection is not a likely confounder for this result.

To validate further the ability of baminercept treatment to affect an IFN signature, we examined by qPCR the expression of SIGLEC1, another IFN induced gene. In contrast to the genes in the 3-gene panel, it is expressed exclusively in monocytes and, moreover, it is a potential marker of SLE disease severity [18]. Analysis of the SIGLEC1 RNA expression using the qPCR data showed that SIGLEC1 expression was elevated in the IFN high group and baminercept treatment reduced its expression confirming the 3-gene signature analysis (Figure 5a,b). Expression (qPCR) of genes specific for monocytes (SLAMF7, SPARC), DC (CD1E) and plasmacytoid DC (pDC) (CLEC4C and LILRA4) was independent of IFN status.

There is considerable overlap in the expression profiles resulting from type 1 (IFNs α, β and ω) and type II IFN (IFNγ) and, furthermore, each IFN is capable in many contexts of inducing the expression of the other IFN class [19]. An 8 gene IFNγ signature was defined based on genes preferentially induced in blood cells by IFNγ [20]. In our data, there was no significant correlation between the basic IFN and IFNγ signatures suggesting that type I IFNs are dominating in RA (Supplemental Figure 3 in File S1). Two genes, GBP1 and GBP2, were induced selectively by IFNγ in salivary gland epithelial cells, yet in our blood data the GBP1/2 score correlated very well with the basic IFN signature (Supplemental Figure 3 in File S1). In other studies, the GBP1/2 genes are induced by type I IFN in blood cells both in vitro and in vivo in IFN treated hepatitis C and melanoma patients. Our data are consistent with exposure to type I IFN in RA.

RA203 "TNF-IR" Flow Diagram

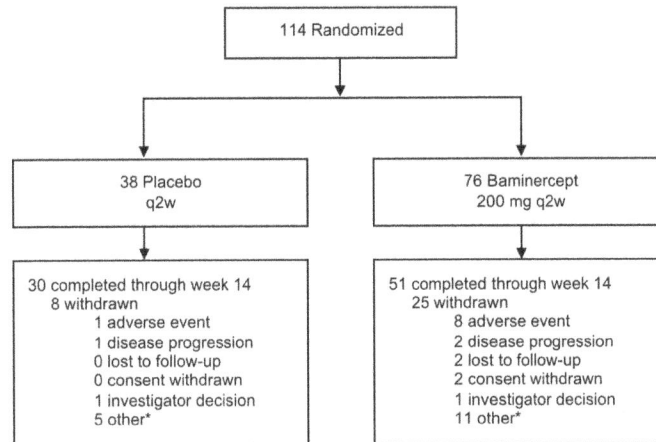

114 Randomized

38 Placebo
q2w

76 Baminercept
200 mg q2w

30 completed through week 14
8 withdrawn
  1 adverse event
  1 disease progression
  0 lost to follow-up
  0 consent withdrawn
  1 investigator decision
  5 other*

51 completed through week 14
25 withdrawn
  8 adverse event
  2 disease progression
  2 lost to follow-up
  2 consent withdrawn
  1 investigator decision
  11 other*

*Trial was stopped early due to failed primary endpoint in the parallel RA202 study, hence high discontinuation rate relative to the RA202.

RA202 "DMARD-IR" Flow Diagram

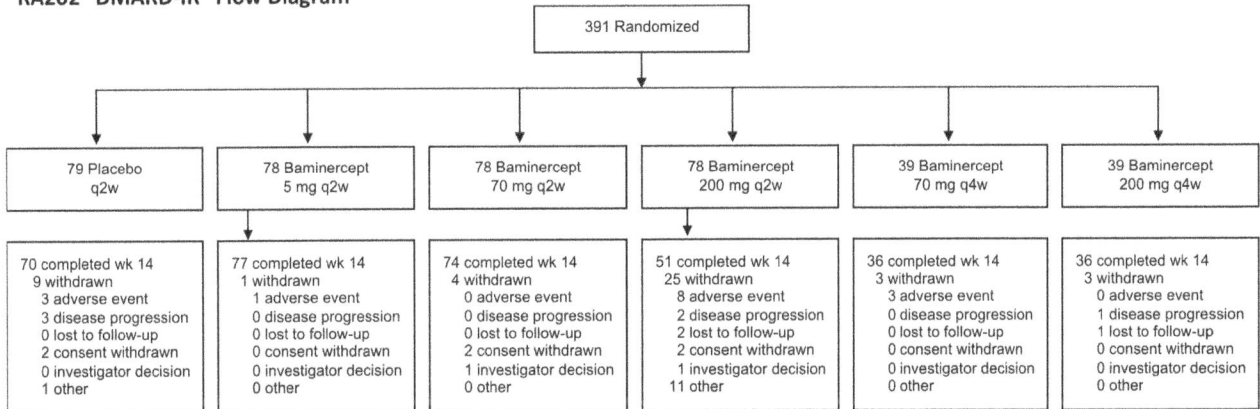

391 Randomized

79 Placebo q2w	78 Baminercept 5 mg q2w	78 Baminercept 70 mg q2w	78 Baminercept 200 mg q2w	39 Baminercept 70 mg q4w	39 Baminercept 200 mg q4w
70 completed wk 14	77 completed wk 14	74 completed wk 14	51 completed wk 14	36 completed wk 14	36 completed wk 14
9 withdrawn	1 withdrawn	4 withdrawn	25 withdrawn	3 withdrawn	3 withdrawn
3 adverse event	1 adverse event	0 adverse event	8 adverse event	3 adverse event	0 adverse event
3 disease progression	0 disease progression	0 disease progression	2 disease progression	0 disease progression	1 disease progression
0 lost to follow-up	0 lost to follow-up	0 lost to follow-up	2 lost to follow-up	0 lost to follow-up	1 lost to follow-up
2 consent withdrawn	0 consent withdrawn	2 consent withdrawn	2 consent withdrawn	0 consent withdrawn	0 consent withdrawn
0 investigator decision	0 investigator decision	1 investigator decision	1 investigator decision	0 investigator decision	0 investigator decision
1 other	0 other	0 other	11 other	0 other	0 other

Figure 1. Flow diagrams for the two clinical trials assessing the effects of baminercept treatment on rheumatoid arthritis patients.

Elevated levels of type I IFN or an IFN-like inducing activity can be found in the sera of a subset of the SLE patients with a transcriptional IFN signature; however, in RA the results range from not detectable to low levels relative to SLE sera [21,22]. We examined serum IFN levels using highly sensitive A549 (more type I IFN selective) or WISH (similar sensitivity to type I and II IFN) cell based reporter assays with an ELISA-based Mx1 protein readout. Analysis of 64 baseline sera from the TNF-IR study including all of the patients with elevated baseline IFN signatures did not reveal IFN activity, whereas substantial activity was readily found in the sera from some SLE patients. Therefore, the blood RNA IFN signature in RA is likely derived from local exposure in organs to IFN.

IFN signature is associated with lymphopenia in both RA and SLE

SLE patients with a high IFN signature tend to be lymphopenic [23]. Using the 15 gene microarray-based IFN signature to group patients at baseline into a high or low IFN status, we observed that both IFN high RA and SLE patients were lymphopenic (Figure 6a). The degree of lymphopenia in IFN high RA patients was not as pronounced as in the comparable SLE group possibly paralleling the relative intensities of the IFN signatures in these two diseases.

In rodents, blockade of the LTBR system leads to lymphocytosis within several weeks most likely due to loss of high endothelial venule addressin expression and reduced entry into the lymph nodes and mucosal environments [24]. Treatment with baminercept led to increased lymphocyte and monocyte counts in the blood of patients with full effect observed within 2–5 weeks (Figure 6b and Supplemental Figures 4 and 5 in File S1). The 5 mg q2w dose was partially active and similar results were seen with both the 70 and 200 mg q2w doses indicating approximate saturation. It is believed that one driver for lymphopenia in SLE may be chronic IFN exposure and prolonged lymphocyte retention within the lymph nodes [25]. To assess whether reduced IFN exposure could contribute to the baminercept induced lymphocytosis, we compared the change in lymphocyte counts in the IFN low and high subsets. Lymphocyte counts increased in both groups following baminercept treatment; however, the magnitude of the change was greater in much of the IFN high subset in the TNF-IR study and trended higher in DMARD-IR

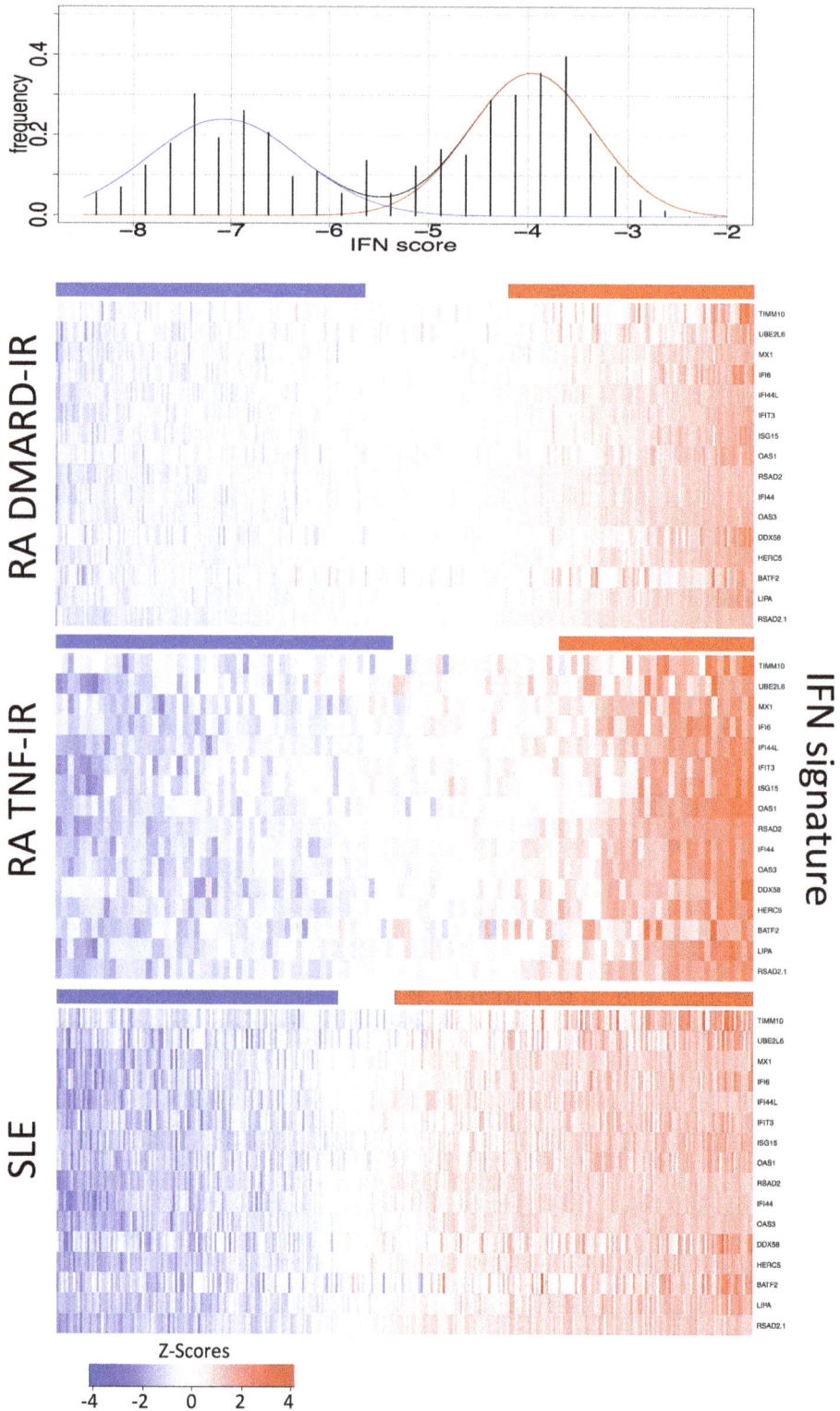

Figure 2. Comparison of the IFN signature in DMARD-IR and TNF-IR RA patients. Baseline heat maps of the RA DMARD-IR, TNF-IR and the SLE cohorts studied in this work. Red indicates increased expression of a panel of 15 IFN inducible genes showing similar percentages of IFN signature positive patients in each RA subgroup (the gene RSAD2 is represented twice). Bars above each map show the clustering as IFN positive (red) or negative (blue) based on assignment to two normal distributions as shown in the top panel with p<0.05. Color bar ranges are as stated for SLE and DMARD-IR, but −3 to 3 for TNF-IR (as per figure 3).

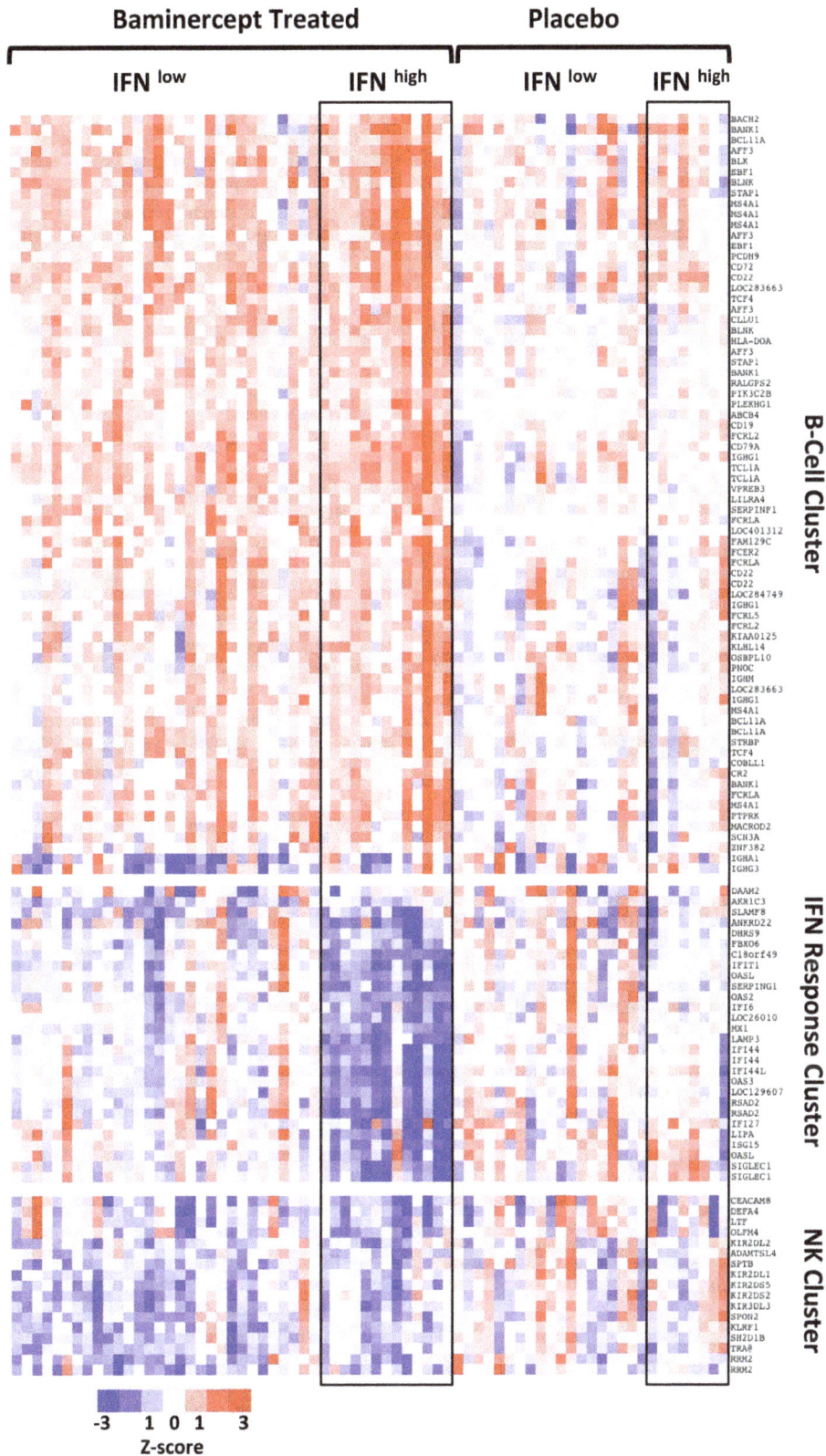

Figure 3. Baminercept induced changes in total blood RNA expression. Heat map showing the change in gene expression after 14 week of either placebo or baminercept treatment. Patients were forced into 4 groups based on treatment and baseline IFN signature. Each of the three gene clusters defined from initial unsupervised clustering are presented separately. The three clusters are characterized by genes associated with B cells, IFN response or NK cells, although some other genes are also present within each category. List only includes genes whose changes were significant (p<0.05), passed FDR and had greater than a 1.5 fold difference in a separate paired sample analysis.

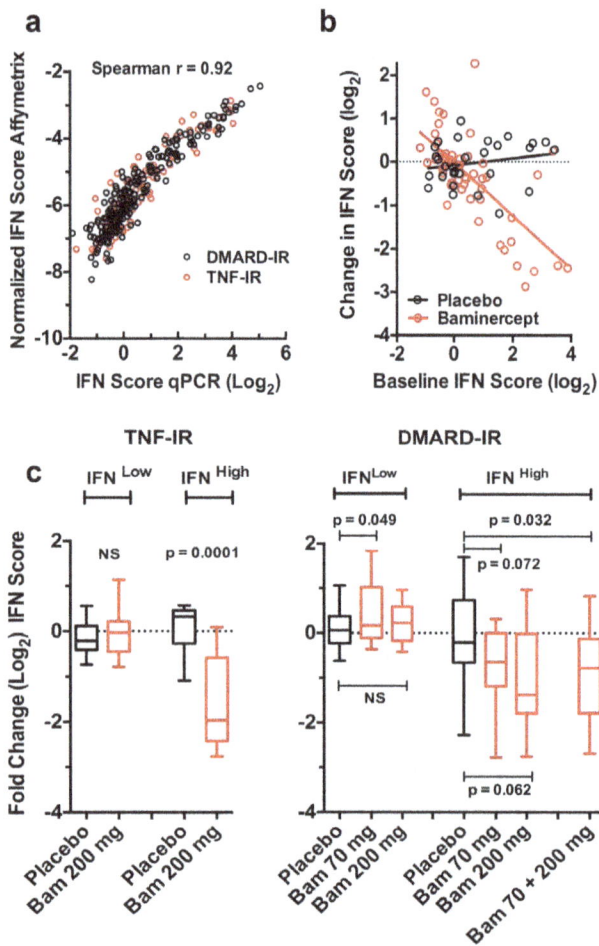

Figure 4. Blockade of the lymphotoxin-LIGHT pathway with baminercept reduces the blood RNA IFN signature in RA patients. a). Analysis of the individual baseline IFN scores as determined using the 15 gene microarray data and a three-gene qPCR score showing excellent correlation. b). Analysis of the change in the 3-gene qPCR IFN score as a function of baseline IFN score following 14 weeks of treatment with 200 mg baminercept q2w in TNF-IR patients, significance is calculated using a linear model of change in IFN score as an interaction of baseline IFN score and treatment (placebo or baminercept). The significance for baseline IFN is $p = 2 \times 10^{-7}$ and for the interaction term $p = 2.3 \times 10^{-7}$. Treatment alone is marginally significant $p = 0.0506$. c). Change in the qPCR-based IFN score at 14 weeks in patients with low vs. high baseline IFN score (low <1, high > 1). Red boxes represent baminercept (Bam) treated patients receiving either 70 or 200 mg q2w (DMARD-IR) or 200 mg q2w (TNF-IR) while black boxes indicate placebo treated patients; n = 20, 50, 11 and 12 (TNF-IR) and 49, 44, 50, 20, 28, 18 and 38 (DMARD-IR) patients in each category in the order listed. P values are from a Mann-Whitney test of placebo vs. baminercept treated patients.

(Figure 6c). These results are consistent with contributions to baminercept induced lymphocytosis from both altered addressin expression and reduced IFN exposure.

In mice, lymphocytosis following LTBR blockade results from elevated T and B cells counts [24]. In these clinical studies, FACS analysis of a small subset of the patients (TNF-IR) showed that B cell numbers were increased roughly 70% over baseline compared to a 24% increase in T cells (Supplemental Figure 6 in File S1). The elevated B cell signature based on the data in figure 3 correlated roughly with the extent of lymphocytosis (r = 0.338, p<

0.0001,) and therefore it is likely that the B cell signature reflects differential lymphocytosis in the baminercept treated cohorts. Furthermore, PCR quantitation of the levels of genes uniquely expressed in lymphocyte subsets revealed some interesting details (Figure 7). RNA levels of CD20 (B cells) increased consistent with the general lymphocytosis, but TCRδ and some natural killer cell specific genes, KLRF1 as well as KLRD1, KIR2DS1 and KIR3DL1 decreased substantially (only a subset of genes identified from the transcriptional profiling were included in the qPCR array). Thus the qPCR data confirmed the decreased NK signature shown in figure 3. Comparison of the change in absolute lymphocyte counts with the change in RNA levels showed a positive correlation with the expression of CD20, TCRα and CD8B RNA (Spearman r values of 0.56, 0.47 and 0.49 respectively), but little correlation with TCRδ (γδ T cells), KLRF1 (NK) and Defensin 3A (immature neutrophils) (r = 0.14, 0.02 and 0.01 respectively). The change in KLRF1 was not coupled to baseline IFN status. In a FACS analysis, B cells and CD4 cell numbers increased, while NK cell numbers trended towards a decrease (Supplemental Figure 6 in File S1). Therefore baminercept appeared to reduce the numbers of immature neutrophils, TCRγδ and NK cells in the blood by a mechanism distinct from the lymphocytosis effects and prior studies in rodents have implicated LTBR in the biology of both TCRγδ and NK cells [26–31]. The decrease in immature neutrophils is intriguing given their propensity to generate chromatin nets and the recent suggestion that nets are a source of citrullinated antigens in RA [32,33].

Given the emphasis on plasmacytoid DC as the source of the IFN signature in SLE, we examined RNA levels in the blood of two known pDC markers, CLEC4C (BDCA2) and LILRA4 (ILT7). LILRA4 levels increased following baminercept treatment, yet CLEC4C levels were unchanged (Supplemental Figure 7 in File S1). CLEC4C appears to be a relatively specific pDC marker, whereas LILRA4 is highly expressed by both pDCs and memory B cells (Immunological Genome). Therefore these data suggest that baminercept does not affect pDC trafficking and increased LILRA4 expression is consistent with the increased numbers of B cells in the blood.

Relationship between IFN status and clinical parameters

After 3 months of treatment, changes in disease status were assessed using the American College of Rheumatology (ACR) scoring system. Overall, baminercept was well tolerated (Supplemental Table 3 in File S1); yet, in neither trial did baminercept treatment substantially increase the ACR scores (Supplemental Table 4 in File S1). Baminercept treatment resulted in a trend towards reduced swollen joint counts (SJC28) in both studies (Supplemental Figure 8 in File S1). Inhibition of TNF or IL-6 significantly decreases ESR and serum CRP levels; however, baminercept did not appreciably lower either serum parameter (Supplemental Figure 9 in File S1).

When patients were grouped based on baseline qPCR IFN status, there was no obvious trend towards a greater reduction in SJC28 in either IFN subgroup in the DMARD-IR study (Supplemental Figure 8 in file S1). The TNF-IR study was too small for such subgrouping. As these studies examined almost 800 patients, an analysis of gender effects was possible and baseline IFN scores were slightly lower in RA males (p = 0.04) and trended slightly lower in males in SLE. No correlation was observed between the IFN high and low groups with baseline swollen joint counts (SJC28), the Disease Activity Score 28 ESR (DAS28 ESR), C-reactive protein, erythrocyte sedimentation rates (ESR), rheumatoid factor titer or anti-CCP positivity (Supplemental Figure 10

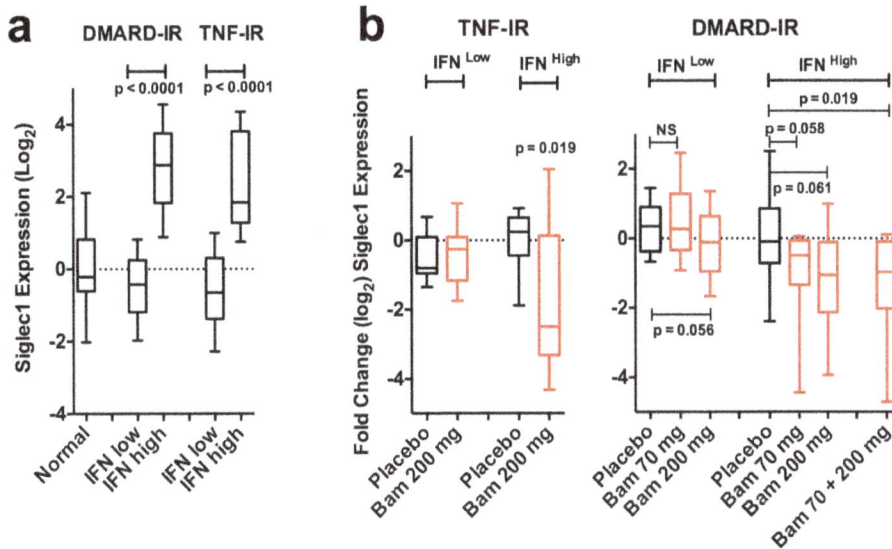

Figure 5. Baminercept treatment lowered RNA expression of the monocyte-associated gene SIGLEC1 in the blood. a). Expression of the monocyte associated gene SIGLEC1 (qPCR determination) is elevated in patients with an elevated IFN signature (qPCR IFN score cut point of 1). b.) SIGLEC1 expression (log$_2$) was reduced by treatment with baminercept (n's and boxes as per figure 4). P values are from a Mann-Whitney test of placebo vs. baminercept treated patients.

in File S1). Baminercept treatment did not affect total serum IgG, IgM and IgA levels nor were preexisting tetanus toxoid titers altered.

Discussion

We show here that inhibition of the LT/LIGHT pathway reduced not only the global IFN signature, but also RNA levels of SIGLEC1, an IFN-regulated gene expressed only in monocytes. RA and SLE patients with an IFN signature were more lymphopenic and baminercept treatment reversed the lymphopenia. These results demonstrate at the clinical level a fundamental linkage between the LT/LIGHT axis and IFN responses as well as between IFN and lymphopenia. To date, only high dose steroids and anti-interferon-α antibodies have been shown to reduce the signature and the inhibition by anti-IFNα antibodies appears to be partial [34–39]. Neither therapy informs on the nature of the underlying IFN biology. Importantly, a reduction in the IFN signature did not result in diminished arthritis suggesting that the pathology driving the IFN signature is not tightly coupled to the local joint disease. This conclusion needs to be qualified because the trials were insufficiently powered for the IFN positive subset, the treatment duration was relatively short and the levels of inflammatory disease were modest as indicated by the low baseline CRP levels.

The question of what biology is being reflected by the blood IFN signature in RA as well as in other autoimmune diseases remains unanswered. In SLE, the IFN signature is correlated in general with a distinct serological profile, renal disease, and progression to atherosclerosis and disease severity, yet its presence is not obviously linked to any particular immunology [23,40]. Our RA studies and those of others did not reveal obvious differences based on IFN status between the DMARD-IR and TNF-IR cohorts or their clinical or serological features [41,42]. A positive IFN signature in RA has been linked to a poor response to rituximab [43] and a weak or variable correlation with response to TNF inhibition [22,44,45]. In both systemic onset juvenile idiopathic arthritis patients and in Sjogren's syndrome, TNF

inhibition led to an increased IFN signature supporting the hypothesis that TNF- and IFN-driven pathologies may lie at opposite poles of the autoimmune disease spectrum [46,47]. The ability of baminercept to dampen an IFN signature may have been a liability in a TNF dominated setting such as RA.

SLE patients are often lymphopenic and lymphopenia correlated with an elevated IFN signature in both SLE and systemic sclerosis patients [23,48]. Here, we confirmed this association in our SLE cohort and extended it to include RA patients. Lymphopenia could reflect perturbed bone marrow hematopoiesis accompanying systemic inflammation and/or increased retention of lymphocytes in the lymph nodes [49,50]. In the latter mechanism, IFN triggers complex formation between CD69 and sphingosine-1-phosphate receptors thereby inhibiting cell egress into the cortical sinuses [25]. Indeed, administration of IFNβ to multiple sclerosis patients or mice results in lymphopenia [51,52]. Increased retention of lymphocytes in the IFN-rich lymphoid microenvironments would allow more dwell time for productive encounters. Baminercept-induced lymphocytosis most likely has a contribution from restricted entry into the LN and mucosal compartments due to loss of addressin positive high endothelial venules. Baminercept could also reduce lymphopenia by shortening retention times in the LN following reduced IFN exposure. Our data are consistent with contributions from both trafficking and retention components and support the hypothesis that IFN-driven lymphocyte retention in the lymphoid tissues is a substantial component of lymphopenia in autoimmune disease.

The effect of baminercept on the blood IFN signature was largely unanticipated; however, observations from several experimental systems demonstrate that the LT/LIGHT network is entwined with IFN responses to infection [53]. First, murine CMV infection of the spleen induces an early IFN response derived from reticular stromal cells in the marginal zone [31,54,55]. Various aspects of lymphoid reticular stroma are critically dependent upon LTBR signaling and loss of LTBR signaling ablated the initial IFN response to murine CMV infection. Second, SIGLEC1-positive sentinel macrophages in both the LN and splenic environments

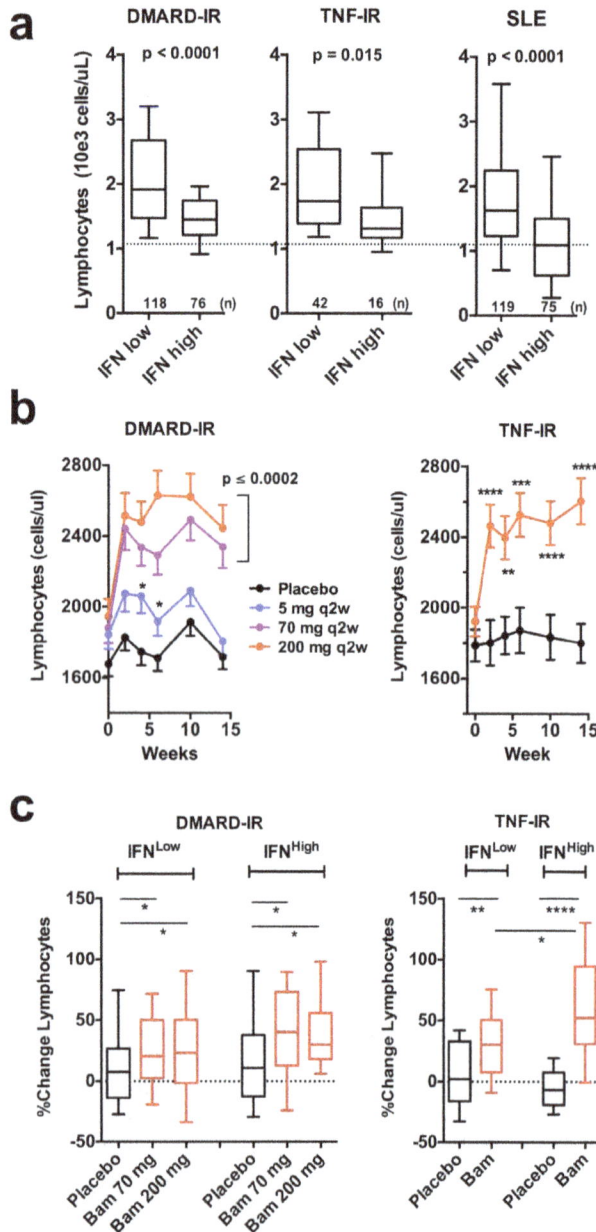

Figure 6. IFN signature positive RA patients are lymphopenic and baminercept treatment resulted in lymphocytosis. a). Patients were segregated based on low and high microarray IFN scores (< -6.5 and > -4.5) and baseline blood lymphocyte counts are plotted. b). Time course of the effects on absolute lymphocyte counts during 14 weeks of baminercept or placebo treatment (means, +/− SEM). All time points in two highest dosed cohorts in DMARD-IR were significant (p< 0.0002), otherwise, significance is indicated by p-values * <0.05, ** < 0.01, *** <0.001 and **** <0.0001. c). Patients were grouped into baseline qPCR IFN signature low or high as in Fig. 1c. Percent change in lymphocyte counts following 14 weeks of treatment with placebo or baminercept is plotted (significance Mann-Whitney in all cases).

survey lymph or blood for immune complexes, lipids, particulates, viruses and sialylated antigens [56–58]. In the case of immune complexes or complement tagged antigens, they capture these elements and route them into the follicle for presentation to B cells.

The differentiation state of these sentinel macrophages is LTBR-dependent [59,60]. Following VSV infection, virus replicates within the LN subcapsular macrophages and the splenic marginal zone metallophilic macrophages triggering IFN production and an effective host response [60–62]. Within the spleen, marginal zone metallophilic macrophages are the major local producers of type I IFN in response to an intravenous HSV challenge [63] and they also generate IFN in response to *Campylobacter jejuni* infection [64]. In a related observation, listeria infection of LTBR-deficient mice failed to generate an IFN response in the spleen [65]. Other LT-dependent sources could include both dendritic cells [11,66–68] as well as follicular dendritic cells where TLRs could be activated following internalization and recycling of antigen [69].

Why is this linkage between the LT and IFN systems manifesting itself in RA? In SLE, a subset of IFN signature high patients has measureable IFN circulating in the blood [21,70]. However, IFN was not detected in the blood of our RA patients and therefore the exposure to IFN must occur while leucocytes traffic through the organs. In RA, robust evidence for a substantial IFN signal in the joints is lacking [3,71,72]. One hypothesis is that lymphocytes become "imprinted" by IFN while trafficking through organized lymphoid microenvironments. Many if not all autoimmune diseases have undercurrents of systemic disease as evidenced by the involvement of additional organ systems, e.g. the lungs in RA, the CNS in SLE, Sjogren's and sarcoidosis, etc. We speculate that LNs draining organs with articular or extra-articular disease, as in lung or glandular involvement in RA, produce IFN as a consequence of sensing signals such as dead cell debris, chromatin complexes, neutrophil nets or antigens as complement tagged or immunoglobulin complexes [69,73]. In this scenario, the amount of IFN exposure would reflect the magnitude of the systemic involvement and may coincide with LN reactivity or even gross lymphadenopathy. Indeed, some association was noted in SLE between lymphoadenopathy and an increased IFN signature [23]. We speculate that baminercept's effects on the IFN signature are due to alteration of the sentinel functions of the lymphoid microenvironments albeit via myeloid or stromal elements.

In conclusion, inhibition of the LTR signaling in RA patients reduced IFN imprinting. The IFN signature is linked to the lymphopenia in RA and SLE supporting a role for IFN in lymphocyte retention in lymphoid organs. Experimentally, the use of viral challenges has revealed much of the linkage between LTBR and IFN responses and, while autoimmune diseases do not have obvious ongoing viral infections, parallels have been drawn between immune responses to virus and chromatin in SLE [74]. Thus, these observations may be highlighting a potential coupling mechanism between tissue damage, debris recognition and an overactive self-reactive immune response. Disruption of LTBR signaling could be a new tool for the investigation and potentially the treatment of certain subgroups in autoimmune diseases.

Experimental Procedures

Patients and Trials

Baminercept is a fusion protein of the extracellular domain of human LTBR coupled to the hinge and Fc domain of human IgG1 [75]. DMARD-IR (104RA202, NCT00664716, EUdraCT 2006-005466-39) was a multicenter, phase IIb, randomized, double-blinded placebo-controlled study of RA patients who had had an inadequate response (IR) to a disease modifying anti-rheumatic drug. In this study 391 RA patients were treated for 14 weeks with subcutaneous injections of placebo q2w (79 patients), 5 mg baminercept (BG9948) q2w (78), 70 mg q2w (78), 70 mg q4w (39), 200 mg q2w (78) or 200 mg q4w (39). 365 patients

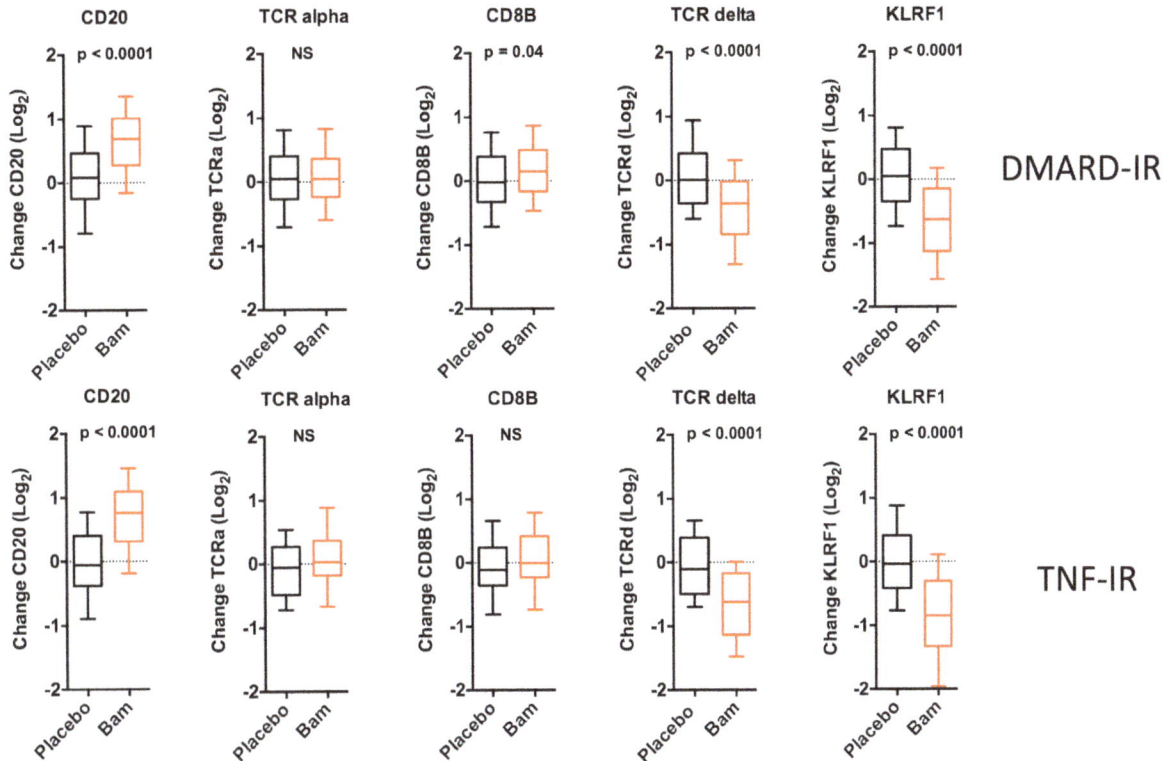

Figure 7. Baminercept alters the levels of RNAs representative of lymphocyte subsets in the blood. Baminercept treatment increased the blood RNA expression (qPCR determination) of genes representing B cells (CD20), T cells (TCRA, CD8B), whereas expression of markers for γδ-T cells (TCRD) and NK cells (KLRF1) decreased. In the DMARD-IR study, data from both 70 and 200 mg 2qw cohorts are pooled.

completed the study. Study was conducted between July 2007 and October 2008 at 58 sites in Argentina, Brazil, Hungary, Mexico, Poland, Romania, Russia and United Kingdom and investigators are listed in the supplemental materials.

TNF-IR (104RA203, NCT00458861, EUdraCT 2006-005467-26) was a multicenter, phase IIb, double-blinded, placebo-controlled study of RA patients who lacked an adequate response to TNF-blocking therapy and had discontinued TNF blocking treatment for at least 90 days. The study dosed 114 patients with subcutaneous injections q2w of either placebo (38) or baminercept 200 mg (76). This study was terminated early due to poor efficacy in the DMARD-IR study; however, 81 patients completed the 3 months of dosing and another 15 patients received at least 2 months of treatment. Study was conducted between March 2007 and October 2008 at 40 sites in the United States, Canada, Belgium and United Kingdom.

Investigators for both baminercept studies are listed in the supplemental materials in File S1. RA patients in both studies were eligible if they met the American College of Rheumatology (ACR) criteria for rheumatoid arthritis and had active RA for at least 6 months. Patients had to have been receiving 10–25 mg methotrexate per week for at least 3 months with a stable dose for the last 4 weeks before entry. Methotrexate therapy was maintained for the duration of the studies. Patients had to have more than 8 swollen and tender joints (66/68 joint count) and either a CRP≥ 1.5 ULN or ESR ≥28 mm/hr at screening. The protocols for these trials re available as supporting information; see Protocol S1 and S2. There is no intent to publish further clinical data from

these studies and the ACR scores (primary trial endpoint) are presented within the supplemental data.

SLE data were from registry (called SPARE) representing a collection of 292 SLE patients from the Hopkins Lupus Center in the US. Patients were eligible if they were aged 18–75 years and met the American College of Rheumatology Revised Criteria for Classification of Systemic Lupus Erythematous. Baseline data were used in this study and patients were under standard clinical practice. Normal controls for RNA analyses were composed of healthy volunteer donors from Biogen Idec. Control group had equal numbers of males and females and was not exactly gender balanced with the predominantly female composition of both the RA and SLE cohorts.

Ethics Statement

The RA studies were approved by the appropriate institutional review boards or ethics committees and all patients provided written informed consent (see supplementary materials in File S1 for a complete listing). All patients from the Hopkins Lupus Center (Johns Hopkins University School of Medicine) provided written informed consent to participate in the SPARE registry and the Johns Hopkins institutional review board approved the study.

Analyses of whole blood RNA

Patient whole blood was collected into PaxGene tubes and analyzed using conventional Affymetrix microarrays and qPCR was performed on the RNA samples using the Fluidigm analyzer. Details for RNA analyses as well as the IFN reporter assays are provided in the Supplemental Materials in File S1. Baseline transcriptional profiling datasets are deposited at GEO, GSE45291.

Supporting Information

File S1   Supporting files. Supplemental Methods and Investigator Listing. Supplemental Table 1, Demographics of the Patients in the RA studies and the SLE registry. Supplemental Table 2, Measurement of IFN signatures. Supplemental Table 3, Incidence of adverse events by preferred term for the combined placebo-controlled studies. Supplemental Table 4, Lack of an appreciable effect of baminercept treatment on ACR scores as assessed at 14 weeks. Supplemental Figure 1, Comparison of IFN signatures in RA and SLE. Supplemental Figure 2, Elevation of serum LIGHT levels in RA patients following baminercept treatment. Supplemental Figure 3, Characteristics of the IFN signatures observed in this study. Elevation of serum LIGHT levels in RA patients following baminercept treatment. Supplemental Figure 4, Characteristics of baminercept induced lymphocytosis in RA patients. Supplemental Figure 5, Relationship between IFN signature and baminercept treatment on blood neutrophil and monocyte counts. Supplemental Figure 6, FACS analysis of the effects of baminercept treatment on peripheral blood lymphocyte subsets. Supplemental Figure 7, Quantitative PCR analysis on whole blood RNA of the effects of baminercept treatment on gene markers of myeloid subsets. Supplemental Figure 8, Effects of baminercept treatment on the Swollen Joint Count 28 (SJC28) scores in the DMARD-IR and TNF-IR studies. Supplemental Figure 9, Little effect of baminercept treatment on CRP levels and Erythrocyte Sedimentation Rates (ESR) in the DMARD-IR and TNF-IR studies. Supplemental Figure 10, The IFN signature

status in RA patients does not correlate with clinical or serological parameters.

Acknowledgments

We thank the patients who participated in the studies; the investigators and personnel at the study sites, and the members of the baminercept project team, including Paul Chen, Niki Cox, Patrick Cullen, Fred D'Amato, Susan Gawlak, Janet Griffiths, Evangelia Hatzis, Bina Keshaven, Megan Lo, Helena Madden, Nick Messinese, Werner Meier, John O'Gorman, Suezanne Parker, Jitesh Rana, Ann Ranger, Joyce Sobolewski, Cynthia Theodos, Miranda Tighe, Melissa Wojcik and Jim Woodworth. We also thank Larrisa Miller for help with the IFN reporter assay, Susan Kalled and Ronenn Rubinoff for major contributions to the SPARE SLE registry and Ian Rifkin, Carl Ware, Jen Gommerman, Peter Lipsky and Peggy Crow for critique of the manuscript.

Author Contributions

Conceived and designed the experiments: JB JG TP AN MW CN MP EB JLB. Performed the experiments: JB NA AT JG TP AN MW CN MP EB JLB. Analyzed the data: JB JG TP JLB. Contributed to the writing of the manuscript: JB JG TP EB JLB.

References

1. Ronnblom L, Eloranta ML (2013) The interferon signature in autoimmune diseases. Current opinion in rheumatology 25: 248–253.
2. Elkon KB, Wiedeman A (2012) Type I IFN system in the development and manifestations of SLE. Current opinion in rheumatology 24: 499–505.
3. Higgs BW, Liu Z, White B, Zhu W, White WI, et al. (2011) Patients with systemic lupus erythematosus, myositis, rheumatoid arthritis and scleroderma share activation of a common type I interferon pathway. Annals of the rheumatic diseases 70: 2029–2036.
4. Crow YJ (2011) Type I interferonopathies: a novel set of inborn errors of immunity. Annals of the New York Academy of Sciences 1238: 91–98.
5. Kirou KA, Gkrouzman E (2013) Anti-interferon alpha treatment in SLE. Clinical immunology 148: 303–312.
6. Browning JL (2008) Inhibition of the lymphotoxin pathway as a therapy for autoimmune disease. Immunological reviews 223: 202–220.
7. Ware CF (2008) Targeting lymphocyte activation through the lymphotoxin and LIGHT pathways. Immunological reviews 223: 186–201.
8. Remouchamps C, Boutaffala L, Ganeff C, Dejardin E (2011) Biology and signal transduction pathways of the Lymphotoxin-alphabeta/LTbetaR system. Cytokine & growth factor reviews 22: 301–310.
9. Lu TT, Browning JL (2014) Role of the Lymphotoxin/LIGHT System in the Development and Maintenance of Reticular Networks and Vasculature in Lymphoid Tissues. Frontiers in immunology 5: 47.
10. Gray EE, Cyster JG (2012) Lymph node macrophages. Journal of innate immunity 4: 424–436.
11. Summers deLuca L, Gommerman JL (2012) Fine-tuning of dendritic cell biology by the TNF superfamily. Nature reviews Immunology 12: 339–351.
12. De Trez C (2012) Lymphotoxin-beta receptor expression and its related signaling pathways govern dendritic cell homeostasis and function. Immunobiology 217: 1250–1258.
13. Upadhyay V, Fu YX (2013) Lymphotoxin signalling in immune homeostasis and the control of microorganisms. Nature reviews Immunology 13: 270–279.
14. Satpathy AT, Briseno CG, Lee JS, Ng D, Manieri NA, et al. (2013) Notch2-dependent classical dendritic cells orchestrate intestinal immunity to attaching-and-effacing bacterial pathogens. Nature immunology 14: 937–948.
15. Wege AK, Huber B, Wimmer N, Mannel DN, Hehlgans T (2013) LTbetaR expression on hematopoietic cells regulates acute inflammation and influences maturation of myeloid subpopulations. Innate immunity ePub.
16. Steinberg MW, Cheung TC, Ware CF (2011) The signaling networks of the herpesvirus entry mediator (TNFRSF14) in immune regulation. Immunological reviews 244: 169–187.

17. Allaire NE, Bushnell SE, Bienkowska J, Brock G, Carulli J (2013) Optimization of a high-throughput whole blood expression profiling methodology and its application to assess the pharmacodynamics of interferon (IFN) beta-1a or polyethylene glycol-conjugated IFN beta-1a in healthy clinical trial subjects. BMC research notes 6: 8.
18. Rose T, Grutzkau A, Hirseland H, Huscher D, Dahnrich C, et al. (2013) IFNalpha and its response proteins, IP-10 and SIGLEC-1, are biomarkers of disease activity in systemic lupus erythematosus. Annals of the rheumatic diseases 72: 1639–1645.
19. Hall JC, Casciola-Rosen L, Berger AE, Kapsogeorgou EK, Cheadle C, et al. (2012) Precise probes of type II interferon activity define the origin of interferon signatures in target tissues in rheumatic diseases. Proceedings of the National Academy of Sciences of the United States of America 109: 17609–17614.
20. Waddell SJ, Popper SJ, Rubins KH, Griffiths MJ, Brown PO, et al. (2010) Dissecting interferon-induced transcriptional programs in human peripheral blood cells. PloS one 5: e9753.
21. Hua J, Kirou K, Lee C, Crow MK (2006) Functional assay of type I interferon in systemic lupus erythematosus plasma and association with anti-RNA binding protein autoantibodies. Arthritis and rheumatism 54: 1906–1916.
22. Mavragani CP, La DT, Stohl W, Crow MK (2010) Association of the response to tumor necrosis factor antagonists with plasma type I interferon activity and interferon-beta/alpha ratios in rheumatoid arthritis patients: a post hoc analysis of a predominantly Hispanic cohort. Arthritis and rheumatism 62: 392–401.
23. Kirou KA, Lee C, George S, Louca K, Peterson MG, et al. (2005) Activation of the interferon-alpha pathway identifies a subgroup of systemic lupus erythematosus patients with distinct serologic features and active disease. Arthritis and rheumatism 52: 1491–1503.
24. Browning JL, Allaire N, Ngam-Ek A, Notidis E, Hunt J, et al. (2005) Lymphotoxin-beta receptor signaling is required for the homeostatic control of HEV differentiation and function. Immunity 23: 539–550.
25. Cyster JG, Schwab SR (2012) Sphingosine-1-phosphate and lymphocyte egress from lymphoid organs. Annual review of immunology 30: 69–94.
26. Silva-Santos B, Pennington DJ, Hayday AC (2005) Lymphotoxin-mediated regulation of gammadelta cell differentiation by alphabeta T cell progenitors. Science 307: 925–928.
27. Elewaut D, Ware CF (2007) The unconventional role of LT alpha beta in T cell differentiation. Trends in immunology 28: 169–175.
28. Vallabhapurapu S, Powolny-Budnicka I, Riemann M, Schmid RM, Paxian S, et al. (2008) Rel/NF-kappaB family member RelA regulates NK1.1- to NK1.1+

transition as well as IL-15-induced expansion of NKT cells. European journal of immunology 38: 3508–3519.

29. Powolny-Budnicka I, Riemann M, Tanzer S, Schmid RM, Hehlgans T, et al. (2011) RelA and RelB transcription factors in distinct thymocyte populations control lymphotoxin-dependent interleukin-17 production in gammadelta T cells. Immunity 34: 364–374.

30. Van Den Broeck T, Van Ammel E, Delforche M, Taveirne S, Kerre T, et al. (2013) Differential Ly49e expression pathways in resting versus TCR-activated intraepithelial gammadelta T cells. Journal of immunology 190: 1982–1990.

31. Verma S, Wang Q, Chodaczek G, Benedict CA (2013) Lymphoid-tissue stromal cells coordinate innate defense to cytomegalovirus. Journal of virology 87: 6201–6210.

32. Knight JS, Kaplan MJ (2012) Lupus neutrophils: 'NET' gain in understanding lupus pathogenesis. Current opinion in rheumatology 24: 441–450.

33. Khandpur R, Carmona-Rivera C, Vivekanandan-Giri A, Gizinski A, Yalavarthi S, et al. (2013) NETs are a source of citrullinated autoantigens and stimulate inflammatory responses in rheumatoid arthritis. Science translational medicine 5: 178ra140.

34. Lepelletier Y, Zollinger R, Ghirelli C, Raynaud F, Hadj-Slimane R, et al. (2010) Toll-like receptor control of glucocorticoid-induced apoptosis in human plasmacytoid predendritic cells (pDCs). Blood 116: 3389–3397.

35. Guiducci C, Gong M, Xu Z, Gill M, Chaussabel D, et al. (2010) TLR recognition of self nucleic acids hampers glucocorticoid activity in lupus. Nature 465: 937–941.

36. Yao Y, Richman L, Higgs BW, Morehouse CA, de los Reyes M, et al. (2009) Neutralization of interferon-alpha/beta-inducible genes and downstream effect in a phase I trial of an anti-interferon-alpha monoclonal antibody in systemic lupus erythematosus. Arthritis and rheumatism 60: 1785–1796.

37. McBride JM, Jiang J, Abbas AR, Morimoto A, Li J, et al. (2012) Safety and pharmacodynamics of rontalizumab in patients with systemic lupus erythematosus: results of a phase I, placebo-controlled, double-blind, dose-escalation study. Arthritis and rheumatism 64: 3666–3676.

38. Petri M, Wallace DJ, Spindler A, Chindalore V, Kalunian K, et al. (2013) Sifalimumab, a Human Anti-Interferon-alpha Monoclonal Antibody, in Systemic Lupus Erythematosus: A Phase I Randomized, Controlled, Dose-Escalation Study. Arthritis and rheumatism 65: 1011–1021.

39. Higgs BW, Zhu W, Morehouse C, White WI, Brohawn P, et al. (2013) A phase 1b clinical trial evaluating sifalimumab, an anti-IFN-alpha monoclonal antibody, shows target neutralisation of a type I IFN signature in blood of dermatomyositis and polymyositis patients. Annals of the rheumatic diseases 78: 256–262.

40. Huang YL, Chung HT, Chang CJ, Yeh KW, Chen LC, et al. (2009) Lymphopenia is a risk factor in the progression of carotid intima-media thickness in juvenile-onset systemic lupus erythematosus. Arthritis and rheumatism 60: 3766–3775.

41. Cantaert T, van Baarsen LG, Wijbrandts CA, Thurlings RM, van de Sande MG, et al. (2010) Type I interferons have no major influence on humoral autoimmunity in rheumatoid arthritis. Rheumatology 49: 156–166.

42. Thurlings RM, Boumans M, Tekstra J, van Roon JA, Vos K, et al. (2010) Relationship between the type I interferon signature and the response to rituximab in rheumatoid arthritis patients. Arthritis and rheumatism 62: 3607–3614.

43. Raterman HG, Vosslamber S, de Ridder S, Nurmohamed MT, Lems WF, et al. (2012) The interferon type I signature towards prediction of non-response to rituximab in rheumatoid arthritis patients. Arthritis research & therapy 14: R95.

44. Reynier F, Petit F, Paye M, Turrel-Davin F, Imbert PE, et al. (2011) Importance of correlation between gene expression levels: application to the type I interferon signature in rheumatoid arthritis. PloS one 6: e24828.

45. van Baarsen LG, Wijbrandts CA, Rustenburg F, Cantaert T, van der Pouw Kraan TC, et al. (2010) Regulation of IFN response gene activity during infliximab treatment in rheumatoid arthritis is associated with clinical response to treatment. Arthritis research & therapy 12: R11.

46. Palucka AK, Blanck JP, Bennett L, Pascual V, Banchereau J (2005) Cross-regulation of TNF and IFN-alpha in autoimmune diseases. Proceedings of the National Academy of Sciences of the United States of America 102: 3372–3377.

47. Mavragani CP, Niewold TB, Moutsopoulos NM, Pillemer SR, Wahl SM, et al. (2007) Augmented interferon-alpha pathway activation in patients with Sjogren's syndrome treated with etanercept. Arthritis and rheumatism 56: 3995–4004.

48. Assassi S, Mayes MD, Arnett FC, Gourh P, Agarwal SK, et al. (2010) Systemic sclerosis and lupus: points in an interferon-mediated continuum. Arthritis and rheumatism 62: 589–598.

49. de Bruin AM, Libregts SF, Valkhof M, Boon L, Touw IP, et al. (2012) IFNgamma induces monopoiesis and inhibits neutrophil development during inflammation. Blood 119: 1543–1554.

50. Cain DW, Snowden PB, Sempowski GD, Kelsoe G (2011) Inflammation triggers emergency granulopoiesis through a density-dependent feedback mechanism. PloS one 6: e19957.

51. Hartrich L, Weinstock-Guttman B, Hall D, Badgett D, Baier M, et al. (2003) Dynamics of immune cell trafficking in interferon-beta treated multiple sclerosis patients. Journal of neuroimmunology 139: 84–92.

52. Gao Y, Majchrzak-Kita B, Fish EN, Gommerman JL (2009) Dynamic accumulation of plasmacytoid dendritic cells in lymph nodes is regulated by interferon-beta. Blood 114: 2623–2631.

53. Gommerman JL, J.L B, C.F W (2014) The Lymphotoxin Network: Orchestrating a Type I Interferon response to optimize adaptive immunity. Cytokine & growth factor reviews in press.

54. Schneider K, Loewendorf A, De Trez C, Fulton J, Rhode A, et al. (2008) Lymphotoxin-mediated crosstalk between B cells and splenic stroma promotes the initial type I interferon response to cytomegalovirus. Cell host & microbe 3: 67–76.

55. Hsu KM, Pratt JR, Akers WJ, Achilefu SI, Yokoyama WM (2009) Murine cytomegalovirus displays selective infection of cells within hours after systemic administration. The Journal of general virology 90: 33–43.

56. Barral P, Polzella P, Bruckbauer A, van Rooijen N, Besra GS, et al. (2010) CD169(+) macrophages present lipid antigens to mediate early activation of iNKT cells in lymph nodes. Nature immunology 11: 303–312.

57. Cyster JG (2010) B cell follicles and antigen encounters of the third kind. Nature immunology 11: 989–996.

58. Klaas M, Crocker PR (2012) Sialoadhesin in recognition of self and non-self. Seminars in immunopathology 34: 353–364.

59. Phan TG, Grigorova I, Okada T, Cyster JG (2007) Subcapsular encounter and complement-dependent transport of immune complexes by lymph node B cells. Nature immunology 8: 992–1000.

60. Moseman EA, Iannacone M, Bosurgi L, Tonti E, Chevrier N, et al. (2012) B cell maintenance of subcapsular sinus macrophages protects against a fatal viral infection independent of adaptive immunity. Immunity 36: 415–426.

61. Honke N, Shaabani N, Cadeddu G, Sorg UR, Zhang DE, et al. (2012) Enforced viral replication activates adaptive immunity and is essential for the control of a cytopathic virus. Nature immunology 13: 51–57.

62. Iannacone M, Moseman EA, Tonti E, Bosurgi L, Junt T, et al. (2010) Subcapsular sinus macrophages prevent CNS invasion on peripheral infection with a neurotropic virus. Nature 465: 1079–1083.

63. Eloranta ML, Alm GV (1999) Splenic marginal metallophilic macrophages and marginal zone macrophages are the major interferon-alpha/beta producers in mice upon intravenous challenge with herpes simplex virus. Scandinavian journal of immunology 49: 391–394.

64. Klaas M, Oetke C, Lewis LE, Erwig LP, Heikema AP, et al. (2012) Sialoadhesin promotes rapid proinflammatory and type I IFN responses to a sialylated pathogen, Campylobacter jejuni. Journal of immunology 189: 2414–2422.

65. Kutsch S, Degrandi D, Pfeffer K (2008) Immediate lymphotoxin beta receptor-mediated transcriptional response in host defense against L. monocytogenes. Immunobiology 213: 353–366.

66. Summers deLuca L, Ng D, Gao Y, Wortzman ME, Watts TH, et al. (2011) LTbetaR signaling in dendritic cells induces a type I IFN response that is required for optimal clonal expansion of CD8+ T cells. Proceedings of the National Academy of Sciences of the United States of America 108: 2046–2051.

67. Lorenzi S, Mattei F, Sistigu A, Bracci L, Spadaro F, et al. (2011) Type I IFNs control antigen retention and survival of CD8alpha(+) dendritic cells after uptake of tumor apoptotic cells leading to cross-priming. Journal of immunology 186: 5142–5150.

68. Spadaro F, Lapenta C, Donati S, Abalsamo L, Barnaba V, et al. (2012) IFN-alpha enhances cross-presentation in human dendritic cells by modulating antigen survival, endocytic routing, and processing. Blood 119: 1407–1417.

69. Heesters BA, Das A, Chatterjee P, Carroll MC (2014) Do follicular dendritic cells regulate lupus-specific B cells? Mol Immunol epub.

70. Yao Y, Liu Z, Jallal B, Shen N, Ronnblom L (2013) Type I interferons in Sjogren's syndrome. Autoimmunity reviews 12: 558–566.

71. Nzeusseu Toukap A, Galant C, Theate I, Maudoux AL, Lories RJ, et al. (2007) Identification of distinct gene expression profiles in the synovium of patients with systemic lupus erythematosus. Arthritis and rheumatism 56: 1579–1588.

72. Yoshida S, Arakawa F, Higuchi F, Ishibashi Y, Goto M, et al. (2012) Gene expression analysis of rheumatoid arthritis synovial lining regions by cDNA microarray combined with laser microdissection: up-regulation of inflammation-associated STAT1, IRF1, CXCL9, CXCL10, and CCL5. Scandinavian journal of rheumatology 41: 170–179.

73. Elkon KB, Santer DM (2012) Complement, interferon and lupus. Curr Opin Immunol 24: 665–670.

74. Migliorini A, Anders HJ (2012) A novel pathogenetic concept-antiviral immunity in lupus nephritis. Nature reviews Nephrology 8: 183–189.

75. Browning JL, Dougas I, Ngam-ek A, Bourdon PR, Ehrenfels BN, et al. (1995) Characterization of surface lymphotoxin forms. Use of specific monoclonal antibodies and soluble receptors. Journal of immunology 154: 33–46.

3

NK Cell Activity Differs between Patients with Localized and Diffuse Cutaneous Leishmaniasis Infected with *Leishmania mexicana:* A Comparative Study of TLRs and Cytokines

Isabel Cristina Cañeda-Guzmán[1], Norma Salaiza-Suazo[1], Edith A. Fernández-Figueroa[1], Georgina Carrada-Figueroa[2], Magdalena Aguirre-García[1], Ingeborg Becker[1]*

1 Unidad de Investigación en Medicina Experimental, Facultad de Medicina, Universidad Nacional Autónoma de México, Hospital General de México, México, D.F., México,
2 Universidad Autónoma Juárez de Tabasco, Villahermosa, Tabasco, México

Abstract

Leishmania mexicana causes localized (LCL) or diffuse cutaneous leishmaniasis (DCL). The cause of dissemination in DCL remains unknown, yet NK cells possibly play a role in activating leishmanicidal mechanisms during innate and adaptive immune responses. We had previously shown that *Leishmania* lipophosphoglycan (LPG) is a ligand for TLR2, activating human NK cells. We have now analyzed NK cells in LCL and DCL patients. NK numbers and effector mechanisms differed drastically between both groups of patients: DCL patients showed reduced NK cell numbers; diminished IFN-γ and TNF-α production; and lower TLR2, TLR1, and TLR6 expression as compared to LCL patients. The altered protein expression found in NK cells of DCL patients correlated with their down-regulation of IFN-γ gene expression in LPG-stimulated and non-stimulated cells as compared to LCL patients. NK cell response was further analyzed according to gender, age, and disease evolution in LCL patients showing that female patients produced higher IFN-γ levels throughout the disease progression, whereas TLR2 expression diminished in both genders with prolonged disease evolution and age. We furthermore show the activation pathway of LPG binding to TLR2 and demonstrated that TLR2 forms immunocomplexes with TLR1 and TLR6. In addition to the reduced NK cell numbers in peripheral blood, DCL patients also showed reduced NK cell numbers in the lesions. They were randomly scattered within the lesions, showing diminished cytokine production, which contrasts with those of LCL lesions, where NK cells produced IFN-γ and TNF-α and were found within organized granulomas. We conclude that in DCL patients the reduced NK-cell numbers and their diminished activity, evidenced by low TLR expression and low cytokine production, are possibly involved in the severity of the disease. Our results provide new information on the contribution of NK cells in *Leishmania* infections of the human host.

Editor: Simona Stager, INRS - Institut Armand Frappier, Canada

Funding: This project was financed by CONACyT-102155 and PAPIIT IN215212. The funders had no role in study design, data collection and analysis, decision to publish, or preparation of the manuscript.

Competing Interests: The authors have declared that no competing interests exist.

* Email: becker@unam.mx

Introduction

Leishmania mexicana causes a wide spectrum of cutaneous diseases, ranging from localized cutaneous leishmaniasis (LCL), characterized by ulcers at sites of parasite inoculation, to diffuse cutaneous leishmaniasis (DCL), where parasites spread throughout the skin forming disfiguring nodules [1]. In Mexico, 400 new patients with cutaneous leishmaniasis are diagnosed each year, where the prevalence of DCL is less than 1% [2]. Although the cause for the uncontrolled parasite spread in DCL patients remains unknown, the early innate immune response against *Leishmania* possibly plays a pivotal role in determining disease evolution. *Leishmania* lipophosphoglycan (LPG) is a major surface molecule that activates TLR2 in cells of the innate immunity [3,4]. The carbohydrate composition of LPG characterizes different

Leishmania species [5,6]. Murine models of leishmaniasis have linked various TLRs (TLR2, TLR3, TLR4 and TLR9) with enhanced IFN-γ and IL-12 production and parasite control [4,7–10]. Among the first innate cells capable of early IFN-γ and TNF-α production are NK cells [11]. They can be divided into 2 subsets: CD56^{dim} and CD56^{bright}, yet the roles of these subsets have not been clearly characterized in leishmaniasis [12,13]. We had previously shown that *Leishmania* LPG activates human NK cells through TLR2 stimulation, leading to IFN-γ and TNF-α production [3]. These cytokines synergize in the macrophage to induce iNOS leading to NO production, one of the molecules responsible for intracellular *Leishmania* destruction [14]. Even though NK cells have been shown to play an important protective role in mouse *Leishmania* infections [11,15], their response has not been analyzed in patients with LCL and DCL.

In the present study, we comparatively analyzed NK-cell activity as well as their response towards the parasite in LCL and DCL patients. We found that peripheral blood and lesional NK cells of DCL patients were severely reduced in number and produced markedly less IFN-γ and TNF-α, as compared to LCL patients. In addition to the reduced cytokine production, NK cells of DCL patients also showed diminished TLR2, TLR1 and TLR6 expression, both in LPG-stimulated and non-stimulated NK cells, which contrasted sharply with the heightened response found in LCL patients. The reduced NK cell cytokine production correlated with a down-regulation of IFN-γ gene expression in DCL patients. We further show the activation pathway of TLR2 by *Leishmania* LPG, and the participation of TLR1 and TLR6 in the binding of LPG.

Materials and Methods

Ethics Statement

The study was reviewed and approved by the Ethics and Research Committees of the Faculty of Medicine of UNAM (Universidad Nacional Autónoma de México) (FMED/CI/RGG/013/01/2008) and guidelines established by the Mexican Health Authorities were strictly followed. All patients and controls were informed and signed a written consent to participate in the study.

Patients and controls

28 patients with LCL and 6 with DCL from La Chontalpa (Tabasco State), an endemic area in southeastern Mexico, were analyzed. Patients were diagnosed by clinical criteria, parasite demonstration in Giemsa-stained smears taken from lesions and intradermal Montenegro hypersensitivity test. LCL patients showed skin ulcers with few parasites, all were positive to the Montenegro test. DCL patients had multiple non-ulcerative nodules covering large areas of the skin that contained heavily parasitized macrophages. All DCL patients were negative for the Montenegro skin test. All patients received anti-*Leishmania* treatment with Glucantime.

Blood samples were taken from 28 LCL patients (17 males and 11 females), which had a mean age of 28 years and a disease duration ranging from 1.5 to 18 months. The LCL patients were divided according to gender, age ($\leq$25 years and $\leq$26 years) and evolution time ($\leq$3 months and $\geq$4 months). The 6 DCL patients (five males and one female) had a mean age of 44 years (24–57 years) with an average disease evolution of 18 years (two patients had 3 years, three had 17 years and one had 35 years). Blood from 21 healthy donors was obtained in a blood bank.

Parasite culture

Leishmania major (MHOM/SU/73/5-ASKH) promastigotes were cultured in RPMI-1640 medium (Gibco, Grand Island, NY, USA) with 10% heat-inactivated FBS (Gibco) and 293 µg/mL L-glutamine (Sigma, St. Louis, MO, USA). Parasite infectivity was maintained through regular passages in BALB/c mice.

Lipophosphoglycan purification

LPG was purified as previously described [3]. Briefly, parasites were sub-cultured every 4–5 days and grown to a density of 2×10^7/mL. Promastigotes were harvested from stationary-phase cultures and centrifuged at $3200 \times g$ for 10 min and washed in PBS. The pellet was extracted with chloroform/methanol/water (4:8:3, v/v) during 30 min at RT. The insoluble material was used for LPG extraction with 9% 1-butanol in water (2×50 mL) and

the pooled supernatants were vacuum dried. LPG was purified from this fraction by HPLC, using an octyl-sepharose column and a 1-propanol gradient (5–60%) in 0.1 M ammonium acetate. Two octyl-sepharose columns were used to optimize LPG purity. The preparations tested negative for endotoxin with the *Limulus* sp. amebocyte lysate assay (E-Toxate Kit; Sigma). Additionally, a sample of LPG was analyzed by SDS-PAGE to verify the absence of protein contaminants. 10 µg/mL LPG was used in all experiments.

NK cell purification

NK cells were purified from PBMC of LCL and DCL patients, as well as from healthy donors. Briefly, PBMC were separated by density gradient (Histopaque-1077, Sigma-Aldrich) at $300 \times g$ for 20 min at 20°C. Cells were obtained from the interface, washed twice in cold PBS and placed in RPMI-1640 (Gibco), supplemented with 10% heat-inactivated FBS, 2 mM L-glutamine, 10 nM HEPES, 100 µg/mL penicillin-streptomycin (Gibco), 17 mM NaHCO$_3$ and seeded in Petri dishes at 37°C, 5% CO$_2$ during 18 h for adherence of monocytes. Non-adherent cells were removed, washed in PBS and NK cells were purified with an NK cell isolation kit II (Miltenyi Biotec, Bergisch Gladbach, Germany). Briefly, 1×10^7 total cells was suspended in 40 µL PBS containing 10 µL of cocktail of biotin-conjugated monoclonal antibodies against CD3, CD4, CD14, CD15, CD19, CD36, CD123 and glycophorin A and incubated for 10 min at 4°C. 30 µL PBS and 20 µL anti-biotin microbeads were added for 15 min at 4°C. The cells were washed with PBS, centrifuged at $300 \times g$ for 10 min and passed through a magnetic separation LS column (Miltenyi). NK cells were isolated by negative selection. The purity of the enriched NK cells was assessed by flow cytometry using anti-CD56-PE, anti-CD3-FITC (Coulter Immunotech) antibodies, achieving 97% purity. NK cells were washed and plated in 24-well culture-plates.

Immunoprecipitation

We further determined whether the recognition of LPG by TLR2 in NK cells also led to binding of TLR1 and/or TLR6 and additionally analyzed the activation pathway of TLR2 in NK cells of control subjects by immunoprecipitation of TLR2-MyD88, MyD88-IRAK-1, MyD88-TRAF-6, IRAK-1-TRAF-6 and TRAF-6-IKK-α. After purification, NK cells were suspended in RPMI-1640 with 10% heat-inactivated FBS and incubated for 2 h at 37°C with 5% CO$_2$. Thereafter, 10×10^6 NK cells were incubated with LPG (10 µg/mL) for 1 h at 37°C, 5% CO$_2$ and the same number of NK cells were incubated in RPMI alone. Cells were washed twice with cold PBS and lysed in 250 µl modified radioimmunoprecipitation (RIPA) buffer (Tris-base, pH 7.4 10 mM, NaCl 150 mM, EDTA 1 mM, NaF 10 mM, NP-40 1%, PMSF 1 mM, aprotinin 10 mg/mL, leupeptin 1 mg/mL, Na$_3$VO$_4$ pH = 10 10 mM, DTT 1 mM) and incubated for 30 min on ice. Cell lysates were centrifuged at $10\,000 \times g$ for 10 min at 4°C and the supernatants were collected. Protein concentration was determined using DC Protein Assay Reagents Package (Bio-Rad Laboratories, Hercules, CA, USA).

For immunoprecipitation assays, 200 µg of supernatants from LPG-activated and non-activated NK cells were pre-cleared with protein G-agarose beads (Life Technologies) for 1 h under agitation at 4°C and centrifuged at $14\,000 \times g$ for 5 min at 4°C. Protein lysates were immunoprecipitated with anti-TLR2, anti-MyD88, anti-IRAK-1 or anti-TRAF-6 1:20 (Santa Cruz antibodies: sc-10739, sc-11356, sc-7883, sc-8409, respectively) under agitation overnight at 4°C. The immunocomplex was captured with protein G-agarose beads for 2 h under agitation at 4°C. Beads were washed ten times in cold washing buffer (Tris-base, pH 7.4 10 mM, NaCl 150 mM, EDTA 1 mM, NP-40 1%) and immunoprecipitated proteins were diluted into 2× reducing Laemmli buffer pH = 6.6 (4 mL 10% SDS; 2.5 mL 0.5 M Tris-HCl, 0.4% (w/v) SDS; 1 mL 2-mercaptoethanol and glycerol 20%), boiled at 95°C for 5 min and stored at −70°C until Western blot assays were done.

Total and nuclear protein extraction

To obtain the total protein extract, 2×10^6 NK cells were incubated with LPG 10 µg/mL for 15, 30, 45 and 60 min or for 15 min with PMA. Cells were washed twice with PBS and lysed in 50 µl of RIPA modified buffer for 30 min. Cellular extracts were centrifuged at 10 000×g for 10 min at 4°C and the supernatants were collected. For nuclear proteins extracts 3×10^6 NK cells were incubated with LPG 10 µg/mL for 1 h. Cells were washed twice with PBS and lysed by incubating them for 10 min in a detergent-free hypotonic buffer (10 mM Tris, pH = 7.6. 10 mM NaCl, 1.5 mM $MgCl_2$, 0.5 mM EDTA, 1 mM DTT, 1.5 µg/mL leupeptin, 0.7 mM PMSF). Extracts were centrifuged at 4°C for 10 min at 956×g. The supernatants were discharged and intact nuclei were incubated in extraction buffer (20 mM Tris, pH = 8.0, 450 mM KCl, 0.05 mM EDTA, 1 mM DTT, 1.5 µg/mL leupeptin, 5 mM spermidine, 25% glycerol) for 45 min under constant agitation at 4°C. DNA pellets were eliminated by centrifugation for 15 min at 13 500×g at 4°C. Total and nuclear protein extracts were quantified with DC Protein Assay Reagents Package.

Immunoblotting

For Western-blotting, 20 µg of total protein or nuclear extracts from non-stimulated and LPG-stimulated NK cells were used. Immunoprecipitates, nuclear and total protein extracts were analyzed by SDS–PAGE in 10% acrylamide gels. The proteins were transferred onto Immobilon-P membranes using a semidry electroblotting apparatus. The membranes were blocked with 5% milk in Tris-buffer saline-Tween 20 (TBST: 10 mM Tris–HCl, pH 7.4, 0.15 M NaCl, and 0.05% Tween 20) for 1 h at RT. Immunoblotting was done with anti-TLR1 (sc-8687), anti-TLR6 (sc-30001), anti-actin (sc-1616), anti-MyD88 (sc-11356), anti-IRAK1 (sc-7883), anti-TRAF6 (sc8409), anti-IKK-γ (sc-7181, 7330 and 8330), anti-pIκB-α (Cell signaling 9246), anti-pIKK-α/β (Cell signaling 2697) and anti-NF-κB p50 and p65 (sc-7178 and sc-372) diluted 1:200 (sc- antibodies) or 1:1000 (Cell signaling antibodies and actin) in TBST at 4°C overnight with constant shaking. HRP anti-rabbit IgG (E22, Biomeda), goat anti-mouse diluted 1:5000 or bovine anti-goat IgG diluted 1:10 000 in 5% non-fat dry milk were used as secondary antibodies, and incubated at RT for 1 h with shaking. Blots were developed using SuperSignal West Pico Chemiluminescent Substrate (Thermo Scientific) and exposed to X-ray films.

Analysis of TLR expression by flow cytometry

NK cells (1×10^6) from LCL and DCL patients as well as from healthy controls were incubated with 10 µg/mL LPG or with other TLR2 agonists such as PGN (10 µg/mL) or Pam$_3$Cys-Ser (10 µg/mL) (EMC Microcollections GmbH, Tübingen, Germany) in 24 well culture-plates during 18 h in RPMI-1640 supplemented with 10% heat inactivated FBS at 37°C with 5% CO_2. After washing with PBS, LPG-stimulated NK cells, as well as non-stimulated cells, were fixed with 2% paraformaldehyde (Merck) and incubated with blocking buffer (PBS containing human IgG, 2% FBS, 5 mM EDTA and 0.1% sodium azide) on ice for 30 min. Afterwards the cells were washed and stained with 2 µL of Ab goat anti-human TLR2, TLR1 or TLR6 (sc- 8680, sc-8687, sc-30001)

and FITC conjugated rabbit anti-goat IgG (Zymed 81-1611) or isotype controls. Additionally, cells were incubated with anti-CD56-PE (BD-Pharmingen).

TLRs were analyzed in 10^4 NK cells by FACS, using CellQuest software (FACScan BD Immunocytometry Systems, Mountain View, CA. USA). Results are expressed in MFI. For some experiments, NK cells were stained with anti-CD56, anti-CD16, anti-TLR2, anti-TLR1 or anti-TLR6 for 30 min at RT. The antibodies used for this analysis included: PE-conjugated anti-CD56, PE-Cy^{TM}5-anti-CD16, PE-Cy^{TM}5 mouse (IgG1k) and PE mouse (IgG1k) for isotype controls, all from BD-Pharmingen; rabbit polyclonal IgG TLR6 (H-90), goat polyclonal IgG TLR1 (N-20), goat polyclonal IgG TLR2 (N-17) all from Santa Cruz Biotechnology; FITC rabbit anti-goat IgG (H+L) conjugated, FITC goat anti-rabbit IgG (H+L) from Zymed and FITC goat IgG isotype control from Coulter.

Immunohistochemistry (IHC) for detection of NK cells, TLRs and cytokines in NK cells from LCL and DCL patients

Skin punch biopsies (4–6 mm) were taken from the lesions of DCL and LCL patients. The tissues were embedded in paraffin, cut into 5-µm thick slices. Some of the slides were stained with H&E to evaluate the inflammatory characteristics. For Immunohistochemistry analysis the slides were hydrated and antigenically reactivated in a citrate buffer (0.01 M citric acid, 0.01 M sodium citrate) for 10 min at 95°C. Endogenous peroxidase was blocked with methanol/H_2O_2 3% for 10 min and nonspecific antigenic sites were blocked with 3% bovine serum albumin dissolved in Tris-HCl pH = 7.6 with 0.1% Triton X-100 for 60 min at RT. Thereafter, samples were stained with mouse anti-CD57 (Zymed 08–0167) overnight at 4°C, washed, incubated with secondary antibody biotin anti-mouse (Zymed 62-6540) for 30 min at RT and with streptavidin AP (AB complex/AP, DAKO K0376,) for 30 min at RT. Tissues were washed and color development was assessed after incubation with AP Red substrate kit (Zymed 00–2203) or Stay Green/AP kit (Abcam antibodies: ab-156428) at RT.

TLRs and cytokines were detected by double staining. For this, the samples were washed and endogenous peroxidase and nonspecific antigens were blocked as described above. Thereafter, the samples were incubated 1:50 with goat anti-TLR1, mouse anti-TLR2, rabbit anti-TLR6, mouse anti-IFN-γ or mouse anti-TNF-α 1:100 (sc-8687, sc-21759, sc-30001, ab-11866 and sc-1350, respectively) for 30 min at RT, washed and secondary antibodies were incubated for 30 min at RT. The secondary antibodies included: mouse and rabbit specific HRP/AEC detection IHC kit (Abcam ab94705) for TLR6, biotin-labelled rabbit anti-goat (Zymed 81–1640) antibodies for TLR1 and TNF-α and biotin-labelled goat anti-mouse (Zymed 62–6540) was used for detecting TLR2 and IFN-γ. Thereafter, tissues were washed and incubated with horseradish peroxidase (Zymed 43–4311) for 30 min at RT. For TLR and IFN-γ detection samples were washed and color development was assessed after incubation with DAB Black kit (Biocare Medical BRI40 H, L). For TNF-α, a DAB Substrate kit was used (Roche Cat. 11718096001). The slides were counterstained with Mayers haematoxylin (Biogenex, CA, USA). Digital images of tissue sections were captured using a light microscope and an AxioCam MRc5 camera (Zeiss, Germany). In order to obtain the number of single and double positive cells in these lesions, cells were counted in 8 pictures of each tissue were taken with a final area corresponding to 1 mm^2 of 3 LCL and 3 DCL patients. Controls for primary and secondary antibodies were negative.

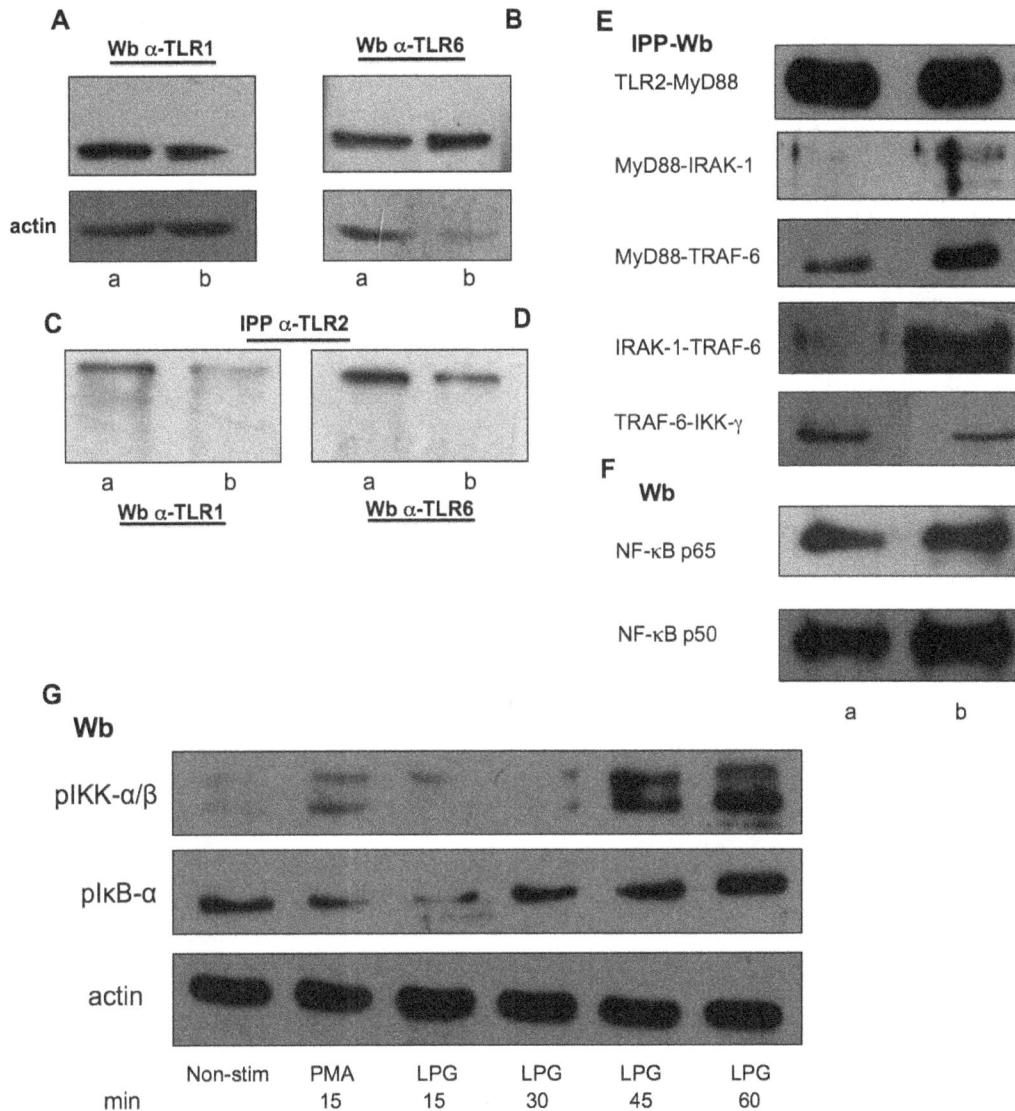

Figure 1. LPG promotes binding of TLR signaling proteins and NF-κB nuclear translocation. (A and B) Western blot shows TLR1 and TLR6 in NK cells. (C and D) Immunoprecipitations were performed with anti-TLR2 in non-stimulated (lane a) and LPG-stimulated NK cells after 1 h of co-incubation (lane b). (C) Immunoprecipitates were subjected to Western blotting and probed with anti-TLR1 and (D) anti-TLR6 antibodies, respectively. A representative immunoblot from four different experiments is shown. (E) NK cell lysates in non-stimulated and LPG-stimulated NK cells were immunoprecipitated with anti-TLR2, anti-MyD88, anti-IRAK-1 and anti-TRAF-6 antibodies and Western blotted with anti-MyD88, anti-IRAK-1, anti-TRAF-6 and anti-IKK-γ antibodies. (F) Nuclear translocation of p50 and p65 NF-κB isoforms were analyzed in non-stimulated and LPG-stimulated NK cells. (G) Phosphorilation of pIKK-α/β and pIκB-α were analyzed in non-stimulated NK cells (Non-stim) or in cells stimulated with PMA (15 min) or LPG (15, 30, 45 and 60 min). A representative immunoblot from two different experiments is show.

IFN-γ and TNF-α production

NK cells (1×10^6) from LCL and DCL patients, as well as from healthy donors were incubated with 10 μg/mL LPG in 1 mL RPMI-1640 with 10% heat-inactivated FBS during 18 h at 37°C and 5% CO_2. IFN-γ and TNF-α were analyzed by ELISA tests in 96-well plates (Costar, Corning, NY). Samples were set up in triplicates. Briefly, microtiter plates were coated with anti-TNF-α (clone MAb1, 6 μg/mL; BD Pharmingen, San Diego, CA) or anti-IFN-γ (clone NIB42, 6 μg/mL; BD Pharmingen) in 100 mM Na_2HPO_4, pH 9.0 during 12 h at 4°C and blocked with PBS containing 0.05% Tween 20 and 10% FBS. The supernatants and recombinant hTNF-α (BD Pharmingen) or recombinant hIFN-γ (R&D Systems) were incubated with RPMI-1640 medium containing 10% FBS during 2 h at RT. Both cytokines were detected with biotinilated anti-hTNF-α (clone MAb11, 2 μg/mL; BD Pharmingen) or anti-hIFN-γ (clone 4S.B3, 2 μg/mL; BD Pharmingen) in 1% BSA for 1 h. The plate was developed using streptavidine-alkaline-phosphatase conjugate (Life Technologies) with p-nitrophenyl phosphate (4 mg/mL, Life Technologies) as substrate. Absorbance was measured at 405 nm with an ELISA reader (BIO-TEK INSTRUMENTS). The detection limits for both cytokines were 15 pg/mL.

Gene expression of TLR2, IFN-γ and TNF-α by Real-time PCR

Gene expression of TLR2, IFN-γ and TNF-α were analyzed by real-time PCR in 5 healthy controls, 6 LCL and 3 DCL patients.

Total RNA from non-stimulated and LPG-stimulated NK cells (18 h) was retro-transcribed using High-Capacity cDNA Archive kit (Applied Biosystems), according to manufacturers instructions. Quantitative Taqman PCR analysis was performed with the ABI PRISM 7900HT Sequence Detection System (Applied Biosystems) containing 1× Taqman Universal Master Mix (Applied Biosystems) and 1× probes and primers sets Hs00610101_m1 (TLR2), Hs00174128_m1 (TNF) and Hs00989291_m1 (IFN). The thermal profile was as follows: 95°C for 10 min and 40 cycles at 95°C for 15 s and 60°C for 1 min. All amplification reactions were done in duplicate and the relative quantification of TLR2, TNF-α and IFN-γ gene expression were calculated using the comparative Ct method ($2^{-\Delta\Delta CT}$) [16]. Levels of mRNA expression were assessed after normalization, using GAPDH as internal control.

Statistical analysis

Statistical differences between groups were obtained using Mann-Whitney U-test or Student's T-test. The Kruskal-Wallis test was used for the comparison of more than two groups of data. Correlation analyses were performed by Spearmans test. Data are presented as mean ±SEM, $p<0.05$ was considered statistically significant. These statistical analyses were done using the Prism 5 software (GraphPad Software, San Diego, CA, USA).

Results

LPG bindsTLR1 and TLR6 and activates the TLR signaling pathway

Both TLR1 and TLR6 proteins are expressed in non-stimulated and LPG-stimulated NK cells from healthy controls (Fig. 1A and 1B). In order to analyze whether TLR2 binds to TLR1 and TLR6 in NK cells, we immunoprecipitated with anti-TLR2 and Western blotted with α-TLR1 or α-TLR6. A recognition band was found both experimental conditions: in non-stimulated and LPG-stimulated NK cells. It is noteworthy, that in both cases, a more intense recognition was observed in non-stimulated NK cells (Fig. 1C and 1D, lane a) as compared to LPG-stimulated NK cells (Fig. 1C and 1D, lane b). We speculate that the reduced binding of TLR1 or TLR6 to TLR2 after incubation with LPG is possibly due to partial obstruction of the docking site after LPG binds to TLR2.

Through immunoprecipitations we analyzed the binding of proteins involved in the TLR signaling pathway in non-stimulated and LPG-stimulated NK cells. The immunoprecipitations included: TLR2-MyD88, MyD88-IRAK-1, MyD88-TRAF-6, IRAK-1-TRAF-6 and TRAF-6-IKK-γ. We observed protein binding in all immunoprecipitations, with an increase when the NK cells were stimulated with LPG (Fig. 1E, second, third and fourth blots). Only the binding of TRAF-6-IKK-γ decreased (Fig. 1E, fifth blot). This decrease in binding was expected, since the kinases need to be degraded to induce NF-κB translocation to the nucleus. To determine whether LPG induces NF-κB nuclear translocation, we used nuclear extracts of NK cells to analyze p50 and p65 isoforms and their nuclear translocation. We found nuclear translocation of both isoforms in LPG-stimulated NK cells (Fig. 1F, lane b).

Finally, we analyzed the kinetics of phosphorylation of the kinases IKK and IκB in non-stimulated NK cells and in cells stimulated with PMA 10 μg/mL or LPG 10 μg/mL during 15, 30, 45 and 60 min. We observed an increase in phosphorylation of these kinases at 45 and 60 min after stimulation with LPG (Fig. 1G). With these data we were able to confirm that LPG activates NK cells through the TLR2 pathway.

NK cells in peripheral blood and lesions of LCL and DCL patients

Quantitation of NK cells in blood and tissues of patients with both clinical forms revealed that LCL patients had more NK cells in blood as well as in lesions, as compared to DCL patients. NK cells in PBMC were analyzed by flow cytometry (Fig. 2A and 2B), showing that the percentage of NK cells in peripheral blood of LCL patients ranged from 1.4–27.8% (mean: 8.43±1.22), whereas in DCL patients they ranged from 0.5–3.1% (Fig. 2C). No correlation was found between the number of NK cells in peripheral blood and disease duration, age or gender.

Immunohistochemical stains of NK cells in skin biopsies showed enhanced numbers of NK cells in lesions of LCL patients, as compared to DCL patients (Fig. 2D images 1 and 3). H&E stains showed granuloma formations in LCL tissues (Fig. 2D, image 2), whereas in DCL patients, a randomly scattered distribution of inflammatory cells was found (Fig. 2D, image 4). NK-cell counts in tissues showed a mean number 210 cells/mm^2 for LCL patients, whereas DCL patients showed 67 cell/mm^2 (Fig. 2E). Taken together, LCL patients had significantly more NK cells as compared to DCL patients, both in peripheral blood as well as in infected lesions.

TLR2 expression on NK cells of peripheral blood

NK cells were isolated by negative selection achieving a purity of 97%, as shown by flow cytometry (Fig. 3A, middle image). TLR2 expression was analyzed in non-stimulated as well as LPG-simulated NK cells of 28 LCL patients, six DCL patients and 21 healthy controls. All NK cells expressed TLR2, albeit with different intensity. NK cells of LCL patients expressed significantly higher levels of TLR2, as compared to DCL cells or to healthy controls (Fig. 3B and 3C), yet no differences were found in TLR2 expression when comparing non-stimulated with LPG-stimulated NK cells within each patient group (Fig. 3C).

To ascertain whether the increased TLR2 expression found in LCL patients was related to gender, disease duration or age, we subdivided the 28 patients according to these parameters. Thus, we analyzed the TLR2 expression in 11 females and 17 males. We found that NK cells of male LCL patients expressed significantly higher levels of TLR2, as compared to females, both in non-stimulated as in LPG-stimulated cells (Fig. 4A). When analyzing TLR2 expression in NK cells according to disease progression, we found that both in males and females the expression of TLR2 diminishes significantly after four months of disease duration (Fig. 4B). The analysis of TLR2 expression according to age revealed that males ≥26 years always express higher levels of TLR2, as compared to female LCL patients of the same age group, both in non-stimulated as well as in LPG-stimulated cells (Fig. 4C).

TLR1, TLR2 and TLR6 expression on purified NK cells of LCL and DCL patients

Having shown that LPG is a ligand for TLR1, TLR2 and TLR6 and that TLR2 can bind with either TLR1 or TLR6, we analyzed whether specific heterodimers could be associated with the clinical forms of the disease. We analyzed the expression of all three TLRs in non-stimulated and LPG-stimulated NK cells in three groups of individuals: nine LCL patients (two females and seven males, who had a mean age 25±5 years, and a mean disease duration of five months); four DCL patients (one female and three males, who had a mean age of 52 years, and a disease duration 19 years), and four healthy controls without a history of leishmaniasis.

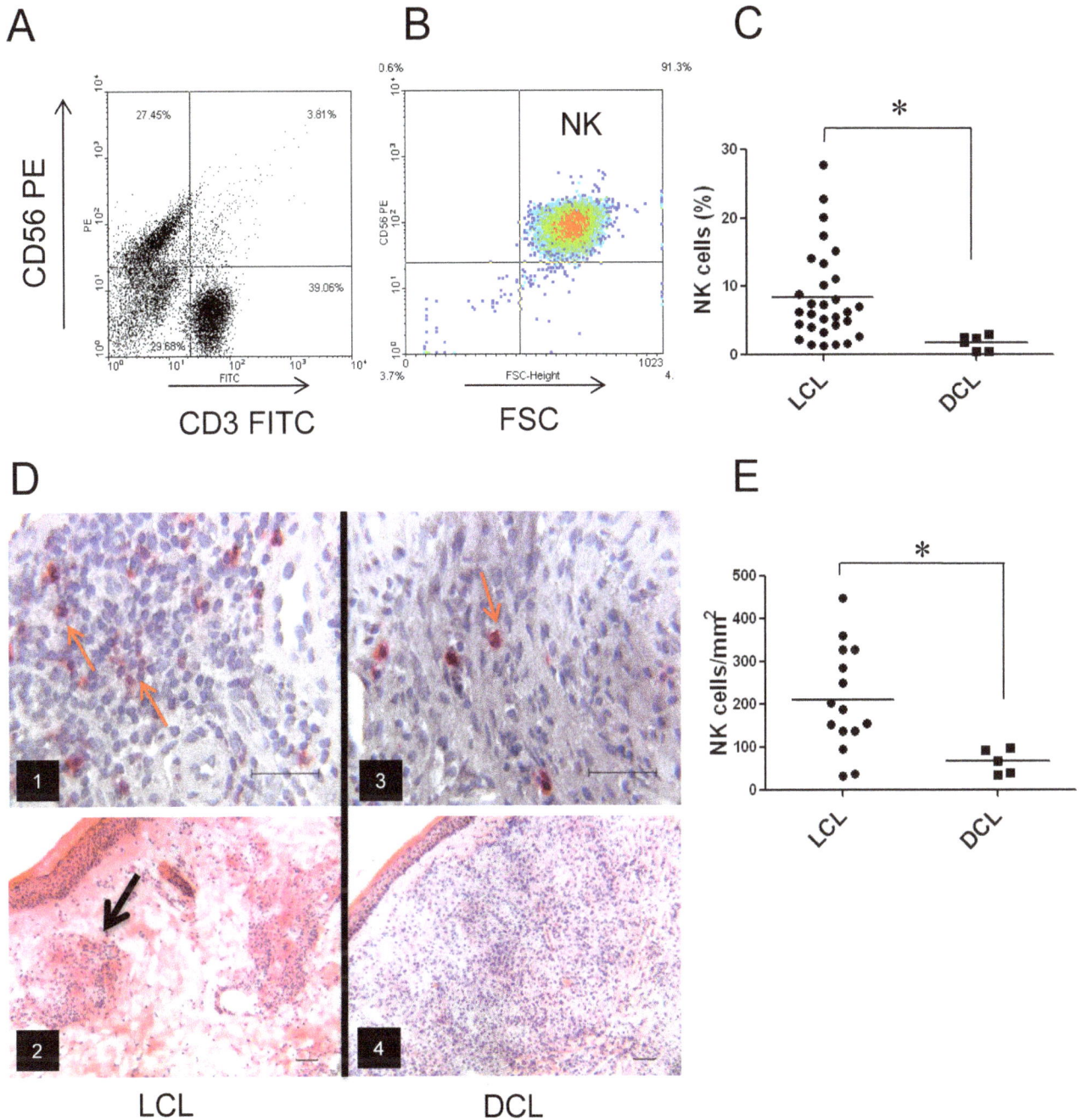

Figure 2. NK cells in patients infected with *Leishmania mexicana*. (A) Representative flow cytometry plots of peripheral blood from patients before separation of NK cells from PBMC. (B) NK cells after purification (CD56+/CD3-). (C) Percentage of NK cells from patients with cutaneous leishmaniasis in peripheral blood [LCL (n = 30) and DCL (n = 6)]. Each dot represents a patient and horizontal line represents the mean of each group. (D) Immunostaining of NK cells in lesions shown NK cells. (D1) NK cells in LCL patients stained in red (CD57+) some of which are marked with red arrows. (D3) NK cells in lesions of DCL patients. (D2) H&E staining of lesions from LCL patients showing granuloma (black arrow). (D4) H&E staining of lesion from DCL patient. (E) Number of NK cells per mm² in lesions. Each dot represents a patient and the horizontal line represents the mean. Images are representative of LCL patients (n = 15) and DCL patients (n = 5). *p≤0.05 was considered significant. Scale bar = 50 μm.

Healthy controls and LCL patients expressed significantly higher levels of all three TLRs, as compared to DCL patients. LPG stimulation showed no significant increase in TLR expression between LCL and DCL patients (Fig. 5A).

Only LCL patients were analyzed for TLR1, TLR2 and TLR6 expression, according to age, due to the reduced number of DCL patients. The nine LCL patients were divided into in two groups:

≤25 years (n = 5) and ≥26 years (n = 4). A significant reduction of all three TLR receptors was observed in patients ≥26 years, as compared to patients ≤25 years, since the later expressed only half the values of TLR1, TLR2 and TLR6, both in non-stimulated as well as in LPG-stimulated NK cells (Fig. 5B).

In an attempt to analyze whether this non-responsiveness of all three receptors was specific for LPG, we analyzed the expression

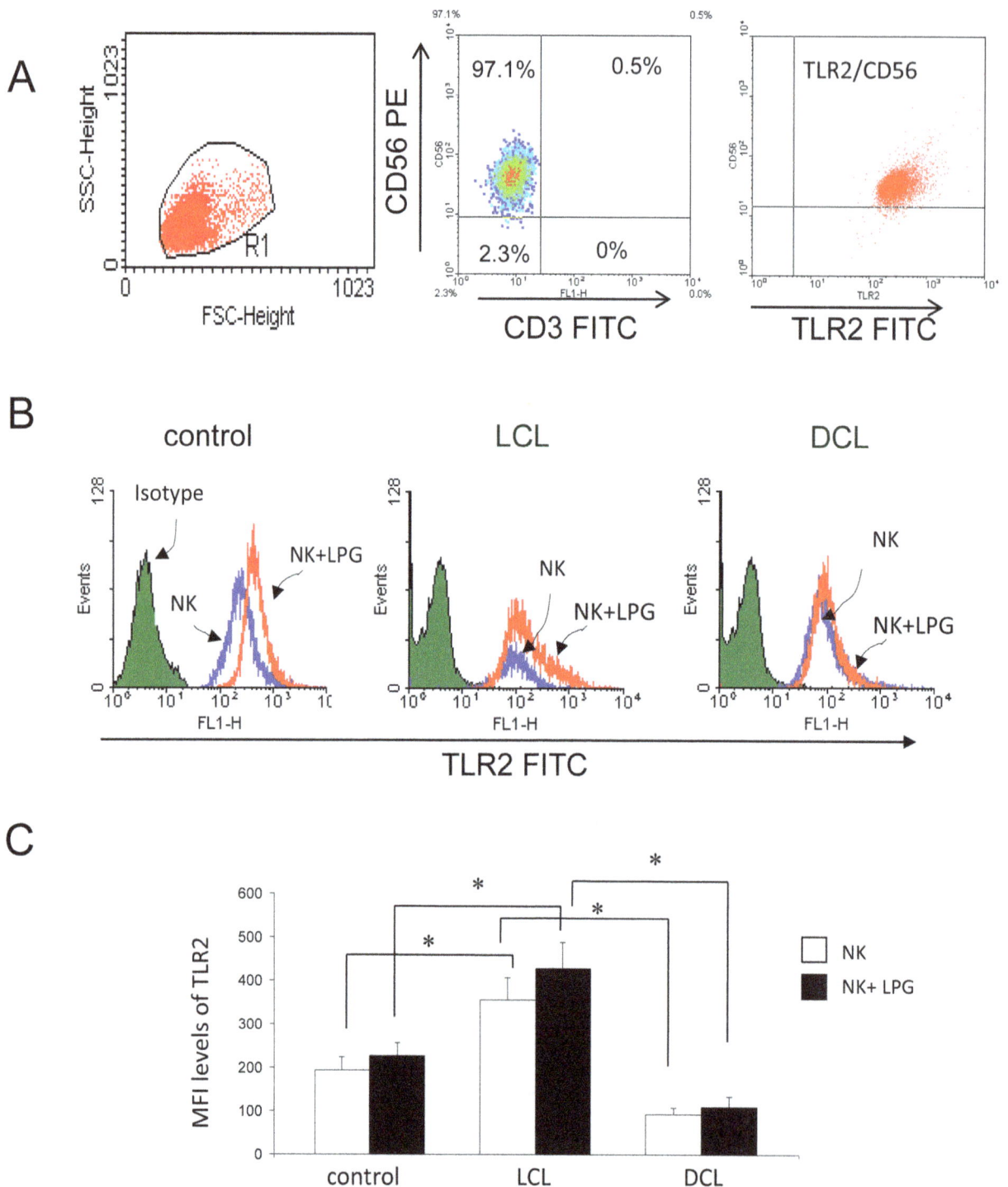

Figure 3. Analysis of TLR2 expression on NK cells. (A) Representative flow CD56+/CD3− expression in membranes of NK cells; right image: NK cells were gated and analyzed for TLR2 (TLR2+/CD56+) expression. (B) Representative histograms showing the MFI levels of TLR2 expression on NK cells from control and patients (LCL and DCL). (C) Quantitation of TLR2 expression on NK cells. □ Non-stimulated cells, ■ LPG-stimulated cells. Data are representative of healthy controls (n = 21), LCL patients (n = 28) and DCL patients (n = 6). These results are the mean ±SEM. *p≤0.05 was considered significant.

of these TLRs in NK cells of both groups of patients after stimulation with additional TLR2 agonists: PGN (peptidoglycan) and Pam3Cys-Ser. Significant differences in the expression of all three receptors on NK cells were observed between the two patient groups: whereas NK cells of LCL patients showed an enhanced

expression of all three TLR receptors, all of which tended to increase with TLR2 agonists, DCL patients showed significantly lower levels of TLR1, TLR2 and TLR6 expression, which remained unchanged despite stimulation with various TLR2 ligands (S1). These data show that the unresponsiveness of NK

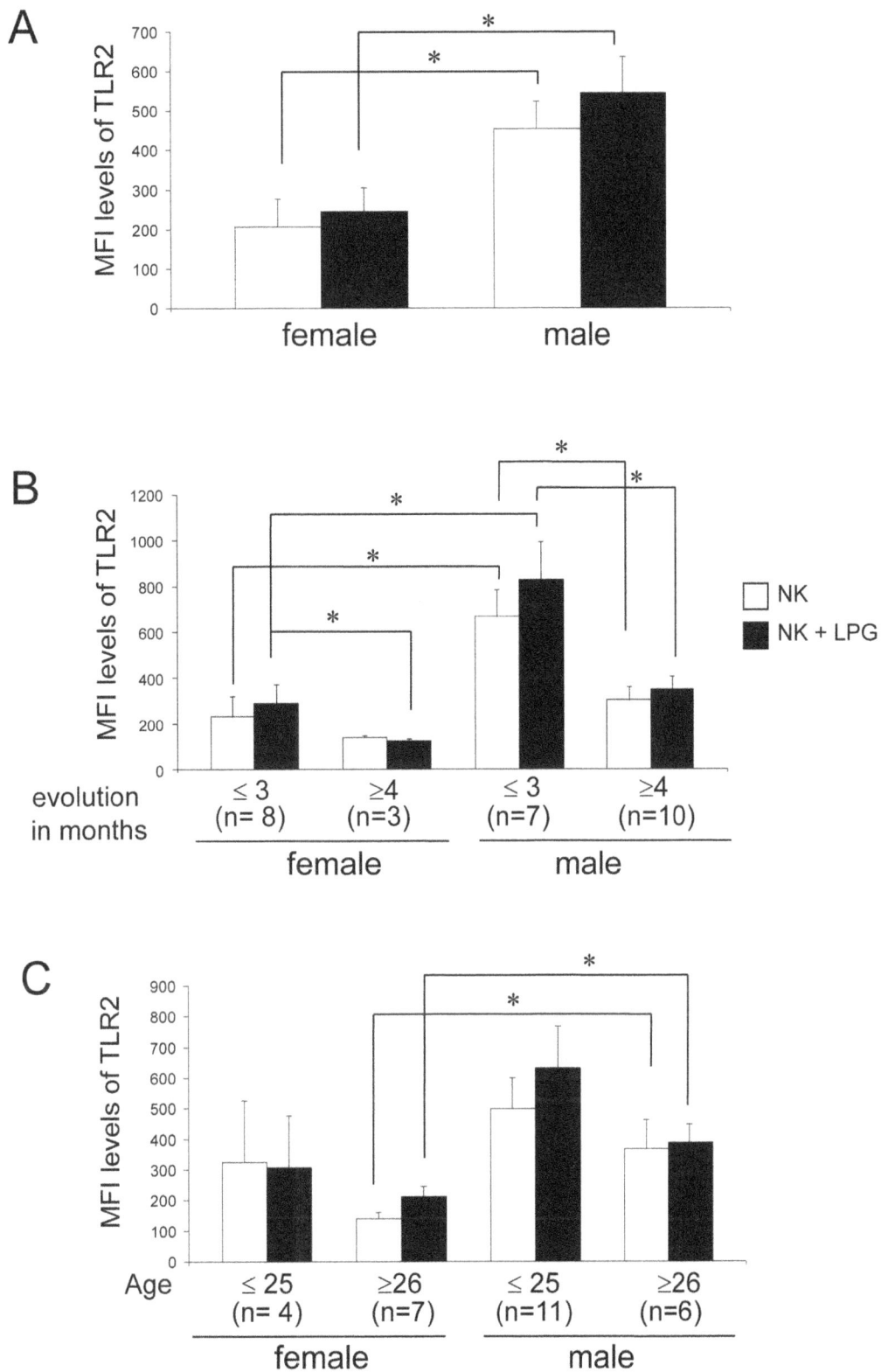

Figure 4. TLR2 expression in NK cells in LCL patients (n = 28). Analysis according to: (A) gender, (B) disease evolution (≤3 or ≥4 months) or (C) age (≤25 or ≥26 years). □ Non-stimulated NK cells, ■ LPG-stimulated NK cells. Cell surface expression is indicated by MFI. These results are the mean ± SEM. *p≤0.05 was considered significant.

A

B

□ NK
■ NK + LPG

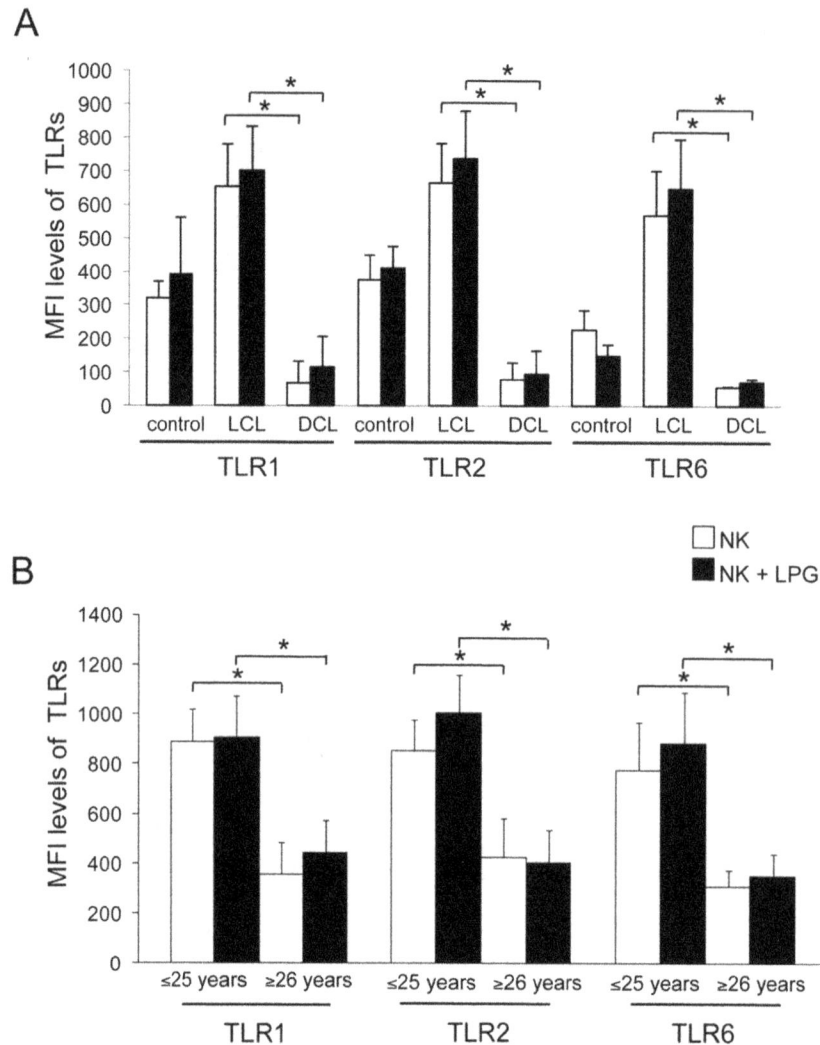

Figure 5. TLR1, TLR2 and TLR6 expression on NK cells from controls and patients (LCL and DCL). (A) Analysis according to disease form. (B) TLR2, TLR1 and TLR6 expression according to age (≤25 or ≥26 years) in LCL patients. □ Non-stimulated NK cells, ■ LPG-stimulated NK cells. Cell surface expression is indicated by MFI. These results are the mean ±SEM. *Significant differences were observed between LCL and DCL patients for all TLRs in LPG-stimulated and non-stimulated cells.

cells of DCL patients is not specific for *Leishmania* LPG, but for the other TLR2 agonists as well.

TLR1, TLR2 and TLR6 expression on NK cells of tissue lesions of LCL and DCL patients

To assess the phenotype and distribution of NK cells expressing these TLRs in the lesions of LCL and DCL patients, we performed double immunostaining: CD57 and TLR1 (or TLR2 or TLR6) (Fig. 6A). The mean number of NK cells expressing TLR1, TLR2 or TLR6 in LCL patients was 115 ± 15, 151 ± 31 and 125 ± 17 cells/mm^2, whereas in DCL patients the mean number was 70 ± 8, 65 ± 8 and 58 ± 20 cells/mm^2, respectively (Fig. 6B). Thus, LCL patients showed significantly higher numbers of NK cells (CD57$^+$/TLR$^+$) expressing TLR2, TLR1 or TLR6 on NK cells, as compared to DCL patients.

TLR1, TLR2 and TLR6 expression in NK subsets CD56^{dim} and CD56^{bright}

Since NK cells are subdivided phenotypically according to their function into CD56^{dim} (cytotoxic) and CD56^{bright} (cytokine

producing) cells, we were interested in analyzing TLR1, TLR2 and TLR6 expression in both NK subsets of LCL and DCL patients (Fig. 7A and 7B). We therefore analyzed the expression of these receptors in 9 LCL and 4 DCL patients, before and after stimulation with LPG. Only NK CD56^{bright} cells expressed high levels of TLR1, TLR2 and TLR6, which were significantly higher in LCL patients (4 to 8-fold), as compared to DCL patients. There were also significant differences in TLRs expression between both NK subsets: CD56^{dim} expressed significantly lower levels of TLRs as compared to CD56^{bright} (Fig. 7C, 7D and 7E). However, no significant differences were found between non-stimulated and LPG-stimulated NK cells in both subsets of NK cells of the different groups.

IFN-γ and TNF-α production by NK cells in blood and tissue lesions

Production of IFN-γ and TNF-α was analyzed in 28 LCL, 6 DCL patients and 21 healthy donors in LPG-stimulated and non-stimulated purified NK cells. Non-stimulated NK cells from healthy subjects and LCL, DCL patients produced similar basal

A

B

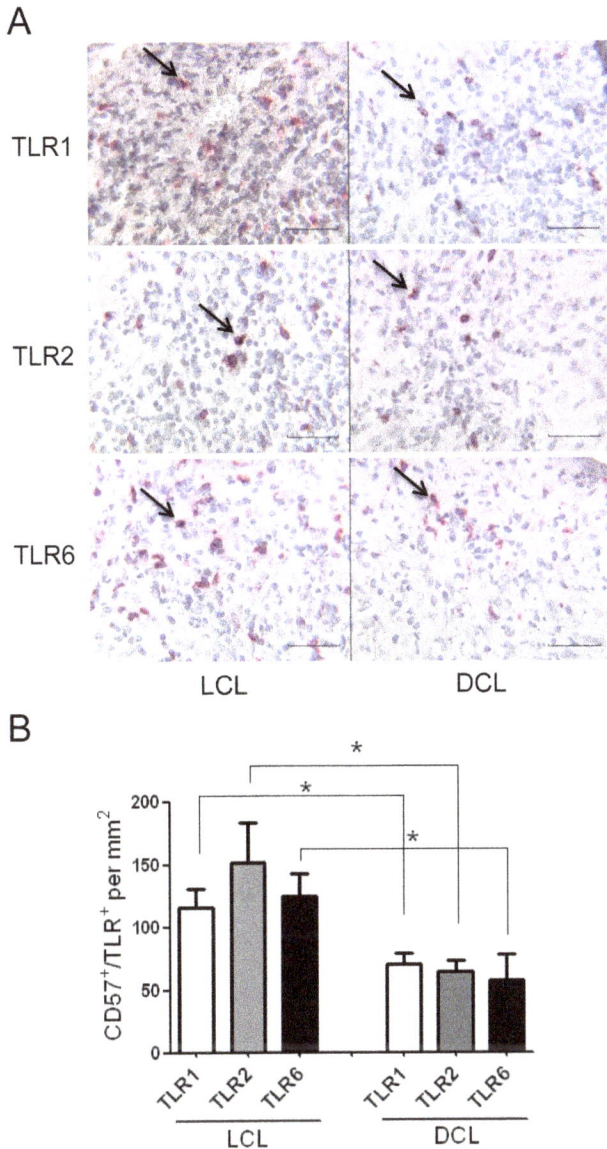

Figure 6. TLR1, TLR2 and TLR6 expression on NK cells in lesions of 3 LCL and 3 DCL patients. (A) Double immunohistochemistry staining of TLR expression (TLR1, TLR2 and TLR6) on NK cells (CD57). (B) Number of NK cells expressing TLRs per mm^2. Results are the mean $\pm$SEM. Scale bar = 50 μm. Black arrows show double positive cells.

IFN-γ production with disease evolution in female and male LCL patients, we further separated the patients into groups according to their disease duration into ≤3 months or ≥4 months. NK cells of female LCL patients with ≥4 months disease duration showed higher IFN-γ production in basal conditions, as well as after LPG stimulation, as compared to those with ≤3 months or to male LCL patients (Fig. 8C). When analyzing IFN-γ production according to age, we found that females, particularly those aged ≤25 (37% of the women) showed a vigorous response (5-fold increase) when NK cells are stimulated with LPG. Although NK cells of female LCL patients aged ≥26 showed a higher IFN-γ production in non-stimulated NK cells, as compared to younger females, these cells responded only slightly to LPG. This stands in contrast to the minimal response towards this parasite antigen found in male patients of any age, who only showed a minimal increase in cytokine production after LPG stimulation (Fig. 8D). Taken together, our data reveal that NK cells of female patients aged ≤25 years, with disease duration of ≥4 months, showed the most vigorous IFN-γ production when the cells are stimulated with LPG, whereas NK cells from female patients aged ≥26 years already come activated and therefore respond only weakly to further stimulus by LPG. This contrasts with the diminished IFN-γ production in male NK cells of all age groups, in both non-stimulated and LPG-stimulated conditions, irrespective of disease duration. When comparing IFN-γ production in NK cells of lesions in LCL and DCL patients, we found that LCL patients showed higher numbers of double positive cells ($CD57^+$/IFN-γ^+), as compared to DCL patients (Fig. 8E). Our data show that IFN-γ production by NK cells in both blood and tissue lesions were markedly reduced in DCL, as compared to LCL patients.

Additionally, we analyzed TNF-α production in NK cells in the same group of subjects and found that LCL patients produced higher levels (mean: 42 pg/mL) as compared to DCL patients (mean: 23 pg/mL), particularly after LPG stimulation, where, instead of enhancing cytokine production as in LCL patients (53 pg/mL), NK cells of DCL patients further reduced their TNF-α production (17 pg/mL). The difference of TNF-α production in LPG-stimulated NK cells between LCL and DCL patients was significant (Fig.9A). We also analyzed TNF-α production in LCL patients according to gender, disease duration and age. NK cells of female LCL patients produced significantly more TNF-α than male LCL patients in non-stimulated (56 vs 32 pg/mL) cells. After LPG stimulation, NK cells of both females and males increased their TNF-α production (64 vs 46 pg/mL), albeit the differences were not statistically significant (Fig. 9B). No significant difference in TNF-α production was found when comparing different age groups or disease duration (data not shown). The analysis of TNF-α production in lesions of both patient groups showed that LCL patients had more double positive cells ($CD57^+$/TNF-α^+), as compared to DCL patients (Fig. 9C, black arrows). Interestingly, many large single positive cells ($CD57^-$/TNF-α^+) are observed in tissues of DCL patients (Fig. 9C, red arrows). Since they are not NK cells, the exact nature of these larger cells with TNF-α^+ staining found in tissues of DCL remains to be determined.

TLR2, IFN-γ and TNF-α gene expression in NK cells in LCL and DCL patients

In order to clarify whether the reduced cytokine production and TLR2 expression in DCL patients was related to reduced gene expression, real-time PCR was done in NK cells of both groups of patients. The gene expression of TLR2, IFN-γ and TNF-α was analyzed in non-stimulated and LPG-stimulated NK cells of 6 LCL and 3 DCL patients as well as 5 healthy controls. DCL vs LCL patients were compared using $2^{-\Delta\Delta CT}$ method and as a

amounts of IFN-γ (with mean values of: 39, 37, 46 pg/mL, respectively). Yet after stimulation with LPG, only NK cells from LCL patients and healthy subjects increased their IFN-γ production (mean values: 60 and 77 pg/mL, respectively). In contrast, NK cells from DCL patients reduced their IFN-γ production to half their basal value (from 46 to 22 pg/mL), when stimulated with LPG (Fig. 8A). To ascertain whether the increased IFN-γ production found in LCL patients was related to gender, disease duration and/or age, we subdivided the 28 patients according to these parameters. Thus, we analyzed the cytokine production in 11 females and 17 males. Female patients produced significantly more IFN-γ in non-stimulated (60 pg/mL) and LPG-stimulated (103 pg/mL) NK cells, as compared to males, which only showed a slight increase in IFN-γ production (21 to 32 pg/mL) after LPG stimulation (Fig. 8B). In an attempt to associate

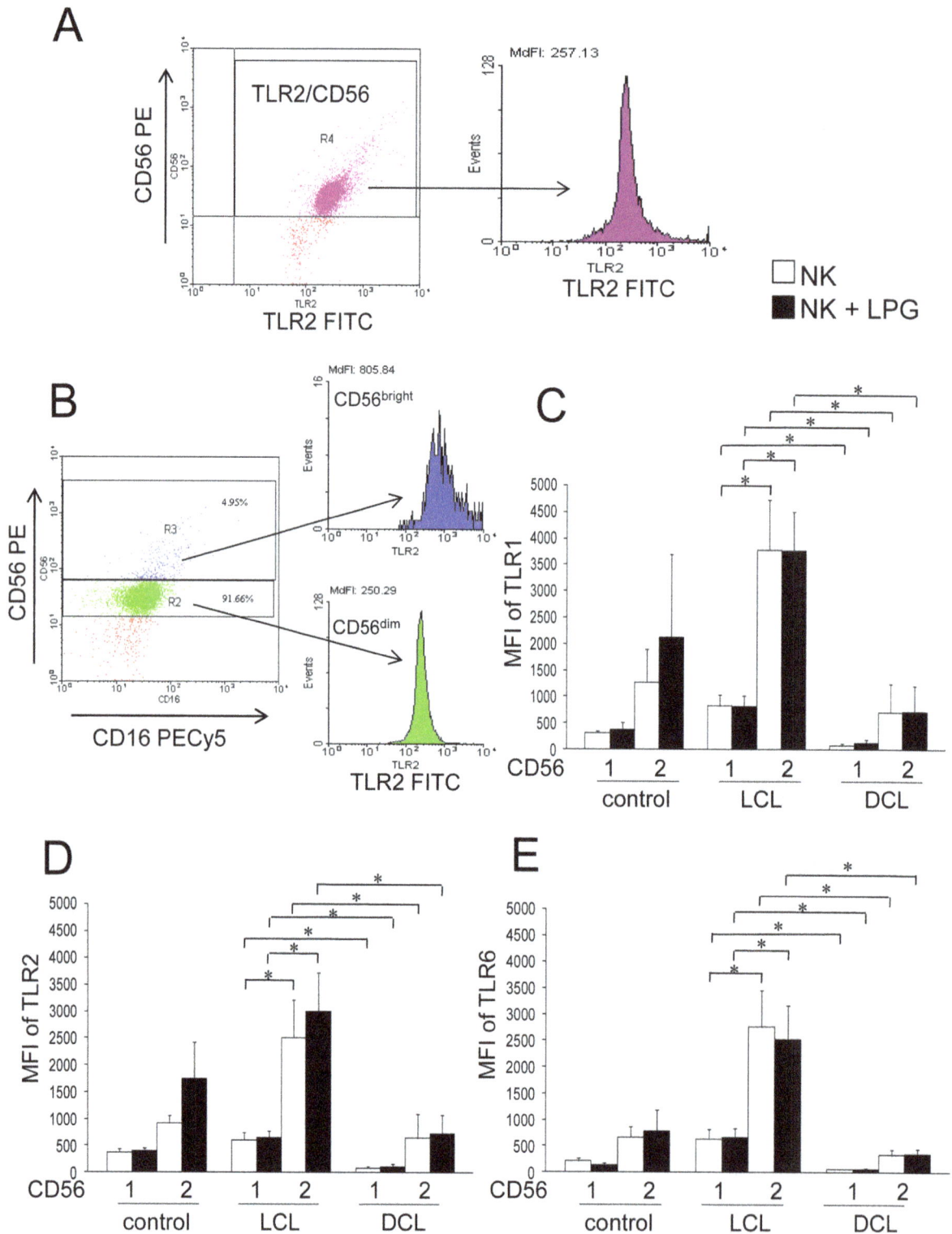

Figure 7. TLR1, TLR2 and TLR6 expression on NK-cell subsets (CD56^bright and CD56^dim) of patients and controls. (A) Representative flow cytometry dot plot (TLR2 vs. CD56) and histogram of TLR2 expression in NK cells. (B) This gate was subsequently analyzed for TLR2 expression on NK-cell subsets. Dot plot (CD16$^+$/CD56$^+$) and histogram for CD56^{bright} (blue box) and CD56^{dim} (green box) NK cells. (C) TLR1 expression. (D) TLR2 expression. (E) TLR6 expression. □ Non-stimulated NK cells; ■ LPG-stimulated NK cells. Lane 1: CD56^{dim}; lane 2: CD56^{bright} NK cells. Cell surface expression is indicated by MFI. Results are the mean ±SEM. *Significant differences were observed between NK cell subsets of LCL and DCL patients for all 3 TLRs in LPG-stimulated and non-stimulated cells. LCL patients (n = 9), DCL patients (n = 4) and controls (n = 4).

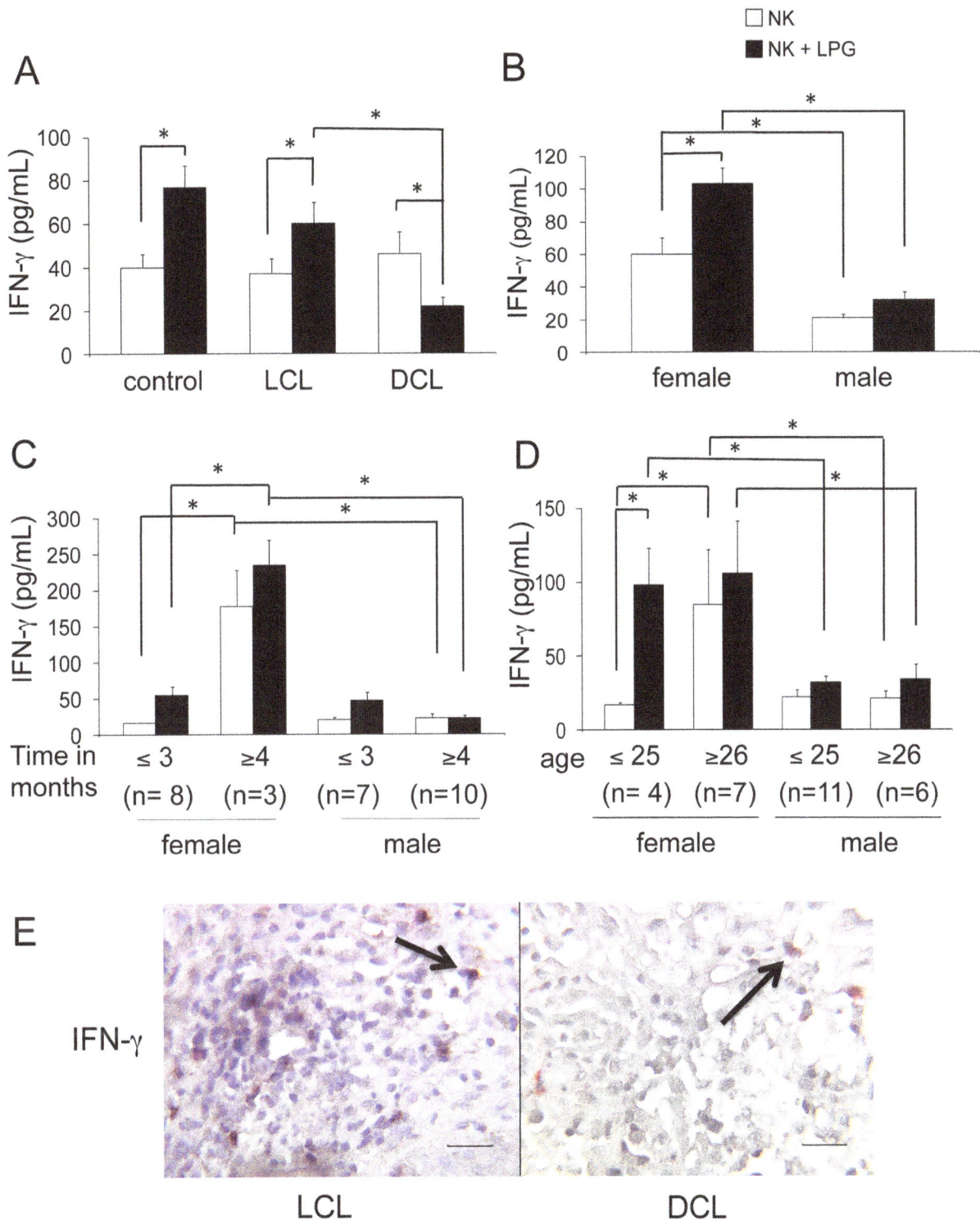

Figure 8. IFN-γ production by NK cells. (A) IFN-γ production of peripheral blood NK cells [control subjects (n = 21), LCL patients (n = 28) and DCL patients (n = 6)]. Analysis in LCL patients [female (n = 11) and male (n = 17)] according to: (B) gender; (C) disease duration; (D) age. (E) Double immunohistochemical labelling (CD57⁺/IFN-γ⁺) in lesions of patients (LCL and DCL) showed redish-brown staining generated by the combination of a red AP substrate used for NK cells and DAB Black used for IFN-γ staining. □ Non-stimulated NK cells. ■ LPG-stimulated NK cells. Mean ±SEM is shown. *p≤0.05 was considered significant. Scale bar = 50 μm. Black arrows show double positive cells.

calibrator, LCL $2^{-\Delta\Delta CT}$ was used. We also compared DCL or LCL vs healthy controls, using controls as calibrators for both studies. The results show a significant up-regulation of IFN-γ gene expression in NK cells of LCL patients after stimulation with LPG, as compared to healthy controls (Table 1, lane 7). In contrast, DCL patients showed a significant down-regulation in IFN-γ gene

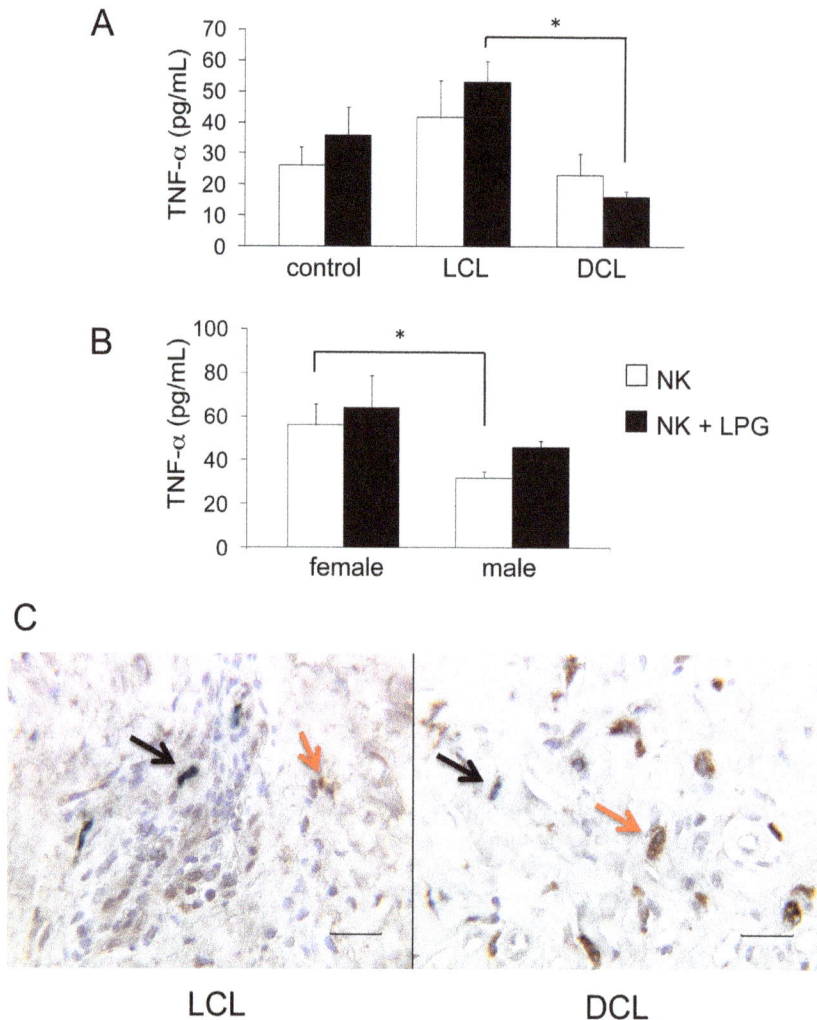

Figure 9. TNF-α production by NK cells. (A) TNF-α production in peripheral blood [control subjects (n = 21), LCL patients (n = 28) and DCL patients (n = 6)]. (B) Analysis of TNF-α production of LCL patients according to gender [female (n = 11) and male (n = 17)]. (C) Double immunohistochemistry (CD57⁺/TNF-α⁺) staining of lesions of LCL and DCL patients showed dark green staining induced by the combination of a green substrate (Stay Green/AP) used for NK cells and DAB (brown) used for TNF-α staining. □ Non-stimulated NK cells, ■ LPG-stimulated NK cells. Mean ±SEM is shown. *p≤0.05 was considered significant. Scale bar = 50 μm. Double positive cells CD57⁺/TNF-α⁺ (black arrows) and single positive cells CD57⁻/TNF-α⁺ (red arrows).

expression both in non-stimulated NK cells (Table 1, lane 6) as well as after LPG-stimulation (Table 1, lane 9), when compared with LCL patients.

DCL patients also showed down-regulation of TLR2 gene expression in non-stimulated as well as in LPG-stimulated NK cells, when compared to LCL patients (Table 1, lane 6 and lane 9) or to healthy controls (Table1, lane 5 and lane 8), albeit these differences were not statistically significant. The same holds true for the expression of TNF-α genes, which also showed a non-significant down-regulation in DCL patients, as compared to LCL patients, both in non-stimulated as in LPG-stimulated NK cells (Table 1, lane 6 and lane 9).

Thus, we were able to show that the reduced protein expression of IFN-γ in NK cells of DCL patients correlated with the down-regulation of its gene expression.

Discussion

The cause of uncontrolled parasite dissemination in DCL patients infected with *Leishmania mexicana* remains an enigma.

Although much insight has been gained on the importance of a Th1 response for parasite control in mouse models [14], these data cannot be extrapolated to the human disease. The molecules and mechanisms of innate and adaptive immunities, particularly the role of inflammation, need to be further assessed in the physiopathology of human leishmaniasis. One of the cells that possibly play a role in defining disease severity is the NK cell, since this innate cell is able to produce IFN-γ and TNF-α, both of which are required to activate the leishmanicidal machinery within macrophages. We had previously shown that *Leishmania* LPG is a ligand for TLR2 leading to IFN-γ and TNF-α production [3]. Our current results show that in addition to TLR2, TLR1 and TLR6 are also present in the binding of LPG.

Most studies of TLRs in leishmaniasis have been done in the murine models, where expression of TLR2, TLR4, TLR7, TLR8 and TLR9 have been analyzed and related to disease outcome, together with other contributing factors such as *Leishmania* species and genetic background. Yet data on the role of TLRs obtained from experimental murine leishmaniasis remain controversial: on

Table 1. Transcript expression by quantitative real time PCR in non-stimulated (NS) and LPG-stimulated NK cells (S).

Gene	1	2	3	4	5	6	7	8	9
	Fold change								
TLR2	0.96	1.06	1.06	0.53	0.09	0.18	0.57	0.10	0.18
IFN-γ	1.04	1.57	1.13	2.80	1.00	0.36*	4.08*	1.09	0.26*
TNF-α	1.00	1.34	2.00	1.05	0.62	0.57	1.34	1.20	0.89

TLR2, IFN-γ and TNF-α gene expression in NK cells of healthy controls (n = 5), LCL (n = 6) and DCL (n = 3) patients. 1. C_S vs C_NS; 2. LCL_S vs LCL_NS; 3. DCL_S vs DCL_NS; 4. LCL_NS vs C_NS; 5. DCL_NS vs C_NS; 6. DCL_NS vs LCL_NS; 7. LCL_S vs C_S; 8. DCL_S vs C_S; 9. DCL_S vs LCL_S. C: healthy controls, LCL: patients with localized cutaneous leishmaniasis, DCL: patients with diffuse cutaneous leishmaniasis. *p<0.05 significant differences.

one hand, enhanced the expression of these TLRs have been related to protection mediated by cytokine production, whereas their absence has been associated with a Th2 response and elevated *Leishmania* numbers [7,10,17–20]. Contrasting results have shown that the absence of TLR2 during the initial stages of the disease lead to reduced parasite burdens in *L. amazonensis* infected mice, which was associated with more organized granuloma formations [21]. This was supported by data of $TLR2^{-/-}$ mice that achieved a better elimination of the parasite due to reduced inflammatory infiltrates [22].

Yet the role of TLRs in human leishmaniasis has not been thoroughly explored. Some studies have shown that patients with leishmaniasis increase their TLR (1, 2, 3, 4 and 9) expression, as compared to healthy or cured subjects [23–29]. Furthermore, TLR expression has been shown to decrease during chronic diseases and with age [29–32]. The expression of TLRs also depends on the cell type [23,30] species/strains and virulence of *Leishmania* parasites [22,33] or TLR polymorphisms [34].

Little is known of TLRs and NK cell activity in patients with different clinical forms of cutaneous leishmaniasis and to what degree these can be related. Previous studies of NK cells in DCL patients have reported a reduction in NK cell numbers that could be restored after treatment and parasite reduction [1,35], suggesting that the parasite is able to regulate NK cells. Lieke et al. demonstrated that NK cells incubated with *L. major* or *L. aethiopica* could lead to death not only of the parasite, but of the NK cell as well [36]. Yet functional modulation of NK cells by this parasite remained to be analyzed. We were therefore interested in analyzing the expression of TLR2, as well as cytokine production by NK cells of patients with LCL and DCL and to evaluate their possible association with disease severity. We were furthermore interested whether specific heterodimers form between TLR2 and TLR1 or TLR6 when binding to LPG and if there is a preferential expression of any of these TLRs in patients with LCL and DCL that could be related to disease severity. We found striking differences in the NK-cell numbers, in the magnitude of TLR expression as well as in IFN-γ and TNF-α productions by NK cells of DCL and LCL patients, which correlated with disease severity: DCL patients showed reduced NK cell numbers (possibly due to NK-cell death), down-regulated TLR2, TLR1 and TLR6 expression as well as reduced cytokine production, as compared to LCL patients. In contrast, LCL patients showed enhanced expression of these TLRs, which correlated with augmented IFN-γ and TNF-α production by their blood NK cells, in addition to enhanced tissue NK cells with IFN-γ and TNF-α staining.

Although tissue lesions of DCL patients showed reduced NK cells with TNF-α staining, they harbored larger NK-negative cells, which stained for TNF-α. Our study did not clarify the nature of these cells, yet due to their size/form, we are tempted to speculate that they could be mast cells, capable of storing preformed TNF-α, that is released upon various stimuli. The elevated amounts of cells containing TNF-α in lesions of DCL patients, possibly account for the intense inflammation and associated tissue damage found in these patients [37]. The tissue damage due to intense inflammation has also been shown in patients with mucocutaneous leishmaniasis [38,39].

A further finding was that the NK cells of LCL patients expressing TLRs were found within granulomas. Highly organized granuloma structures have been related to host resistance during hepatic leishmaniasis of patients with visceral leishmaniasis caused by *Leishmania donovani* [40]. Within the protective microenvironment created by granuloma formations, NK cells possibly contribute to anti-leishmanial mechanisms by secreting IFN-γ and TNF-α, leading to macrophage activation and helping to create a protective Th-1 environment together with CD4+ cells, both of which are significantly enhanced in LCL, as compared to DCL patients [1,41]. Our data on TLRs in granulomas in patients with cutaneous leishmaniasis are in accordance with the literature, where TLR9 and TLR2 have been reported [21,24]. In contrast to the enhanced numbers of NK cells within granulomas found in tissue lesions of LCL patients, DCL lesions show reduced numbers of NK cells scattered within lesions showing no cellular organization, both of which possibly contribute to lack of disease control in these patients.

The enhanced IFN-γ and TNF-α production observed in LCL patients corresponded to females, which showed a more pronounced increase of their IFN-γ production upon prolonged disease evolution (≥4 months). We propose that our results possibly give a new insight into the mechanisms involved in conferring a higher resistance to female patients towards *Leishmania* infections, as has been reported in the literature [37,42]. Our observations on the lower IFN-γ production in female LCL patients during the first 3 months after infection and the subsequent increase of these cytokine as disease progresses has also been reported by other groups [43–46]. IFN-γ production seems to depend on the patient's background, clinical form, age and gender [47]. We hypothesize that this continuous increase in cytokine production in female patients is possibly due to enhanced IFN-γ receptors in their NK cells that ensure autocrine activation and further cytokine production.

In accordance, down-regulation of TLR1, TLR2 and TLR6 expression on NK cells of DCL patients and their diminished IFN-γ and TNF-α cytokine production possibly contributes to disease progression due to their inability to induce leishmanicidal mechanisms of macrophages. The significantly reduced IFN-γ gene expression, and to a lesser extent those of TLR2 and TNF-α, in NK cells of DCL patients, indicates that *Leishmania mexicana* possibly modulates the host immune response through epigenetic mechanisms. This modulation seems not only related to NK cells since reduced levels of IFN-γ and TNF-α have also been reported in other cells of DCL patients [48–50]. It is not clear whether the phenotypical and functional modifications of NK cells are the consequence or the cause of *Leishmania* infections, yet it is noteworthy that these patients are not prone to other microbial infections. We are tempted to propose that *Leishmania mexicana* is capable of an epigenetic modulation of the host's transcriptional program, reducing TLR2 expression and cytokine production. If this were the case, the molecular basis of this epigenetic variation remains to be analyzed. The analysis of genes and proteins of the TLR2 signal transduction pathway in NK cells of DCL patients could also add further insight into the cause of disease progression of these patients. Additionally, an analysis of HLA and other susceptibility genes are warranted in DCL patients to shed further light into their enhanced disease severity.

In conclusion, we here present novel information on NK-cell functions in human leishmaniasis. To the best of our knowledge, this is the first report that not only shows the complete activation pathway of LPG binding to TLR2 in NK cells, but also shows that TLR2 can bind to either TLR1 or TLR6. Furthermore our comparative results on NK-cell numbers, phenotypical characteristics and cytokine production in LCL and DCL patients possibly shed new light into the physiopathological mechanisms of the disease. Disease susceptibility of DCL patients is possibly linked to reduced NK cell numbers and reduced activity based on diminished TLR2, TLR1 and TLR6 expression, which in turn reduces their ability to detect *Leishmania* LPG, thus rendering them unable to secrete IFN-γ and TNF-α that are needed to induce leishmanicidal effector mechanisms within phagocytic cells.

The phenotypic and functional alterations in NK cells are most probably not the sole cause responsible of parasite dissemination in DCL patients, yet their contribution cannot be ruled out. It remains to be established whether expression of these TLRs are also modified in other cells of DCL patients in order to more clearly establish the role of NK cells in disease susceptibility during *Leishmania mexicana* infections.

Accession Numbers

Accession links for numbers/ID numbers for genes and proteins mentioned in the text:

TLR1
Gene: http://www.ncbi.nlm.nih.gov/gene/7096
Protein: http://www.uniprot.org/uniprot/Q15399
TLR2
Gene: http://www.ncbi.nlm.nih.gov/gene/7097
Protein: http://www.uniprot.org/uniprot/O60603
TLR6
Gene: http://www.ncbi.nlm.nih.gov/gene/10333
Protein: http://www.uniprot.org/uniprot/Q9Y2C9
CD16
Gene: http://www.ncbi.nlm.nih.gov/gene/2214
Protein: http://www.uniprot.org/uniprot/Q9UPY7
CD56
Gene: http://www.ncbi.nlm.nih.gov/gene/4684
Protein: http://www.uniprot.org/uniprot/P13591
MyD88
Gene: http://www.ncbi.nlm.nih.gov/gene/4615
Protein: http://www.uniprot.org/uniprot/Q99836
IRAK1
Gene: http://www.ncbi.nlm.nih.gov/gene/3654
Protein: http://www.uniprot.org/uniprot/P51617
TRAF6
Gene: http://www.ncbi.nlm.nih.gov/gene/7189
Protein: http://www.uniprot.org/uniprot/Q9Y4K3
IKK-α
Gene: http://www.ncbi.nlm.nih.gov/gene/1147
Protein: http://www.uniprot.org/uniprot/O15111
IKK-β
Gene: http://www.ncbi.nlm.nih.gov/gene/3551
Protein: http://www.uniprot.org/uniprot/O14920
IKK-γ
Gene: http://www.ncbi.nlm.nih.gov/gene/8517
Protein: http://www.uniprot.org/uniprot/Q9Y6K9
IκB-α
Gene: http://www.ncbi.nlm.nih.gov/gene/4792
Protein: http://www.uniprot.org/uniprot/P25963
NF-κB p50
Gene: http://www.ncbi.nlm.nih.gov/gene/4790
Protein: http://www.uniprot.org/uniprot/P19838
NF-κB p65
Gene: http://www.ncbi.nlm.nih.gov/gene/5970
Protein: http://www.uniprot.org/uniprot/Q04206
TNF-α
Gene: http://www.ncbi.nlm.nih.gov/gene/7124
Protein: http://www.uniprot.org/uniprot/Q9UBM5
IFN- γ
Gene: http://www.ncbi.nlm.nih.gov/gene/3458
Protein: http://www.uniprot.org/uniprot/P01579

Supporting Information

Figure S1 Expression of TLR1, TLR2 and TLR6 in NK cells stimulated with different TLR2 ligands (LPG, PGN

and Pam₃Cys). Cell surface expression is indicated by the geometric mean of fluorescence intensity (MIF). These results are the mean $\pm$SEM. *$p \leq 0.05$ was considered statistically significant.

Acknowledgments

Isabel Cristina Cañeda-Guzmán was supported by a PhD fellowship from CONACyT and is a doctoral student of Programa de Doctorado en Ciencias Biológicas, Universidad Nacional Autónoma de México (UNAM).

We are grateful to PhD. José Sotero Delgado-Domínguez and MSc. Adriana Ruiz-Remigio for their support.

Author Contributions

Conceived and designed the experiments: ICCG IB. Performed the experiments: ICCG EAFF NSS. Analyzed the data: ICCG EAFF IB. Contributed reagents/materials/analysis tools: GCF MAG. Wrote the paper: ICCG EAFF IB.

References

1. Salaiza-Suazo N, Volkow P, Pérez-Tamayo R, Moll H, Gillitzer R, et al. (1999) Treatment of two patients with diffuse cutaneous leishmaniasis caused by *Leishmania mexicana* modifies the immunohistological profile but not the disease outcome. Trop Med Int Health 4: 801–811.
2. MEXICO World Health Organization website. Available: www.who/int/leishmaniasis/resources/MEXICO.pdf. Accessed December 5, 2013.
3. Becker I, Salaiza N, Aguirre M, Delgado J, Carrillo-Carrasco N, et al. (2003) *Leishmania* lipophosphoglycan (LPG) activates NK cells through toll-like receptor-2. Mol Biochem Parasitol 130: 65–74.
4. de Veer MJ, Curtis JM, Baldwin TM, DiDonato JA, Sexton A, et al. (2003) MyD88 is essential for clearance of *Leishmania major*: possible role for lipophosphoglycan and Toll-like receptor 2 signaling. Eur J Immunol 33: 2822–2831.
5. Kamhawi S (2006) Phlebotomine sand flies and *Leishmania* parasites: friends or foes? Trends Parasitol 22: 439–445.
6. Tuon FF, Amato VS, Bacha HA, AlMusawi T, Duarte MI (2008) Toll-like receptors and leishmaniasis. Infect Immun 76: 866–872.
7. Kropf P, Freudenberg MA, Modolell M, Price HP, Herath S, et al. (2004) Toll-like receptor 4 contributes to efficient control of infection with the protozoan parasite *Leishmania major*. Infect Immun 72: 1920–1928.
8. Schleicher U, Liese J, Knippertz I, Kurzmann C, Hesse A, et al. (2007) NK cell activation in visceral leishmaniasis requires TLR9, myeloid DCs, and IL-12, but is independent of plasmacytoid DCs. J Exp Med 204: 893–906.
9. Liese J, Schleicher U, Bogdan C (2008) The innate immune response against *Leishmania* parasites. Immunobiology 213: 377–387.
10. Abou Fakher FH, Rachinel N, Klimczak M, Louis J, Doyen N (2009) TLR9-dependent activation of dendritic cells by DNA from *Leishmania major* favors Th1 cell development and the resolution of lesions. J Immunol 182: 1386–1396.
11. Scharton-Kersten TM, Sher A (1997) Role of natural killer cells in innate resistance to protozoan infection. Curr Opin Immunol 9: 44–51.
12. Moretta L (2010) Dissecting CD56^dim human NK cells. Blood 116: 3689–3691.
13. Cooper MA, Fehniger TA, Caligiuri MA (2001) The biology of human natural killer-cell subsets. Trends Immunol 22: 633–640.
14. Bogdan C (2012) Natural killer cells in experimental and human leishmaniasis. Front Cell Infect Microbiol 2: 69. doi: 10.3389/fcimb.2012.00069.
15. Nylén S, Maasho K, Söderström K, Ilg T, Akuffo H (2003) Live *Leishmania* promastigotes can directly activate primary human natural killer cells to produce interferon-gamma. Clin Exp Immunol 131: 457–467.
16. Schmittgen TD, Livak KJ (2008) Analyzing real-time PCR data by the comparative C_T method. Nat protocols 3: 1101–1108.
17. Faria MS, Reis FC, Lima AP (2012) Toll-like receptors in *Leishmania* infections: guardians or promoters? J Parasitol Res: 930257. doi: 10.1155/2012/930257.
18. Liese J, Schleicher U, Bogdan C (2007) TLR9 signaling is essential for the innate NK cell response in murine cutaneous leishmaniasis. Eur J Immunol 37: 3424–3434.
19. Cezario GA, de Oliveira LR, Peresi E, Nicolete VC, Polettini J, et al. (2011) Analysis of the expression of toll-like receptors 2 and 4 and cytokine production during experimental *Leishmania chagasi* infection. Mem Inst Oswaldo Cruz 106: 573–583.
20. Srivastava A, Singh N, Mishra M, Kumar V, Gour JK, et al. (2012) Identification of TLR inducing Th1-responsive *Leishmania donovani* amastigote-specific antigens. Mol Cell Biochem 359: 359–368.
21. Guerra CS, Silva RM, Carvalho LO, Calabrese KS, Bozza PT, et al. (2010) Histopathological analysis of initial cellular response in TLR2 deficient mice experimentally infected by *Leishmania (L.) amazonensis*. Int J Exp Pathol 91: 451–459.
22. Srivastava S, Pandey SP, Jha MK, Chandel HS, Saha B (2013) *Leishmania* expressed lipophosphoglycan interacts with Toll-like receptor (TLR)-2 to decrease TLR-9 expression and reduce anti-leishmanial responses. Clin Exp Immunol. 172: 403–409. doi: 10.1111/cei.12074.
23. Tuon FF, Fernandes ER, Duarte MI, Amato VS (2010) The expression of TLR2, TLR4 and TLR9 in the epidermis of patients with cutaneous leishmaniasis. J Dermatol Sci 59: 55–57.
24. Tuon FF, Fernandes ER, Pagliari C, Duarte MI, Amato VS (2010) The expression of TLR9 in human cutaneous leishmaniasis is associated with granuloma. Parasite Immunol 32: 769–72.
25. Tuon FF, Fernandes ER, Duarte MI, Amato VS (2012) Expression of TLR2 and TLR4 in lesions of patients with tegumentary American leishmaniasis. Rev Inst Med Trop Sao Paulo 54: 159–163.
26. Nicodemo AC, Amato VS, Miranda AM, Floeter-Winter LM, Zampieri RA, et al. (2012) Are the severe injuries of cutaneous leishmaniasis caused by an exacerbated Th1 response? Parasite Immunol 34: 440–443.
27. Vieira ÉL, Keesen TS, Machado PR, Guimarães LH, Carvalho EM, et al. (2013) Immunoregulatory profile of monocytes from cutaneous leishmaniasis patients and association with lesion size. Parasite Immunol 35: 65–72.
28. Mukherjee AK, Gupta G, Adhikari A, Majumder S, Kar Mahapatra S, et al. (2012) Miltefosine triggers a strong proinflammatory cytokine response during visceral leishmaniasis: role of TLR4 and TLR9. Int. Immunopharmacol 12: 565–572.
29. Tolouei S, Hejazi SH, Ghaedi K, Khamesipour A, Hasheminia SJ (2013) TLR2 and TLR4 in cutaneous leismaniasis caused by *Leishmania major*. Scand J Immunol 78: 478–484.
30. Krutzik SR, Ochoa MT, Sieling PA, Uematsu S, Ng YW, et al. (2003) Activation and regulation of Toll-like receptors 2 and 1 in human leprosy. Nat Med 9: 525–532.
31. van Duin D, Mohanty S, Thomas V, Ginter S, Montgomery RR, et al. (2007) Age-associated defect in human TLR-1/2 function. J Immunol 178: 970–975.
32. Renshaw M, Rockwell J, Engleman C, Gewirtz A, Katz J, et al. (2002) Cutting edge: impaired Toll-like receptor expression and function in aging. J Immunol 169: 4697–4701.
33. Chandra D, Naik S (2008) *Leishmania donovani* infection down-regulates TLR2-stimulated IL-12p40 and activates IL-10 in cells of macrophage/monocytic lineage by modulating MAPK pathways through a contact-dependent mechanism. Clin Exp Immunol 154: 224–234.
34. Ajdary S, Ghamilouie MM, Alimohammadian MH, Riazi-Rad F, Pazkad SR (2011) Toll-like receptor 4 polymorphisms predispone to cutaneous leishmaniasis. Microbes Infect 13: 226–231.
35. Pereira LI, Dorta ML, Pereira AJ, Bastos RP, Oliveira MA, et al. (2009) Increase of NK cells and proinflammatory monocytes are associated with the clinical improvement of diffuse cutaneous leishmaniasis after immunochemotherapy with BCG/*Leishmania* antigens. Am J Trop Med Hyg 81: 378–383.
36. Lieke T, Nylén S, Eidsmo L, Schmetz C, Berg L, et al. (2011) The interplay between *Leishmania* promastigotes and human natural killer in vitro leads to direct lysis of *Leishmania* by NK cells and modulation of NK cell activity by *Leishmania* promastigotes. Parasitology 138: 1898–1909.
37. Mendes DS, Dantas ML, Gomes JM, Santos WL, Silva AQ, et al. (2013) Inflammation in disseminated lesions: an analysis of CD4⁺, CD20⁺, CD68⁺, CD31⁺ and vW⁺ cells in non-ulcerated lesions of disseminated leishmaniasis. Mem Inst Oswaldo Cruz 108: 18–22.
38. Nylén S, Eidsmo L (2012) Tissue damage and immunity in cutaneous leishmaniasis. Parasite Immunol 34: 551–561.
39. Carvalho LP, Passos S, Schriefer A, Carvalho EM (2012) Protective and pathologic immune responses in human tegumentary leishmaniasis. Front Immunol 3: 301. doi: 10.3389/fimmu.2012.00301.
40. Moore JW, Moyo D, Beattie L, Andrews PS, Timmis J, et al. (2013) Functional complexity of the *Leishmania* granuloma and the potential of in silico modeling. Front Immunol 4: 35. doi: 10.3389/fimmu.2013.00035.
41. Ritter U, Moll H, Laskay T, Bröcker E, Velazco O, et al. (1996) Differential expression of chemokines in patients with localized and diffuse cutaneous American leishmaniasis. J Infect Dis 173: 699–709.
42. Guerra-Silveira F, Abad-Franch F (2013) Sex bias in infectious disease epidemiology: patterns and processes. PLoS One 8: e62390. doi: 10.1371/journal.pone.0062390.
43. Rocha PN, Almeida RP, Bacellar O, De Jesus AR, Filho DC, et al. (1999) Down-regulation of Th1 type of response in early human American cutaneous leishmaniasis. J Infect Dis 180: 1731–1734.
44. Ajdary S, Alimohammadian MH, Eslami MB, Kemp K, Kharazmi A (2000) Comparison of the immune profile of nonhealing cutaneous Leishmaniasis patients with those who have active lesions and those who have recovered from infection. Infect Immun 68: 1760–1764.
45. Alimohammadian MH, Jones SL, Darabi H, Riazirad F, Ajdary S, et al. (2012). Assessment of interferon-γ levels and leishmanin skin test results in persons recovered for leishmaniasis. Am J Trop Med Hyg 87: 70–5. doi: 10.4269/ajtmh.2012.11-0479.

46. Kima PE, Soong L (2013) Interferon gamma in leishmaniasis. Front Immunol 4: 156. doi: 10.3389/fimmu.2013.00156.

47. Matos GI, Fernandes Covas C, Cássia Bittar R, Gomes-Silva A, Marques F. et al. (2007) IFNG+874T/A polymorphism is not associated with American tegumentary leishmaniasis susceptibility but can influence *Leishmania* induced IFN-γ production. Infect Dis 7: 33.

48. Carrada G, Cañeda C, Salaiza N, Delgado J, Ruiz A, et al. (2007) Monocyte cytokine and costimulatory molecule expression in patient infected with *Leishmania mexicana*. Parasite Immunol 29: 117–126.

49. Leopoldo PT, Machado PR, Almeida RP, Schriefer A, Giudice A, et al. (2006) Differential effects of antigens from *L. braziliensis* isolates from disseminated and cutaneous leishmaniasis on in vitro cytokine production. BMC Infect Dis 6: 75.

50. Galindo-Sevilla N, Soto N, Mancilla J, Cerbulo A, Zambrano E, et al. (2007) Low serum levels of dehydroepiandrosterone and cortisol in human diffuse cutaneous leishmaniasis by *Leishmania mexicana*. Am J Trop Med Hyg 76: 566–572.

4

Filament-Producing Mutants of Influenza A/Puerto Rico/8/1934 (H1N1) Virus Have Higher Neuraminidase Activities than the Spherical Wild-Type

Jill Seladi-Schulman, Patricia J. Campbell, Suganthi Suppiah, John Steel, Anice C. Lowen*

Department of Microbiology and Immunology, Emory University School of Medicine, Atlanta, Georgia, United States of America

Abstract

Influenza virus exhibits two morphologies – spherical and filamentous. Strains that have been grown extensively in laboratory substrates are comprised predominantly of spherical virions while clinical or low passage isolates produce a mixture of spheres and filamentous virions of varying lengths. The filamentous morphology can be lost upon continued passage in embryonated chicken eggs, a common laboratory substrate for influenza viruses. The fact that the filamentous morphology is maintained in nature but lost in favor of a spherical morphology *in ovo* suggests that filaments confer a selective advantage within the infected host that is not necessary for growth in laboratory substrates. Indeed, we have recently shown that filament-producing variant viruses are selected upon passage of the spherical laboratory strain A/Puerto Rico/8/1934 (H1N1) [PR8] in guinea pigs. Toward determining the nature of the selective advantage conferred by filaments, we sought to identify functional differences between spherical and filamentous particles. We compared the wild-type PR8 virus to two previously characterized recombinant PR8 viruses in which single point mutations within M1 confer a filamentous morphology. Our results indicate that these filamentous PR8 mutants have higher neuraminidase activities than the spherical PR8 virus. Conversely, no differences were observed in HAU:PFU or HAU:RNA ratios, binding avidity, sensitivity to immune serum in hemagglutination inhibition assays, or virion stability at elevated temperatures. Based on these results, we propose that the pleomorphic nature of influenza virus particles is important for the optimization of neuraminidase functions *in vivo*.

Editor: Ralph Tripp, University of Georgia, United States of America

Funding: This work was funded by the National Institutes of Health/National Institute of Allergy and Infectious Disease under Centers for Excellence in Influenza Research and Surveillance (CEIRS) contract number HHSN266200700006C (http://www.niaid.nih.gov/labsandresources/resources/ceirs). The funders had no role in study design, data collection and analysis, decision to publish, or preparation of the manuscript.

Competing Interests: The authors have declared that no competing interests exist.

* Email: anice.lowen@emory.edu

Introduction

Influenza A virus (IAV) is an enveloped virus containing eight negative-sense RNA gene segments [1]. It is the causative agent of seasonal epidemics of respiratory illness as well as occasional pandemics, the most recent of which occurred in 2009 [2]. IAV is pleomorphic, producing virions of spherical and filamentous morphology [3]. Strains that produce predominantly spherical or ovoid virions have typically been passaged many times within laboratory substrates, while filament-producing strains occur in primary or low passage isolates [4,5]. Filaments are of variable length and can be up to 30 μm long [6]. Herein, we define filaments as any virion 300 nm in length or longer (≥3x the diameter of a typical spherical virion). Studies performed using reverse genetics systems have identified the M1 matrix protein as the major genetic determinant of virion morphology, however portions of the viral nucleoprotein (NP) as well as the cytoplasmic tails of the M2 ion channel, hemagglutinin (HA) and neuraminidase (NA) proteins have been shown to affect virion morphology as well [7–13].

Early observations showed that the filamentous morphology is gradually lost upon continued passage in embryonated chicken eggs in favor of a more spherical morphology [14,15]. We also observed that filaments could be lost following ten passages in eggs or MDCK cells, but that this phenotypic change was not required for robust adaptation to either substrate [5]. The fact that filaments are maintained in nature while dispensable for growth in laboratory substrates suggests that the filamentous morphology provides a selective advantage within the infected host that is not necessary for growth in the laboratory. Previously, we showed that passaging of the spherical laboratory strain A/Puerto Rico/8/1934 (H1N1) [PR8] twelve times in guinea pigs led to the emergence of virions that are filamentous in morphology [5]. Through sequencing of the M1 matrix gene of the passage 12 (P12) virus pool, we identified several coding mutations within M1. Individual introduction of four of these amino acid changes using reverse genetics yielded mutant viruses that produced significantly more filaments than the wild-type [p<0.05; difference in proportions test] [5].

While selection for a filamentous morphology through passaging in an animal host confirms an advantage of filamentous virions *in vivo*, the nature of the selective advantage remains unclear. To determine the advantage filament-producing viruses have over their spherical counterparts, we used recombinant wild-type PR8 (rPR8wt) and two previously characterized filamentous M1 mutants – rPR8 M1 N87S (N87S) and rPR8 M1 R101G (R101G) [5]. Our published particle counts showed that 16% and 41% of virions were filamentous for N87S and R101G viruses, respectively, compared to 4% for PR8wt [5]. These three viruses present an ideal system in which to address the differences between exclusively spherical and filament-producing IAV, for the following reasons: i) the mutant strains are highly similar genetically to the rPR8wt, simplifying the interpretation of results; ii) the mutations used arose naturally, minimizing the likelihood of disrupting viral functions through their introduction; and iii) the mutant viruses differ significantly from rPR8wt in terms of filament production. Thus, rPR8wt, N87S, and R101G viruses were analyzed in a series of *in vitro* assays. We hypothesized that functional differences between spherical and filamentous virions might arise due to their differing surface areas, and therefore focused our efforts on the two surface glycoproteins of IAV, HA and NA. We tested whether the HA avidity or NA activity per virion differed between the spherical rPR8wt virus and filament producing strains. In addition, the ratio of hemagglutination units (HAU) to plaque forming units (PFU), the ratio of HAU to RNA copies, and virion stability at elevated temperatures were investigated. Our findings suggest a role of the viral NA protein in the fitness advantage conferred by filamentous virion morphology: by two independent measures, the two filamentous rPR8 mutants displayed higher neuraminidase activities compared to rPR8wt, but did not differ significantly in binding avidity, inhibition of binding by antiserum, infectivity or thermostability.

Material and Methods

Ethics statement

This study was performed in accordance with the recommendations in the Guide for the Care and Use of Laboratory Animals of the National Institutes of Health. Animal husbandry and experimental procedures were approved by the Emory University Institutional Animal Care and Use Committee (IACUC protocol #2000719).

Viruses and cells

The rPR8wt, rPR8 M1 N87S, and rPR8 M1 R101G viruses were generated using reverse genetics as previously described [16–18]. Briefly, rPR8-based viruses were recovered following eight (pDZ) plasmid transfection of 293T cells and subsequent inoculation of transfected cells and culture medium into 9–11 day old embryonated chicken's eggs. Stocks of the rPR8 wild-type virus and mutants were generated in 9–11 day old embryonated chicken's eggs. Influenza A/Udorn/301/1972 (H3N2) virus was grown in MDCK cells. Influenza A/Anhui/1/2013 (H7N9) virus was grown in eggs under enhanced BSL3 containment and inactivated by addition of beta-propiolactone (BPL) prior to removal from the BSL3 facility.

Washed chicken red blood cells from Lampire Biological were used for all hemagglutination-based assays. MDCK cells, a kind gift of Peter Palese, were maintained in minimal essential medium supplemented with 10% fetal bovine serum and penicillin/streptomycin. 293T cells (ATCC), used for virus rescue by reverse genetics, were maintained in Dulbecco's minimal essential medium supplemented with 10% fetal bovine serum. Embryonated chickens' eggs were obtained from Hy-Line International and

incubated at 37°C, with rocking, for 9–11 days prior to inoculation with IAV.

Infectious titer comparison

Viruses were diluted to concentration of 128 HAU. Hemagglutination units, or HAU, are defined as the reciprocal of the highest dilution of virus still allowing agglutination of red blood cells. After confirming the HA titer, viruses were titrated in triplicate by plaque assay of 10-fold serial dilutions on MDCK cells. A Student *t*-test was used to compare the infectious titers of each mutant virus to rPR8wt virus.

C_q value comparison

Viruses were diluted to concentration of 128 HAU. After confirming the HA titer, RNA was extracted from 160 μl of each diluted virus sample using the QIAamp Viral RNA Mini Kit (QIAGEN), according to the manufacturer's instructions. cDNA was generated using Maxima reverse transcriptase (Thermo Scientific) and a universal forward primer (GGCCAGCAAAAG-CAGG). Quantitative PCR was then performed on a Bio-Rad CFX384 thermocycler using the cDNA as template, SsoFast EvaGreen Supermix (Bio-Rad), and primers specific for the NP segment (F: TATTCGTCTCAGGGAGCAAAAGCAGG [19] and R: CTGATTTCAGTGGCATTCTGGC). Each cDNA was analyzed in triplicate and the resulting cycle threshold (C_q) values were recorded. Average C_q values shown in Table 1 were calculated by first converting each C_q value to $2^{(-C_q)}$, calculating the arithmetic mean, and then taking the $-\log_2$ of the arithmetic mean.

Red blood cell elution assay

Each virus was standardized to a concentration of 128 HAU. Duplicate HA assays were then set up in parallel using 1:2 serially diluted viruses and allowed to develop at 4°C. One set of plates was then transferred to 37°C (t = 0 hours) to trigger neuraminidase activity, while the second set of plates was left at 4°C to act as a negative control. Red blood cells were monitored for elution (visible as the formation of a red blood cell pellet at the bottom of the well) at the following time points: 1, 2, 3, 4, 6, and 8 hours.

MUNANA neuraminidase activity assay

Neuraminidase activity assays using the soluble substrate methylumbelliferyl N-acetylneuraminic acid (MUNANA) were performed as previously described by Campbell et al. [20]. Virus was diluted to 5×10^5 PFU/ml and 80 μl was added to each well of a black 96-well plate (CoStar). A sample of each diluted virus preparation was retained for quantification of viral RNA therein by RT-qPCR. Concentrations of MUNANA substrate ranging from 1.17 μM to 150 μM were used. When cleaved by the viral NA, MUNANA produces a fluorescent product. Fluorescence was quantified using a Biotek Synergy H1 plate reader every minute over the course of an hour. Fluorescence curves were then fitted to the Michaelis-Menton equation to determine values of V_{max} (maximal enzyme velocity) and K_m (the Michaelis constant, the substrate concentration at which the reaction rate is half of V_{max}). Each experiment included triplicate samples of each virus.

Virus concentration for Western blot analysis

Each virus was purified from allantoic fluid collected from 9–11 day embryonated chicken eggs infected with 250 PFU of virus. Allantoic fluid was spun at 3,000 rpm for 10 minutes at 4°C in a Sorvall tabletop centrifuge after which the supernatant was transferred to ultracentrifuge tubes (Beckman Coulter). Samples

Table 1. 128 HAU of rPR8wt, rPR8 M1 N87S and rPR8 M1 R101G viruses comprise comparable infectious titers and genome copies.

Virus	Infectious titer (PFU/ml)[a]	Average infectious titer (PFU/ml)	C_q value[b]	Average C_q value
rPR8wt	6.00×10^7	1.15×10^8	19.06	19.16
	1.55×10^8		19.37	
	1.30×10^8		19.08	
rPR8 M1 N87S	5.00×10^7	7.60×10^7	19.23	19.32
	5.00×10^7		19.42	
	1.30×10^8		19.32	
rPR8 M1 R101G	4.00×10^7	7.80×10^7	18.86	18.94
	6.50×10^7		18.92	
	1.30×10^8		19.04	

[a]rPR8wt to rPR8 M1 N87S comparison (p = 0.38), rPR8wt to rPR8 M1 R101G comparison (p = 0.40). A two-tailed Student t-test was used to assess significance.
[b]rPR8wt to rPR8 M1 N87S comparison (p = 0.23), rPR8wt to rPR8 M1 R101G comparison (p = 0.10). To assess significance, a two-tailed Student t-test was applied to values of $2^{(-Cq)}$.

were spun in an SW32 rotor at 10,000 rpm for 30 minutes at 4°C and supernatant was then transferred to a fresh tube where a 5-ml 30% sucrose cushion was added. Samples were spun in an SW32 rotor at 25,000 rpm for 1.5 hours at 4°C. All supernatant was removed and 100 μl of PBS was added to the virus pellet and allowed to resuspend at 4°C overnight.

NP normalization and Western blot

Concentrated virus samples were denatured by boiling for 10 minutes and treated with PNGaseF (New England Biolabs) for 1 hour at 37°C to allow for deglycosylation. The amount of NP in each virus sample was quantified by polyacrylamide gel electrophoresis followed by Coomassie staining (GelCode Blue – Thermo Scientific) and analysis with Image Lab software (Bio-Rad). The volume of each sample used for western blotting was then normalized based on NP content. Samples were loaded on a 4–15% SDS gradient gel (Bio-Rad Mini Protean) and electrophoresed at 130 V for 1 hour and 5 minutes. Protein was transferred (semi-dry) onto nitrocellulose membrane for 1 hour at 100 mA and blocking was performed overnight. NA was detected using a goat anti-NA primary antibody (BEI NR-9598) and a donkey anti-goat alexa 647-conjugated secondary antibody. NP was detected using a rabbit anti-NP primary antibody (a kind gift of Peter Palese) and a donkey anti-rabbit alexa 488-conjugated secondary antibody. Band intensity was quantified using Image Lab software (Bio-Rad).

Red blood cell-based avidity assay

The red blood cell-based avidity assay was performed similarly to those described in [21]. Briefly, a 1.3% solution of red blood cells in PBS was treated with a series of dilutions of *C. perfringens* neuraminidase (Sigma) for 30 minutes at 37°C. Neuraminidase concentrations incremented by 5 mU/ml for the PR8-based viruses and 10 mU/ml for the H3 and H7 subtype viruses. Treated red blood cells were then added to virus at a standardized concentration of 8 HAU in a v-bottom, 96-well plate. Hemagglutination was assessed after 2 hours at 4°C. To rule out the activity of the viral NA in interpreting results, virus was diluted in PBS containing oseltamivir carboxylate (GS4071) and the assay was allowed to develop at 4°C.

Trypsin-heat-periodate treatment

In order to remove nonspecific inhibitors of hemagglutination, serum treatment was performed as outlined in [22]. Briefly, serum was treated with L-1-Tosylamide-2-phenylethyl chloromethyl ketone (TPCK) trypsin for 30 minutes at 56°C. After cooling to room temperature, serum was then treated with 0.011 M metapotassium periodate (KIO$_4$) for 15 minutes at room temperature. After KIO$_4$ treatment, serum was treated with 1% glycerol in PBS for 15 minutes at room temperature after which an 85% PBS solution was added to reach a final serum dilution of 1:10.

Hemagglutination inhibition (HI) assay

Trypsin-heat-periodate-treated anti-PR8 guinea pig serum was diluted in PBS either 1:2 or 1:1.5 across a v-bottom, 96-well plate. Each virus was standardized to a concentration of 8 HAU and was then added to the diluted serum. Serum and virus were incubated together at 4°C for 30 minutes after which 0.5% red blood cells in PBS were added to each well. The assay was allowed to develop at 4°C. Naïve guinea pig serum was used as a negative control. The HI titers reported reflect HI activity above background levels.

Plaque reduction assay

Each virus was diluted to approximately 250 PFU. Trypsin-heat-periodate treated anti-PR8 guinea pig serum was serially diluted 1:80, 1:160, 1:320, and 1:640 in PBS. Control serum obtained from a naïve guinea pig was also used. Virus was added to the diluted serum and incubated for 30 minutes at 37°C. The infectious titer of each serum/virus sample then quantified by plaque assay in MDCK cells. This assay was performed in triplicate.

Thermostability assay

Each virus was diluted to approximately 1×10^6 PFU. Fifteen 120 μl aliquots of each virus were incubated at 50°C and three aliquots of each virus were removed at 0, 15, 30, 60, and 120 minutes. Titers for each sample were quantified via plaque assay on MDCK cells.

Results

Equivalent HAU of the rPR8wt, rPR8 M1 N87S, and rPR8 M1 R101G viruses do not differ in infectivity or RNA copy number

Each of the functional assays that we applied to our spherical and filamentous PR8 viruses required normalization of the input of each virus. Ideally, this normalization would be achieved by counting virus particles in transmission electron micrographs, but this approach was not practical given that the preparations used were relatively dilute and concentration by centrifugation can alter virus morphology. We therefore performed the following experiment to determine the relationships between the hemagglutination-based titer, infectious (PFU) titer and RNA copy number for each virus. rPR8wt, N87S, and R101G viruses were diluted to 128 HAU and HA titers were confirmed. Diluted virus samples were then titrated in triplicate by plaque assay. The mutant viruses showed lower PFU titers compared to rPR8wt, but the differences were not statistically significant (Table 1). RNA was extracted from 160 μl of each diluted virus and quantified by reverse transcription followed by quantitative PCR. C_q values obtained were consistent across all three viruses (Table 1). Thus, for all three viruses, the HAU to PFU and HAU to RNA copy number ratios were comparable. To assess the precision and consistency of the hemagglutination assay, we furthermore evaluated the PFU titers and relative RNA copy numbers of three 128 HAU samples of rPR8wt virus that had been obtained through independent dilution series. The average PFU titers obtained ranged from 1.66 to 1.78×10^8 PFU/ml (n = 3 per 128 HAU sample). The average C_q values were also very similar, ranging from 18.64 to 18.85. Taken together, these results indicate that similar results would be expected following normalization of rPR8wt, N87S, and R101G viruses by PFU, HAU or RNA copy number.

The rPR8 M1 N87S and rPR8 M1 R101G filamentous mutants have higher neuraminidase activity than rPR8wt virus

The NA activities of the spherical and filament-producing viruses were assessed by comparing rPR8wt, N87S, and R101G viruses in a red blood cell elution assay. To test our hypothesis that filamentous and spherical virions differ at the level of the whole virus particle, due to differing surface areas, we aimed to evaluate NA activity per virion rather than per NA protein. We therefore normalized virus input by hemagglutination titer rather than protein levels. Briefly, HA assays were set up in parallel using a standardized amount of virus (128 HAU) and allowed to develop at 4°C. At that point, one set of plates was transferred to 37°C. At this temperature, the viral NA is active and begins cleaving the sialic acids on the surface of the red blood cells, causing them to drop to the bottom of the well (elution). We monitored the plates for elution over the course of 8 hours. Progressive elution was observed at 37°C, while no elution was seen over the same time period at 4°C. We found that, when incubated with the R101G mutant virus, red blood cells eluted at a faster rate compared to those incubated with rPR8wt (Figure 1A). The N87S mutant had a less marked phenotype than the R101G mutant, but also eluted red blood cells at a faster rate than the rPR8wt – particularly at the later time points (Figure 1B).

The rPR8 M1 N87S and rPR8 M1 R101G filamentous mutants have higher neuraminidase activity in the MUNANA assay than rPR8wt virus

To confirm that the differing elution phenotypes observed were due to differing NA activities, we compared the spherical and filamentous rPR8 viruses using a MUNANA-based assay. MUNANA (methylumbelliferyl N-acetylneuraminic acid) is a soluble substrate that produces a fluorescent product when cleaved by the viral NA. For this assay, viruses were standardized to equivalent PFU and RNA titers and concentrations of MUNANA substrate ranging from 1.17 μM to 150 μM were used. Levels of fluorescence were measured every minute over a sixty-minute

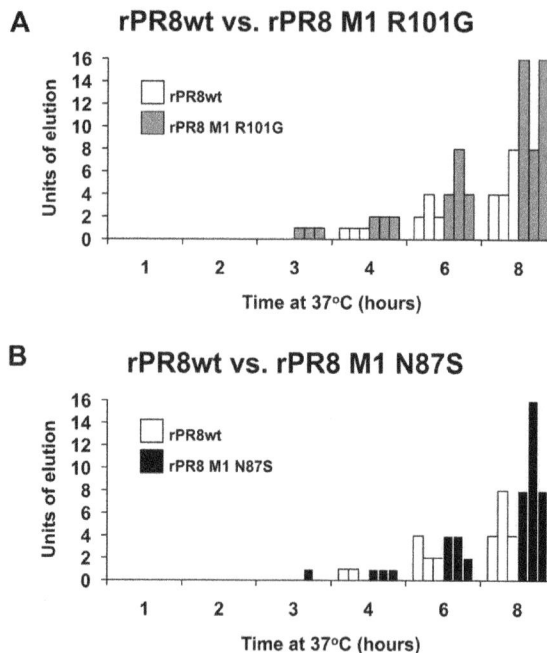

Figure 1. rPR8 M1 R101G and rPR8 M1 N87S viruses elute red blood cells at a faster rate than rPR8wt virus. HA assays were set up using virus diluted to a concentration of 128 HAU. After the assays had developed, plates were transferred to 37°C to allow for red blood cell elution by the viral neuraminidase. A second set of plates remained at 4°C where no elution occurred (not shown). The results of three independent experiments are shown, with each experiment represented by a separate bar. Within each experiment, viruses were analyzed in triplicate (standard deviation for each virus = 0). "Units of elution" is defined as the reciprocal of the highest virus dilution showing elution. A) Elution of rPR8 M1 R101G virus is compared to that of rPR8wt virus. B) Elution of rPR8 M1 N87S virus is compared to that of rPR8wt virus.

period. The resulting fluorescence curves were then fitted to the Michaelis-Menton equation for calculation of K_m and V_{max} values associated with each virus. It is important to note that, in line with our aim of evaluating NA enzyme kinetics per virion, NA protein levels contained within each virus sample were not normalized for this assay.

The results obtained correlated well with those observed from the red blood cell elution assay (Figure 2). We confirmed that equivalent amounts of each virus were assayed by performing RT-qPCR on viral RNA extracted from the same diluted virus preparations employed in the MUNANA assay (Figure 2B). The R101G mutant virus displayed the highest V_{max}, followed by the N87S mutant. rPR8wt had the lowest V_{max} (Table 2). The K_m for all three viruses was found to be consistent, as expected considering the NA protein is the same for all three viruses (Table 2). Based on the results of both the elution assay and the MUNANA assay, we concluded that the filament-producing M1 mutant viruses had a higher neuraminidase activity per virion than the spherical wild-type virus.

When standardized to NP protein levels, NA and M1 protein incorporation among rPR8wt, rPR8 M1 N87S, and rPR8 M1 R101G is similar

Because filamentous virions can be much greater in size than spherical virions, a logical explanation for our NA activity results is that filamentous virions have more NA adorning their surface. Indeed, the consistent K_m values across all three viruses obtained

A

B

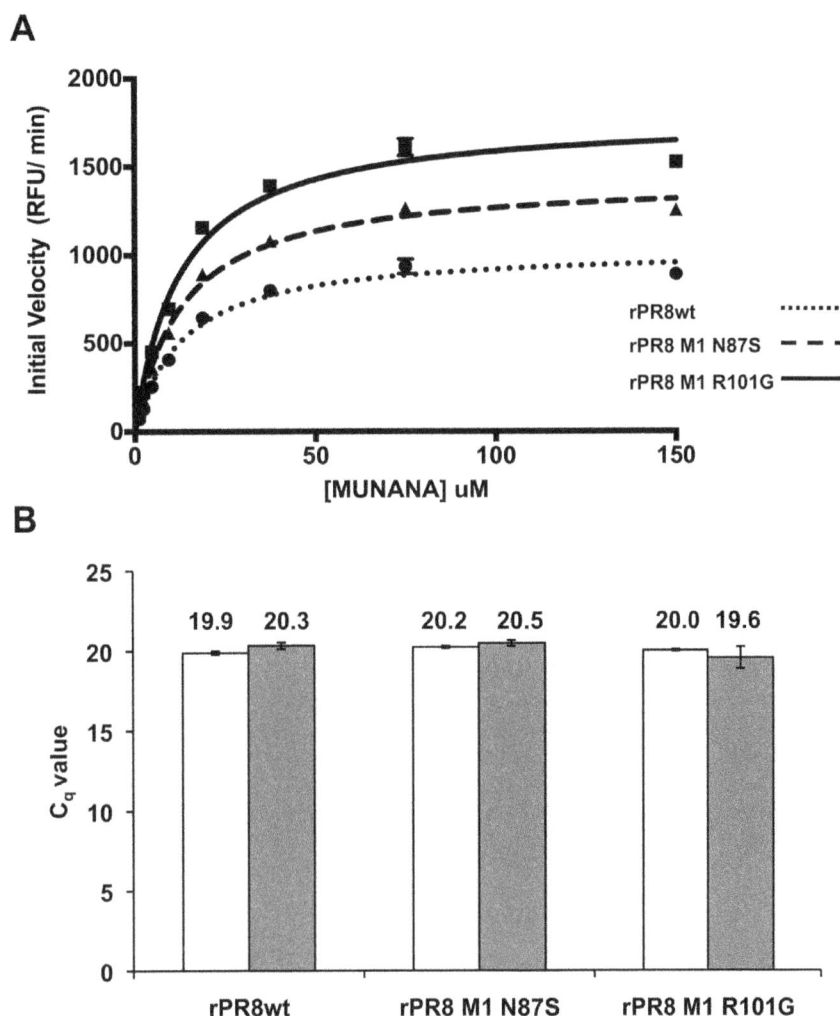

Figure 2. rPR8 M1 R101G and rPR8 M1 N87S viruses have higher neuraminidase activity than rPR8wt virus. A) Neuraminidase enzyme kinetics. Virus input was standardized to 5×10^5 PFU and concentrations of MUNANA substrate ranging from 1.17 µM to 150 µM were used. Fluorescence generated at each time point (every minute over the course of 1 hour) was detected using a Biotek Synergy H1 plate reader. The resulting fluorescence curves were then fitted to the Michaelis-Menton equation. B) That equivalent amounts of each virus were used in the MUNANA assay was confirmed by RT-qPCR for the viral NP segment. The arithmetic mean (n = 3) and standard deviation of $2^{(-Cq)}$ values were calculated and then converted back to a C_q scale by taking the $\log_2$. Two biological replicates of each virus are included in white and grey bars; each biological replicate comprised three technical replicates.

from the MUNANA assay suggest that the intrinsic NA activity is unaffected. To test this hypothesis, we performed Western blots on concentrated virus preparations of rPR8wt, N87S, and R101G, and probed for NP, NA, and M1 proteins. The fluorescence intensity of bands was quantified using a Bio-Rad Chemidoc imager. NP and M1 were included as controls: due to its association with the viral genome, NP levels would be expected to be constant among viruses of differing morphology, while M1 levels would be expected to increase with surface area. For a given amount of NP, the filamentous mutant viruses did not show increased quantities of NA or M1 proteins in virions (Figure 3A and 3B). Similar results were obtained when egg-grown virus

Table 2. rPR8 M1 N87S and rPR8 M1 R101G viruses have a higher neuraminidase activity than rPR8 wt virus in a MUNANA-based assay.

Virus	V_{max}	V_{max} 95% confidence interval	K_m	K_m 95% confidence interval
rPR8wt	1040	978–1101	13.02	10.41–15.63
rPR8 M1 N87S	1434	1370–1497	13.15	11.17–15.14
rPR8 M1 R101G	1785	1669–1901	15.52	10.60–20.44

stocks were analyzed directly (rather than concentrating them first), and when inputs were normalized by viral RNA content, rather than normalization to NP (data not shown). Based on our inability to detect increases in M1:NP ratios for the filament-producing viruses relative to rPR8wt, we concluded that the Western blot assay used was not sufficiently sensitive to detect differences (or lack thereof) in NA or M1 incorporation. The preponderance of spherical viruses present in the N87S and R101G virus stocks most likely obscures any differences in protein content between spherical and filamentous particles.

No difference in binding avidity is observed between rPR8wt, rPR8 M1 N87S, and rPR8 M1 R101G

After assessing the NA activity between spherical and filamentous viruses, we compared the function of the viral HA in a red blood cell-based avidity assay. We treated chicken red blood cells with a series of dilutions of *C. perfringens* neuraminidase. This treatment removes alpha 2,3-, alpha 2,6- and alpha 2,8-linked sialic acids. Thus, red blood cells treated with higher concentrations of neuraminidase had fewer sialic acids on their surface than those treated with lower concentrations of neuraminidase. We then added a standardized amount of virus (8 HAU) to the treated red blood cells and allowed agglutination to occur. We found that the neuraminidase concentration that prevented agglutination was the same for the rPR8wt, N87S, and R101G viruses, indicating that red blood cell binding avidity is not affected by the changes in morphology seen with these viruses (Figure 4). Additionally, to validate that the assay was sufficiently sensitive to detect differences in red blood cell binding avidity, we compared avidity of the rPR8-based viruses to those of viruses with differing HA

types (specifically, H3 and H7). We found that A/Udorn/301/1972 (H3N2) and BPL-inactivated A/Anhui/1/2013 (H7N9) virus had higher red blood cell binding avidities than the PR8-based viruses. From these results, we concluded that the changes in virion morphology mediated by the N87S and R101G mutations do not affect the binding avidity of rPR8 virus.

No difference in hemagglutination inhibition and little difference in plaque reduction was observed among rPR8wt, rPR8 M1 N87S, and rPR8 M1 R101G

Next, we compared hemagglutination inhibition (HI) between rPR8wt, N87S, and R101G viruses, reasoning that, due to their increased size, filaments may be more difficult to neutralize than spheres. Using 1:2 dilutions of trypsin-heat-periodate treated anti-PR8 guinea pig immune serum and virus standardized to 8 HAU, we found no difference in HI among rPR8wt, N87S, and R101G (Table 3). Since we were working with populations of mixed morphology, which may make differences between filaments and spheres difficult to detect, we sought to improve the sensitivity of the assay by using a series of 1:1.5 serum dilutions. Similar to the assays utilizing 1:2 dilutions, we observed little difference in HI between the spherical wild-type and filamentous mutants (Table 3).

To substantiate the relationship between particle morphology and sensitivity of virus to immune serum, we also performed a plaque reduction assay. Briefly, trypsin-heat-periodate treated anti-PR8 guinea pig serum was diluted to 1:80, 1:160, 1:320, or 1:640 in PBS. The same dilutions of a naïve guinea pig serum were used as controls. Virus was diluted to approximately 250 PFU and incubated with the diluted serum for 30 minutes at 37°C.

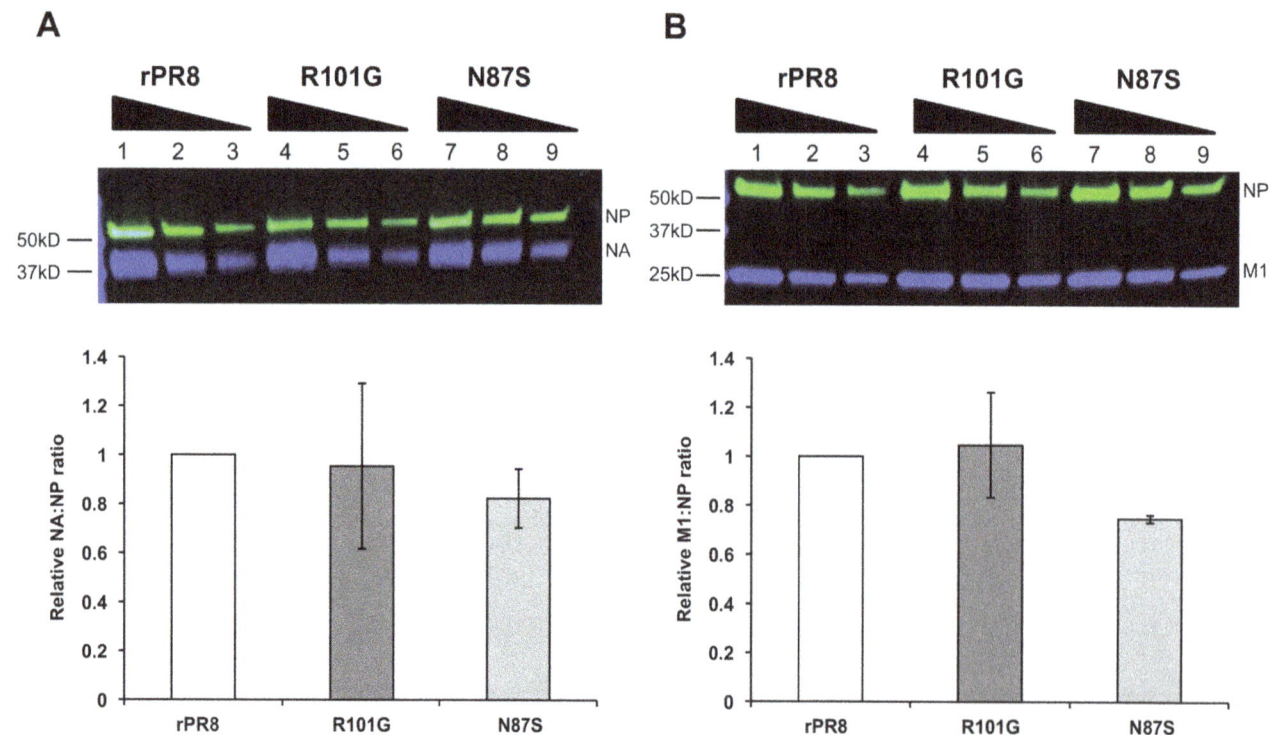

Figure 3. NA and M1 protein levels between rPR8wt, rPR8 M1 N87S, and rPR8 M1 R101G are similar when normalized to NP protein levels. Virus samples were concentrated via ultracentrifugation through a 30% sucrose cushion and resuspended in PBS. Samples were then deglycosylated and denatured, after which NP protein levels were standardized via Coomassie. For the Western blot, protein was detected using primary antibodies specific for NA, M1, and NP and fluorophore-conjugated secondary antibodies. All bands were quantified using Image Lab software (Bio-Rad). Error bars represent standard deviation.

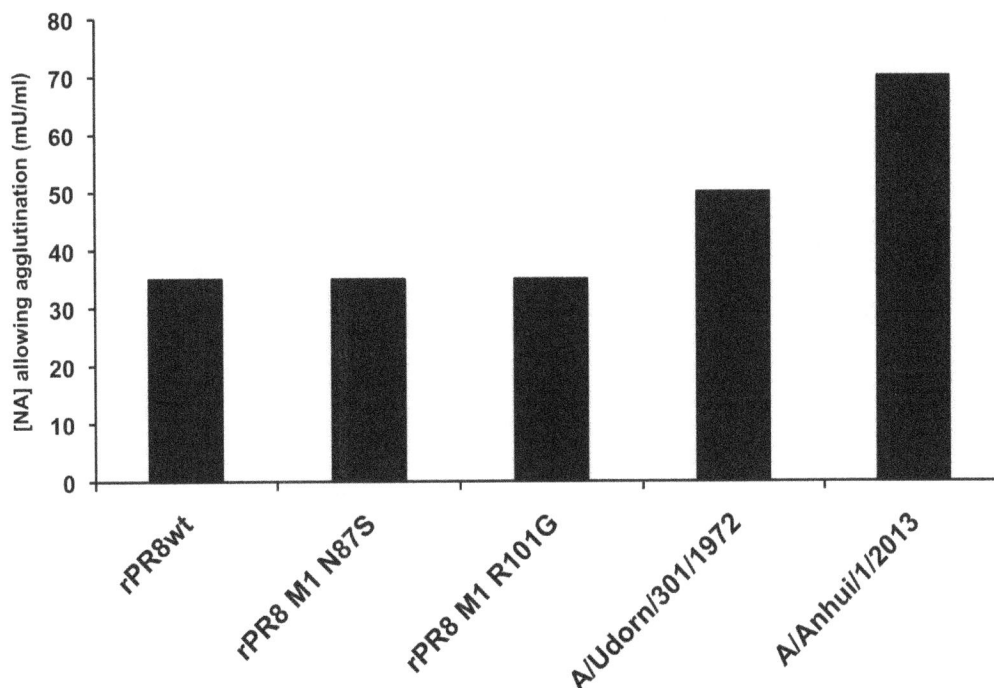

Figure 4. rPR8wt, rPR8 M1 N87S, and rPR8 M1 R101G viruses have the same red blood cell binding avidity. Chicken red blood cells were treated with a series of dilutions of *C. perfringens* neuraminidase. Treated red blood cells were then added to a standardized amount of each virus (8 HAU) and allowed to develop at 4°C. The assay was run in triplicate (standard deviation for each virus = 0). The highest concentration of neuraminidase that still allowed agglutination by each virus is plotted.

Following the incubation period, virus titer was determined in triplicate for each serum/virus sample by plaque assay on MDCK cells. Plaque numbers were compared to those obtained when virus was incubated with the control serum. All three viruses showed reductions in titer with immune serum diluted 1:80 and 1:160, but not with immune serum diluted 1:320 or 1:640 (Figure 5). The extent of reduction seen with the wt vs. mutant viruses at the 1:160 dilution was found to be significantly different for both mutants (p<0.05, t-test) and suggested that the two filamentous viruses are slightly more sensitive to antibody neutralization than is the spherical PR8wt strain (Figure 5). We interpret these results with caution, however, since the number of plaques remaining after incubation with 1:160 diluted immune serum was near the limit of detection. Overall, the results from the HI assays and the plaque reduction assay indicate that the greater surface area of filamentous compared to a spherical viruses does not confer resistance to antibody neutralization.

No difference in virion stability is observed between rPR8wt, rPR8 M1 N87S, and rPR8 M1 R101G

Due to potential differences in the structure of the matrix layer [23], we hypothesized that filamentous and spherical viruses might differ in their sensitivity to environmental stresses, such as fluctuations in temperature. To test this hypothesis, we evaluated virion stability at high temperatures. Each virus was diluted to a concentration of 1×10^6 PFU and incubated at 50°C for one of the following lengths of time: 0, 15, 30, 60, or 120 minutes. Following heat exposure, the titer of each sample was quantified in triplicate via plaque assay in MDCK cells. All three viruses had similar infectious titers remaining at each time point, indicating that the observed changes in virion morphology do not affect virion stability at elevated temperatures (Figure 6).

Table 3. There are no differences in hemagglutination inhibition among rPR8wt, rPR8 M1 N87S, rPR8 M1 R101G viruses.

Virus	1:2 serum dilutions HI titer[a]			1:1.5 serum dilutions HI titer[a]		
	A	B	C	A	B	C
rPR8wt	160	160	320	256	256	384
rPR8 M1 N87S	160	160	160	256	256	384
rPR8 M1 R101G	160	160	320	171	256	384

[a]The reciprocal of the highest dilution of serum that prevented hemagglutination is shown for three replicates (A, B and C).

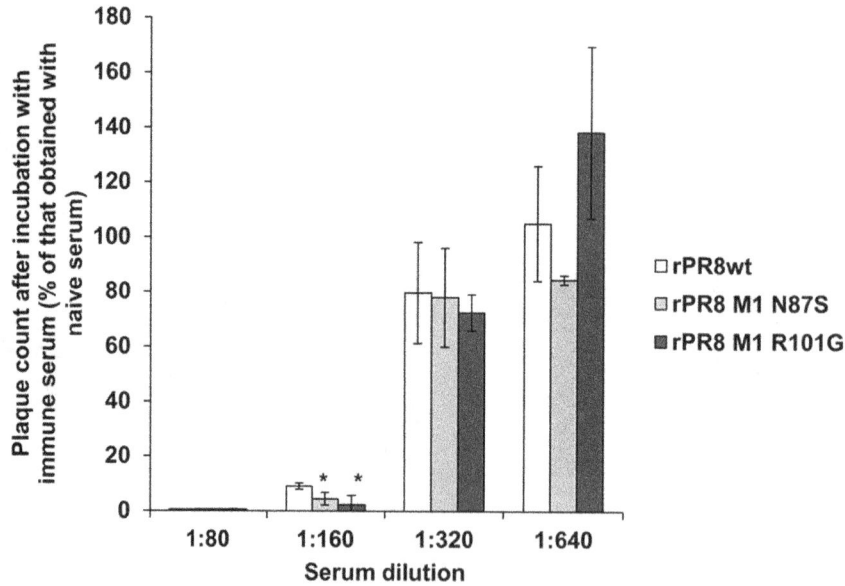

Figure 5. There is little difference in plaque reduction among rPR8wt, rPR8 M1 N87S, and rPR8 M1 R101G viruses. Each virus was diluted to approximately 250 PFU. Trypsin-heat-periodate treated serum was diluted 1:80, 1:160, 1:320, and 1:640 in PBS. Virus was added to serum dilutions and incubated for 30 minutes at 37°C. Virus titer for each serum/virus sample was then quantified by plaque assay on MDCK cells. The number of plaques obtained following incubation with immune serum is plotted as a percentage of the plaques obtained following incubation with naïve serum. The mean of three replicates is plotted, and error bars indicate standard deviation. *p<0.05 compared to rPR8wt virus. The limit of detection for the plaque assays was 5 PFU/ml.

Discussion

The fact that the filamentous morphology of IAV is maintained in nature but not in the laboratory suggests that filaments have a functional significance within the infected host. Due to the greater surface area of filaments relative to spheres, we hypothesized that functional differences between the two morphologies may lie with the HA and NA surface glycoproteins. We therefore focused our study on the HA and NA functions of strains with differing morphological phenotypes. We took advantage of two M1 point mutants selected during serial adaptation of rPR8 virus to an

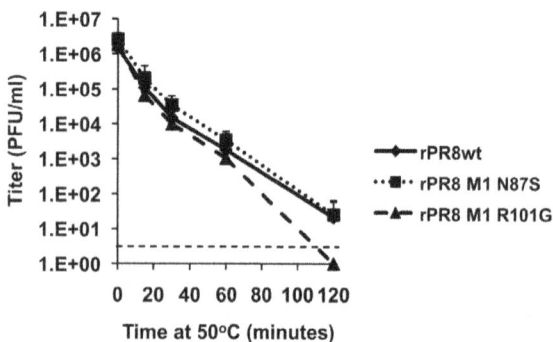

Figure 6. No difference in virion stability at an elevated temperature was observed between rPR8wt, rPR8 M1 N87S, and rPR8 M1 R101G viruses. Each virus was diluted to 1×10⁶ PFU and incubated in triplicate at 50°C for one of the following lengths of time: 0, 15, 30, 60, and 120 min. Results shown are the average of four separate assays performed in triplicate (thus n=12). The titers of each mutant virus were compared to that of the wt virus at each time point using Student's t test. All p values were >0.05 except that obtained for wt vs. N87S viruses at the 0 h time point (p=0.0094). The dotted line indicates the limit of detection.

animal host [5]. By measuring particles in electron micrographs, the R101G mutant was previously shown to comprise 41% filamentous particles, while the N87S had 16% filaments and the rPR8wt virus had 4% filaments [5].

Our approach, focused on the surface of the virion, assumes that the internal components of spherical and filamentous particles are similar. Our results indicating comparable infectivity and RNA content per HAU for spherical and filament-producing strains supports this assumption. Similar results were also reported by Roberts et al. for the A/Udorn/301/1972 (H3N2) strain [10]. Nevertheless, the literature contains conflicting reports on the genomic content of filaments versus spheres. Early studies suggested that filamentous virions could be polyploid (containing more than one copy of the genome) or contain more RNA than their spherical counterparts [24,25]. In contrast, a recent cryo-electron tomography study has shown that many longer filaments produced by A/Udorn/301/1972 (H3N2) virus lack RNPs [26]. Lastly, sectioning TEM and cryo-electron tomography studies have shown that filamentous virions contain a single copy of the viral genome located at the apical tip of the budding virion [23,27]. These apparently contradictory results can be partially reconciled by noting that the absence of genomes from filamentous particles appears to apply mainly to very long filaments [26]. In some cases, IAV strain specific differences in the properties of filaments may also play a role.

Our observations through two independent functional assays show that the two filament-producing rPR8 mutants have higher NA activities than the spherical rPR8wt virus. Replacement of the PR8 M segment with that of the filamentous 2009 pandemic strain A/Netherlands/602/2009 (H1N1) was also shown to increase both filament production and NA activity compared to the rPR8wt virus [20]. Now we show that significant increases in NA activity can be conferred through a single point mutation that changes virion morphology, thereby strengthening the causal link between morphology and NA activity. We predict that the increased NA activities associated with filament-containing virus preparations are due to greater numbers of NA proteins adorning the surface of filaments compared to spheres. We were not able to test this prediction robustly, however, due to limitations in the sensitivity of our Western blot assay. An alternative mechanism by which morphology could impact NA activity relates to the distribution of NA molecules on the virion surface. If filaments and spheres differ in terms of the positioning of NA on the particle, increased neuraminidase activity could be due to a cooperative effect mediated by greater NA protein clustering on filamentous virions. Consistent with this idea, clustering of NA at the tip of the virus particle proximal to the cell membrane has been reported [23,28,29]. Such an arrangement was suggested to promote destruction of host cell receptors as the virus is budding.

Contrary to what was observed for NA activity, we found no difference in binding avidity to red blood cells between the spherical and filamentous rPR8 viruses. Similarly, we did not observe marked differences in HI titer or in plaque reduction between spherical and filamentous viruses. These results suggest that the mechanism by which NA activity is increased for filament-producing viruses does not apply to HA. For example, if incorporation of both glycoproteins increases with filament size, then our data would suggest that avidity does not increase linearly with the valency of the virus particle. Lastly, we did not observe a difference in thermostability between spherical and filamentous viruses. Thus our data suggest that, at least in the PR8 background and in a guinea pig host, the selective advantage of a filamentous morphology lies with increased NA activity.

Enhanced NA activity could be advantageous to the virus by promoting release from infected cells and/or spread within the respiratory tract to new target cells [30]. Indeed, Roberts et al. suggested that increased amounts of NA protein per virion could aid movement through the mucus lining the airway [31].

Additionally, increased NA activity was shown to improve transmission in guinea pigs [20,32]. Importantly, the M segment has been shown to affect virus transmission as well [20,33]. Whether this effect on transmission is directly mediated by viral morphology has not yet been established. However, the fact that a single point mutation in the M1 matrix protein can both significantly alter virion morphology and confer increased NA activity suggests a mechanism by which the M segment may affect transmission. We know from previous work that the rPR8 M1 N87S mutant virus, which has both a significantly more filamentous morphology as well as a higher NA activity than rPR8wt, is not transmissible by a contact route in the guinea pig transmission model [5]. It is likely that N87S and the other point mutations identified in M1 following serial passage need to be coupled with additional permissive mutations on the M segment and/or elsewhere in the genome to promote transmission [34].

In summary, we have shown that filament-producing viruses have a higher neuraminidase activity than their spherical counterparts. Other properties such as HA binding avidity, HI titer, and thermostability were unaffected by changes in virion morphology. The viruses used herein were single M1 point mutants generated on a PR8 background and produced significantly more filaments than rPR8wt. The fact that these point mutations, when introduced individually, confer both a filamentous morphology and increased NA activity further strengthens the idea that the selective advantage conferred by filamentous virions lies in their increased NA activity over spherical virions.

Author Contributions

Conceived and designed the experiments: AL JSS JS. Performed the experiments: JSS PJC SS. Analyzed the data: AL JSS JS. Contributed to the writing of the manuscript: JSS AL JS.

References

1. Palese P, Shaw ML (2007) Orthomyxoviridae: the viruses and their replication. In: Knipe DM, Howley PM, editors. Fields Virology 5th edition Philadelphia: Lippincott Williams & Wilkins. pp 1647–1689.
2. Novel Swine-Origin Influenza A (H1N1) Virus Investigation Team, Dawood FS, Jain S, Finelli L, Shaw MW, Lindstrom S, et al. (2009) Emergence of a novel swine-origin influenza A (H1N1) virus in humans. N Engl J Med. 360: 2605–2615.
3. Chu CM, Dawson IM, Elford WJ (1949) Filamentous forms associated with newly isolated influenza virus. Lancet. 1: 602.
4. Itoh Y, Shinya K, Kiso M, Watanabe T, Sakoda Y, et al. (2009) In vitro and in vivo characterization of new swine-origin H1N1 influenza viruses. Nature. 460: 1021–1025.
5. Seladi-Schulman J, Steel J, Lowen AC (2013) Spherical influenza viruses have a fitness advantage in embryonated eggs, while filament-producing strains are selected in vivo. Journal of Virol. 87: 13343–13353.
6. Mosley VM, Wyckoff RW (1946) Electron micrography of the virus of influenza. Nature. 157: 263.
7. Burleigh LM, Calder LJ, Skehel JJ, Steinhauer DA (2005) Influenza A viruses with mutations in the M1 helix six domain display a wide variety of morphological phenotypes. J Virol. 79: 1262–1270.
8. Bourmakina SV, Garcia-Sastre A (2003) Reverse genetics studies on the filamentous morphology of influenza A virus. J Gen Virol. 84: 517–527.
9. Elleman CJ, Barclay WS (2004) The M1 matrix protein controls the filamentous phenotype of influenza A virus. Virology. 321: 144–153.
10. Roberts PC, Lamb RA, Compans RW (1998) The M1 and M2 proteins of influenza A virus are important determinants in filamentous particle formation. Virology. 240: 127–137.
11. Jin H, Leser GP, Zhang J, Lamb RA (1997) Influenza virus hemagglutinin and neuraminidase cytoplasmic tails control particle shape. EMBO J. 16: 1236–1247.
12. Bialas KM, Bussey KA, Stone RL, Takimoto T (2014) Specific nucleoprotein residues affect influenza virus morphology. J Virol. 88: 2227–2234.
13. Mitnaul LJ, Castrucci MR, Murti KG, Kawaoka Y (1996) The cytoplasmic tail of influenza A virus neuraminidase (NA) affects NA incorporation into virions, virion morphology, and virulence in mice but is not essential for virus replication. J Virol. 70: 873–879.
14. Kilbourne ED, Murphy JS (1960) Genetic studies of influenza viruses. I Viral morphology and growth capacity as exchangeable genetic traits Rapid in ovo adapation of early passsage Asian strain isolates by combination with PR8. J Exp Med. 111: 387–406.
15. Choppin PW, Murphy JS, Tamm I (1960) Studies of two kinds of virus particles which comprise influenza A2 virus strains. III. Morphological characteristics: independence to morphological and functional traits. J Exp Med. 112: 945–952.
16. Fodor E, Devenish L, Engelhardt OG, Palese P, Brownlee GG, et al (1999) Rescue of influenza A virus from recombinant DNA. J Virol 73: 9679–9682.
17. Steel J, Lowen AC, Mubareka S, Palese P (2009) Transmission of influenza virus in a mammalian host is increased by PB2 amino acids 627K or 627E/701N. PLoS Pathog. 5: e100052.
18. Quinlivan M, Zamarin D, Garcia-Sastre A, Cullinane A, Chambers T, et al. (2005) Attenuation of equine influenza viruses through truncations of the NS1 protein. J Virol. 79: 8431–8439.
19. Hoffmann E, Stech J, Guan Y, Webster RG, Perez DR (2001) Universal primer set for the full-length amplification of all influenza A viruses. Arch Virol. 146: 2275–2289.
20. Campbell PJ, Danzy S, Kyriakis CS, Deymier MJ, Lowen AC, et al (2014) The M segment of the 2009 pandemic influenza virus confersincreased NA activity, filamentous morphology, and efficient contact transmissibility to A/Puerto Rico/8/1934-based reassortant viruses Journal of Virol. 88: 3802–3814.
21. Hensley SE, Das SR, Bailey AL, Schmidt LM, Hickman HD, et al (2009) Hemagglutinin receptor binding avidity drives influenza A virus antigenic drift. Science. 326: 734–736.
22. Webster RG, Cox NJ, Sthor K (2002) WHO manual on animal influenza diagnosis and surveillance. World Health Organization, Geneva, Switzerland. Available: http://www.who.int/csr/resources/publications/influenza/en/wh ocdscsrncs20025rev.pdf.
23. Calder LJ, Wasilewski S, Berriman JA, Rosenthal PB (2010) Structural organization of a filamentous influenza A virus. Proc Natl Acad Sci USA 107: 10685–10690.
24. Ada GL, Perry BT (1958) Properties of the nucleic acid of the Ryan strain of filamentous influenza virus. J Gen Virol. 19: 40–54.
25. Smirnov YA, Kuznetsova MA, Kaverin NV (1991) The genetics aspects of influenza virus filamentous particle formation. Arch Virol. 118: 279–284.

26. Vijayakrishnan S, Loney C, Jackson D, Suphamungmee W, Rixon FJ, et al. (2013) Cryotomography of budding influenza A virus reveals filaments with diverse morphologies that mostly do not bear a genome at their distal end. PLoS Pathog. 9: e1003413.

27. Noda T, Sagara H, Yen A, Takada A, Kida H, et al. (2006) Architecture of ribonucleoprotein complexes in influenza A virus particles. Nature. 439: 490–492.

28. Murti KG, Webster RG (1986) Distribution of hemagglutinin and neuraminidase on influenza virions as revealed by immunoelectron microscopy. Virology. 149: 36–43.

29. Harris A, Cardone G, Winkler DC, Heymann JB, Brecher M, et al. (2006) Influenza virus pleiomorphy characterized by cryoelectron tomography. Proc Natl Acad Sci USA. 103: 19123–19127.

30. Matrosovich MN, Matrosovich TY, Gray T, Roberts NA, Klenk HD. (2004) Neuraminidase is important for the initiation of influenza virus infection in human airway epithelium. J Virol. 78: 1265–1267.

31. Roberts PC, Compans RW (1998) Host cell dependence of viral morphology. Proc Natl Acad Sci USA. 95: 5746–5751.

32. Bouvier NM, Lowen AC, Palese P (2008) Oseltamivir-resistant influenza A viruses are transmitted efficiently among guinea pigs by direct contact but not by aerosol. J Virol. 82: 10052–10058.

33. Chou YY, Albrecht RA, Pica N, Lowen AC, Richt JA, et al. (2011) The M segment of the 2009 new pandemic H1N1 influenza virus is critical for its high transmission efficiency in the guinea pig model J Virol. 85: 11235–11241.

34. Gong LI, Suchard MA, Bloom JD (2013) Stability-mediated epistatis constrains the evolution of an influenza protein. Elife. 2: e00631.

5

Galectin-1 Exerts Inhibitory Effects during DENV-1 Infection

Karina Alves Toledo[1⑨], **Marise Lopes Fermino**[2⑨], **Camillo del Cistia Andrade**[2], **Thalita Bachelli Riul**[2], **Renata Tomé Alves**[2], **Vanessa Danielle Menjon Muller**[2], **Raquel Rinaldi Russo**[2], **Sean R. Stowell**[3], **Richard D. Cummings**[3], **Victor Hugo Aquino**[2], **Marcelo Dias-Baruffi**[2]*

1 Department of Biological Sciences, Universidade Estadual Paulista – UNESP (FCL-Assis), Assis, Brazil, 2 Departamento de Análises Clínicas, Toxicológicas e Bromatológicas, Faculdade de Ciências Farmacêuticas de Ribeirão Preto, Universidade de São Paulo, Ribeirão Preto, Brazil, 3 Emory University School of Medicine, Atlanta, Georgia, United States of America

Abstract

Dengue virus (DENV) is an enveloped RNA virus that is mosquito-transmitted and can infect a variety of immune and non-immune cells. Response to infection ranges from asymptomatic disease to a severe disorder known as dengue hemorrhagic fever. Despite efforts to control the disease, there are no effective treatments or vaccines. In our search for new antiviral compounds to combat infection by dengue virus type 1 (DENV-1), we investigated the role of galectin-1, a widely-expressed mammalian lectin with functions in cell-pathogen interactions and immunoregulatory properties. We found that DENV-1 infection of cells in vitro exhibited caused decreased expression of Gal-1 in several different human cell lines, suggesting that loss of Gal-1 is associated with virus production. In test of this hypothesis we found that exogenous addition of human recombinant Gal-1 (hrGal-1) inhibits the virus production in the three different cell types. This inhibitory effect was dependent on hrGal-1 dimerization and required its carbohydrate recognition domain. Importantly, the inhibition was specific for hrGal-1, since no effect was observed using recombinant human galectin-3. Interestingly, we found that hrGal-1 directly binds to dengue virus and acts, at least in part, during the early stages of DENV-1 infection, by inhibiting viral adsorption and its internalization to target cells. To test the in vivo role of Gal-1 in DENV infection, Gal-1-deficient-mice were used to demonstrate that the expression of endogenous Galectin-1 contributes to resistance of macrophages to in vitro-infection with DENV-1 and it is also important to physiological susceptibility of mice to in vivo infection with DENV-1. These results provide novel insights into the functions of Gal-1 in resistance to DENV infection and suggest that Gal-1 should be explored as a potential antiviral compound.

Editor: Tian Wang, University of Texas Medical Branch, United States of America

Funding: This work was supported by Fundação de Coordenação de Aperfeiçoamento de Pessoal de Nível Superior (CAPES - Grant 23038.039425–42/2008), Conselho Nacional de Pesquisa e Desenvolvimento Científico e Tecnológico (CNPq – Grants: 576322/2008–3 and 487351/2012–6) and Fundação de Amparo à Pesquisa do Estado de São Paulo (FAPESP – Grant 2013/07340–1) to MDB. The funders had no role in study design, data collection and analysis, decision to publish, or preparation of the manuscript.

Competing Interests: The authors have declared that no competing interests exist.

* Email: mdbaruff@fcfrp.usp.br

⑨ These authors equally contributed to this work.

Introduction

Dengue is a mosquito-borne viral disease of expanding geographical range and incidence, it is estimated that up to 3.6 billion people live in endemic regions [reviewed in reference 1]. Recent estimates indicated that the number of infections worldwide is 400 million with ~500,000 episodes of severe dengue, and <20,000 dengue related deaths per year [1].

Dengue is predominantly transmitted by the mosquito *Aedes agypti* and is caused by dengue viruses (DENV), a group of four serologically distinct positive strand RNA viruses: DENV-1, DENV-2, DENV-3, and DENV-4. They belong to the Flaviviridae family and genus Flavivirus (reviewed in [2]). Infection with any serotype can induce a range of disease from sub-clinical to a severe disorder. The severe disorder is associated with hemorrhage and plasma leakage which are recognized as dengue hemorrhagic fever (DHS) or dengue shock syndrome (DSS) [3,4]. There are currently no specific treatments for dengue disease [5], and therefore, only supportive care is given [6]. Thus, antiviral compounds need to be identified in view of the spread of dengue disease throughout the world [5].

To identify control mechanisms for Dengue disease, we investigated the physiological functions of an endogenous innate immune protein named galectin-1 (Gal-1), a β-galactoside-binding lectin, in controlling infection caused by dengue virus (DENV-1). Galectin-1 is a ubiquitously expressed lectin, and can occur in both intracellular (cytoplasm and nucleus) as well as extracellular (cell surface and serum) compartments, despite the lack of a signal peptide for classical secretion [7]. Galectin-1 is differentially expressed by various normal and pathological tissues, including muscle, heart, liver, kidney, prostate, lymph nodes, spleen, thymus, placenta, testis, retina and also in immune and non-immune cells [8]. For instance, during infection or inflammation, Gal-1 may be released by infected epithelium, activated macrophages, and endothelial cells [8]. In fact, concerning endothelial cells, it has been extensively demonstrated that Gal-1 contributes to multiple steps of the angiogenesis cascade and then it has pro-angiogenic activity (reviewed in [9]).

Gal-1 exists in a monomer-dimer equilibrium, and in its dimeric form, the lectin can mediate cell-cell or host-pathogen interactions [10,11,12], similar to other members of the galectin family [13,14] and other mammalian lectin families [15]. It has been extensively shown that it presents an immunomodulatory effect on microbial infections [16]. This lectin has a role in viral infections but its mechanisms and physiological functions are not clear. While some groups have reported an antiviral activity of Gal-1 during infections caused by Nipah virus [17,18], Nodavirus [19], Influenza virus [20] and human simplex virus 1 (HSV-1) [21], other groups have reported that Gal-1 promotes infections caused by human immunodeficiency virus 1 (HIV-1) [22-27], HSV-1 [28] and human T-lymphotropic virus 1 HTLV-1 [29].

To our knowledge, the role of Gal-1 in DENV infection is yet to be evaluated. Here we show that both endogenous and exogenous Gal-1 inhibits DENV-1 infectivity, both in *in vitro* and *in vivo* infection in mice. Our results suggest that recombinant Gal-1 might have potential use as a novel approach to control DENV-1-induced pathology.

Materials and Methods

Cell lineages

The mosquito cell lineage from *Aedes albopictus* (C6/36) was cultivated at 28°C in L-15 medium (Leibovitz) (Cultilab, Campinas, Brazil) supplemented with 0.3% tryptose phosphate broth, 0.02% glutamine, 1% minimum essential medium (MEM) non-essential amino acids solution and 5% fetal bovine serum (Hyclone, Logan, USA). Vero-E6 (African green monkey kidney, ATCC CCL-81) cells were grown at 37°C in DMEM (Gibco, Life Technologies, Gaithersburg, MD, USA) supplemented with 10% fetal bovine serum. The human urinary bladder carcinoma cells (ECV-304, ATCC CRL-1998) were maintained at 37°C in RPMI-1640 medium (Gibco). Human lung microvascular endothelial cell lineage (HMVEC-L; ATCC CC2527) was cultivated in EC growth medium (EBM-2; Cambrex, Walkersville, MD, USA) containing 5% fetal bovine serum, human recombinant epidermal growth factor, human recombinant insulin-like growth factor-1, human basic fibroblast growth factor, vascular endothelial growth factor, hydrocortisone, ascorbic acid, gentamicin, and amphotericin B.

DENV-1

The stock of the DENV-1 (strain Mochizuki, GenBank: AB074760.1) was prepared in C6/36 cells and titrated by plaque formation on Vero-E6 cells, as described previously [30]. Supernatants containing virus were collected and stored at −80°C for use in *in vitro* assays. *In vivo* assays were performed with the DENV-1 mouse brain-adapted strain, generated from Mochizuki strain in the same manner as described in reference [31]. Mouse-brain adapted DENV-1 was used on in vivo assays because non-adapted mouse strains do not readily replicate or cause pathology in immunocompetent mice, which is the case of mice used in the present study. Therefore, mouse-adapted DENV is lethal after intracranial challenge, and this severity parameter was used here to assess the physiological impact of Gal-1.

Mice and survival study

Gal-1-deficient (*Lgals1*$^{-/-}$) mice and age-matched wild-type (WT) mice on a C57Bl-6 background were used in experimental DENV-1 infections. For mortality assays, groups ranging from six to eight 3-day-old mice from both WT and *Lgals1*$^{-/-}$ lineages were infected with mouse-brain adapted DENV-1 as previously described, with modifications [31,32]. Briefly, mice were intracerebrally injected with 10^6 virions diluted in a total volume of 10 μl of phosphate buffer after anesthetization with a mixture of 10 mg/Kg of xylasine (Dopalen Vetbrands) and 100 mg/Kg of ketamine (Dopaser Hertap Caller). The brain macerates from non-infected mice were used for mock infection. The brains from non-infected and infected mice were collected after animals were euthanized by inhalation of carbon dioxide. Subsequent to the intracranial inoculation mice were examined daily, and mortality rates, as a direct result of the infection, were recorded up to 10 days post-infection. After this period, the surviving animals were euthanized by inhalation of carbon dioxide.

Macrophage cultures

Resident macrophages were obtained from peritoneal washouts of 4–6 weeks-old WT and *Lgals1*$^{-/-}$ mice, after euthanasia by inhalation of carbon dioxide. Cells were suspended in RPMI-1640 medium supplemented with 10% of fetal bovine serum and allowed to attach onto 24-well plates. After an overnight incubation period, unattached cells were removed and adherent cells (macrophages) were used for *in vitro* infection with DENV-1 or submitted to Gal-1 expression analysis using Western Blot assay or conventional PCR methods.

Ethical aspects

The present study uses death endpoint as a direct result from infection with DENV-1 and without humane euthanasia. This choice was strongly justified based on the following reasons: 1) the alternative use of humane endpoints based on clinical criteria was not possible since the earlier and reliable indicators of disease severity biomarkers had not been established or validated at the times the experiments were performed; 2) Our study was designed so that the survival assay consisted of a total of 35 mice from each lineage. If we had proposed to establish and validate biomarkers for severity, in order to use a humane endpoint, we would have had to use a much larger number of mice, which in our view would be unnecessary and raise other ethical concerns; 3) The mouse strain C57BL-6 was used in our study because its genetic counterpart, the *Lgals1*$^{-/-}$ mice, is naturally resistant to infection with DENV-1, so it was necessary to use a high inoculum in newborn mice, which promotes death during the acute infection; 4) All mouse experiments were performed under approved conditions in accordance to Faculdade de Ciências Farmacêuticas de Ribeirão Preto – Universidade de São Paulo (USP) Institutional Animal Care and User Committee approved protocols. The Ethics Committee on Animal Research of the University of São Paulo approved all the procedures described (Protocol Number: 10.1.1300.53.0).

Human recombinant Galectin-1 (hrGal-1) and Galectin-3 (hrGal-3)

Recombinant forms (dimeric and monomeric) of human galectin-1 (hrGal-1) and human galectin-3 were prepared based on procedures previously described [33–36]. In addition, purified hrGal-1 was treated with 100 mM iodoacetamide (Sigma-Aldrich, MO, USA) in 100 mM lactose/PBS overnight at 4°C, as described [10,18,22,33]. To ensure that hrGal-1 and hrGal-3 samples were endotoxin free, Detoxi-Gel Endotoxin removing gel (Pierce Biotechnology, Rockford, IL) was used. The activity of all produced galectins was assessed by hemagglutination. Biotinylation of hrGal-1 was performed using sulfo-NHS-LC-biotin (sulfosuccinimidyl 6-[biotinamido] hexanoate) (Pierce), according to the manufacturer's recommendations.

In vitro viral infection

Indicated cell lineages were inoculated with DENV-1 (MOI 0.5) or vehicle solution (supernatant from non infected cells) and cultivated for 24, 48, 72, 96 or 120 hours, as indicated, at 37°C in a humidified, CO_2-controlled atmosphere in appropriate medium supplemented with 10% FBS. Following, supernatants of culture were recovered for determination of viral load. Gal-1 effects were assessed by incubating cells, virus or both with the indicated concentrations of this lectin for 1 hour at 37°C before viral inoculum, as indicated. To evaluate the involvement of Gal-1 CRD in its antiviral activity the treatments were done in the presence of 10 mM lactose or sucrose.

Adsorption and Internalization assays

Adsorption and internalization assays were performed as described previously [37] with modifications. For adsorption assays, ECV-304 cells were seeded in 24-well plates and infected with DENV-1 with a MOI of 10, in the presence or absence of 10 μM of hrGal-1, for 1 hour at 4°C. Following, cells were washed twice with PBS and immediately submitted to total RNA extraction or stored at −80°C until the time of use. For the internalization assays, cells were seeded in 24-well plates and inoculated with DENV-1 (MOI 10), for 1 hour at 4°C. After the incubation period, the inoculum was removed by 2 washes with PBS. The cells were then incubated with medium containing or not 10 μM of hrGal-1, for additional 1 hour at 37°C. The cells were then washed with PBS and treated with citrate buffer for 1 min to inactivate the adsorbed but not internalized virus. Finally, cells were washed with PBS to remove citrate buffer and stored at −80°C for subsequent quantification of viral load.

Real-Time and conventional PCR

Viral loads were quantified in the culture supernatants using a one-step quantitative Real-Time PCR [38]. The total viral RNA purified from 1×10^7 PFU of DENV-1 were 10-fold serially diluted to generate a standard curve. The viral RNA was purified using the QIAamp Viral RNA minikit (QIAGEN; Hamburg, Germany). Quantitative PCR reaction was carried out with the SuperScript III Platinum SYBR Green One-Step qRT-PCR kit (Invitrogen, Life Technologies) in a One-Step Real-Time PCR RT-PCR (Applied Biosystems, Life Technologies). Triplicate reactions were performed for each sample, and a no template control was included as a negative control. The primer sequences used for DENV-1 detection were RNC5-S: 5′-3′AGTTGTTAGTC-TACGTGGACCGA and RNC5-C: 5′-3′CGCGTTTCAGCA-TATTGAAAG.

Qualitative analysis of Gal-1 mRNA expression on WT and $Lgals1^{-/-}$ cells was performed using conventional RT-PCR. Total RNA was purified using RNeasy Protect Mini Kit (QIAGEN) and cDNA obtained using M-MLV reverse transcriptase (1U) and oligo dT primers (both from Invitrogen, Life Technologies). PCR amplification was performed with primers for mouse Gal-1 (pFBNdgal-1: 5′-3′CGGATCCCATATGGCCTGTGGTCTG and pRHXgal-1: 5′-3′GCTCG AGAAGCTTTCACTCAA-AGGCC) and β-actin (Fb-actin: 5′-3′CCCTAGGC ACCA-GGGTGTGA and Rb-actin 5′-3′:GCCATGTTCAATGGGG-TACTTC).

Virucidal assay

The virucidal activity of hrGal-1 was assessed as described in reference [37], with modifications. Briefly, DENV-1 (2×10^5 PFU) was incubated at 37°C for 1 hour in presence or absence of 10 μM of hrGal-1. The incubation was performed in presence of absence of RNAse A (150 mg/mL, Sigma-Aldrich). After one hour, the viral RNA was purified using QIAamp Viral RNA minikit and the samples were subjected to Real-Time PCR as described above. Purified viral RNA, treated or not with RNAse A, was used as positive control of reaction.

Enzyme-linked Immunosorbent Assay

Soluble Gal-1 present in the culture supernatants was quantified by ELISA. Briefly, 96-well microplates were coated with rabbit polyclonal anti-Gal-1 antibody (1 μg/ml, produced in our laboratory). Plates were washed (PBS-Tween 0.05%) and incubated for 2 h at 37°C with blocking buffer (PBS/FBS 3%). Next, supernatant samples were added to plates and incubated at room temperature for 2 hours. After extensive washing, a chicken polyclonal anti-Gal-1 antibody (2 μg/ml; produced in our laboratory), diluted in PBS/FBS 3%, was added to each well and incubated for 1 h, at 37°C. After washing, wells were incubated with HRP-conjugated donkey anti-chicken IgY (Jackson ImmunoResearch, West Grove, PA, USA) for 1 h, at 37°C. Subsequently; substrate solution (substrate buffer, 1% TMB and 1% H_2O_2) was added. After a 20 min incubation period at room temperature, the reaction was stopped by addition of stop solution (5.5% H_2SO_4). Absorbance was determined at 450 nm using an ELISA reader (Thermo Labsystems, Franklin, MA, USA). A standard curve ranging from 20 to 20,000 pg/ml of hrGal-1 was generated for each ELISA.

The ability of hrGal-1 to bind DENV-1 was also tested by ELISA. Each well in 96-well microtiter plates was coated with 1 μg of hrGal-1 or 1% BSA overnight at 4°C. Plates were then rinsed once with PBS-Tween 0.05% and incubated with blocking buffer (PBS-Tween 0.05%, BSA 3%) for 2 hours at room temperature. After washing, serial two-fold dilutions of DENV-1 were added to each well and plates were incubated for 2 hours at room temperature. After three washes with PBS-Tween 0.05%, each well was incubated with mouse anti-E protein IgG (AbD Serotec, Raleigh, NC, USA) for 1 h, at 37°C. Following this incubation step, plates were washed and incubated with HRP-conjugated donkey anti-mouse IgG (Jackson IR) for 1 h, at 37°C. The development of peroxidase reaction was performed with TMB substrate, as describe above. To assess the participation of Gal-1 CRD on viral-lectin interactions, different concentrations of lactose or sucrose were added to wells before the addition of virus dilutions.

Flow cytometry

Measurement of free ligands for Gal-1 on ECV-304 cells surface was performed by incubating ECV-304 cells with 10 μM biotinylated-hrGal-1 for 1 hour at 4°C, in presence or absence of 40 mM lactose or sucrose (Sigma-Aldrich). After washing, cells were incubated with streptavidin-FITC (Jackson IR) for 30 minutes at 4°C, washed and fixed. Labeled cells were acquired on a FACS Canto (Becton Dickinson, Mountain View, CA, USA) and analyzed in the DIVA software (Becton Dickinson).

Cell death assay

Apoptosis and necrosis signals were investigated through propidium iodide (PI) and Annexin-V staining. Membrane permeability was evaluated in fresh ECV-304 cells, after immediate addition of propidium iodide (2 mg). DNA degradation was detected in ECV-304 cells gently resuspended in 0.3 ml hypotonic PI solution (PI, 50 µg/ml in 0.1% sodium citrate plus 0.1% Triton X-100; Sigma-Aldrich). Tubes were kept at 4°C for 16 hours in the dark. Cells treated with Camptothecin (CPT – 10 µM – Sigma-Aldrich) were used as positive inducer of cellular death.

Cell viability assay

Cell viability was measured by the colorimetric MTT (1-(4,5-Dimethylthiazol-2-yl)-3,5-diphenylformazan, Sigma-Aldrich) assay as previously described [39].

Western blot assay

Cells were lysed in sample buffer (62.5 M Tris, pH 6.8, 2% SDS (w/v), 5% glycerol (v/v), 30 µM phenol red and 0.9% β-mercaptoethanol) and incubated for 5 min at 100°C. Samples were resolved in 15% polyacrylamide gels and transferred onto nitrocellulose membranes (Amersham Biosciences, Uppsala, Sweden). After saturation with 5% non-fat dry milk, membranes were probed with mouse monoclonal anti-Gal-1 or mouse monoclonal anti-β-actin (Abcam, MA, EUA) for 2 hours at room temperature. After washing, membranes were incubated with HRP-conjugated donkey anti-mouse IgG (Jackson IR) for 45 minutes at room temperature. Bound antibodies were revealed by enhanced chemiluminescence using the ECL kit (Pierce).

Data Analysis

Statistically significant differences among groups were assayed using analysis of variance (ANOVA) (Bonferroni Dunn test). Values of $p<0.05$ were considered significant results.

Results

Reduced expression of endogenous Gal-1 results in increased permissiveness to DENV-1 infection

To investigate the role of endogenous Gal-1 in the course of DENV infection, we infected three different cell lines with DENV. Vero-E6 cells are known to be permissive to all four dengue virus serotypes [40–42], while ECV-304 (a carcinoma cell lineage with endothelial characteristics) and lung microvascular endothelial cells (HMVEC-L) are known to be permissive to dengue virus serotype-2 [24,43–45]. Interestingly, ECV-304 and Vero-E6 cells express similar levels of Gal-1 protein, while HMVEC-L expressed somewhat higher levels of Gal-1 when compared to other cell lines tested (Figure 1A) and quantified by ImageJ program (Figure 1A). Next, cells were inoculated with DENV-1 (MOI 0.5) and cultivated for 72 hours, and the viral load was quantified from the culture supernatants by One Step Real-Time PCR. We found that Vero-E6 cells, which displayed the lowest Gal-1 expression level (Figure 1A), were highly permissive to DENV-1 infection (Figure 1B). In sharp contrast, we detected the lowest level of viral load in the supernatants of HMVEC-L cells (Figure 1B), which displayed the highest Gal-1 expression level (Figure 1A). To further investigate the relationship between Gal-1 levels and permissiveness to DENV infection, we infected the ECV-304 cells with DENV-1 for 72 h and evaluated Gal-1 expression by western blot. As shown in Figure 1C, the presence of DENV-1 decreased the expression of endogenous Gal-1 in comparison to that cells maintained in medium alone. In addition, ECV-304-infected cells secreted more Gal-1 to culture supernatants (Figure 1D), which could explain at least in part the reduction of cell-associated Gal-1 protein after infection (Figure 1C).

Treatment with recombinant hrGal-1 reduces viral production in DENV-1 virus-infected cells

Since Gal-1 expression levels seemed to be inversely correlated to DENV permissiveness, we therefore evaluate whether the addition of exogenous Gal-1 could interfere with DENV infection in vitro. First, we demonstrated that ECV-304 cells display Gal-1-specific binding sites because human recombinant Gal-1 (hrGal-1) was able to bind ECV-304 cell surfaces, and this binding is abrogated in the presence of lactose, a weak but effective inhibitor of Gal-1, but not by sucrose, an isomeric sugar that does not bind galectins (Figure 2A). Similar results were obtained using HMVEC-L and Vero-E6 cells (data not shown). Monolayers of ECV-304, Vero-E6 and HMVEC-L cells were treated with 10 µM of hrGal-1 for 1 hour at 37°C, followed by addition DENV-1 virus (MOI 0.5) for 72 hours, and the viral load was quantified from the culture supernatants. As demonstrated before (Figure 1B), EVC-304 and Vero-E6 cells are much more permissive to DENV-1 infection than HMVEC-L cells; however, all the three cell lines had a significant reduction in viral load (35% in Vero-E6 cells, 60% in ECV-304 cells and 65% HMVEC-L cells) when pre-treated with hrGal-1 (Figure 2B). The kinetics of DENV-1 infection was also monitored in EVC-304 cells, pretreated or not with hrGal-1, during a period of 120 hours after infection. As shown in (Figure 2C), at 48, 72, 96 and 120 hours postinfection, the viral loads detected in the supernatant of DENV-1-infected ECV-304 cells pre-treated with hrGal-1 were significantly lower compared with viral load recovered from the supernatants of Gal-1-untreated cells. We also found a dose-dependent inhibition of DENV-1 infection when ECV-304 cells were pretreated with increasing hrGal-1 concentrations for 1 hour before the infection (Figure 2D).

It has been shown that Gal-1 exists in a monomer-dimer equilibrium, and several important functions of this protein have been shown to be dependent on Gal-1 dimerization [8,36]. Therefore, we tested whether the inhibitory effect of Gal-1 on DENV-1 infection was dependent on its capacity to form dimers. Using a mutant Gal-1, which is unable to form dimers, we showed that the monomeric form of hrGal-1(m) had no capacity to reduce DENV-1 viral loads in the supernatant of EVC-304-infected cells compared with the hrGal-1 (d), indicating that dimerization is important for the inhibitor effects of Gal-1 on DENV-1 infection (Figure 2D). Importantly, we observed that this inhibitory effect was specific for hrGal-1 since galectin-3, another galectin binding protein from galectin family, and one which naturally occurs in multimeric forms, showed no inhibitory effect on vital load (Figure 2D).

To assess the involvement of the carbohydrate-recognition domain (CRD) of Gal-1 in this inhibitory effect, ECV-304 cells were pre-treated or not with hrGal-1 in presence or absence of a specific sugar inhibitor (lactose). Lactose blocked the inhibitory effect of hrGal-1 on DENV-1 infection, whereas sucrose did not block (Figure 2E), indicating a dependence of the Gal-1 CRD for these functions.

Inhibitory effect of Gal-1 on DENV-1 release is not associated with induction of cell death

We explored whether the antiviral effect of Gal-1 could be due to induction of cell death. Thus, we evaluated the apoptosis and necrosis of ECV-304 cells pre-treated or not with hrGal-1 and infected with DENV-1 virus. As can be seen in the Figure 3A, DENV-1-infected ECV-304 cells (pretreated or not with hrGal-1) did not show significant staining with either PI or Annexin-V-FITC, in contrast to cells treated with camptothecin, a positive

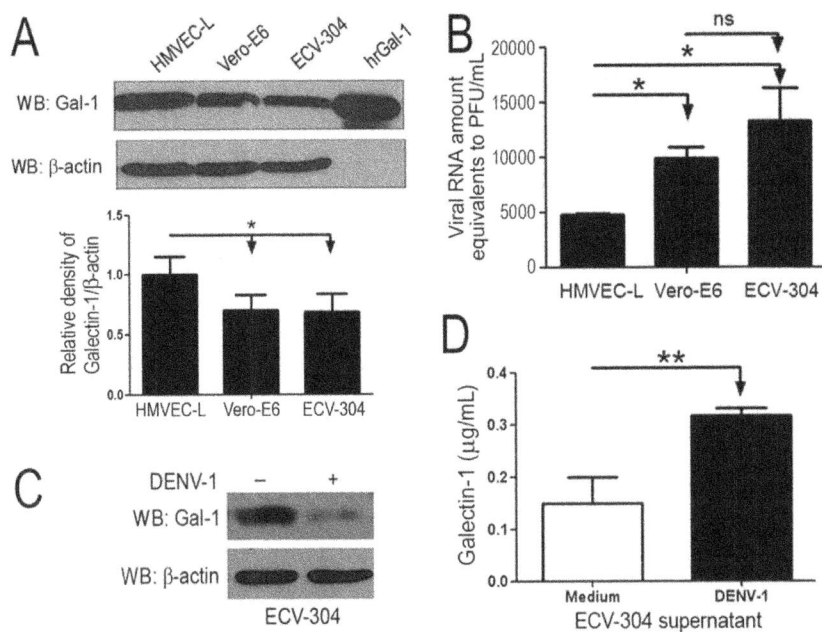

Figure 1. Lower expression of Gal-1 is correlated with higher viral loads produced by DENV-1-infected cells. (A) Gal-1 expression on HMVEC-L, Vero-E6 and ECV-304 cells was assessed by western blot method and normalized by β-actin endogenous control. The relative density of Gal-1 was determined by ImageJ software. (B) HMVEC-L, Vero-E6 and ECV-304 cells (2.5×10^4) were incubated with DENV-1 (MOI 0.5) for 72 hours at 37°C. At the end of incubation period, the total amounts of viral RNA in the cell-free supernatants were determined by Real-Time PCR, using a standard curve constructed from DENV-1 RNA purified from 1×10^7 PFU (PFU: plate formed units). Results are shown as Viral RNA amount equivalents to PFU/ml±SD from 3 independent assays performed in triplicates. (C) ECV-304 cells were inoculated with DENV-1 (MOI 0.5) or only with medium and cultivated for 72 hours at 37°C. Cells were analyzed for Gal-1 expression by western blot assay. (D) Soluble Gal-1 was detected in the supernatants from cell cultures using ELISA method (N = 3). *$p < 0.01$; **$p < 0.001$.

inducer of cell death. In order to confirm this result, we also checked the degradation of chromosomal DNA and cell viability by using the MTT assay. Corroborating our previous result using Annexin-V/PI staining, pretreatment of cells with hrGal-1 before DENV-1 infection did not cause any effect on DNA degradation and cell viability (Figure 3B and C, respectively). Cell viability and apoptosis assays performed in Vero-E6 and HMVEC-L cell lineages infected with DENV-1 in presence or absence of hrGal-1 provided similar results (data not shown). Altogether, these data indicate that Gal-1 inhibits DENV-1 infection without inducing cell death in infected cells.

hrGal-1 binds to DENV-1 and inhibits its adsorption and internalization processes in ECV-304 cells

To further investigate the inhibitory effect of exogenous Gal-1 on DENV-1 infection, we first checked whether Gal-1 was able to bind directly to the virus and exert any *direct virucidal* activity against DENV-1. As shown in Figure 4A, DENV-1 bound to immobilized hrGal-1 in a dose-dependent manner, whereas the virus failed to bind to BSA-coated wells. Unexpectedly, the binding of DENV-1 to hrGal-1 was not abolished by the addition of lactose, an inhibitor of carbohydrate binding (Figure 4A). This may mean that the affinity of binding between hrGal-1 and DENV-1 is extremely high toward immobilized hrGal-1, and thus not readily reversible by lactose, or binding occurs through a non-carbohydrate interaction to hrGal-1. We next evaluated whether hrGal-1 could affect virus adsorption and/or virus internalization. As shown in Figure 4B, hrGal-1 significantly inhibited virus adsorption at 4°C for 1 hour (Figure 4B) when hrGal-1 was present during the incubation. If adsorption took place in a hrGal-1-free medium, and the lectin was added at culture supernatants

when the temperature was raised at 37°C and maintained only additional 1 h of incubation, the virus yield also significantly decreased in comparison with untreated cultures (Figure 4B). A possible virucidal effect of hrGal-1 on DENV-1 was discarded by a virucidal assay (Figure 4C). Altogether, these results suggest that hrGal-1 may influence the early steps of DENV-1 infection. Finally, we investigated whether the inhibitory effects exerted by Gal-1 also depended on its interaction with the target cells. The pretreatment of DENV-1 with hrGal-1 [(DENV1+rhGal-1)+ECV] led to a significant decrease in viral load in the culture supernatants (Figure 4D). However, when ECV-304 cells were treated with hrGal-1 before DENV infection [(ECV+rhGal-1)+DENV1] or ECV-304 cells were treated concomitantly with hrGal-1 and DENV-1 (ECV+rhGal-1+DENV1), we observed an even greater reduction in the viral load in the culture supernatants (Figure 4D).

Absence of endogenous Gal-1 leads to early mortality of mice to DENV-1 infection

Based on the results presented so far and to better demonstrate the role of Gal-1 in controlling DENV-1 infection, we next infected newborn Gal-1-deficient ($Lgals1^{-/-}$) and wild-type mice with mouse-brain adapted DENV-1 virus and analyzed host survival for 10 days (Figure 5A). Although mice from both lineages displayed similar overall mortality rate, $Lgals1^{-/-}$ mice began to succumb earlier than WT mice: within the first 4 days post-infection, almost 60% of $Lgals1^{-/-}$ mice died, while 90% of WT mice survived up to 5 days past challenge (Figure 5A).

Since macrophages are important target for DENV virus in mouse models of dengue infection [46,47] and we demonstrated above that there is an inverse correlation between DENV

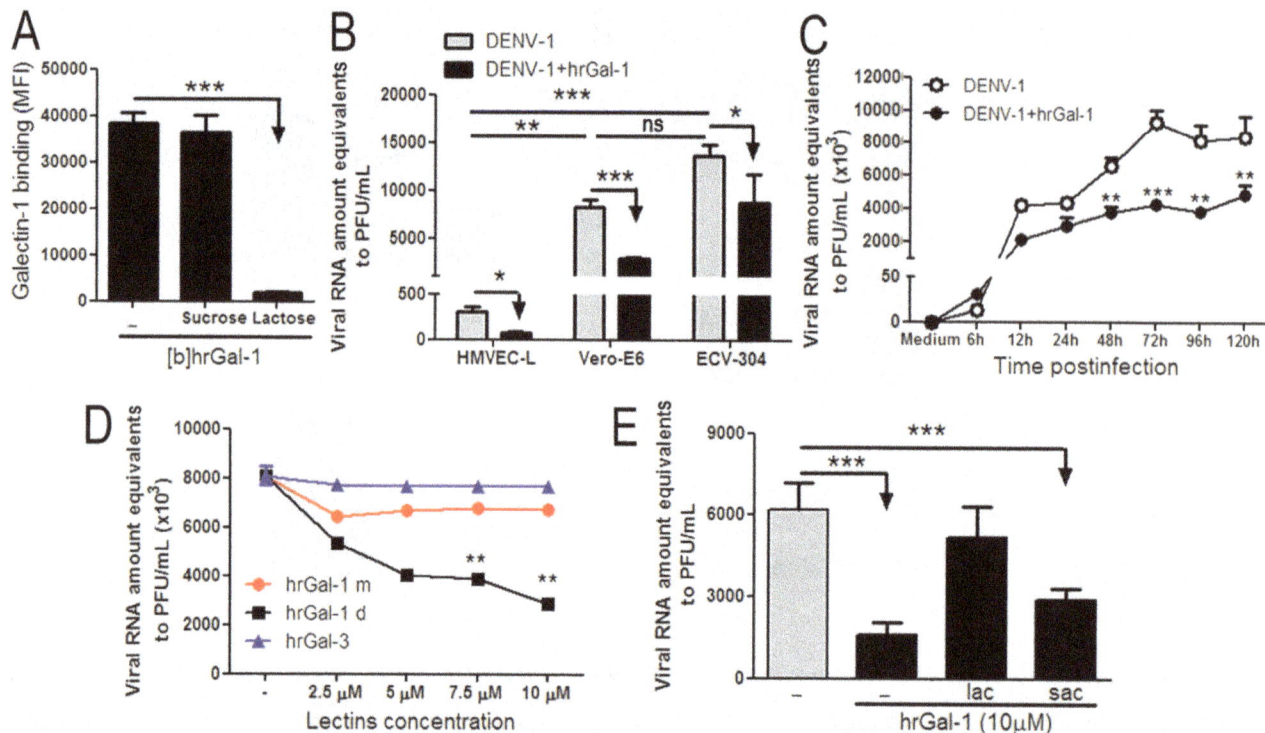

Figure 2. Treatment with human recombinant Gal-1 inhibits DENV-1 in vitro infection. (A) Biotinylated-hrGal-1 (20 µg/mL) was incubated with ECV-304 cells in presence or absence of 40 mM lactose or sucrose for 1 hour at 4°C. The binding of biotinylated-hrGal-1 to ECV-304 cells surfaces was detected by staining with streptavidin-FITC and measured by flow cytometry. The analysis was performed using a Diva software (Becton Dickson) and results are expressed as mean mean fluorescence intensity (MFI)±SD. Tests were performed in triplicates. **(B)** HMVEC-L, Vero-E6 and ECV-304 cells were incubated with 10 µM hrGal-1 or only medium for 1 hour at 37°C. Following, cells were inoculated with DENV-1 at a MOI of 0.5 and cultivated for 72 hours. At 72 hours postinfection the supernatants were collected and the viral RNA amounts were quantified by Real-Time PCR. Results are shown as Viral RNA amounts equivalent to PFU/ml±SD from 3 assays performed in triplicates. **(C)** ECV-304 cells were treated with hrGal-1 and infected with DENV-1 as described in (B) for 120 hours. The supernatants were collected at the indicated times postinfection and the viral loads were quantified by Real-Time PCR as described in (B). (N=3) **(D)** ECV-304 cells were incubated with increased concentrations of monomeric-Gal-1 (hrGal-1 m), dimeric-Gal-1 (hrGal-1 d) or galectin-3 (hrGal-3) for 1 hour at 37°C before inoculation with DENV-1 (MOI 0.5). Cells were cultivated for 72 hours at 37°C and viral load was quantified as described in (A). (N=3). **(E)** ECV-304 cells were treated with hrGal-1 (10 µM) in the presence of 40 mM lactose (LAC) or 40 mM sucrose (SUC) and then infected with DENV-1 as described in (B), for 72 hours. The viral load was quantified as described in (B). Data are representative from three independent experiments. *p<0.01; **p<0.001; ***p<0.0001.

permissiveness and Gal-1 expression level, we evaluate the susceptibility of macrophages isolated from $Lgals1^{-/-}$ to DENV infection. As expected, macrophages from $Lgals1^{-/-}$ mice did not express Gal-1 mRNA or protein levels (Figure 5B). Corroborating the data obtained with endothelial cells (Figure 1A and 1B), we detected much higher viral load in the supernatant of $Lgals1^{-/-}$ macrophages than in the supernatants from WT macrophages (Figure 5C). This result suggests that endogenous Gal-1 contributes to mice resistance during infection with DENV-1.

Discussion

Here we demonstrated that both endogenous and exogenous Gal-1 reduces DENV-1 infection by inhibiting virus infection of mammalian cells. Our results show that, at least in part, the inhibition by Gal-1 involves the prevention of adsorption and internalization of dengue virus into target cells. Also, the inhibitory effect of Gal-1 on DENV-1 infection depends on carbohydrate recognition and Gal-1 dimerization.

Gal-1 is widely expressed in animal cells and tissues; it is expressed in the thymus and by lymphoid parenchymal epithelial cells, endothelial cells, trophoblasts, activated T and B cells, macrophages, follicular DCs, and CD4+CD25+ regulatory T cells

[12]. Gal-1 has an important immunomodulatory activity, playing essential roles during microbial infection by modulating both innate and adaptive immunity [16]. However, the role of Gal-1 in the context of viral infections is less clear. Gal-1 has an anti-viral effect on infections by Nipah virus [17,18], Nodavirus [19], Influenza virus [20] and HSV-1 [21]. In such cases, Gal-1 negatively controls the infection by both directly interacting with viral glycoproteins, and thus inhibiting their mobility, maturation and functions [18,40], and by affecting the immune response of the target cells after infection [17,19]. However, Gal-1 can also promote the infectivity of cells by HSV-1 [28], HIV-1 [22–27] and HTLV-1 [29]. In such cases Gal-1 acts as a soluble adhesion molecule that stabilizes virus attachment to host cells and facilitates their entry [20]. Concerning DENV, there are no data in the literature exploring the role of Gal-1 in the infection caused by any of the four DENV-serotypes.

The initial steps leading to DENV entry into the host cells for primary infection are very poorly understood. Here we demonstrated that ECV-304, Vero-E6 and HMVEC-L cell lineages and WT murine macrophages are permissive to DENV-1 infection, and all of them constitutively express Gal-1 (Figure 1A and 5B). However, Gal-1 expression on HMVEC-L cells is higher when compared with the other two cell lineages, and interestingly, the

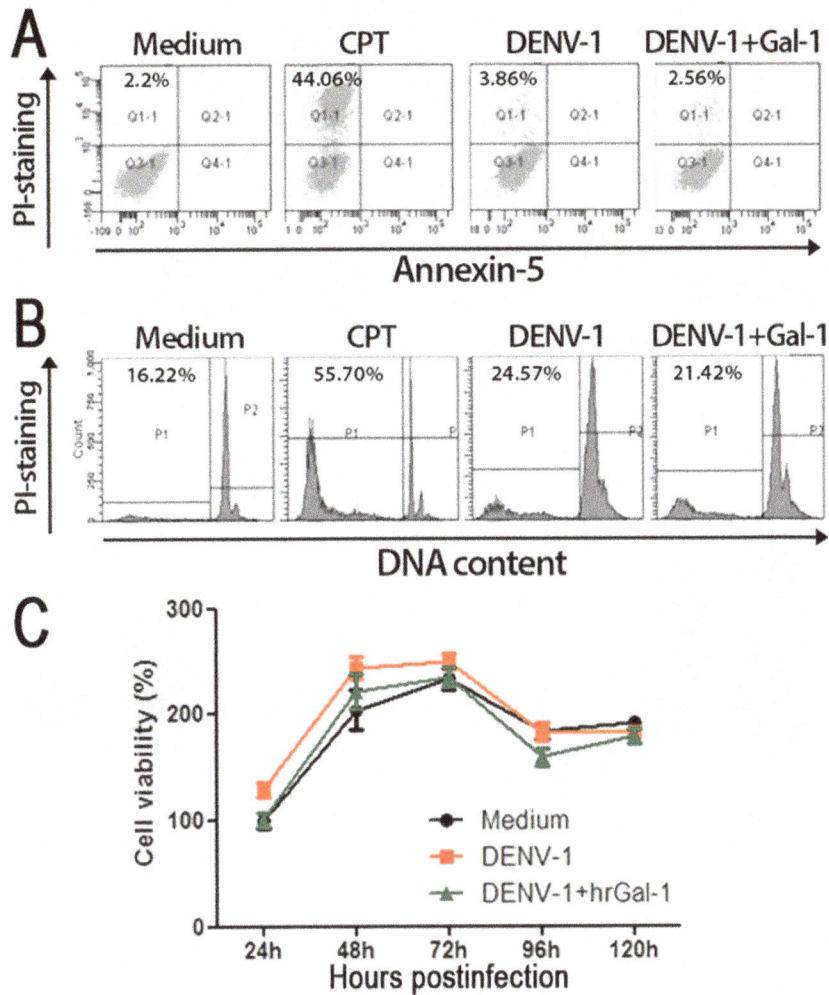

Figure 3. Gal-1 does not induce cell death during DENV-1 infection. (A and B) ECV-304 cells (2.5×10^4) were treated with hrGal-1 (10 μM) and infected with DENV-1 (MOI 0.5). At 72 hours postinfection, PI staining was used to evaluate the membrane permeability (A) and DNA degradation (B). For these purposes, PI was added to fresh cells or to permeabilized cells, respectively. Samples were acquired and analyzed by flow cytometry. Data is representative from three experiments with similar results. **(C)** ECV-304 cells were treated or not with 10 μM of hrGal-1 and infected with DENV-1 as described in (A). At the indicated times postinfection, cell viability was examined by MTT assay. Cells cultivated only with medium at 24 hours were designated as 100% of cell viability. Data is representative of 3 independent experiments performed in triplicates.

permissiveness of HMVEC-L cells to DENV-1 is lower than ECV-304 and Vero-E6 cells. On the other hand, macrophages with no expression of Gal-1 (*Lgals1*$^{-/-}$) are more permissive to DENV-1 infection. These data suggest an inverse correlation between Gal-1 expression and permissiveness to DENV-1 infection. It has been shown that dengue virus can interact with a large number of proteins [48], including the heat-shock protein 70 and DC-SIGN (a C-type mannose-binding lectin) [49]. It is also known that the galectins may form glycoprotein lattices on the cell surface [8,23], directly affecting their distribution, functions and endocytosis [18]. Since HMVEC-L cells present higher expression of Gal-1 compared with ECV-304 and Vero-E6, it is tempting to speculate that the membrane-associated Gal-1 may interact with DENV glycoprotein E to form lattices, and thus inhibit DENV-1 infectivity by reducing the entry of virus particles. It is also possible that Gal-1 could inhibit subsequent virus maturation, similar to the observed for Nipah virus [18].

Although we can not rule out that other factors could be also affecting HMVEC-L susceptibility, the possibility that Gal-1 might restricts viral entry is corroborated by our findings, showing that addition of exogenous Gal-1 inhibits virus adsorption to ECV-304 cells and its internalization during *in vitro* infection (Figure 4B). This inhibitory effect is reflected on the decreased virus release at 72 hours postinfection, and it is observed not only in ECV-304 cells, but also in Vero-E6 and HMVEC-L cell lineages (Figure 2B). In this set of experiments we demonstrated that the inhibitory effect of Gal-1 on DENV-1 release depends on protein dimerization, previously demonstrated to be required for efficient cross-linking of functional receptors or for the formation of signaling lattices [50–52]. Also, hrGal-1 inhibitory effect was dependent on carbohydrate recognition as is specifically impaired by the presence of lactose (Figure 2E). Together, these findings support the idea that the inhibitory effect of Gal-1 partly involves extracellular activities of this protein, which may include the lattice-formation (which is CRD-dependent) and interferes with virus adsorption and internalization.

Gal-1 may also exert an inhibitory effect on DENV-1 release by affecting the host cell responses. It has been reported that Gal-1

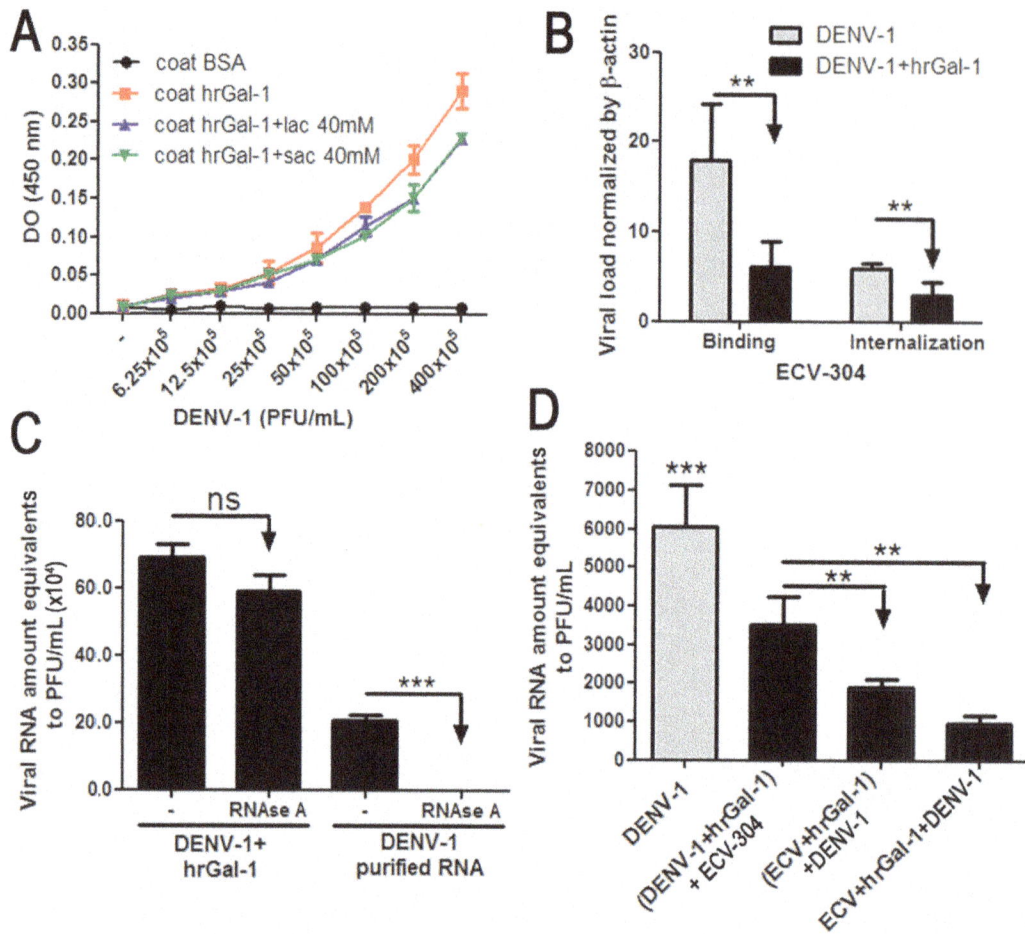

Figure 4. Gal-1 acts at early stages during DENV-1 infection. (A) Binding of DENV-1 to hrGal-1 in a dose-dependent manner. Serial two-fold dilutions of DENV-1 were applied to 96-well plates coated with 1 µg of hrGal-1 per well, and the bound virus particles were detected by ELISA with mouse anti-E protein antibody. BSA-coated wells served as the negative control. To assess the involvement of Gal-1 CRD, the assay was performed in presence of 40 mM lactose or sucrose. Each value represents the mean±the SD from 4 assays performed in duplicates. **(B)** Adsorption and internalization assays: for adsorption assay, ECV-304 cells were infected with DENV-1 at MOI of 10 in presence or absence of 10 µM hrGal-1 during 1 h at 4°C and then washed to remove viral inoculum. Cells were collected and the viral RNA was quantified by Real-Time PCR. Data was normalized by host β-actin expression. For internalization assay, ECV-304 cells were inoculated with DENV-1 (MOI of 10) at 4°C for 1 hour. Then, cells were washed and transferred to 37°C and hrGal-1 (10 µM) or only medium were added to culture. After 1 hour of incubation, non-internalized viruses were inactivated with citrate buffer and viral loads were quantified by Real-Time PCR. Data is presented as Viral RNA amount equivalents to PFU/mL±SD from 3 experiments assessed in triplicates. **(C)** For virucidal assay, DENV-1 was incubated with hrGal-1, in the presence or absence of RNAse. After 1 h incubation at 37°C, RNA was isolated and subjected to RT-Real-Time PCR. Purified viral RNA incubated or not with RNAse was used as control (N=3). **(D)** ECV-304 cells were infected with DENV-1 at a MOI of 0.5 (DENV-1). For the treatments, hrGal-1 was incubated with ECV-304 and DENV-1 simultaneously (ECV+Gal-1+DENV), or hrGal-1 (10 µM) was pre-incubated with either ECV-304 cells or with DENV-1 (MOI 0.5) for 60 minutes before the inoculation (ECV+hrGal-1)+DENV versus (DENV+hrGal-1)+ECV, respectively. At 72 hours postinfection, supernatants were collected and the viral loads were quantified by Real-Time PCR (N=3). **p<0.001; ***p<0.0001.

expression is altered after viral infections (*Helicobacter pylori* [53] e HTLV-1 [29]. We found decreased cellular Gal-1 expression accompanied of accentuated levels of Gal-1 in the supernatants from DENV1-infected ECV-304 cells at 72 hours postinfection (Figure 1C and 1D). It is possible that once released to the extracellular milieu, Gal-1 could act as an autocrine regulatory factor for endothelial cells to limit viral spread or act as potential damage-associated molecular pattern (DAMP) [54,55], thus interfering with the immune responses arising after DENV-1 infection.

It has been demonstrated that intracranial infection of mice on a C57Bl-6 background results in neurological abnormalities and death, but these mice does not show the most usual clinical signs observed in humans [30–33]. However, although we can not

extrapolate our data concerning the impact of Gal-1 in in vivo DENV-1 infection of mice to DENV-1 infection in humans, this approach allowed us to develop insights into the mechanisms behind Gal-1 effects.

The lethality of mice infected with DENV-1 is also associated with increased vascular permeability induced by an uncontrolled release of pro-inflammatory cytokines known as "Cytokine storm" [49,56]. Herein we demonstrated that newborn *Lgals1*−/− mice infected with DENV-1 start dying earlier than WT mice. This condition seems to be associated with the evidence that the *Lgals1*−/− macrophages (and probably other cell types as well) release higher amounts of virus particles at 72 hours postinfection, compared with the WT macrophages. Interestingly, there is uncertainty in the scientific community concerning DENV

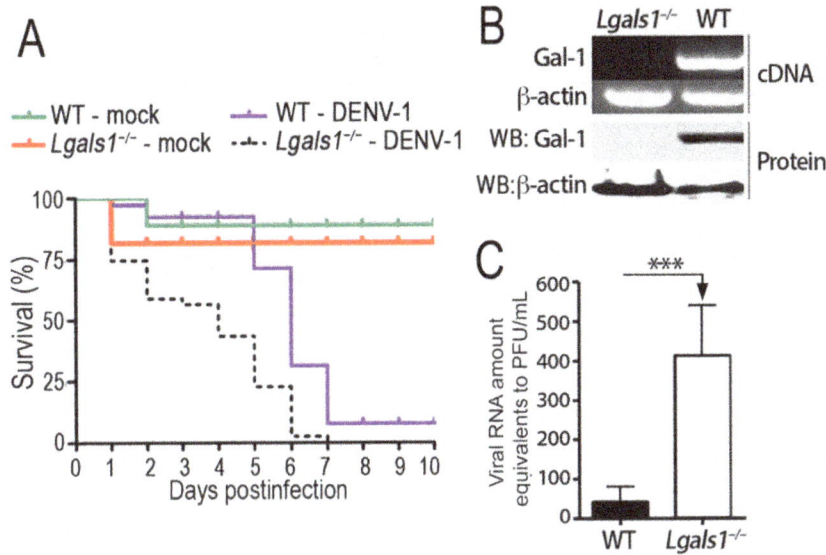

Figure 5. Gal-1 is physiologically relevant to in vivo infection with DENV-1. (A) Newborn WT and *Lgals1*[-/-] mice were intracerebraly infected with 10^6 PFU/ml of DENV-1 mouse-brain adapted or mock (supernatant from mouse brain not infected with DENV-1) and their mortality was monitored for 10 days. Results are shown as the percentage survival from five independent assays performed with 6–8 mice per group. **(B)** Total mRNA isolated from resident peritoneal macrophages of Gal-1-deficient (*Lgals1*[-/-]) and wild-type (WT) mice was converted into cDNA and the Gal-1 expression was analyzed using conventional PCR. The β-actin gene was used as an endogenous control. Alternatively, total protein from *Lgals1*[-/-] and WT macrophages were isolated and Gal-1 expression was quantified by western blot assay and normalized to β-actin expression. **(C)** Peritoneal resident macrophages from *Lgals1*[-/-] or WT mice were cultivated (5×10^5/well) in 24-well plates and inoculated with DENV-1 at a MOI of 0.5. After 72 hours at 37°C, cell-free supernatants were recovered and the viral loads were determined by Real-Time PCR. Results are showed as Viral RNA amounts equivalent to PFU/ml±SD from three experiments assessed in triplicates. ***$p < 0.0001$.

infectivity on macrophages. Some groups have noted that human and mouse macrophages are major cellular targets for DENV infection [46,49,57,58], but others suggests that the virus does not efficiently infect these cells in the absence of sub-neutralizing antibodies [59]. In our system, macrophages from WT mice were infected with DENV-1, however, the viral load from these cells was very low (viral RNA amount equivalent to 50 PFU/mL, Figure 5C), compared to viral load from other cell lineages (between 5,000 and 20,000 PFU/mL, Figure 1B). Nevertheless, the viral load in macrophages from *Lgals1*[-/-] animals was about eight times higher than that from WT macrophages, suggesting that endogenous Gal-1 contributes to resistance of mice to DENV-1 infection. The absence of Gal-1 in newborn *Lgals1*[-/-] mice may favor the establishment of a stronger cytokine storm in these mice later in the infection, since Gal-1 is classically known as an important anti-inflammatory factor [8,60]. Altogether, these conditions may contribute to the faster mortality observed in *Lgals1*[-/-] mice. Our results are in accordance to previous report showing that *Lgals1*[-/-] mice were also more susceptible to influenza virus infection compared with their WT counterparts [20].

Despite the increasing incidence of DENV as a human pathogen, there are no antiviral agents or vaccines for treatment or prevention [61]. Data presented here show that both endogenous and exogenous Gal-1 are inhibitory to DENV-1 infection. The differences between dengue pathogenesis in mouse and humans should be taken into account, but our results raise the possibility of using recombinant Gal-1 of as an additional/alternative method of treatment for dengue disease. This concept has also been advanced by others for the development of

therapeutic treatments for pathogenic and non-pathogenic diseases [8,62–64]. It has been shown that prophylactic or therapeutic administration of Gal-1 in animal experimental models of inflammatory diseases; cancer or neurodegeneration can ameliorate the disease symptoms or even the mice survival (reviewed in [8]). In the case of pathogenic diseases, the effects of recombinant Gal-1 administration are not well defined and have been shown to be context-dependent, since it can restrict or facilitate the infection [18,22,65]. Despite the difficulties in this field, the potential use of galectins as therapeutic targets has advanced. In the present work, we have shown that Gal-1 may interfere with the course of dengue virus infection probably through several mechanisms, including its participation in DENV-1 entry and cellular responses. Our future investigations aimed to elucidate the molecular mechanisms behind Gal-1 effects and also its roles during dengue human pathogenesis. Together, our study may promote the development of new drugs to combat the pathogenesis caused by this virus.

Acknowledgments

We thank Rubens Eduardo da Silva and Fabiana Rossetto de Morais for their excellent technical assistance with in vivo experiments and cytometry analysis, respectively.

Author Contributions

Conceived and designed the experiments: KAT MLF VHA MDB. Performed the experiments: KAT CDCA MLF RTA TBR VDMM RRR. Analyzed the data: KAT MLF CDCA TBR VDMM RRR VHA SRS RDC MDB. Contributed reagents/materials/analysis tools: VHA MDB. Wrote the paper: KAT MLF MDB.

References

1. Murray NE, Quam MB, Wilder-Smith A (2013) Epidemiology of dengue: past, present and future prospects. Clin Epidemiol 5: 299–309.

2. Beaumier CM, Gillespie PM, Hotez PJ, Bottazzi ME (2013) New vaccines for neglected parasitic diseases and dengue. Transl Res 162: 144–155.

3. Guzman MG, Kouri G (2002) Dengue: an update. Lancet Infect Dis 2: 33–42.

4. Halstead SB (2002) Dengue hemorrhagic fever: two infections and antibody dependent enhancement, a brief history and personal memoir. Rev Cubana Med Trop 54: 171–179.

5. Whitehorn J, Yacoub S, Anders KL, Macareo LR, Cassetti MC, et al. (2014) Dengue Therapeutics, Chemoprophylaxis, and Allied Tools: State of the Art and Future Directions. PLoS Negl Trop Dis 8: e3025.

6. NaTHNaC (2009) Dengue Fever. Health Protection Agency. Natural Travel Health Network and Centre.

7. Hughes RC (1997) The galectin family of mammalian carbohydrate-binding molecules. Biochem Soc Trans 25: 1194–1198.

8. Camby I, Le Mercier M, Lefranc F, Kiss R (2006) Galectin-1: a small protein with major functions. Glycobiology 16: 137R–157R.

9. Thijssen VL, Griffioen AW (2014) Galectin-1 and -9 in angiogenesis: A sweet couple. Glycobiology 24: 915–920.

10. Stowell SR, Cho M, Feasley CL, Arthur CM, Song X, et al. (2009) Ligand reduces galectin-1 sensitivity to oxidative inactivation by enhancing dimer formation. J Biol Chem 284: 4989–4999.

11. Barondes SH, Cooper DN, Gitt MA, Leffler H (1994) Galectins. Structure and function of a large family of animal lectins. J Biol Chem 269: 20807–20810.

12. Sato S, Ouellet M, St-Pierre C, Tremblay MJ (2012) Glycans, galectins, and HIV-1 infection. Ann N Y Acad Sci 1253: 133–148.

13. Stowell SR, Arthur CM, Dias-Baruffi M, Rodrigues LC, Gourdine JP, et al. (2010) Innate immune lectins kill bacteria expressing blood group antigen. Nat Med 16: 295–301.

14. Stowell SR, Arthur CM, McBride R, Berger O, Razi N, et al. (2014) Microbial glycan microarrays define key features of host-microbial interactions. Nat Chem Biol 10: 470–476.

15. Arthur CM, Cummings RD, Stowell SR (2014) Using glycan microarrays to understand immunity. Curr Opin Chem Biol 18: 55–61.

16. Cedeno-Laurent F, Dimitroff CJ (2012) Galectin-1 research in T cell immunity: past, present and future. Clin Immunol 142: 107–116.

17. Levroney EL, Aguilar HC, Fulcher JA, Kohatsu L, Pace KE, et al. (2005) Novel innate immune functions for galectin-1: galectin-1 inhibits cell fusion by Nipah virus envelope glycoproteins and augments dendritic cell secretion of proinflammatory cytokines. J Immunol 175: 413–420.

18. Garner OB, Aguilar HC, Fulcher JA, Levroney EL, Harrison R, et al. (2010) Endothelial galectin-1 binds to specific glycans on nipah virus fusion protein and inhibits maturation, mobility, and function to block syncytia formation. PLoS Pathog 6: e1000993.

19. Poisa-Beiro L, Dios S, Ahmed H, Vasta GR, Martínez-López A, et al. (2009) Nodavirus infection of sea bass (Dicentrarchus labrax) induces up-regulation of galectin-1 expression with potential anti-inflammatory activity. J Immunol 183: 6600–6611.

20. Yang ML, Chen YH, Wang SW, Huang YJ, Leu CH, et al. (2011) Galectin-1 binds to influenza virus and ameliorates influenza virus pathogenesis. J Virol 85: 10010–10020.

21. Rajasagi NK, Suryawanshi A, Sehrawat S, Reddy PB, Mulik S, et al. (2012) Galectin-1 reduces the severity of herpes simplex virus-induced ocular immunopathological lesions. J Immunol 188: 4631–4643.

22. Ouellet M, Mercier S, Pelletier I, Bounou S, Roy J, et al. (2005) Galectin-1 acts as a soluble host factor that promotes HIV-1 infectivity through stabilization of virus attachment to host cells. J Immunol 174: 4120–4126.

23. Mercier S (2008) Galectin-1 promotes HIV-1 infectivity in macrophages through stabilization of viral adsorption. Virology 371: 121–129.

24. St-Pierre C, Manya H, Ouellet M, Clark GF, Endo T, et al. (2011) Host Soluble Galectin-1 Promotes HIV-1 Replication through a Direct Interaction with Glycans of Viral gp120 and Host CD4. J Virol 85: 11742–11751.

25. St-Pierre C, Ouellet M, Giguère D, Ohtake R, Roy R, et al. (2012) Galectin-1-specific inhibitors as a new class of compounds to treat HIV-1 infection. Antimicrob Agents Chemother 56: 154–162.

26. Reynolds JL, Law WC, Mahajan SD, Aalinkeel R, Nair B, et al. (2012a) Morphine and galectin-1 modulate HIV-1 infection of human monocyte-derived macrophages. J Immunol 188: 3757–3765.

27. Reynolds JL, Law WC, Mahajan SD, Aalinkeel R, Nair B, et al. (2012b) Nanoparticle based galectin-1 gene silencing, implications in methamphetamine regulation of HIV-1 infection in monocyte derived macrophages. J Neuroimmune Pharmacol 7: 673–685.

28. Gonzalez MI, Rubinstein N, Ilarregui JM, Toscano MA, Sanjuan NA, et al. (2005) Regulated expression of galectin-1 after in vitro productive infection with herpes simplex virus type 1: implications for T cell apoptosis. Int J Immunopathol Pharmacol 18: 615–623.

29. Gauthier S, Pelletier I, Ouellet M, Vargas A, Tremblay MJ, et al. (2008) Induction of galectin-1 expression by HTLV-I Tax and its impact on HTLV-I infectivity. Retrovirology 5: 105.

30. Muller VD, Russo RR, Cintra AC, Sartim MA, Alves-Paiva Rde M, et al. (2012) Crotoxin and phospholipases A$_2$ from Crotalus durissus terrificus showed antiviral activity against dengue and yellow fever viruses. Toxicon 59: 507–515.

31. Gualano RC, Pryor MJ, Cauchi MR, Wright PJ, Davidson AD (1998) Identification of a major determinant of mouse neurovirulence of dengue virus type 2 using stably cloned genomic-length cDNA. J Gen Virol 79: 437–446.

32. Ip PP, Liao F (2010) Resistance to dengue virus infection in mice is potentiated by CXCL10 and is independent of CXCL10-mediated leukocyte recruitment. J Immunol 184.: 5705–5714.

33. Stowell SR, Qian Y, Karmakar S, Koyama NS, Dias-Baruffi M, et al. (2008) Differential roles of galectin-1 and galectin-3 in regulating leukocyte viability and cytokine secretion. J Immunol 180: 3091–3102.

34. Stowell SR, Karmakar S, Arthur CM, Ju T, Rodrigues LC, et al. (2009) Galectin-1 induces reversible phosphatidylserine exposure at the plasma membrane. Mol Biol Cell 20: 1408–1418.

35. Cho M, Cummings RD (1995) Galectin-1, a beta-galactoside-binding lectin in Chinese hamster ovary cells. I. Physical and chemical characterization. J Biol Chem 270: 5198–5206.

36. Cho M, Cummings RD (1996) Characterization of monomeric forms of galectin-1 generated by site-directed mutagenesis. Biochemistry 35: 13081–13088.

37. Koishi AC, Zanello PR, Bianco ÉM, Bordignon J, Nunes Duarte dos Santos C (2012) Screening of Dengue virus antiviral activity of marine seaweeds by an in situ enzyme-linked immunosorbent assay. PLoS One 7: e51089.

38. dos Santos HW, Poloni TR, Souza KP, Muller VD, Tremeschin F, et al. (2008) A simple one-step real-time RT-PCR for diagnosis of dengue virus infection. J Med Virol 80: 1426–1433.

39. Mosmann T (1983) Rapid colorimetric assay for cellular growth and survival: application to proliferation and cytotoxicity assays. J Immunol Methods 65: 55–63.

40. Lee JY, Kim JY, Lee YG, Byeon SE, Kim BH, et al. (2007) In vitro immunoregulatory effects of Korean mistletoe lectin on functional activation of monocytic and macrophage-like cells. Biol Pharm Bull 30: 2043–2051.

41. Agis-Juárez RA, Galván I, Medina F, Daikoku T, Padmanabhan R, et al. (2009) Polypyrimidine tract-binding protein is relocated to the cytoplasm and is required during dengue virus infection in Vero cells. J Gen Virol 90: 2893–2901.

42. Mosso C, Galván-Mendoza IJ, Ludert JE, del Angel RM (2008) Endocytic pathway followed by dengue virus to infect the mosquito cell line C6/36 HT. Virology 378: 193–199.

43. Warke RV, Xhaja K, Martin KJ, Fournier MF, Shaw SK, et al. (2003) Dengue virus induces novel changes in gene expression of human umbilical vein endothelial cells. J Virol 77: 11822–11832.

44. Warke RV, Becerra A, Zawadzka A, Schmidt DJ, Martin KJ, et al. (2008) Efficient dengue virus (DENV) infection of human muscle satellite cells upregulates type I interferon response genes and differentially modulates MHC I expression on bystander and DENV-infected cells. J Gen Virol 89: 1605–1615.

45. Vervaeke P, Alen M, Noppen S, Schols D, Oreste P, et al. (2013) Sulfated Escherichia coli K5 Polysaccharide Derivatives Inhibit Dengue Virus Infection of Human Microvascular Endothelial Cells by Interacting with the Viral Envelope Protein E Domain III. PLoS ONE 8(8): e74035.

46. Kyle JL, Beatty PR, Harris E (2007) Dengue virus infects macrophages and dendritic cells in a mouse model of infection. J Infect Dis 195: 1808–1817.

47. Prestwood TR, May MM, Plummer EM, Morar MM, Yauch LE, et al. (2012) Trafficking and replication patterns reveal splenic macrophages as major targets of dengue virus in mice. J Virol 86: 12138–12147.

48. Mairiang D, Zhang H, Sodja A, Murali T, Suriyaphol P, et al. (2013) Identification of new protein interactions between dengue fever virus and its hosts, human and mosquito. PLoS One 8: e53535.

49. Rodenhuis-Zybert IA, Wilschut J, Smit JM (2010) Dengue virus life cycle: viral and host factors modulating infectivity. Cell Mol Life Sci 67: 2773–2786.

50. Demetriou M, Granovsky M, Quaggin S, Dennis JW (2001) Negative regulation of T-cell activation and autoimmunity by Mgat5 N-glycosylation. Nature 409: 733–739.

51. Nieminen J, Kuno A, Hirabayashi J, Sato S (2007) Visualization of galectin-3 oligomerization on the surface of neutrophils and endothelial cells using fluorescence resonance energy transfer. J Biol Chem 282: 1374–1383.

52. Brewer CF, Miceli MC, Baum LG (2002) Clusters, bundles, arrays and lattices: novel mechanisms for lectin-saccharide-mediated cellular interactions. Curr Opin Struct Biol 12: 616–623.

53. Lim JW, Kim H, Kim KH (2003) Cell adhesion-related gene expression by Helicobacter pylori in gastric epithelial AGS cells. Int J Biochem Cell Biol 35: 1284–1296.

54. Sato S, St-Pierre C, Bhaumik P, Nieminen J (2009) Galectins in innate immunity: dual functions of host soluble beta-galactoside-binding lectins as damage-associated molecular patterns (DAMPs) and as receptors for pathogen-associated molecular patterns (PAMPs). Immunol Rev 230: 172–187.

55. Vasta GR (2009) Roles of galectins in infection. Nat Rev Microbiol 7: 424–438.

56. Munoz-Jordan JL, Sanchez-Burgos GG, Laurent-Rolle M, Garcia-Sastre A (2003) Inhibition of interferon signaling by dengue virus. Proc Natl Acad Sci USA 100: 14333–14338.

57. Kyle JL, Beatty PR, Harris E (2007) Dengue virus infects macrophages and dendritic cells in a mouse model of infection. J Infect Dis 195: 1808–1817.

58. Moreno-Altamirano MM, Sánchez-García FJ, Legorreta-Herrera M, Aguilar-Carmona I (2007) Susceptibility of mouse macrophage J774 to dengue virus infection. Intervirology 50: 237–239.

59. Wahala WM, Silva AM (2011) The human antibody response to dengue virus infection. Viruses 3: 2374–2395.

60. Salatino M, Croci DO, Bianco GA, Ilarregui JM, Toscano MA, et al. (2008) Galectin-1 as a potential therapeutic target in autoimmune disorders and cancer. Expert Opin Biol Ther 8: 45–57.

61. Acosta EG, Castilla V, Damonte EB (2009) Alternative infectious entry pathways for dengue virus serotypes into mammalian cells. Cell Microbiol 11: 1533–1549.

62. Horie H, Kadoya T, Sango K, Hasegawa M (2005) Oxidized galectin-1 is an essential factor for peripheral nerve regeneration. Curr Drug Targets 6: 385–394.

63. Kami K, Senba E (2005) Galectin-1 is a novel factor that regulates myotube growth in regenerating skeletal muscles. Curr Drug Targets 6: 395–405.

64. Kato T, Ren CH, Wada M, Kawanami T (2005) Galectin-1 as a potential therapeutic agent for amyotrophic lateral sclerosis. Curr Drug Targets 6: 407–418.

65. Zúñiga E, Gruppi A, Hirabayashi J, Kasai KI, Rabinovich GA, et al. (2001) Regulated expression and effect of galectin-1 on Trypanosoma cruzi-infected macrophages: modulation of microbicidal activity and survival. Infect Immun 69: 6804–6812

6

Niacin Activates the PI3K/Akt Cascade via PKC- and EGFR-Transactivation-Dependent Pathways through Hydroxyl-Carboxylic Acid Receptor 2

Huawang Sun[1,9], Guo Li[2,3,9], Wenjuan Zhang[1], Qi Zhou[1], Yena Yu[1], Ying Shi[2], Stefan Offermanns[4], Jianxin Lu[1]*, Naiming Zhou[2]*

1 Zhejiang Provincial Key Laboratory of Medical Genetics, School of Laboratory Medicine and Life Science, Wenzhou Medical University, Wenzhou, Zhejiang, China, **2** College of Life Sciences, Zijingang Campus, Zhejiang University, Hangzhou, Zhejiang, China, **3** Institute of Aging Research, Hangzhou Normal University, Hangzhou, Zhejiang, China, **4** Department of Pharmacology, Max-Planck-Institute for Heart and Lung Research, Bad Nauheim, Germany

Abstract

Niacin has been demonstrated to activate a PI3K/Akt signaling cascade to prevent brain damage after stroke and UV-induced skin damage; however, the underlying molecular mechanisms for HCA_2-induced Akt activation remain to be elucidated. Using CHO-K1 cells stably expressing HCA_2 and A431 cells, a human epidermoid cell line with high levels of endogenous expression of functional HCA_2 receptors, we first demonstrated that niacin induced a robust Akt phosphorylation at both Thr^{308} and Ser^{473} in a time-dependent fashion, with a maximal activation at 5 min and a subsequent reduction to baseline by 30 min through HCA_2, and that the activation was significantly blocked by pertussis toxin. The HCA_2-mediated activation of Akt was also significantly inhibited by the PKC inhibitors GF109203x and Go6983 in both cell lines, by the PDGFR-selective inhibitor tyrphostin A9 in CHO-HCA_2 cells and by the MMP inhibitor GM6001 and EGFR-specific inhibitor AG1478 in A431 cells. These results suggest that the PKC pathway and PDGFR/EGFR transactivation pathway play important roles in HCA_2-mediated Akt activation. Further investigation indicated that PI3K and the $G_{\beta\gamma}$ subunit were likely to play an essential role in HCA_2-induced Akt activation. Moreover, Immunobloting analyses using an antibody that recognizes p70S6K1 phosphorylated at Thr^{389} showed that niacin evoked p70S6K1 activation via the PI3K/Akt pathway. The results of our study provide new insight into the signaling pathways involved in HCA_2 activation.

Editor: Ferenc Gallyas Jr., University of Pecs Medical School, Hungary

Funding: This work was supported by grants from the Ministry of Science and Technology of China (2012CB910402 and 2012AA020303), the National Natural Science Foundation of China (81173106) and the Zhejiang Natural Science Foundation (Z2080207). Dr. S. Offermanns was supported by the German Research Foundation. The funders had no role in study design, data collection and analysis, decision to publish, or preparation of the manuscript.

Competing Interests: The authors have declared that no competing interests exist.

* Email: znm2000@yahoo.com (NZ); jxlu313@163.com (JL)

9 These authors contributed equally to this work.

Introduction

Nicotinic acid has long been believed to have a favorable effect on plasma lipids, lowering plasma LDL-cholesterol and raising HDL-cholesterol [1]. Previous clinical data have also demonstrated its beneficial effects in reducing cardiovascular events and mortality in patients with coronary heart disease [2–5]. The discovery of G protein-coupled receptor GPR109A (HM74a), recently designated hydroxyl-carboxylic acid receptor 2 (HCA_2) because the ketone body β-hydroxybutyrate has been identified as its endogenous ligand [6], as a high-affinity receptor for nicotinic acid [7–9] has drawn significant attention to the potential development of novel agonists with antilipolytic activity.

HCA_2 is a G_i protein-coupled receptor. Upon activation by niacin, HCA_2 evokes an inhibitory effect on adenylate cyclase, leading to a decrease in the intracellular cAMP, and meanwhile also elicits a transient rise in the intracellular Ca^{2+} level in a pertussis toxin (PTX)-sensitive manner [7,8,10]. In adipocytes, the reduction in intracellular cAMP results in the decreased activity of

protein kinase A (PKA), leading to the decreased activity of hormone-sensitive lipase and a reduced triglyceride hydrolysis to free fatty acids [11]. A recent study using LDL-receptor knockout mice lacking the HCA_2 receptor demonstrated that niacin did not cause a decrease in the plasma free fatty acid level, but retained its effect on the plasma HDL and triglycerides, suggesting that the lipid-modifying properties of niacin are not mediated through HCA_2 [12]. However, niacin exhibited beneficial effects on the progression of atherosclerosis via HCA_2 expressed in bone marrow-derived immune cells, but without affecting the plasma lipid profile [13]. Moreover, accumulating evidence convincingly illustrated that niacin mediates its anti-inflammatory effects via HCA_2-dependent mechanisms in monocytes and macrophages [14,15], adipose tissue [16], and vascular endothelium [16].

It is well known that extracellular signals transduced by both receptor tyrosine kinases (RTKs) and GPCRs converge upon the activation of a family of phosphoinositide 3-kinases (PI3Ks), followed by the initiation of a phosphorylation cascade leading to the activation of Akt, also known as protein kinase B [17]. The

PI3K/Akt signaling pathway plays a major role in the control of cell proliferation, survival, metabolism and nutrient uptake in a cell-type-specific manner through a variety of downstream targets [18,19]. A growing body of evidence suggests a role for PI3K/Akt signaling in the regulation of the inflammatory response in diseases including rheumatoid arthritis [20], multiple sclerosis [21], asthma [22], and atherosclerosis [23]. Niacin has been shown to exert its protective effects on stroke [24] and UV-induced skin damage [25] via PI3K/Akt-mediated anti-apoptotic pathways. However, the mechanism(s) underlying the regulation of the PI3K/Akt pathway by HCA_2 is poorly understood.

Our previous data have shown that upon stimulation by niacin, activated HCA_2 results in the dissociation of G_i proteins from $G_{\beta\gamma}$-subunit, causing the PKC pathway to couple to ERK1/2 phosphorylation at early time points (≤ 2 min), and the MMP/EGFR transactivation pathway to act at both early and later time points (2–5 min) [26]. We also present evidence that the $\beta\gamma$-subunit plays a critical role in HCA_2-activated ERK1/2 phosphorylation. In the present study, we used Chinese hamster ovary (CHO) cells recombinantly expressing human HCA_2 receptors (CHO-HCA_2), and A431 cells, a human epidermoid carcinoma cell line that endogenously express functional HCA_2 receptors [27], to characterize the regulation of the PI3K/Akt signaling pathway mediated by the human HCA_2. We found that niacin-mediated activation of human HCA_2 signals to the PI3K/Akt cascade via the G_i protein-initiated PKC and PDGFR/EGFR transactivation-dependent pathways. We also demonstrate that the $G_{\beta\gamma}$ subunit plays a key role in the HCA_2-mediated activation of the PI3K/Akt pathway via interaction with RTK signaling. The results of our study add new understanding to the roles of the HCA_2 receptor in its beneficial effects on the progression of atherosclerosis.

Materials and Methods

Materials

Opti-MEM I reduced serum medium and G418 were purchased from Invitrogen (Carlsbad, CA, USA) and the X-tremeGENE HP reagent was purchased from Roche (Basel, Switzerland). Cell culture medium and fetal bovine serum were obtained from Hyclone (Beijing, China). Alternative Thioglycollate Medium, Pertussis toxin (PTX), GF109203X (bisindolylmaleimide), Go6983, and tyrphostin A9 were obtained from Sigma (St. Louis, MO, USA), while U0126, tyrphostin AG1478, GM6001, PP2 and Wortmannin were from Calbiochem (La Jolla, CA, USA). Anti-phospho-Akt (Ser473), Anti-phospho-Akt(Thr 308), Anti-Akt, Anti-EGFR, Anti-PDGFR, Anti-phospho-EGFR (Tyr1173), Anti-phospho-PDGFR (Tyr1018) and the horseradish peroxidase substrate were bought from Cell Signaling Technology (Danvers, MA, USA). Horseradish peroxidase-conjugated goat anti-rabbit secondary antibody and anti-β-actin antibody were obtained from HuaAn Biotechnology (Hangzhou, China). RIPA lysis buffer and a BCA kit were bought from Beyotime (Haimen, China).

Mice

$Hca_2^{+/-}$ mice were maintained in specific pathogen-free husbandry. Wild-type and $Hca_2^{-/-}$ mice were obtained by intercrossing $Hca_2^{+/-}$ mice. Genotyping of the Hca_2 alleles and the inactivated alleles were performed as described [8]. All animal work was conducted in accordance with the Guide for the Care and Use of Laboratory Animals as adopted and promulgated by the United States National Institutes of Health. The protocol was approved by the research ethics committee of Zhejiang University.

Cell lines and cell culture

CHO-K1 cells (from the American Type Culture Collection) [28] were kindly provided by Dr. Jeffrey Benovic (Thomas Jefferson University, Philadelphia, USA), and were grown in 50:50 Dulbecco's modified Eagle's medium (DMEM)/Ham's F-12 medium supplemented with 10% fetal bovine serum (FBS) and 2 mM glutamine. A431 cells were obtained from Type Culture Collection of Chinese Academy of Sciences (Shanghai, China) and were cultured in DMEM medium supplemented with 10% FBS and 2 mM glutamine. Cells were maintained at 37°C in a humidified incubator containing 5% CO_2. Stable cell lines were produced by transfection of CHO-K1 cells with pCDNA3.1-HCA_2 or pCDNA3.1-HCA_3 using the X-tremeGENE HP reagent according to the manufacturer's instructions and selected using G418 [26]. Surviving cells were cloned by limiting dilution, and cell clones were tested for receptor expression by functional analysis using a CRE-driven luciferase activity reporter gene assay. When needed to overexpress a function-deficient protein to detect receptor signaling, 0.6 μg HCA_2 plasmids plus 2.4 μg Gα-transducin were transiently transfected into CHO-K1 cells or 3 μg βARK1-CT into CHO-HCA_2 stable cells. pCDNA3.1 was used as a control plasmid.

Macrophage isolation

4 to 6 weeks old mice were injected with 1 ml 4% Alternative Thioglycollate Medium for three days and macrophages were isolated according to the standard methods [29]. The primary mouse macrophages were maintained in Modified Roswell Park Memorial Institute (RPMI)-1640 medium supplemented with 10% FBS and 2 mM glutamine.

Immunoblotting assay

CHO-K1 cells or A431 cells were seeded in 24-well plates, rinsed with serum-free DMEM/F-12 or DMEM when grown to 80% confluence and incubated overnight in serum-free medium. After treatment with niacin, the cells were lysed with RIPA buffer. When needed, the cells were preincubated with inhibitors (PTX overnight or other inhibitors for 1 h) prior to treatment with niacin. Total protein was determined using a BCA kit. Equal amounts of total cell lysate were size-fractionated by SDS-PAGE (10–12%) and transferred to a PVDF membrane (Millipore). Membranes were blocked in blocking buffer (TBS containing 0.05–0.1% Tween-20 and 5% nonfat dry milk) for 1 h at room temperature and incubated overnight at 4°C with rabbit monoclonal antibody to Phospho-Akt(Ser473), Phospho-Akt(Thr308), Phospho-p70S6K1, Phospho-ERK, or β-Actin followed by incubation with an anti-rabbit HRP-conjugated secondary antibody according to the manufacturer's protocols. The chemiluminescence was detected with a HRP substrate using a film-based system and quantified using the Bio-Rad Quantity One Imaging system (Bio-Rad Laboratories).

Data analysis

All results are expressed as the mean ± S.E. Data were analyzed using either non-linear curve fitting (GraphPad PRISM version 5.0) or a two-way ANOVA in grouped analysis. Statistical significance was determined using Student's t test. Probability values less than or equal to 0.05 were considered significant.

Results

Niacin induces Akt phosphorylation on both residue Thr^{308} and Ser^{473} through HCA_2

Our previous study has demonstrated that niacin induces ERK1/2 activation via PKC- and EGFR-dependent pathways through HCA_2 in CHO-K1 and A431 cells [26]. In this study, the same CHO-K1 cell line stably expressing the human HCA_2 was used to determine whether HCA_2 regulates Akt phosphorylation. As shown in Figs. 1A, 1B, and Fig. S1A, niacin induced robust Akt phosphorylation in both the activation loop within the kinase domain [A-loop (Thr^{308})] and the hydrophobic motif in the C-terminal region [HM (Ser^{473})] in a concentration-dependent manner. Akt phosphorylation in response to niacin was undetectable in $CHO-HCA_3$ cells (Fig. 1C), suggesting a specific activation of Akt via HCA_2 by niacin. Using A431 cells endogenously expressing HCA_2, niacin-induced Akt phosphorylation on both Thr^{308} and Ser^{473} was observed at comparable levels to that in $CHO-HCA_2$ cells (Figs. 1A and 1B, and Fig. S1A and S1B). We next utilized primary macrophages from Alternative Thioglycollate Medium-pretreated HCA_2-deficient mice or their wild-type littermates to further assess the role of HCA_2 in niacin-mediated Akt activation. As indicated in Fig. 1D, niacin was found to significantly induce Akt phosphorylation in wild-type macrophages. In contrast, no activation of Akt in HCA_2-deficient macrophages was detected in the presence of niacin. Taken together, these data suggest that niacin triggers Akt activation through HCA_2.

HCA_2 activates the Akt signaling pathway via a PTX-sensitive G_i protein-dependent pathway

HCA_2 is associated with G_i protein, and upon activation by niacin, acts to inhibit adenylyl cyclase, resulting in the inhibition of forskolin-induced cAMP accumulation. To explore the role of G_i protein in the niacin-mediated activation of Akt, $CHO-HCA_2$ and A431 cells were cultured in the presence or absence of 100 ng/ml pertussis toxin (PTX) in serum-free medium overnight, followed by stimulation with 1 μM niacin for $CHO-HCA_2$ cells and 100 μM niacin for A431 cells. As shown in Fig. 2, niacin evoked significant Akt phosphorylation on both Thr^{308} and Ser^{473} in a time-dependent fashion, with maximal activation at 5 min and with a subsequent reduction to baseline by 30 min. This activation in both $CHO-HCA_2$ (Figs. 2A and 2C) and A431 (Figs. 2B and 2D) was remarkably inhibited by pretreatment with PTX, suggesting that HCA_2 signals through the Akt pathway via a PTX-sensitive G_i protein-dependent mechanism.

Involvement of PKC in HCA_2-mediated Akt activation

Our previous studies have shown that PKC plays a determinant role in HCA_2-mediated ERK1/2 activation at early time points (≤ 2 min) [26]. To investigate whether PKC plays a role in niacin-stimulated Akt phosphorylation via HCA_2, $CHO-HCA_2$ and A431 cells were pretreated with the PKC inhibitors GF109203x (10 μM) or Go6983 (10 μM) for 1 h, followed by niacin stimulation for the indicated time. Both PKC inhibitors exhibited inhibitory effects on niacin-induced Akt phosphorylation at Thr^{308} and Ser^{473} in both $CHO-HCA_2$ (Figs. 3A and 3C, and Fig. S2D) and A431 cells (Figs. 3B, 3D, and 3E, Fig. S2C, and S2E). Collectively, these data clearly show that PKC plays a critical role in HCA_2-mediated Akt activation.

HCA_2-induced Akt activation is dependent on a growth factor receptor-involved transactivation mechanism

It is generally accepted that the transactivation of growth factor receptors participates in the GPCR-mediated activation of the ERK/MAPK pathway and phosphorylation of Akt/PKB, induction of cell proliferation and migration [30,31]. CHO-K1 cells are known to endogenously express PDGF receptor-β but lack EGFR [32]; however, A431 cells have been shown to express EGFR and

be devoid of endogenous α- and β-PDGF receptors [33]. CHO-HCA_2 and A431 cells were preincubated with the PDGF receptor-selective receptor tyrosine kinase inhibitor tyrphostin A9 (1 μM) for 1 h followed by niacin stimulation for different lengths of time. As shown in Fig. 4A, in the tyrphostin A9-pretreated $CHO-HCA_2$ cells, there was approximately 60% inhibition of Akt phosphorylation compared with cells treated with agonist alone, whereas there was no inhibition of Akt phosphorylation in the tyrphostin A9-pretreated A431 cells (data not shown). These data demonstrate that PDGFR transactivation is involved in HCA_2-induced Akt activation in CHO-K1 cells, but not in A431 cells.

To assess the role of EGFR transactivation in niacin-induced Akt activation in cells that endogenously express HCA_2, A431 cells were utilized for further investigation. Serum-starved A431 cells were treated with AG1478 (100 nM), an EGFR-specific tyrosine kinase inhibitor, for 1 h before exposing them to 100 μM niacin. As shown in Fig. 4B, Fig. S2C, S2D, and S2E, AG1478 dramatically inhibited (>80%) niacin-induced Akt phosphorylation. Several studies have shown that transactivation of EGFR is sensitive to matrix metalloproteinase (MMP) inhibitors [34,35]. To define the mechanism underlying niacin-induced transactivation of the EGFR, A431 cells were treated with the MMP inhibitor GM6001 (10 μM) for 1 h before niacin stimulation. GM6001 treatment led to a significant reduction (>70%) in Akt activation when induced by niacin (Fig. 4B).

We next examined whether HCA_2 is able to induce EGFR phosphorylation in A431 cells and PDGFR phosphorylation in $CHO-HCA_2$. As shown in Fig. 4C and 4D, niacin stimulated EGFR and PDGFR phosphorylation in a time-dependent manner. Moreover, using specific inhibitors GM6001 and AG1478, EGFR phosphorylation was significantly blocked in A431 cells, and about 50% PDGFR phosphorylation was inhibited in CH0-HCA_2 cells by pretreatment with A9. These results demonstrate that HCA_2 evokes Akt activation via the PDGFR transactivation pathway in $CHO-HCA_2$ cells and the EGFR transactivation pathway in A431 cells.

Involvement of PI3K but not Src in HCA_2-mediated Akt activation

Our previous studies have reported that PI3K and Src are involved in ERK1/2 activation in response to HCA_2 receptors [26]. Using $CHO-HCA_2$ and A431 cells treated with the PI3K inhibitor Wortmannin (1 μM) and the Src inhibitor PP2 (10 μM), we observed that Wortmannin abolished niacin-stimulated Akt phosphorylation in both $CHO-HCA_2$ and A431 cells (Figs. 5A and 5B, Fig. S2C, S2D, and S2E), while PP2 had no inhibitory effect on niacin-stimulated Akt activation in either cell line (Figs. 5C and 5D). Collectively, these results show that niacin-induced Akt phosphorylation is PI3K-dependent and Src-independent.

$G_{\beta\gamma}$ plays an essential role in HCA_2-induced Akt activation

For most G_i protein-coupled receptors, signaling from the activated receptor to PI3K/Akt involves the $G_{\beta\gamma}$ subunit of heterotrimeric G proteins [36,37]. Our previous study has demonstrated a critical role for the βγ-subunit in HCA_2-activated ERK1/2 phosphorylation [26]. Accordingly, we sought to further define the role of the $G_{\beta\gamma}$ subunit in HCA_2-induced Akt activation. β-adrenergic receptor kinase COOH domain (495–689aa) (βARK1-CT) and Gα subunit of transducin, both of which are scavengers of $G_{\beta\gamma}$-subunit [38–40], were transfected into CHO-HCA_2 cells and CHO-K1 cells with HCA_2, respectively. Upon transfection, a significant inhibition in HCA_2-mediated Akt phosphorylation was observed (Fig. 6A and 6B), suggesting that

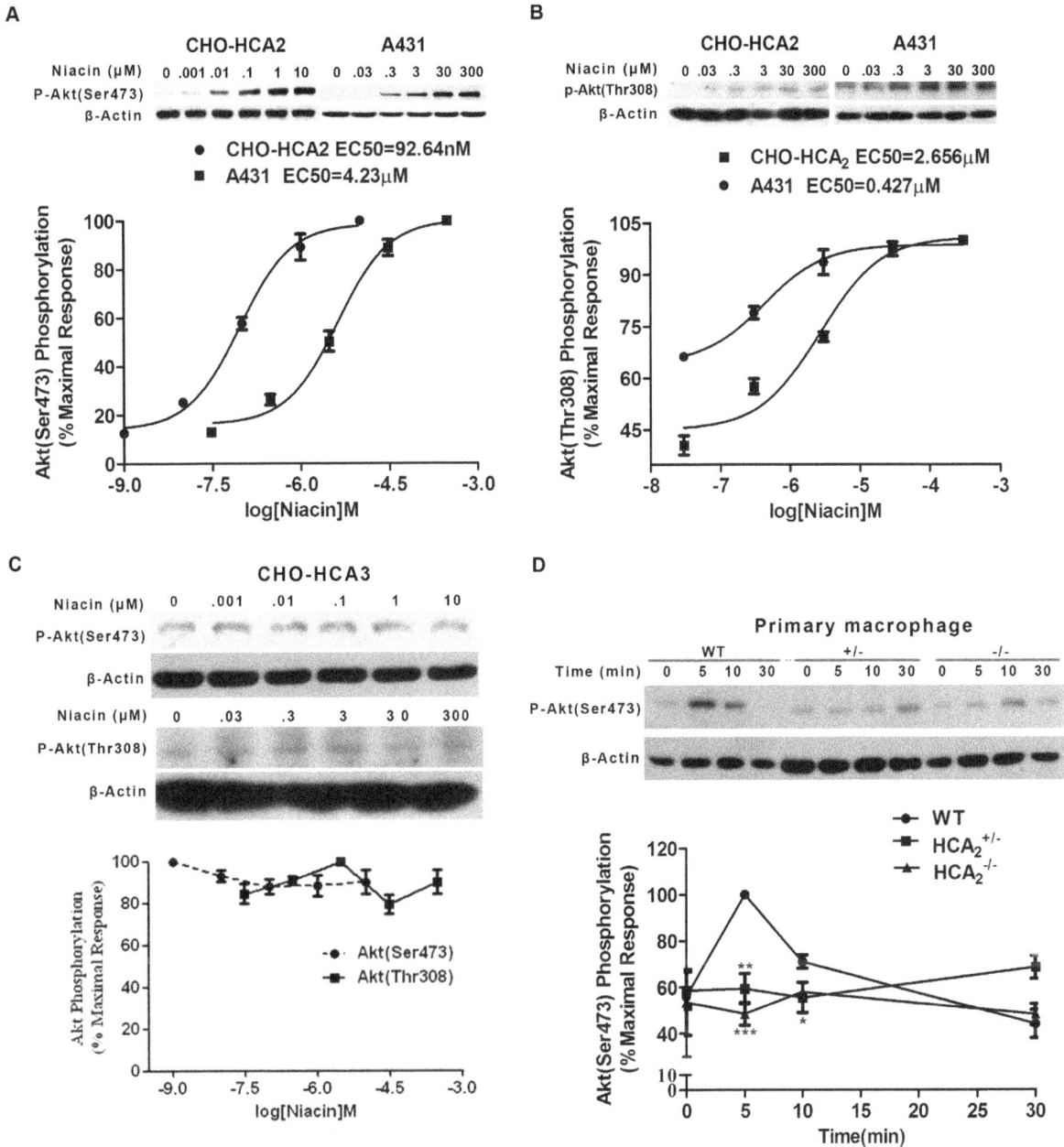

Figure 1. Dynamics of Akt phosphorylation under different concentrations of niacin. CHO-HCA$_2$ (A), A431 (B) or CHO-HCA$_3$(C) cells were plated on 24-well plates with DMEM/F-12 or DMEM. 12 hours later, the medium was changed to serum-free DMEM/F-12 or DMEM. After overnight starvation, all the cells were treated with different concentrations of niacin for 5 min. Akt phosphorylation at both Ser^{473} and Thr^{308} were detected by Immunobloting. Primary macrophages (D), isolated from 4–6 week old mice, were plated on 24-well plates with modified (RPMI)-1640 medium overnight. Cells were then starved for 3 h and stimulated with 400 μM niacin for different times. Akt phosphorylation at Ser^{473} was detected by Immunobloting. WT: wild type mouse. The data shown are representative of at least three independent experiments. The data were analyzed using Student's t test (*, $p < 0.05$; **, $p < 0.01$; ***, $p < 0.001$).

the G$_{\beta\gamma}$ subunit is likely to play a central role in HCA$_2$-induced Akt activation. To investigate the role of G$_{\beta\gamma}$ and G$_{i/o}$ in the regulation of phosphorylation of EGFR and PDGFR, G$_{i/o}$ inhibitor PTX and G$_{\beta\gamma}$ dominant-negative construct Gα-transducin were used. As shown in Fig. S2A and S2B, in both A431 and CHO-HCA2 cells, pretreatment with PTX or transfection with Gα-transducin resulted in a significant inhibition of niacin-induced EGFR or PDGFR phosphorylation. These results demonstrate

that HCA$_2$-mediated activation of EGFR or PDGFR is both G$_{i/o}$ and G$_{\beta\gamma}$-dependent.

Next, we further explored the pathways of HCA$_2$-mediated Akt activation in primary macrophage which express lower level of HCA$_2$ compared to A431 cells, as shown in Fig. S2C, HCA$_2$ caused Akt activation mainly through PKC and EGFR transactivation-dependent pathways, as the same as observed in A431 cells.

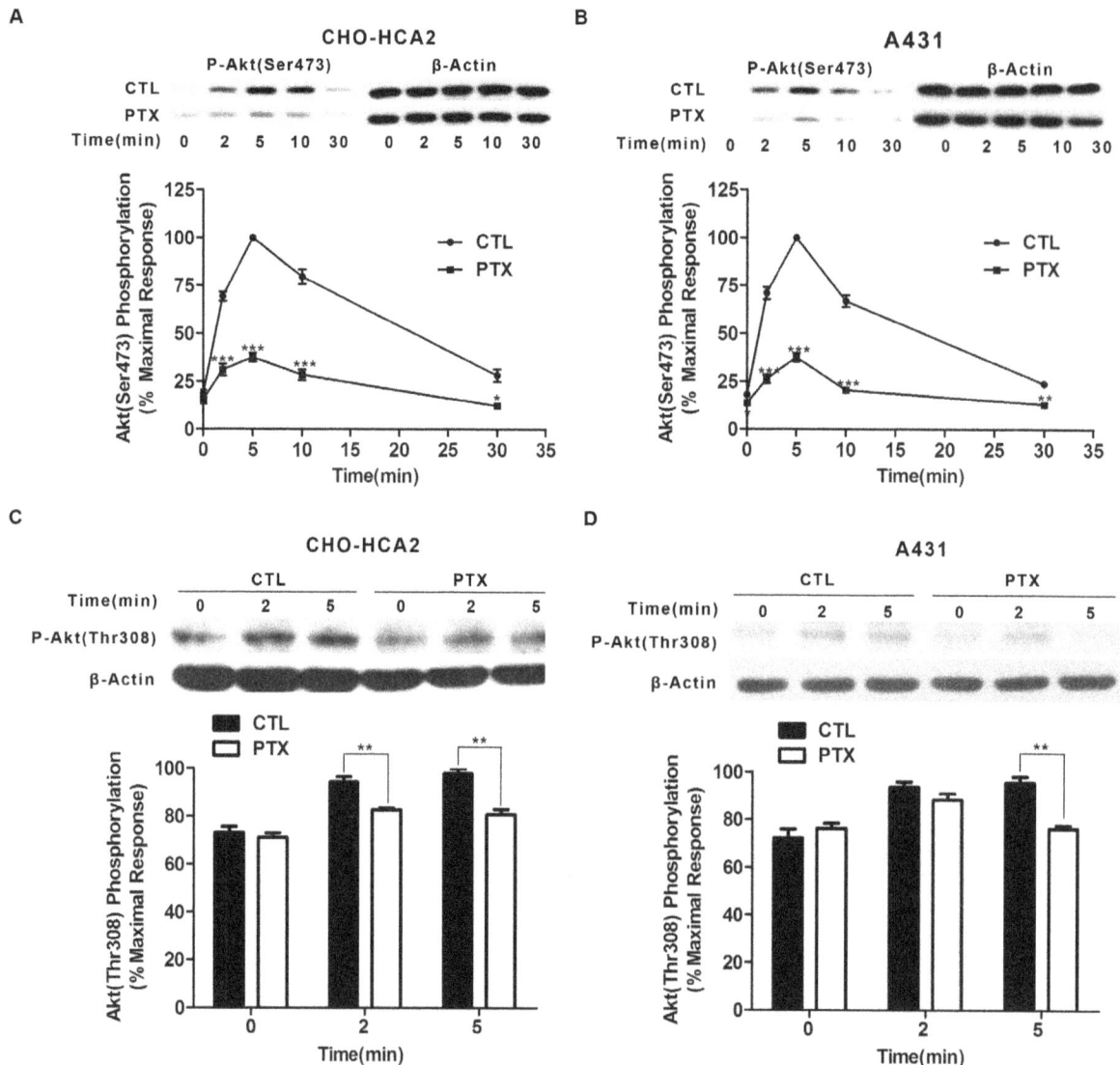

Figure 2. Akt phosphorylation at both Ser^{473} and Thr^{308} was decreased after PTX treatment. Both CHO-HCA$_2$ cells (A and C) and A431 cells (B and D) were treated with 100 ng/ml PTX overnight before niacin stimulation (1 μM niacin for CHO-HCA$_2$ cells and 100 μM niacin for A431 cells when Akt phosphorylation at Ser^{473} was detected, while 300 μM niacin was used for stimulation for both cell lines when Akt phosphorylation at Thr^{308} was detected) for the indicated time and Akt phosphorylation at Ser^{473} (A and B) and Thr^{308} (C and D) were detected by Immunobloting. The data shown are representative of at least three independent experiments. The data were analyzed using Student's t test (*, $p<0.05$; **, $p<0.01$; ***, $p<0.001$).

Niacin stimulates Akt-dependent and ERK1/2-independent p70S6K1 activation

The 70 kDa ribosomal S6 kinase 1 (P70S6K1) is an important regulator for mediating cell growth by inducing protein synthesis and G1 cell cycle progression [41]. Previous studies have reported that P70S6K1 can be activated through the PI3K [42] and MAPK pathways [43]. To determine whether niacin can activate p70S6K1 in A431 cells, a human epidermoid cancer cell, serum-starved A431 cells were stimulated with 100 μM niacin for various times (0–30 min) and lysed, and the extracts were subjected to Immunobloting analyses using an antibody that recognizes p70S6K1 phosphorylated at Thr^{389}, a major phosphorylation site that correlates closely with kinase activity [44]. As shown in Fig. 7A, HCA$_2$-initiated activation of p70S6K1 occurred in a time-dependent manner, with a maximal activation at 5 min

and with a subsequent reduction to 40–50% of the maximal response by 30 min in A431 cells after stimulation with niacin.

To investigate whether HCA$_2$-induced p70S6K1 phosphorylation is mediated by ERK1/2 activation or Akt activation, U0126, a highly selective inhibitor of both MEK1 and MEK2, and Wortmannin, a highly selective inhibitor of PI3K, were analyzed for their effect on the activation of p70S6K1. As shown in Fig. 7B, ERK1/2 activation stimulated by niacin was significantly inhibited by preincubation with U0126 (>75%) or Wortmannin (>50%), whereas the Akt phosphorylation stimulated by niacin was only inhibited by preincubation with Wortmannin (>80%), but not U0126. Further, the p70S6K1 phosphorylation mediated by HCA$_2$ was also only inhibited by preincubation with Wortmannin (>75%), but not U0126. Taken together, these results demonstrate that HCA$_2$ evokes p70S6K1 activation via the PI3K-Akt pathway in A431 cells in response to niacin.

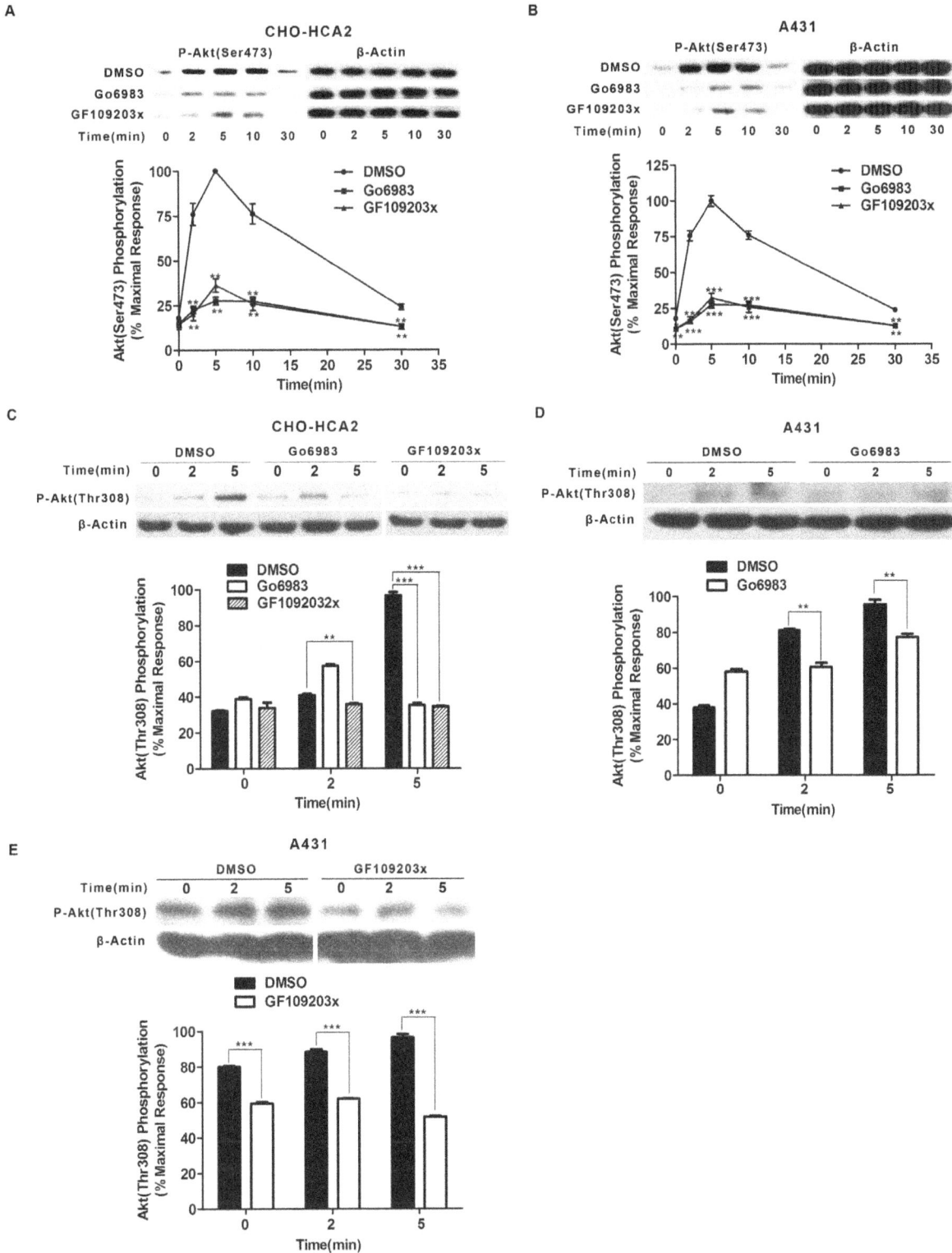

Figure 3. Go6983 and GF109203x decreased Akt phosphorylation at both Ser^{473} and Thr^{308} in CHO-HCA$_2$ and A431 cells. Both CHO-HCA$_2$ cells (A and C) and A431 cells (B, D and E) were treated with either 10 µM Go6983 or 10 µM GF109203x for 1 h and Akt phosphorylation at Ser^{473} (A and B) and Thr^{308} (C–E) were detected. The data shown are representative of at least three independent experiments. The data were analyzed using Student's t test (**, p<0.01; ***, p<0.001).

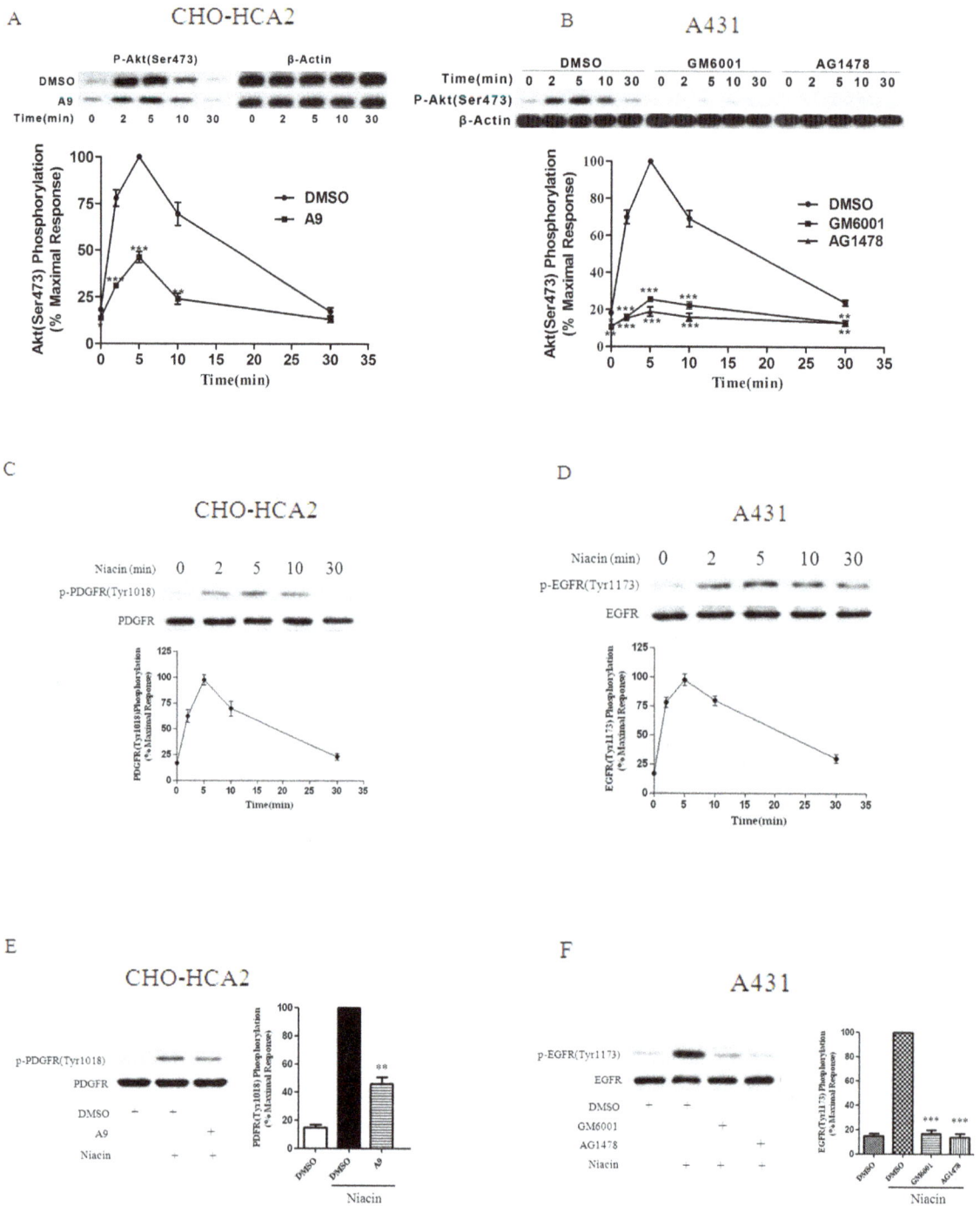

Figure 4. Akt phosphorylation was reduced by A9 treatment in CHO-HCA₂ cells and by GM6001 and AG1478 treatment in A431 cells. CHO-HCA₂ cells (A) were treated with 1 μM A9 for 1 h, while A431 cells (B) were treated with 10 μM GM6001 and 100 nM AG1478 for 1 h, then cells were stimulated with 1 μM or 100 μM niacin for indicated time, Akt phosphorylation at Ser^{473} was detected. C and D, Serum-starved CHO-HCA₂ (C) or A431 (D) cells were stimulated with 1 μM or 100 μM niacin for 5 min, and PDGFR phosphorylation at Tyr^{1018} (C) and EGFR phosphorylation at Tyr^{1173} (D) were detected. E and F, CHO-HCA₂ cells (E) were treated with 1 μM A9 for 1 h, while A431 cells (F) were treated with 10 μM GM6001 and 100 nM AG1478 for 1 h, then cells were stimulated with 1 μM or 100 μM niacin for 5 min, PDGFR phosphorylation at Tyr^{1018} (E) and EGFR phosphorylation at Tyr^{1173} (F) were detected. The data shown are representative of at least three independent experiments. The data were analyzed using Student's t test (**, p<0.01; ***, p<0.001).

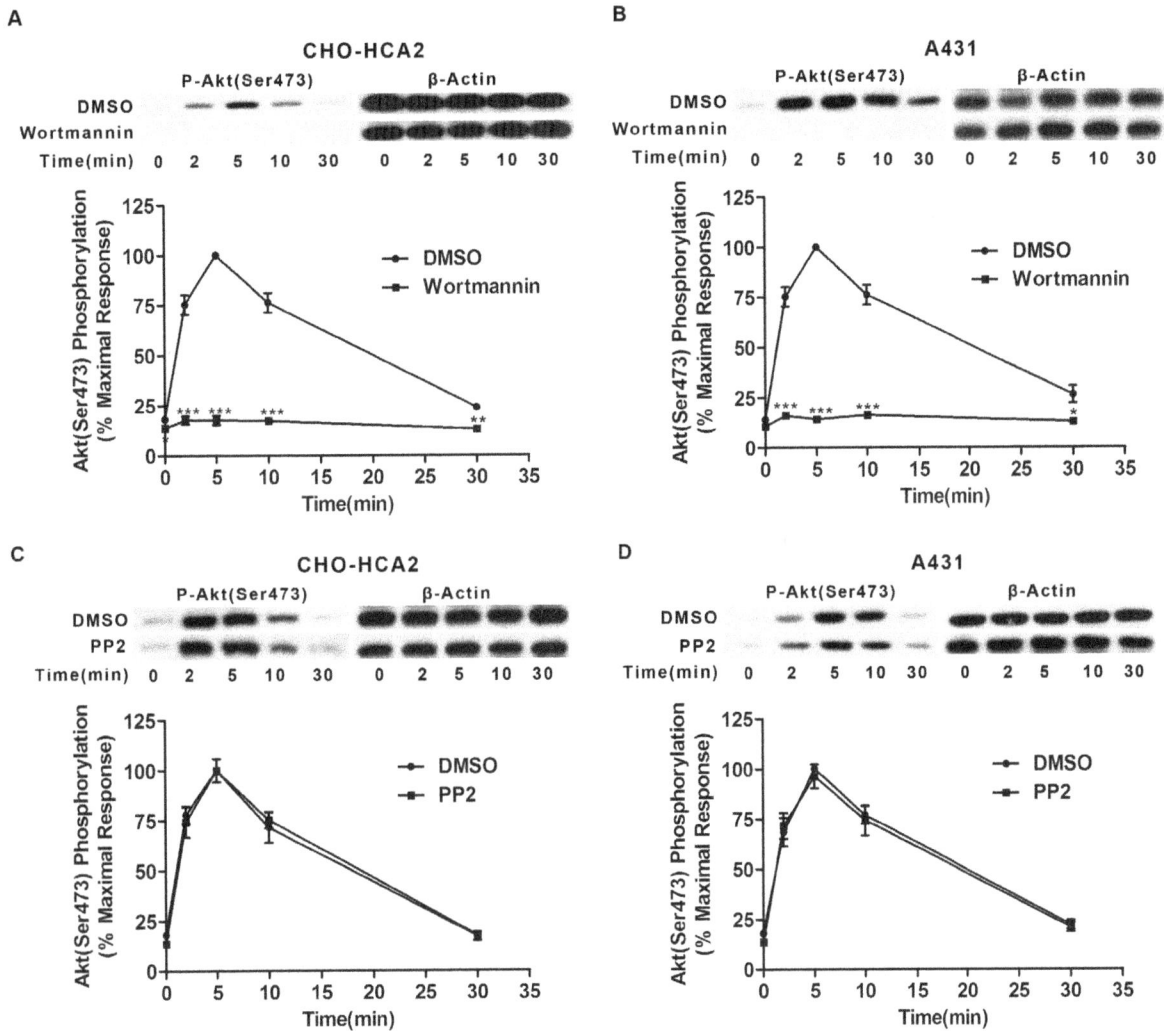

Figure 5. Akt phosphorylation was abolished by Wortmannin treatment, but not by PP2 treatment. Both CHO-HCA$_2$ cells (A and C) and A431 cells (B and D) were treated with either 1 μM Wortmannin or 10 μM PP2 for 1 h and Akt phosphorylation at Ser^{473} was detected. The data shown are representative of at least three independent experiments. The data were analyzed using Student's t test (*, p<0.05; **, p<0.01; ***, p< 0.001).

Discussion

The serine/threonine protein kinase Akt has been shown to play a central role in the regulation of cell survival and proliferation, metabolism, and inflammation in different cell systems through a variety of down-stream effectors [19]. It is generally accepted that Akt, when recruited to the plasma membrane from the cytosol through the binding of its PH domain to the second messenger PIP3 generated by PI3K, is activated by phosphorylation at Thr^{308} in the activation loop and at Ser^{473} within the carboxy-terminus by PDK1 and mTORC2 [19,45,46]. Previous studies showed that niacin exerts its protective effects on stroke- [24] and UV-induced skin damage [25] via PI3K/Akt-mediated anti-apoptotic pathways. Therefore, in the present study, to better delineate the signaling pathways linking the HCA$_2$ receptor to the PI3K/Akt cascade, we used CHO-K1 cells that were stably or transiently transfected with human HCA$_2$ receptors and A431 cells that endogenously express functional human HCA$_2$ to characterize HCA$_2$-mediated Akt activation through visualization of increases in phosphorylation at both Ser^{473} and Thr^{308} using site-specific

antibodies. Our results clearly showed that niacin triggered Akt phosphorylation at both the A-loop (T308) and the HM (S473) in a dose-dependent manner though HCA$_2$, leading to the activation of p70S6K1.

The present study determined the roles of various molecular components in the niacin-elicited activation of Akt by HCA$_2$ receptors stably or transiently expressed in the CHO-K1 cell line, a cellular model system for investigating GPCR coupling to various signaling pathways. In addition, complementary experiments were performed to further evaluate the effects of niacin in the A431 cell line, a human epidermoid cell line natively expressing functional HCA$_2$ [27]. A431 cells have been shown to also express the HCA$_3$ receptor, which shares a high degree of similarity with HCA$_2$, displaying 96% identity to HCA$_2$ but with a 24 amino acid extension at its carboxyl terminus [7,8], and there are no specific antagonists against HCA$_2$ or HCA$_3$ available to discriminate between HCA$_2$ and HCA$_3$ in A431 cells. However, a previous study has revealed that the amount of HCA$_2$ mRNA is approximately 1.5-fold more than that of HCA$_3$ in A431 cells, supporting the proposition that HCA$_2$, rather than HCA$_3$,

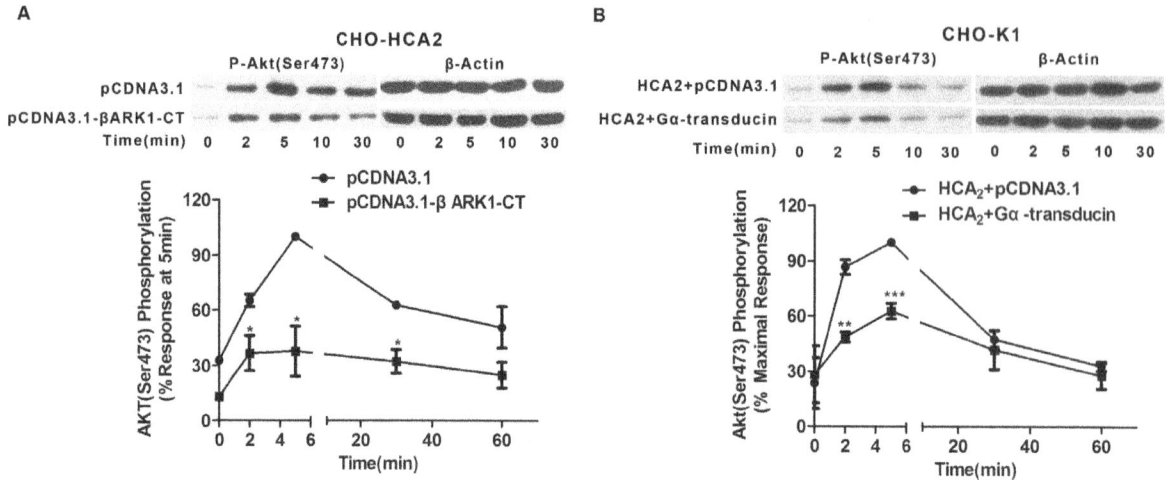

Figure 6. The G$_{\beta\gamma}$ subunit involved in HCA$_2$ signaling mediates Akt phosphorylation. CHO-HCA$_2$ cells (A) were transfected with β-ARK1-CT for 48 h and CHO-K1 cells (B) were co-transfected with Gα-transducin and either pCDNA3.1 or HCA$_2$ for 48 h, followed by niacin stimulation and Akt (Ser^{473}) phosphorylation detection. The data shown are representative of at least three independent experiments. The data were analyzed using Student's t test (*, p<0.05; **, p<0.01; ***, p<0.001).

mediates the major effects of niacin on lipolysis [7]. In addition, a recent study has demonstrated that HCA$_3$ expressed in CHO-K1 cells failed to evoke Ca^{2+} mobilization in response to stimulation with high concentrations of niacin (up to 1 mM) [47]. Our previous results using concentration curve analysis and siRNA-mediated knockdown of HCA$_2$ and HCA$_3$ indicated that the role of HCA$_3$ in ERK1/2 activation in A431 cells that are stimulated by less than 100 μM of niacin is likely to be negligible or

nonexistent [26]. Therefore, it is likely that niacin-induced Akt phosphorylation in A431 cells was mediated by HCA$_2$. Moreover, using primary macrophages isolated from Alternative Thioglycollate Medium-treated HCA$_2$-KO mice, our data confirmed that niacin triggered Akt phosphorylation through the HCA$_2$ receptor.

HCA$_2$ is a G$_i$ protein-coupled receptor. Upon stimulation by niacin, HCA$_2$ inactivates adenylyl cyclase, leading to a decrease in intracellular cAMP levels. Niacin-mediated inhibition of

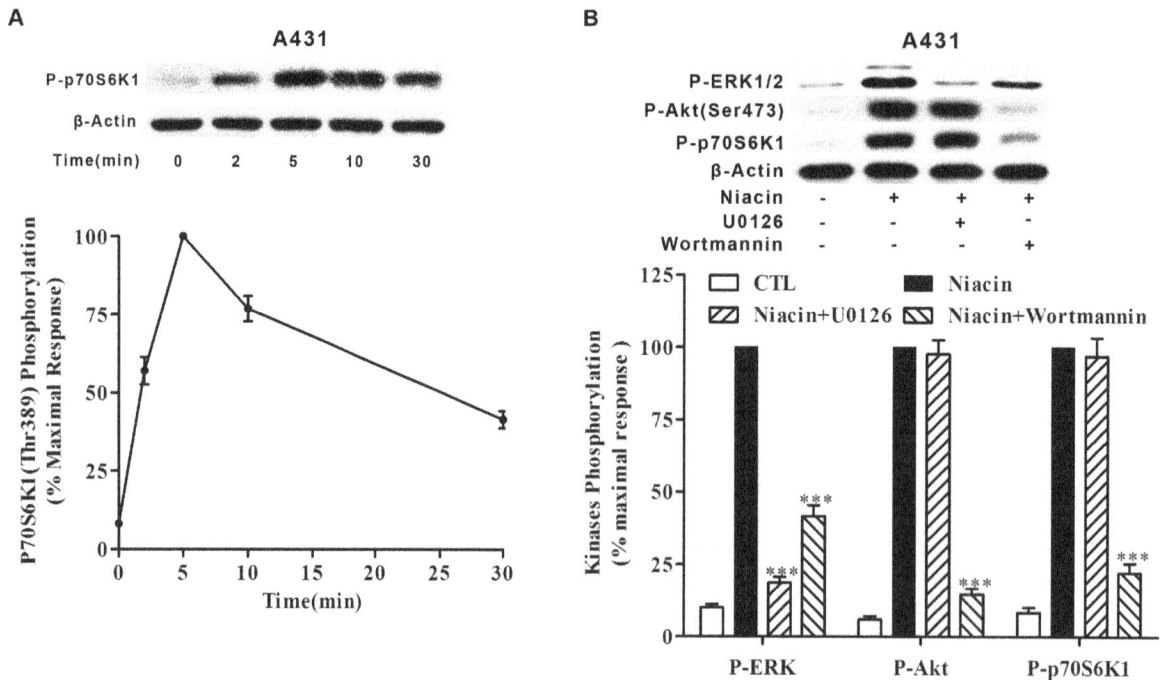

Figure 7. Niacin promotes p70S6K1 phosphorylation through an Akt-dependent but ERK1/2-independent pathway. (A) A431 cells were plated on 24-well plates and were treated with 100 μM niacin for the indicated time after 12 h culture and overnight starvation. p70S6K1 phosphorylation at Thr^{389} was detected by Immunobloting. (B) A431 were treated with either U0126 or Wortmannin with or without niacin stimulation and phosphorylation of Akt (Ser^{473}), ERK and p70S6K1 were detected. The data shown are representative of at least three independent experiments. The data were analyzed using Student's t test (***, p<0.001).

forskolin-evoked cAMP accumulation [7], stimulation of $[^{35}S]GTP\gamma S$ binding [9], Ca^{2+} mobilization and ERK1/2 activation [8,26,48], and anti-lipolytic effects [49] are sensitive to PTX. To determine whether the dominant pathway for HCA_2-mediated Akt phosphorylation is through G protein activation, we first examined the role of the G_i protein in the activation of the Akt signaling cascade. Both CHO-HCA_2 cells and A431 cells exhibited time-dependent activation of Akt in response to niacin, peaking at approximately 5 min and returning to basal levels at 30 min, but this Akt activation was completely attenuated in the presence of PTX. These results indicate that the heterotrimeric G_i protein is essentially involved in the regulation of Akt phosphorylation in both CHO-HCA_2 and A431 cells. Furthermore, although there is evidence that Akt activation occurs in neural and epithelial cells independently of PI3K [50], it is generally accepted that Akt activation is dependent on PI3K, and inhibition of PI3K activity impairs Akt phosphorylation and Akt-mediated cell functions [19,45]. Our results showed that HCA_2-mediated Akt activation was completely blocked in the presence of Wortmannin, a PI3K inhibitor, suggesting that PI3K is an upstream regulator of Akt activation induced by HCA_2.

The agonist-activated HCA_2 receptor elicits a rapid increase in intracellular Ca^{2+} in a PTX-sensitive manner [48]. Our previous data have also demonstrated that HCA_2 couples to ERK1/2 phosphorylation at early time points (≤ 2 min) via the Go6983 and GF109203x-sensitive PKC-dependent pathway [26]. We thus assess the role of PKC in the regulation of HCA_2-induced Akt phosphorylation using specific inhibitors. Our data showed that the HCA_2-elicited Akt phosphorylation was significantly blocked by the broad spectrum PKC inhibitors Go6983 and GF109203x, suggesting that the PKC pathway participates in the activation of Akt, but this activation is distinct from the PKC pathway-mediated ERK1/2 phosphorylation that occurs at early time points (≤ 2 min) in response to niacin. Previous studies have indicated that both conventional and novel PKC isoforms are found to positively and negatively regulate the activation of Akt [51–53]. It is likely for niacin to induce Akt activation via a HCA_2-mediated PKC-dependent pathway. However, more experiments are necessary to further clarify the exact role of conventional and novel PKC isoforms in the regulation of Akt activation though HCA_2.

The crosstalk with receptor tyrosine kinases (RTKs), also termed transactivation, has emerged as a common mechanism linking GPCRs to the MAPK and Akt signaling cascades [31,35]. The role of RTK transactivation is cell-specific; for example, COS-7 cells express the EGF receptor [54], whereas CHO-K1 cells express the PDGF receptor but lack endogenous EGFR [55]. Therefore, experiments using the RTK-selective inhibitors tyrphostin A9 for the PDGF receptor and AG1478 for the EGF receptor were performed to evaluate the role of RTK in the regulation of Akt activation by HCA_2 in both CHO-HCA_2 cells and A431 cells. The significant blocking effect of tyrphostin A9 and AG1478 strongly suggested that HCA_2-mediated Akt phosphorylation required PDGFR-dependent transactivation in CHO-HCA_2 cells and EGFR-dependent transactivation in A431 cells. Additional data derived from experiments using the MMP inhibitor GM6001 demonstrated that the inhibition of matrix metalloproteinase activity attenuated the HCA_2-induced activation of Akt, defining the important role of the proteolytic release of heparin-binding EGF-like growth factor (HB-EGF) in the regulation of EGFR transactivation-dependent Akt phosphorylation by HCA_2 in A431 cells. This is in agreement with our previous evidence that the HCA_2 receptor induced ERK1/2 activation via a MMP-mediated EGFR transactivation pathway [26]. HB-EGF is synthesized as a membrane-anchored form (pro-HB-EGF) in the cell and is proteolyzed by a metalloproteinase of the zinc-dependent "a disintegrin and metalloproteinase" (ADAM) family to form a soluble growth factor, acting on EGFR as a potent ligand [56,57]. Different members of the ADAM family, including ADAM10, ADAM12, and ADAM17, mediate GPCR-induced EGFR trans-activation in different model systems [58]. The precise mechanism(s) that link GPCRs and their effectors for MMPs activation remain(s) largely unknown. Several kinases, such as Src, PKC and PYK2, were found to regulate MMP activity through direct interaction with MMPs [30]. In the present study, we observed that PKC is involved in the regulation of Akt phosphorylation, whereas the Src kinase is not required for HCA_2-induced EGFR transactivation in either CHO-HCA_2 or A431 cells.

In the current study, our results demonstrate that PKC and RTK transactivation are essentially involved in the HCA_2-mediated PI3K/Akt cascade. This activation is abolished by pretreatment with PTX. In addition, we also observed that overexpression of the $G_{\beta\gamma}$ subunit scavenger $G\alpha$-transducin effectively attenuated the Akt activation triggered by HCA_2. This is highly consistent with a model in which G_i-coupled receptors activate the Akt cascade using $G_{\beta\gamma}$-subunit released from $G_{i/o}$ proteins [59–61]. There is a growing body of evidence to conclusively suggest that the $G_{\beta\gamma}$ subunit from $G_{i/o}$ and G_q proteins can directly interact with a selected set of effector molecules, including PLCβ and PI3K [62]. Taken together, our results suggest that activation of the Akt pathway initiated by HCA_2 is likely to be dependent on $G_{\beta\gamma}$-subunit released from G_i proteins in a PI3K-dependent manner.

In conclusion, we present evidence that HCA_2-induced PI3K/Akt activation requires PKC activity and MMP-dependent EGFR transactivation in A431 cells or PDGFR transactivation in CHO-HCA_2 cells through a mechanism that involves $G_{\beta\gamma}$ subunit in a PTX-sensitive manner. However, more research must be performed to fully understand the impact of human HCA_2 receptor signaling to the PI3K/Akt cascade for niacin in the modulation of atherosclerosis and anti-inflammation.

Supporting Information

Figure S1 A. Serum-starved CHO-HCA2 and A431 cells were stimulated with 100 μM niacin for 5 min, B. Serum-starved A431 cells were stimulated with various concentrations of niacin for 5 min, cells were harvested, and equal amounts of total cellular lysate were separated by 10% SDS-PAGE, transferred to a PVDF membrane, and incubated with anti-p-Akt(Ser308) antibody. Blots were stripped and reprobed for T-Akt andβ-Actin to control for loading. The data shown are representative of at least three independent experiments.

Figure S2 A and B, CHO-HCA2 cells (A) and A431 cells(B) were treated with 100 ng/ml PTX overnight or transfection of Ga-transducin, then cells were stimulated with 1 μM or 100 μM niacin for 5 min, and PDGFR phosphorylation at Tyr1018 (A) and EGFR phosphorylation at Tyr1173 (B) were detected. Primary macrophage cells (C) and A431 cells (E) were treated with 1 μM wortmannin, 10 μM Go6983, 100 nM AG1478, while CHO-HCA2 cells (D) were treated with 1 μM wortmannin, 10 μM Go6983, 1 μM A9, cells were then stimulated with 1 μM (CHO-HCA2) or 100 μM (A431) or 400 μM (Primary macrophage) niacin for 5 min, and Akt phosphorylation at Ser473 was detected. The data shown are representative of at least three independent experiments. The data were analyzed using Student's t test (***, p<0.001).

Acknowledgments

The authors of this paper would like to thank Aiping Shao for her technical assistance and equipment usage.

Author Contributions

Conceived and designed the experiments: HS GL JL NZ. Performed the experiments: HS GL WZ QZ YY. Analyzed the data: HS GL YS NZ. Contributed reagents/materials/analysis tools: SO YS. Contributed to the writing of the manuscript: HS GL YS JL NZ.

References

1. Altschul R, Hoffer A, Stephen JD (1955) Influence of nicotinic acid on serum cholesterol in man. Arch Biochem Biophys 54: 558–559.
2. Brown BG, Zhao XQ (2008) Nicotinic acid, alone and in combinations, for reduction of cardiovascular risk. Am J Cardiol 101: 58B–62B.
3. Canner PL, Berge KG, Wenger NK, Stamler J, Friedman L, et al. (1986) Fifteen year mortality in Coronary Drug Project patients: long-term benefit with niacin. J Am Coll Cardiol 8: 1245–1255.
4. Cashin-Hemphill L, Mack WJ, Pogoda JM, Sanmarco ME, Azen SP, et al. (1990) Beneficial effects of colestipol-niacin on coronary atherosclerosis. A 4-year follow-up. JAMA 264: 3013–3017.
5. Taylor AJ, Sullenberger LE, Lee HJ, Lee JK, Grace KA (2004) Arterial Biology for the Investigation of the Treatment Effects of Reducing Cholesterol (ARBITER) 2: a double-blind, placebo-controlled study of extended-release niacin on atherosclerosis progression in secondary prevention patients treated with statins. Circulation 110: 3512–3517.
6. Taggart AK, Kero J, Gan X, Cai TQ, Cheng K, et al. (2005) (D)-beta-Hydroxybutyrate inhibits adipocyte lipolysis via the nicotinic acid receptor PUMA-G. J Biol Chem 280: 26649–26652.
7. Soga T, Kamohara M, Takasaki J, Matsumoto S, Saito T, et al. (2003) Molecular identification of nicotinic acid receptor. Biochem Biophys Res Commun 303: 364–369.
8. Tunaru S, Kero J, Schaub A, Wufka C, Blaukat A, et al. (2003) PUMA-G and HM74 are receptors for nicotinic acid and mediate its anti-lipolytic effect. Nat Med 9: 352–355.
9. Wise A, Foord SM, Fraser NJ, Barnes AA, Elshourbagy N, et al. (2003) Molecular identification of high and low affinity receptors for nicotinic acid. J Biol Chem 278: 9869–9874.
10. Zhang Y, Schmidt RJ, Foxworthy P, Emkey R, Oler JK, et al. (2005) Niacin mediates lipolysis in adipose tissue through its G-protein coupled receptor HM74A. Biochem Biophys Res Commun 334: 729–732.
11. Digby JE, Lee JM, Choudhury RP (2009) Nicotinic acid and the prevention of coronary artery disease. Curr Opin Lipidol 20: 321–326.
12. Lauring B, Taggart AK, Tata JR, Dunbar R, Caro L, et al. (2012) Niacin lipid efficacy is independent of both the niacin receptor GPR109A and free fatty acid suppression. Sci Transl Med 4: 148ra115.
13. Lukasova M, Malaval C, Gille A, Kero J, Offermanns S (2011) Nicotinic acid inhibits progression of atherosclerosis in mice through its receptor GPR109A expressed by immune cells. J Clin Invest 121: 1163–1173.
14. Digby JE, Martinez F, Jefferson A, Ruparelia N, Chai J, et al. (2012) Anti-inflammatory effects of nicotinic acid in human monocytes are mediated by GPR109A dependent mechanisms. Arterioscler Thromb Vasc Biol 32: 669–676.
15. Lukasova M, Hanson J, Tunaru S, Offermanns S (2011) Nicotinic acid (niacin): new lipid-independent mechanisms of action and therapeutic potentials. Trends Pharmacol Sci 32: 700–707.
16. Digby JE, McNeill E, Dyar OJ, Lam V, Greaves DR, et al. (2010) Anti-inflammatory effects of nicotinic acid in adipocytes demonstrated by suppression of fractalkine, RANTES, and MCP-1 and upregulation of adiponectin. Atherosclerosis 209: 89–95.
17. New DC, Wong YH (2007) Molecular mechanisms mediating the G protein-coupled receptor regulation of cell cycle progression. J Mol Signal 2: 2.
18. Franke TF, Yang SI, Chan TO, Datta K, Kazlauskas A, et al. (1995) The protein kinase encoded by the Akt proto-oncogene is a target of the PDGF-activated phosphatidylinositol 3-kinase. Cell 81: 727–736.
19. Manning BD, Cantley LC (2007) AKT/PKB signaling: navigating downstream. Cell 129: 1261–1274.
20. Camps M, Ruckle T, Ji H, Ardissone V, Rintelen F, et al. (2005) Blockade of PI3Kgamma suppresses joint inflammation and damage in mouse models of rheumatoid arthritis. Nat Med 11: 936–943.
21. Sospedra M, Martin R (2005) Immunology of multiple sclerosis. Annu Rev Immunol 23: 683–747.
22. Busse WW, Lemanske RF Jr (2001) Asthma. N Engl J Med 344: 350–362.
23. Fernandez-Hernando C, Ackah E, Yu J, Suarez Y, Murata T, et al. (2007) Loss of Akt1 leads to severe atherosclerosis and occlusive coronary artery disease. Cell Metab 6: 446–457.
24. Shehadah A, Chen J, Zacharek A, Cui Y, Ion M, et al. (2010) Niaspan treatment induces neuroprotection after stroke. Neurobiol Dis 40: 277–283.
25. Lin F, Xu W, Guan C, Zhou M, Hong W, et al. (2012) Niacin protects against UVB radiation-induced apoptosis in cultured human skin keratinocytes. Int J Mol Med 29: 593–600.
26. Li G, Deng X, Wu C, Zhou Q, Chen L, et al. (2011) Distinct kinetic and spatial patterns of protein kinase C (PKC)- and epidermal growth factor receptor (EGFR)-dependent activation of extracellular signal-regulated kinases 1 and 2 by human nicotinic acid receptor GPR109A. J Biol Chem 286: 31199–31212.
27. Zhou L, Tang Y, Cryan EV, Demarest KT (2007) Human epidermoid A431 cells express functional nicotinic acid receptor HM74a. Mol Cell Biochem 294: 243–248.
28. Parent JL, Labrecque P, Driss Rochdi M, Benovic JL (2001) Role of the differentially spliced carboxyl terminus in thromboxane A2 receptor trafficking: identification of a distinct motif for tonic internalization. J Biol Chem 276: 7079–7085.
29. Zhang X, Goncalves R, Mosser DM (2008) The isolation and characterization of murine macrophages. Curr Protoc Immunol Chapter 14: Unit 14 11.
30. Ohtsu H, Dempsey PJ, Eguchi S (2006) ADAMs as mediators of EGF receptor transactivation by G protein-coupled receptors. Am J Physiol Cell Physiol 291: C1–10.
31. Rozengurt E (2007) Mitogenic signaling pathways induced by G protein-coupled receptors. J Cell Physiol 213: 589–602.
32. Shi W, Fan H, Shum L, Derynck R (2000) The tetraspanin CD9 associates with transmembrane TGF-alpha and regulates TGF-alpha-induced EGF receptor activation and cell proliferation. J Cell Biol 148: 591–602.
33. Assefa Z, Valius M, Vantus T, Agostinis P, Merlevede W, et al. (1999) JNK/SAPK activation by platelet-derived growth factor in A431 cells requires both the phospholipase C-gamma and the phosphatidylinositol 3-kinase signaling pathways of the receptor. Biochem Biophys Res Commun 261: 641–645.
34. Gschwind A, Zwick E, Prenzel N, Leserer M, Ullrich A (2001) Cell communication networks: epidermal growth factor receptor transactivation as the paradigm for interreceptor signal transmission. Oncogene 20: 1594–1600.
35. Pierce KL, Luttrell LM, Lefkowitz RJ (2001) New mechanisms in heptahelical receptor signaling to mitogen activated protein kinase cascades. Oncogene 20: 1532–1539.
36. Billington CK, Kong KC, Bhattacharyya R, Wedegaertner PB, Panettieri RA Jr, et al. (2005) Cooperative regulation of p70S6 kinase by receptor tyrosine kinases and G protein-coupled receptors augments airway smooth muscle growth. Biochemistry 44: 14595–14605.
37. Kong KC, Billington CK, Gandhi U, Panettieri RA Jr, Penn RB (2006) Cooperative mitogenic signaling by G protein-coupled receptors and growth factors is dependent on G(q/11). FASEB J 20: 1558–1560.
38. Koch WJ, Hawes BE, Allen LF, Lefkowitz RJ (1994) Direct evidence that Gi-coupled receptor stimulation of mitogen-activated protein kinase is mediated by G beta gamma activation of p21ras. Proc Natl Acad Sci U S A 91: 12706–12710.
39. Lopez-Ilasaca M, Crespo P, Pellici PG, Gutkind JS, Wetzker R (1997) Linkage of G protein-coupled receptors to the MAPK signaling pathway through PI 3-kinase gamma. Science 275: 394–397.
40. Punn A, Levine MA, Grammatopoulos DK (2006) Identification of signaling molecules mediating corticotropin-releasing hormone-R1alpha-mitogen-activated protein kinase (MAPK) interactions: the critical role of phosphatidylinositol 3-kinase in regulating ERK1/2 but not p38 MAPK activation. Mol Endocrinol 20: 3179–3195.
41. Pullen N, Thomas G (1997) The modular phosphorylation and activation of p70s6k. FEBS Lett 410: 78–82.
42. Chung J, Grammer TC, Lemon KP, Kazlauskas A, Blenis J (1994) PDGF- and insulin-dependent pp70S6k activation mediated by phosphatidylinositol-3-OH kinase. Nature 370: 71–75.
43. Martin KA, Blenis J (2002) Coordinate regulation of translation by the PI 3-kinase and mTOR pathways. Adv Cancer Res 86: 1–39.
44. Weng QP, Kozlowski M, Belham C, Zhang A, Comb MJ, et al. (1998) Regulation of the p70 S6 kinase by phosphorylation in vivo. Analysis using site-specific anti-phosphopeptide antibodies. J Biol Chem 273: 16621–16629.
45. Brazil DP, Yang ZZ, Hemmings BA (2004) Advances in protein kinase B signalling: AKTion on multiple fronts. Trends Biochem Sci 29: 233–242.
46. Sarbassov DD, Guertin DA, Ali SM, Sabatini DM (2005) Phosphorylation and regulation of Akt/PKB by the rictor-mTOR complex. Science 307: 1098–1101.
47. Tunaru S, Lattig J, Kero J, Krause G, Offermanns S (2005) Characterization of determinants of ligand binding to the nicotinic acid receptor GPR109A (HM74A/PUMA-G). Mol Pharmacol 68: 1271–1280.
48. Li G, Shi Y, Huang H, Zhang Y, Wu K, et al. (2010) Internalization of the human nicotinic acid receptor GPR109A is regulated by G(i), GRK2, and arrestin3. J Biol Chem 285: 22605–22618.
49. Kather H, Aktories K, Schulz G, Jakobs KH (1983) Islet-activating protein discriminates the antilipolytic mechanism of insulin from that of other antilipolytic compounds. FEBS Lett 161: 149–152.
50. Deb TB, Coticchia CM, Dickson RB (2004) Calmodulin-mediated activation of Akt regulates survival of c-Myc-overexpressing mouse mammary carcinoma cells. J Biol Chem 279: 38903–38911.
51. Kroner C, Eybrechts K, Akkerman JW (2000) Dual regulation of platelet protein kinase B. J Biol Chem 275: 27790–27798.

52. Resendiz JC, Kroll MH, Lassila R (2007) Protease-activated receptor-induced Akt activation–regulation and possible function. J Thromb Haemost 5: 2484–2493.

53. Yano S, Tokumitsu H, Soderling TR (1998) Calcium promotes cell survival through CaM-K kinase activation of the protein-kinase-B pathway. Nature 396: 584–587.

54. Shah BH, Yesilkaya A, Olivares-Reyes JA, Chen HD, Hunyady L, et al. (2004) Differential pathways of angiotensin II-induced extracellularly regulated kinase 1/2 phosphorylation in specific cell types: role of heparin-binding epidermal growth factor. Mol Endocrinol 18: 2035–2048.

55. Antonelli V, Bernasconi F, Wong YH, Vallar L (2000) Activation of B-Raf and regulation of the mitogen-activated protein kinase pathway by the G(o) alpha chain. Mol Biol Cell 11: 1129–1142.

56. Prenzel N, Zwick E, Daub H, Leserer M, Abraham R, et al. (1999) EGF receptor transactivation by G-protein-coupled receptors requires metalloproteinase cleavage of proHB-EGF. Nature 402: 884–888.

57. Riese DJ 2nd, Komurasaki T, Plowman GD, Stern DF (1998) Activation of ErbB4 by the bifunctional epidermal growth factor family hormone epiregulin is regulated by ErbB2. J Biol Chem 273: 11288–11294.

58. Schafer B, Marg B, Gschwind A, Ullrich A (2004) Distinct ADAM metalloproteinases regulate G protein-coupled receptor-induced cell proliferation and survival. J Biol Chem 279: 47929–47938.

59. Murga C, Laguinge L, Wetzker R, Cuadrado A, Gutkind JS (1998) Activation of Akt/protein kinase B by G protein-coupled receptors. A role for alpha and beta gamma subunits of heterotrimeric G proteins acting through phosphatidylinositol-3-OH kinasegamma. J Biol Chem 273: 19080–19085.

60. Schwindinger WF, Robishaw JD (2001) Heterotrimeric G-protein betagamma-dimers in growth and differentiation. Oncogene 20: 1653–1660.

61. Wu EH, Wong YH (2006) Activation of muscarinic M4 receptor augments NGF-induced pro-survival Akt signaling in PC12 cells. Cell Signal 18: 285–293.

62. Hamm HE (1998) The many faces of G protein signaling. J Biol Chem 273: 669–672.

7

CD137 Expression Is Induced by Epstein-Barr Virus Infection through LMP1 in T or NK Cells and Mediates Survival Promoting Signals

Mayumi Yoshimori[1,2], Ken-Ichi Imadome[3], Honami Komatsu[1,2], Ludan Wang[1], Yasunori Saitoh[4], Shoji Yamaoka[4], Tetsuya Fukuda[1], Morito Kurata[5], Takatoshi Koyama[2], Norio Shimizu[6], Shigeyoshi Fujiwara[3], Osamu Miura[1], Ayako Arai[1]*

1 Department of Hematology, Graduate School of Medical and Dental Sciences, Tokyo Medical and Dental University, Tokyo, Japan, 2 Department of Laboratory Molecular Genetics of Hematology, Graduate School of Health Care Sciences, Tokyo Medical and Dental University, Tokyo, Japan, 3 Department of Infectious Diseases, National Research Institute for Child Health and Development, Tokyo, Japan, 4 Department of Molecular Virology, Graduate School of Medical and Dental Sciences, Tokyo Medical and Dental University, Tokyo, Japan, 5 Department of Comprehensive Pathology, Graduate School of Medical and Dental Sciences, Tokyo Medical and Dental University, Tokyo, Japan, 6 Department of Virology, Division of Medical Science, Medical Research Institute, Tokyo Medical and Dental University, Tokyo, Japan

Abstract

To clarify the mechanism for development of Epstein-Barr virus (EBV)-positive T- or NK-cell neoplasms, we focused on the costimulatory receptor CD137. We detected high expression of *CD137* gene and its protein on EBV-positive T- or NK-cell lines as compared with EBV-negative cell lines. EBV-positive cells from EBV-positive T- or NK-cell lymphoproliferative disorders (EBV-T/NK-LPDs) patients also had significantly higher *CD137* gene expression than control cells from healthy donors. In the presence of IL-2, whose concentration in the serum of EBV-T/NK-LPDs was higher than that of healthy donors, CD137 protein expression was upregulated in the patients' cells whereas not in control cells from healthy donors. *In vitro* EBV infection of MOLT4 cells resulted in induction of endogenous CD137 expression. Transient expression of *LMP1*, which was enhanced by IL-2 in EBV-T/NK-LPDs cells, induced endogenous *CD137* gene expression in T and NK-cell lines. In order to examine *in vivo* CD137 expression, we used EBV-T/NK-LPDs xenograft models generated by intravenous injection of patients' cells. We identified EBV-positive and CD8-positive T cells, as well as CD137 ligand-positive cells, in their tissue lesions. In addition, we detected CD137 expression on the EBV infected cells from the lesions of the models by immune-fluorescent staining. Finally, CD137 stimulation suppressed etoposide-induced cell death not only in the EBV-positive T- or NK-cell lines, but also in the patients' cells. These results indicate that upregulation of CD137 expression through LMP1 by EBV promotes cell survival in T or NK cells leading to development of EBV-positive T/NK-cell neoplasms.

Editor: Joseph S. Pagano, The University of North Carolina at Chapel Hill, United States of America

Funding: This work was supported by a grant from the Ministry of Health, Labor, and Welfare of Japan (H22-Nanchi-080) as well as a grant from the Ministry of Education, Culture, Sports, Science, and Technology of Japan (23591375). The funders had no role in study design, data collection and analysis, decision to publish, or preparation of the manuscript.

Competing Interests: The authors have declared that no competing interests exist.

* Email: ara.hema@tmd.ac.jp

Introduction

Epstein-Barr virus (EBV) infection can be found in lymphoid malignancies not only of B-cell lineage, but also of T- or NK-cell lineages. These EBV-positive T or NK-cell neoplasms, such as extranodal NK/T-cell lymphoma nasal type (ENKL), aggressive NK-cell leukemia (ANKL), and EBV-positive T- or NK- cell lymphoproliferative diseases (EBV-T/NK-LPDs), are relatively rare but lethal disorders classified as peripheral T/NK-cell lymphomas according to the WHO classification of tumors of hematopoietic and lymphoid malignancies. ENKL is a rapidly progressive lymphoma characterized by extranodal lesions with vascular damage and severe necrosis accompanied by infiltration of neoplastic NK or cytotoxic T cells [1]. ANKL is a markedly aggressive leukemia with neoplastic proliferation of NK cells [2]. EBV-T/NK-LPDs is a fatal disorder presenting sustained infectious mononucleosis-like symptoms, hypersensitivity to mos-

quito bites, or hydroa vacciniforme-like eruption accompanied by clonal proliferation of EBV-infected cells [3,4]. Because most reported cases were children or young adults, and were mainly of the T-cell-infected type, the disorders were designated "EBV-positive T-cell lymphoproliferative diseases of childhood" in the WHO classification, although adult and NK-cell types have been reported [4–6]. The common clinical properties of EBV-T/NK-neoplasms are the presence of severe inflammation, resistance to chemotherapy, and a marked geographic bias for East Asia and Latin America, suggesting a genetic context for disease development [4]. Since these EBV-T/NK-neoplasms overlap [4], common mechanisms are thought to exist in the background and contribute to disease development.

It is well known that EBV infects B cells and makes the infected cells immortal resulting in B-cell lymphomas. Similarly it is suspected that EBV may also cause T- or NK-cell neoplasms. However, why and how EBV latently infects T or NK cells, whether or not EBV directly causes these malignancies, and the mechanism of action responsible for the disease development remain to be clarified. Although new chemotherapy and stem cell transplantation have achieved good results for EBV-T/NK neoplasms recently [7–9], prognosis of the diseases is still poor. The mechanisms for development of the disease need to be determined to establish an optimal treatment.

To clarify the molecular mechanism underlying the development of EBV-T/NK-neoplasms, we focused on the costimulatory receptor CD137. CD137, also known as 4-1BB, is a member of the tumor necrosis factor (TNF) receptor superfamily, and expressed on the surface of activated T and NK cells [10]. In association with TCR stimulation, it plays a pivotal role in proliferation, survival, and differentiation of these cells as a costimulatory molecule [11]. Recently, it was reported that CD137 is expressed on tumor cells from adult T-cell leukemia/lymphoma (ATLL) and from T-cell lymphomas [12,13]. Here we found CD137 expression on EBV-positive cells in EBV-T/NK-neoplasms and investigated its role for the lymphomagenesis using established cell lines as well as cells from EBV-T/NK-LPDs patients.

Results

CD137 expression in EBV-T/NK-cell lines

Six EBV-positive T- and NK-cell lines, SNT8, SNT15, SNT16, SNK1, SNK6, and SNK10 had been established from primary lesions of ENKL patients (SNT8 and SNK6) and PB of EBV-T/NK-LPDs patients (SNT15, SNT16, SNK1, and SNK10) [14]. We investigated CD137 mRNA expression in the cell lines by RT-PCR. CD137 mRNA was expressed in all of them, whereas EBV-negative T-cell lines (Jurkat, MOLT4, and HPB-ALL) and NK-cell line (KHYG1) were negative for the expression (Figure 1A). The mRNA was detected but weak in an EBV-negative NK-cell line, MTA, and in EBV-negative B-cell lines, BJAB, Ramos, and MD901. We also investigated 3 EBV-positive B cell lines, Raji, a lymphoblastoid cell line (LCL), and HS-sultun. The expression was detected in Raji. The expression was weak in LCL, and negative in HS-Sultan. We next investigated CD137 protein expression on the cell surface. Figure 1B shows that CD137 protein was expressed on the cell surface of all EBV-positive T- or NK-cells. In contrast, EBV-negative T-, NK-, and B-cell lines were negative for CD137 expression. On the basis of these results, we concluded that CD137 expression was induced at the mRNA and protein levels in EBV-T/NK cell lines. The expression was detected in 2 of 3 examined EBV-positive B cell lines, Raji and LCL, whereas negative in HS-Sultan. The expression in EBV-positive B cells was insignificant in comparison with EBV-positive T or NK cells. We were unable to detect CD137L expression on the surface these EBV-positive T- or NK-cells lines. The expression was negative on them (Figure S1).

EBV induces CD137 expression in T and NK cells

To clarify whether EBV could directly induce CD137 expression, we performed in vitro EBV infection of an EBV-negative cell line MOLT4. EBV DNA copy number of EBV-infected MOTL4 cells was 8.8×10^5 copies/μgDNA. EBV infection was verified by the presence of EBV nuclear antigen (EBNA) 1 protein expression (Figure 2A). Most cells were positive for EBNA1. The infection was also confirmed by the presence of the viral mRNA, LMP1 and EBNA1, and the absence of EBNA2 by RT-PCR (Figure 2B). This expression pattern was classified as latency type 2. CD137 mRNA was also expressed in EBV-infected MOTL4 cells (Figure 2B and 2C). In addition, Figure 2D showed that CD137 protein expression was detected on EBV-infected

MOLT4 cells. We therefore concluded that EBV infection induced mRNA and surface protein expression of CD137 in MOLT4 cells.

CD137 expression in cells from EBV-T/NK-LPDs patients

The above results were validated using EBV-T/NK cells derived from patients. In EBV-T/NK-LPDs, EBV infection could be detected in a particular fraction of PBMCs and isolated at high purity using antibody-conjugated magnetic beads as described in "Materials and Methods". Seventeen patients (aged 8–72 years; 7 males, 10 females; 10 T- and 7 NK-cell types; CD4 type n = 4, CD8 type n = 5, γδ type n = 1, and CD56 type n = 7) were diagnosed with EBV-T/NK-LPDs according to the criteria as described in "Materials and Methods". We determined the EBV-positive fraction of the lymphocytes in the PB at the diagnosis. The phenotype of the infected cells and EBV DNA load of them were presented in Table 1. EBV DNA was negative or relatively low in CD19-positive cell which EBV can infect (Table 1).

To examine CD137 expression in the EBV-positive fraction, the fractions were isolated by the magnetic beads and obtained for CD137 mRNA detection in 10 patients. Figure 3A shows the CD137 mRNA levels in the freshly isolated cells of EBV-positive cell fraction in PBMCs of each patient. CD137 mRNA levels in CD4-, CD8-, and CD56-positive cell fractions of 5 healthy donors' PBMCs were also demonstrated. The mRNA levels in the patients' cells were significantly higher than those in the cells of healthy donors. Next we examined the expression of CD137 protein by flow cytometry. It showed low expression in freshly isolated PBMCs from both patients and 5 healthy donors (data not shown). However, after culture with IL-2 for 3 days, the expression was increased on the surface of PBMCs from 15 patients but still low on the cells isolated from 5 healthy donors (Figure 3B). The average of CD137 protein levels of EBV-T/NK-LPDs patients was significantly higher than that of healthy donors (Figure 3C). Two-color flow cytometry using antibodies to CD137 and to surface proteins expressed on EBV-positive cells could be performed in 7 patients, and a double-staining pattern was observed in them, whereas fractions from a healthy donor barely expressed the CD137 protein. (Figure S2).

EBV LMP1 induces CD137 expression in T and NK cells through LMP1 induced by IL-2

We investigated the mechanism of enhanced-CD137 expression by IL-2. First we performed luciferase reporter assay with a plasmid containing the CD137 gene promoter. As shown in Figure 2A, EBV-infected MOLT4 cells were shown to express EBV-encoded proteins including LMP1, and EBNA1, considered to be latency type 2. So, MOLT4 cells were cotransfected with expression plasmids capable of expressing either of EBV-encoded proteins, LMP1, LMP2A, LMP2B or EBNA1. As shown in Figure 4A, LMP1 induced significant upregulation of CD137 promoter activity, whereas the other molecules did not. Furthermore, in a transient expression assay with these viral proteins in MOLT4 cells, transcription of endogenous CD137 mRNA was detected only in the LMP1-transfected cells (Figure 4B). These results indicated that, among the EBV proteins, LMP1 transactivated CD137 expression in T and NK cells. Next we examined whether LMP1 expression was enhanced by IL-2 and might contribute to upregulation of CD137 expression in patients' cells. We isolated PBMCs from EBV-T/NK-LPDs patient (CD4-1) and cultured them with or without IL-2. As shown in Figure 4C, semi-quantitative RT-PCR demonstrated that LMP1 mRNA was increased in IL-2-treated PBMCs. CD137 mRNA was also increased in the IL-2-treated cells (Figure 4D). To confirm the

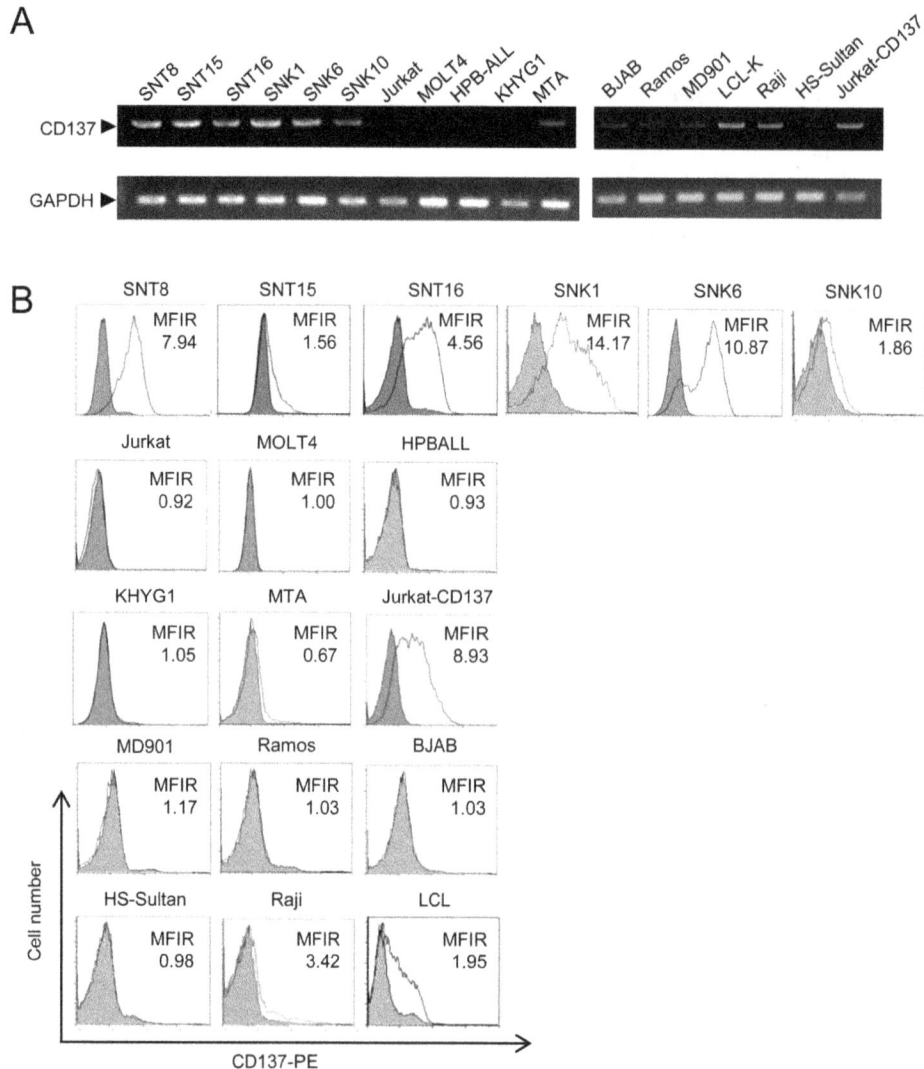

Figure 1. CD137 expression in Epstein-Barr virus (EBV)-positive T- or NK-cell lines. (A) Transcripts of *CD137* (the upper panel) and *GAPDH* (the lower panel) in EBV- positive T- or NK-cell lines were examined by RT-PCR. EBV negative T-, NK, B-cell lines, and EBV-positive B-cell lines were also obtained for the examination. (B) Surface expression of CD137 was examined by flow cytometry using an antibody to CD137 (open histogram) or isotype-matched control immunoglobulin (gray, shaded histogram). The mean fluorescent intensity of CD137 was normalized by that of isotype-matched control and expressed as mean fluorescence intensity rate (MFIR). Each experiment was independently performed more than 3 times and their average data are presented.

in vivo contribution of IL-2 for CD137 expression, we examined the serum concentration of IL-2 in 7 EBV-T/NK-LPDs patients and 5 healthy donors. The concentration in the patients was 0.9-2.4 U/mL in 6 of 7 patients, whereas it was undetectable in 4 of 5 healthy donors (Table 2). These results suggested that CD137 expression was enhanced in the presence of IL-2 most likely through enhanced-expression of LMP1 in EBV-T/NK-LPDs patient cells.

CD137 was detected in EBV-positive cells infiltrating in the tissue lesion of EBV-T/NK-LPDs xenograft model

Next, we examined the CD137 expression on the EBV-positive cells infiltrating into the tissue of EBV-T/NK-LPDs. Since we could not perform the examination for human specimen due to difficulty of obtaining the samples, we used the xenograft models generated by intravenous injection of PBMCs from CD8-3 patient [15]. The injected cells were 2×10^6 in number for each mouse and

include CD8-positive EBV-infected cells with clonally proliferation from CD8-3 patient. EBV DNA load of the infected cells were more than 1.0×10^4 copies/μgDNA. After engraftment, which was defined as detection of EBV DNA in the PB of the model, we performed autopsy. Nine mice were examined and the representative data were shown. As shown in Figure 5A–D, infiltration of EBV-positive and CD8-positive cells into the periportal regions in the liver was detected. 79.2% (396/500) of the infiltrating cells were EBER-positive, and 77.4% (387/500) of the cells were CD8-positive. These results indicated that most infiltrating cells were both positive for CD8 and EBER. Although CD137L-positive cells were also detected in the lesion, the number was markedly smaller than that of EBV-positive cells (Figure 5D). In order to determine CD137 expression on EBV-infected cells, we performed immune-fluorescent staining for the infiltrating cells in the lesions. As shown in Figure 5E, EBNA1-positive and CD137-positive cells were detected in the cells isolated from the lesions. LMP1 expression

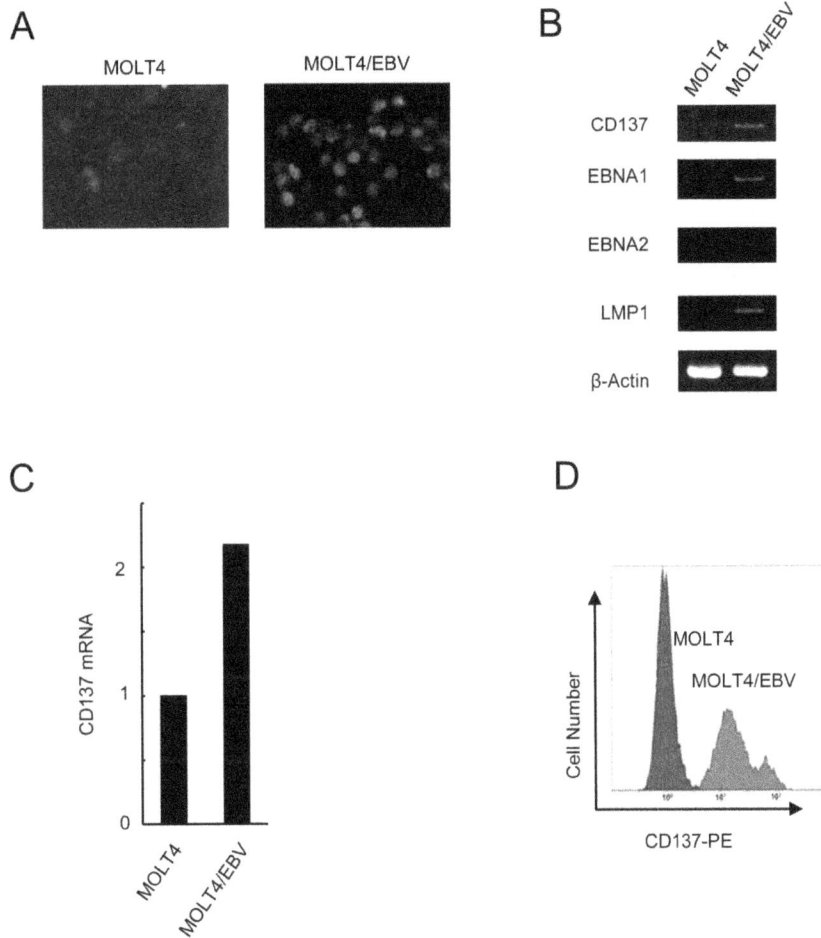

Figure 2. EBV induces CD137 expression in T cells. *In vitro* EBV infection assay performed in MOLT4 cells. (A) EBNA1 protein expression was examined by immune fluorescence staining, 48 hours after the infection, the time when CD137 expression was examined. (B) Expression of the *CD137* gene was examined by RT-PCR. The infection was confirmed by detecting mRNAs of the viral proteins, EBNA1 and LMP1. (C) Transcripts of *CD137* and *GAPDH* were quantified by real time RT-PCR. Relative copy number was obtained by normalizing the *CD137* transcripts to those of those of *GAPDH*. (D) Surface expression of CD137 of MOLT4 cells and EBV-infected MOLT4 cells was examined by flow cytometry.

was confirmed in them (Figure S3). These results indicated that the infiltrating EBV-positive cells were both CD8- and CD137-positive.

Stimulation of CD137 decreases etoposide–induced cell death of EBV-T/NK cells

To explore the contribution of CD137 expression on EBV-T/NK cells to the development of EBV-T/NK-LPDs, we investigated the effects of CD137 on the survival. CHO-CD137L cells with stable expression of human CD137L on their surface were prepared for CD137 stimulation of EBV-T/NK cells (Figure 6A).

First we performed the assay for EBV-positive T- and NK-cell lines. We cocultured the cells with PKH-26-stained CHO cells in the presence of IL-2 with or without etoposide. Jurkat cells were used as a negative control. After the time indicated, we removed the cells and determined the number of living cells by detecting PKH-26 and DiOC6. PKH-26-negative cells were EBV-positive T/NK-cells and Jurkat cells. DiOC6-positive cells were living cells. In the presence of etoposide, the relative number of living EBV-positive T/NK-cells cultured with CHO-CD137L cells was significantly higher than that cultured with control CHO cells (Figure 6B). In contrast, T-cell line Jurkat cells, on which CD137

was not detected (Figure 1B), did not show a difference when cocultured with the 2 types of CHO cells (Figure 6B). In the absence of etoposide, CD137L had no significant effect on the viability of these cells (Figure 6B).

Next we performed the same assay for the primary cells from EBV-T/NK-LPDs patients. We cocultured PBMCs from 2 patients, CD4-2 and CD56-7 with PKH-26-stained CHO cells in the presence of IL-2 with or without etoposide. In the presence of etoposide, the relative number of living cells from EBV-T/NK-LPDs patients cultured with CHO-CD137L cells was significantly higher than that cultured with control CHO cells (Figure 6C). In contrast, cells form a healthy donor did not show a difference when cocultured with the 2 types of CHO cells (Figure 6C). These findings indicated that stimulation of CD137 significantly suppressed etoposide-induced cell death of the EBV-T/NK-LPDs cells.

Discussion

CD137 is expressed following activation of T or NK cells and mediates molecular signals for proliferation, survival, and cytokine production by acting as a costimulatory molecule of the CD3-TCR complex [11,16,17]. However, few data for its roles in

Table 1. Clinical information of the patients' samples subjected to the assay.

Case	Gender	Age	Infected cell	Clinical findings	EBV-DNA (copies/µgDNA) of PB (whole blood)	EBV-DNA (copies/µgDNA) of the EBV-infected cells fraction in PB	EBV-DNA (copies/µgDNA) of CD19-positive cells fraction in PB
CD4-1	M	45	CD4	sCAEBV	3.1×10^2	4.4×10^4 (CD4)	4.4×10^2
CD4-2	F	25	CD4	HMB	7.0×10^4	2.2×10^5 (CD4)	N.D.
CD4-3	F	62	CD4	sCAEBV	3.2×10^4	4.6×10^5 (CD4)	N.D.
CD4-4	F	72	CD4	sCAEBV	9.4×10^4	6.4×10^5 (CD4)	N.D.
CD8-1	F	38	CD8	sCAEBV	1.4×10^5	3.9×10^5 (CD8)	N.D.
CD8-2	F	21	CD8	sCAEBV	1.9×10^3	4.2×10^4 (CD8)	N.D.
CD8-3	F	64	CD8	sCAEBV	2.6×10^5	1.2×10^6 (CD8)	4.6×10^5
CD8-4	M	28	CD8	sCAEBV	1.9×10^3	4.1×10^5 (CD8)	2.0×10^4
CD8-5	M	13	CD8	sCAEBV	2.1×10^3	6.4×10^4 (CD8)	N.D.
γδ	M	9	γδ	HV	8.0×10^3	2.6×10^4 (γδ)	N.D.
CD56-1	F	18	CD56	sCAEBV	2.5×10^2	5.0×10^4 (CD56)	N.D.
CD56-2	F	13	CD56	HMB	5.2×10^4	1.6×10^6 (CD56)	7.5×10^4
CD56-3	F	23	CD56	sCAEBV	1.0×10^4	1.1×10^5 (CD56)	N.D.
CD56-4	F	48	CD56	sCAEBV	8.6×10^4	1.6×10^5 (CD56)	N.D.
CD56-5	M	9	CD56	sCAEBV	1.1×10^4	5.2×10^5 (CD56)	N.D.
CD56-6	M	8	CD56	sCAEBV	5.1×10^2	3.5×10^4 (CD56)	N.D.
CD56-7	M	24	CD56	sCAEBV	2.3×10^3	2.1×10^4 (CD56)	N.D.

M: Male, F: Female.
EBV: Epstein-Barr virus, PB: peripheral blood.
sCAEBV: systemic chronic active Epstein-Barr virus infection, HMB: hypersensitivity to mosquito bites (HMB), HV: hydroa vacciniforme-like eruption.
*The clonality was detected by Southern blotting for EBV terminal repeat.

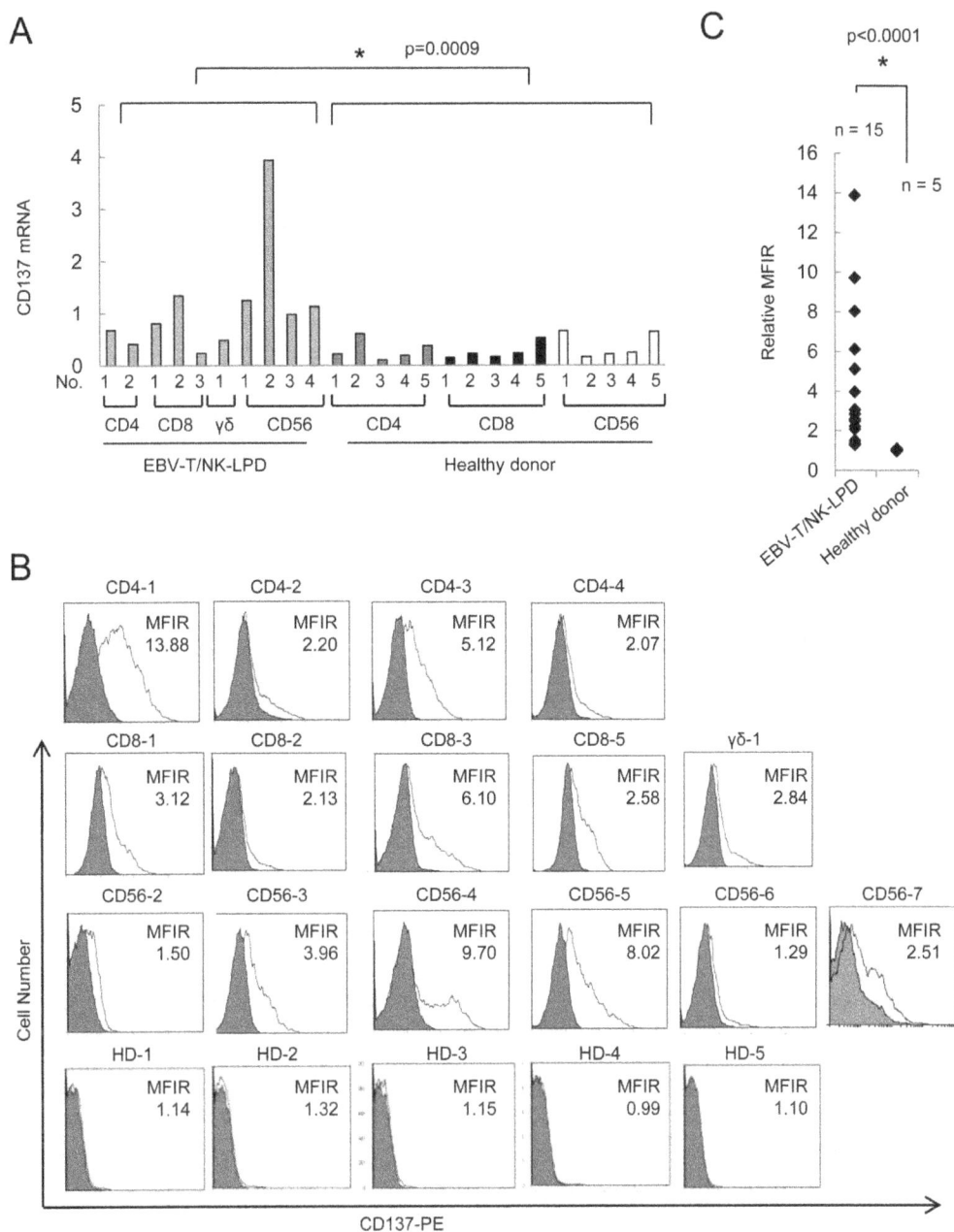

Figure 3. CD137 expression in EBV-positive T or NK cells of patients with EBV-T/NK-lymphoproliferative disorders (EBV-T/NK-LPDs). (A) Transcripts of *CD137* and *GAPDH* of freshly isolated EBV-positive cell fractions from 9 EBV-T/NK-LPDs patients, or cells of the same fractions from healthy donors were quantified by real-time RT-PCR. Relative copy number was obtained by normalizing the *CD137* transcripts to those of *GAPDH*. The relative copy number of the EBV-T/NK-LPDs patients' cells and healthy donor cells were compared. (B) CD137 protein expression in peripheral blood mononuclear cells (PBMCs) from 15 EBV-T/NK-LPDs patients or 5 healthy donors. PBMCs were cultured with IL-2 for 3 days and examined by flow cytometry. The mean fluorescent intensity of CD137 was normalized by that of isotype-matched control and expressed as MFIR (mean fluorescence intensity rate). (C) A bar graph for the relative MFIRs. Each point represents the MFIR of each sample.

development of T or NK cell neoplasms have been reported to date. In this study we examined EBV-positive T or NK cells, and demonstrated that not only the cell lines but also freshly isolated cells of EBV-positive fractions from EBV-T/NK-LPDs patients expressed high levels of *CD137* mRNA. CD137 expression was also detected in EBV-positive cells isolated from the tissue lesions of EBV-T/NK-LPDs xenograft models. We demonstrated that EBV could directly induce CD137 expression most likely through LMP1 in T and NK cells. In addition, stimulation of CD137 by its

ligand could suppress etoposide-induced cell death in EBV-positive and CD137-expressing T or NK cells. These results suggested that EBV could promote survival of T and NK cells by inducing CD137 and might be a cause for EBV-T/NK-neoplasms.

In the present study, *CD137* gene expression was significantly higher in freshly isolated EBV-positive T or NK cells from PB of patients compared with lymphocytes from healthy donors. *In vitro* IL-2 treatment enhanced CD137 expression in the EBV-infected

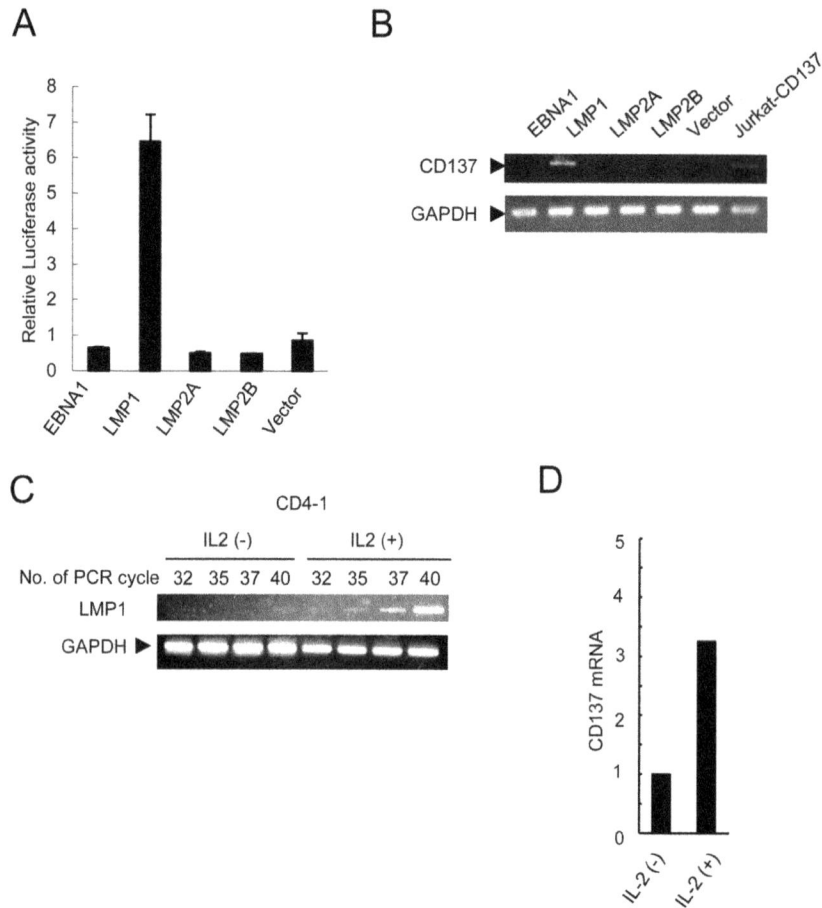

Figure 4. CD137 expression was upregulated by LMP1 whose expression was enhanced by IL-2 in EBV-T/NK-LPDs cells. (A) *CD137* transcription was examined using the assay described. Briefly, MOLT4 cells were transfected with 10 μg of the expression plasmids of the viral proteins, EBNA1, LMP1, LMP2A, LMP2B, or an empty vector as indicated, along with 10 μg of PGL3-4-1BB and 1 μg of pRLSV40. Twelve hours after transfection, the cells were harvested for a dual luciferase assay. Luciferase activity was normalized by *Renilla* luciferase activity and expressed in arbitrary units. The data are expressed as mean ± S.D. of 3 independent experiments. (B) MOLT4 cells were transfected with 10 μg of the expression plasmids of the viral proteins, EBNA1, LMP1, LMP2A, LMP2B, or an empty vector. Transcripts of CD137 (the upper panel) and GAPDH (the lower panel) in these cells were examined by RT-PCR. Jurkat-CD137 cells were used as a positive control. (C) RNAs were obtained from PBMCs from a EBV-T/NK-LPDs patient (CD4-1) which had been cultured with or without IL-2 for 3 days. Semi-quantitative RT-PCR assay for *LMP* was performed. Transcripts of *LMP1* (the upper panel) and *GAPDH* (the lower panel) were presented. (D) Transcripts of *CD137* and *GAPDH* were quantified by real time RT-PCR for the sample of 4C. Relative copy number was obtained by normalizing the *CD137* transcripts to those of *GAPDH*.

Table 2. IL-2 concentration of the serum from EBV-T/NK-LPD patients.

EBV-T/NK-LPD (U/ml)		Healthy donor IL-2 (U/ml)
Case	IL-2 (U/ml)	
CD4-2	<0.8	<0.8
CD4-3	1.9	<0.8
CD4-5	0.9	<0.8
CD4-6	2.4	<0.8
CD8-2	2.1	1
CD8-3	1.1	
CD56-2	0.9	
CD56-3	0.9	

The concentration of IL-2 of the serum from EBV-T/NK-LPDs patients and from healthy donors. The lowest detection limit was 0.8 U/ml.

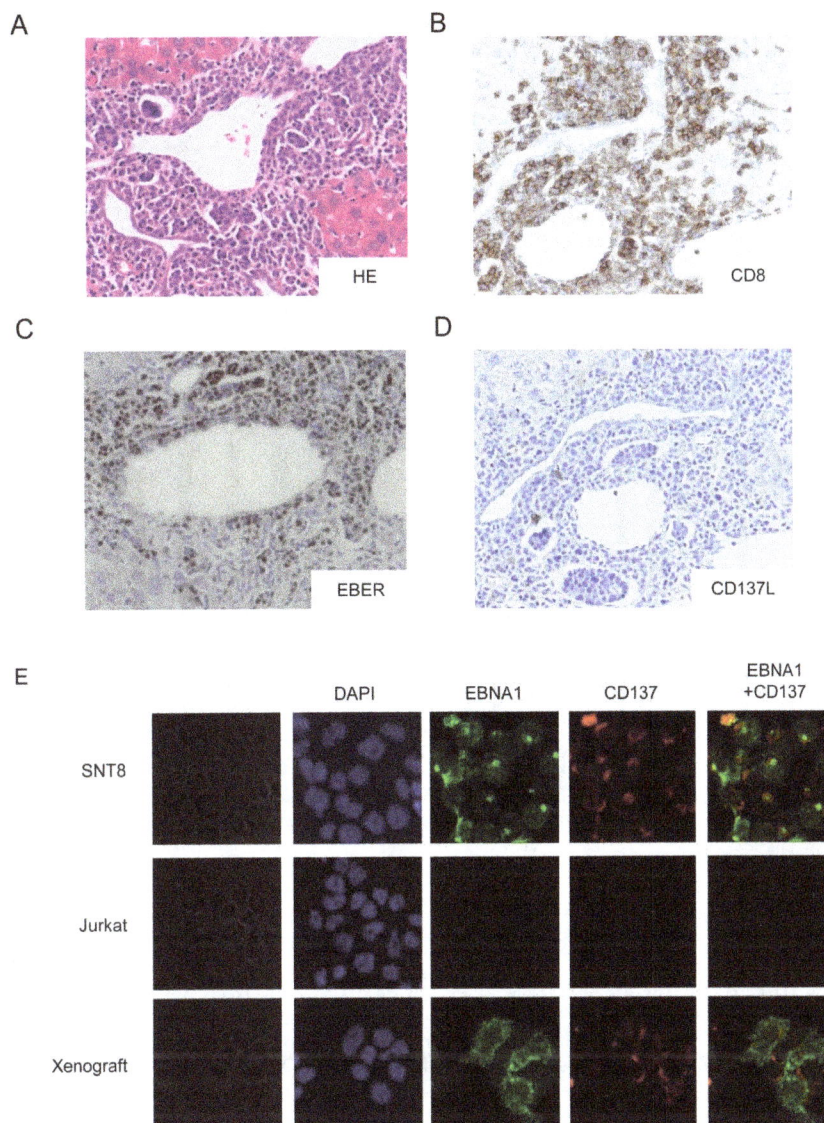

Figure 5. Histopathological specimen from the liver of the xenograft models. We generated the models by transplanting the cells from CD8-3 patient. Nine mice were examined and the representative data were shown. (A) Hematoxylin and eosin staining showed periportal infiltration of lymphocytes. (B) Immunochemical staining with anti-CD8 antibody (brown) showed that the infiltrating lymphocytes were positive for CD8. (C) *In situ* hybridization of Epstein–Barr virus-encoded mRNA (EBER) (brown). Infiltration of EBV-positive cells was detected in the periportal space. (D) Immunochemical staining with anti-CD137L antibody (brown) showed that CD137L-positive cells existed in the periportal space although the number of the cells was smaller than that of EBER positive cells. (original magnification, ×400). (E) Immune-fluorescent staining with anti-EBNA1 and anti-CD137 antibodies of cells isolated from the lesions. Mononuclear cells were obtained from the tissue lesions of a model mouse, stained with the antibodies. The cells were analyzed by confocal microscopy.

cells of the patients, whereas not in control cells of the healthy donors. IL-2 treatment also increased *LMP1* gene expression in EBV-positive cells of EBV-T/NK-LPDs. Takahara and colleagues previously reported that IL-2 enhanced LMP1 expression in EBV-positive ENKL cell lines [18]. Since *CD137* promoter activity was enhanced by LMP1, we suggested that IL-2-induced CD137 protein expression was mediated by LMP1. In addition, the concentration of IL-2 in the serum of EBV-T/NK-LPDs patients was higher than that of healthy donors. Actually the concentration was lower than that of the culture medium, which we used in the assay. Ohga and colleagues, however, reported that the transcription of *IL-2* gene was upregulated in EBV-positive T- or NK-cells [19]. This finding suggested that the level might be high in the tissue lesion where large amount of EBV-positive T- or NK-cell were infiltrating. We detected CD137 protein expression in EBV-positive cells isolated from the lesion. The high expression level of *CD137* mRNA in the circulating EBV-positive cells may contribute to rapid and strong induction of the protein expression in the lesions.

We suggested that EBV enhanced *CD137* mRNA expression through LMP1. Expression level of LMP1 in ENKL is actually variable and other factors, such as miRNA, may play roles for lymphomagenesis in EBV-positive T- or NK-neoplasms [20]. However, all EBV-positive T- or NK-cell lines examined in the present study, expressed LMP1 according to our results (data not shown) and the report [14]. LMP1 activates c-JUN N-terminal

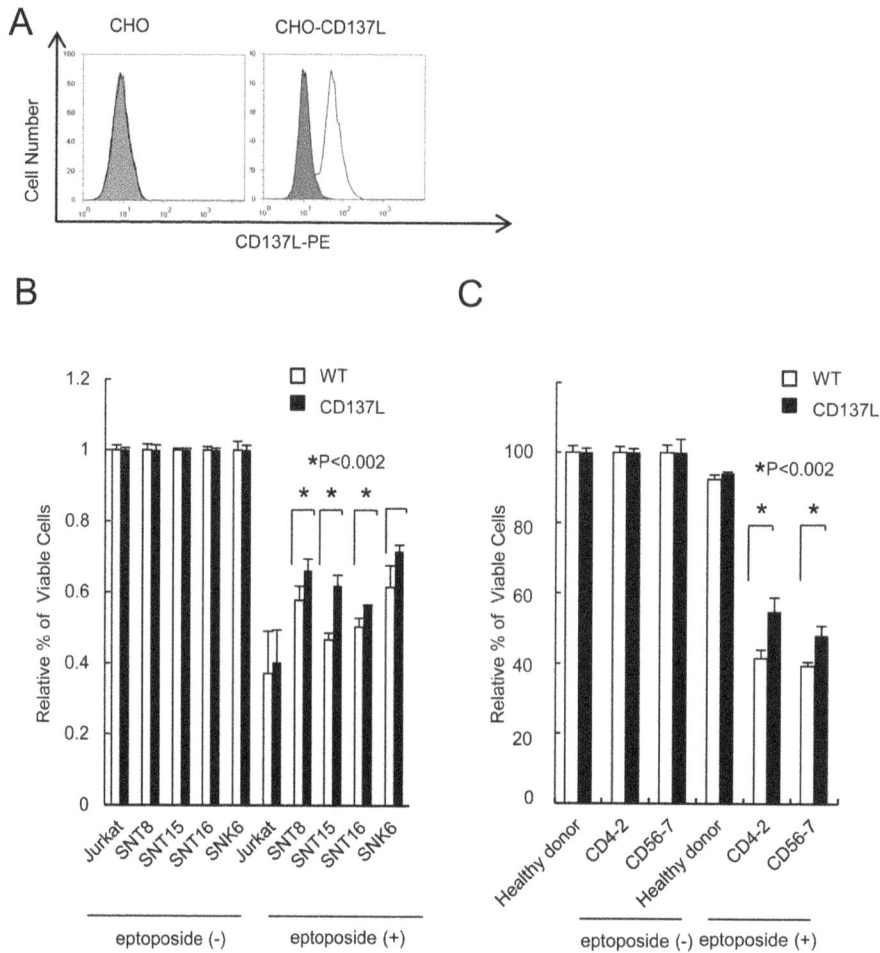

Figure 6. Stimulation of CD137 decreases etoposide-induced cell death of cells from patients with EBV-T/NK-LPDs. (A) CD137L expression on control Chinese Hamster Ovary (CHO) and CHO-CD137L cells. The expression was analyzed by flow cytometry using an antibody to CD137L (open histogram) or isotype-matched control immunoglobulin (gray, shaded histogram). (B) Jurkat cells and EBV- positive T- or NK-cell lines were cultured with 175 U/ml of IL-2 for 48 hours. Then they were cultured on control CHO or CHO-CD137L cells, which had been stained with PKH-26, with or without 2 μM of etoposide for 48 hours. They were then removed for assessment of viability. The cells were stained with DiOC6 and living EBV-T/NK-LPDs cells were detected as PKH-26-negative and DiOC6-positive cells by flow cytometry. The graph chart represents the relative numbers of living cells normalized by those of control cells which were cultured without etoposide. The data are expressed as mean ± S.D. of 3 independent experiments. (C) The PBMCs of EBV-T/NK-LPDs patients and healthy donors were cultured with 175 U/ml of IL-2 for 48 hours. Then they were cultured on control CHO or CHO-CD137L cells. They were then removed for assessment of viability as in B. The graph chart represents the relative numbers of living cells normalized by those of control cells which were cultured without etoposide. The data are expressed as mean ± S.D. of 3 independent experiments.

kinase (JNK) [21], p38 mitogen-activated kinase (p38) [22], and Erk [23], which mediate the AP-1-activating pathway, and also activates NF-κB [24]. It was reported that CD137 expression was regulated by AP-1 and NF-κB in activated T cells [25]. LMP1 can, therefore, induce CD137 expression through AP-1 and NF-κB in T cells. In addition, we reported previously that EBV infection induced ectopic CD40 expression in T-cells [26,27]. CD40 is known to activate NF-κB, JNK, p38 and Erk [28,29]. Also, CD40-induced CD137 expression was recently reported [30]. These results indicate that EBV-induced CD137 expression can be mediated by LMP1, directly as well as through CD40.

Some questions, however, remain to be answered. The first concerns the localization of the CD137L. CD137L expression is induced in T cells when they are activated. [10] Its expression is also detected on various cancer cells [31]. Furthermore, expression of CD137 and CD137L is induced by the viral protein, Tax in ATLL cells and mediates autocrine survival signals, leading to

proliferation of the infected cells and tumor development [12]. We therefore investigated CD137L expression on EBV-T/NK-cells themselves. However, we could not detect CD137L expression clearly on the surface of EBV-T/NK-LPDs cells. CD137L expression is usually detected not only on the surface of activated B and T cells, but also on antigen-presenting cells (APCs) such as dendritic cells, monocytes, and macrophages [32,33]. EBV-negative cells, including histiocytes and macrophages are detected in EBV-T/NK-LPDs lesions surrounding EBV-infected cells [3]. These cells may express CD137L on their surface. Interestingly, CD137L-positive cells were certainly present in the lesions of EBV-T/NK-LPDs (Figure 5D). Since the number of CD137L-positive cells was markedly smaller than that of EBV-positive cells, they were considered to be different cell types. As we previously described, we generated the models by injection of the PBMCs from the patients [15]. Further investigations is required to determine the phenotype of the CD137L-positive cells in the lesions and to clarify whether these cells have some effects on EBV-positive cells, thereby contributing to disease progression. In addition, soluble CD137L (sCD137L) needs to be investigated. sCD137L is produced by lymphocytes or monocytes, with studies showing that it is present in PB of healthy donors and its level is increased in that of patients with hematological malignancies [34] and autoimmune diseases [35]. sCD137L may also have a role in hematopoietic neoplasm development, with its serum levels potentially being a prognostic factor in acute myeloid leukemia and myelodysplastic syndrome [36].

The next question is the actual role of CD137 in the disorders. EBV-T/NK neoplasms are not only lymphoid malignancies, but also have aspects of severe inflammatory diseases accompanied by high fever, cytokinemia, hemophagocytic syndrome and so on [3,18,37-39]. As CD137 mediates survival, proliferation, and cytokine production of CD137-expressing T cells, it may cause inflammation associated with the disease. In addition, CD137 acts as a "ligand" for CD137L. CD137L stimulation by CD137 also mediates intracellular signaling in CD137L-expressing cells [40]. In monocytes expressing CD137L, stimulation of the molecule induces proliferation and differentiation into DCs [41,42]. In B cells expressing CD137L, the stimulation induces proliferation, differentiation and production of immunoglobulins [43,44]. EBV-T/NK-neoplasms are associated with local and systemic inflammation, cytokinemia, or polyclonal gammopathy [38,39]. CD137 may therefore contribute to disease development by inducing not only survival of the infected cells but also inflammation. Inhibition of CD137-mediating signals by targeting CD137 or CD137L should be conducted in order to clarify their roles.

It is well known that CD137 activates survival-promoting molecules including NF-kB in activated T cells [10]. However, the role of the CD137-CD137L interaction *in vivo* is still controversial. Recently, an agonistic CD137 antibody was created and used for xenograft models of human disease, cancer, or autoimmune diseases. In some mouse cancer models, agonistic CD137 antibody induces tumor suppression by upregulating the immune reaction of cytotoxic T-cells against tumor cells [45,46]. On the other hand, in disease models of hyperimmune reactions such as asthma, GVHD, and autoimmune disease, the same antibody had the effect of suppressing T cells [47]. These findings show that CD137 regulates T-cell reactions both positively and negatively, and that the mechanism of the action *in vivo* is extremely complicated. As mentioned previously, EBV-T/NK-LPDs have two aspects: suppressed immune-reaction against EBV-T/NK-cells and a hyper-immune reaction as an inflammatory disease. The conflicting roles of the CD137–CD137L axis may be compatible with these clinical findings of EBV-T/NK-LPDs.

Our results indicate that upregulation of CD137 expression through LMP1 by EBV promotes cell survival in T or NK cells. This effect may contribute to the development of EBV-T/NK-neoplasms and suggests an attractive therapeutic target for the diseases.

Materials and Methods

Cells and reagents

The EBV-positive T/NK-cell (EBV-T/NK cell) lines SNT8, SNT15, SNT16, SNK1, SNK6, and SNK10 were cultured in RPMI containing 10% FCS and 175 U/ml of human IL-2 [14]. The EBV-negative T- and NK-cell lines, Jurkat, MOLT4, HPB-ALL, and MTA were cultured in RPMI containing 10% fetal calf serum (10% FCS-RPMI), whereas the EBV-negative NK-cell line, KHYG1 was cultured in 10% FCS-RPMI containing 175 U/ml of human interleukin-2 (IL-2). The B- cell lines, BJAB, Ramos, Raji,

MD901 [48], HS-Sultan, and LCL were cultured in RPMI containing 10% FCS-RPMI. Jurkat, MOLT4, BJAB, Ramos, HS-Sultan and Raji cells were obtained from the American Type Culture Collection. LCL was established as previously described [26]. The expression of the viral proteins in LCL was demonstrated in Figure S4. MTA cells were obtained from Japanese Collection of Research Bioresources Cell Bank. Jurkat-CD137 and Chinese Hamster Ovary (CHO)-CD137L were generated as previously described [30]. Human recombinant IL-2 was purchased from R&D systems (Abington, UK) and etoposide from Wako (Osaka, Japan).

PCR assay for CD137

The sequences of the PCR primers used for detection of the CD137 gene were as follows: forward, 5′-GTGCCAGATTT-CATCATGGG-3′ (exon 2 of CD137) and reverse, 5′-CAA-CAGCCCTATTGACTTCC-3′ (exon 9 of CD137). The expression levels of the CD137 gene were determined by quantitative PCR, as described previously [13].

Diagnosis of EBV-T/NK-LPDs

EBV-T/NK-LPDs was diagnosed according to the following criteria: the presence of characteristic symptoms, an increase in EBV DNA load in peripheral blood (PB), and the detection of clonally proliferating EBV-positive T or NK cells [4,49].

Detection and isolation of EBV-positive cells in EBV-T/NK-LPDs patients

Detection and isolation of EBV-infected cells were performed as described previously [27]. Briefly, peripheral blood mononuclear cells (PBMCs) from EBV-T/NK-LPDs patients were isolated by density gradient centrifugation using Separate-L (Muto Pure Chemical, Tokyo, Japan) and sorted into CD19-, CD4-, CD8-, or CD56-positive fractions by antibody-conjugated magnetic beads (IMag Human CD19, 4, 8, and 56 Particles-DM; BD Biosciences, Sparks, MD, USA). The fraction which was negative for these markers was considered γδ T cell fraction. The EBV DNA load in each fraction was then measured by the real-time RT-PCR [50] on the basis of the TaqMan system (Applied Biosystems, Foster City, CA, USA). The fraction with the highest titer was assumed to be that with EBV-positive cells. In order to examine *CD137* mRNA expression in the infected cell, we isolated EBV-positive cells from PBMCs by magnetic beads conjugating antibodies for the surface markers of the infected cells.

Antibodies

Mouse antihuman CD137-PE, CD4-FITC, CD8-FITC, CD56-FITC and CD137L-PE as well as their control isotype antibodies were purchased from Becton, Dickinson and Company (Franklin Lakes, NJ, USA).

In vitro EBV infection assay

MOLT4 cells were infected with EBV as described previously [26]. Briefly, EBV was prepared from culture medium of B95-8 cells as described [51], and then concentrated (200-fold) in RPMI medium 1640 supplemented with 10% FCS. The virus suspension was filtered (0.45 μm) and the recipient cells (2×10^6 to 1×10^7) were incubated in 1 or 5 ml of the suspension for 1 h, and then rinsed twice with culture medium (10% RPMI). The efficiency of infection was >90% as judged by EBNA1 staining. For inactivation of the EBV genome, 1 ml of virus suspension in a 100-mm dish was irradiated with UV (254 nm) at 1 J μcm^2 using a FUNA-UV-LINKER FS-800 (Funakoshi, Tokyo). Infection was verified by EBV DNA quantification, and immune fluorescence staining of EBNA1 staining of the cells as described using Polyclonal Rabbit Anti-Human C3c Complement/FITC antibody (Dako, Glostrup, Denmark) [52].

PCR assay for EBV proteins

RT-PCR for detection of mRNA for the viral proteins, *LMP1*, *LMP2A*, *LMP2B* and *EBNA1* was performed according to the previous report [15].

Plasmids

The reporter plasmid PGL3-4-1BB for the detection of *CD137* promoter activation was kindly provided by Dr. Pichler [12]. The reporter plasmid for detection of NF-κB activation, pNF-κB-Luc, was purchased from Stratagene (Santa Clara, CA, USA), and the control *Renilla* luciferase plasmid pRL-SV40 from Promega (Madison, WI, USA). Plasmids containing EBV-encoded proteins, LMP1, LMP2A, LMP2B and EBNA1 were generated from the EBV-infected cell line B95-8 [53].

Luciferase reporter assays

The assays of transiently transfected cells were performed as described previously [54].

Measurement of serum IL-2

The concentration of IL-2 in the serum was examined by SRL, Inc. (Tokyo, Japan) using enzyme-linked immunosorbent assay (ELISA). The lowest detection limit was 0.8 U/ml.

Generation of the xenograft model of EBV-T/NK-LPDs

Male NOD/Shi-scid/IL-2Rγnull (NOG) mice were obtained from the Central Institute for Experimental Animals (Kawasaki, Japan) and maintained under specific pathogen-free conditions. The model was generated by injection of PBMCs from patients to six weeks old mice through the tail vein as described previously [15]. Intravenous anesthesia by tribromoethanol was performed in order to minimize suffering. Engraftment was determined by detecting EBV DNA in the peripheral blood. After engraftment, mice were euthanized via CO_2 inhalation and applied for pathological and virological analyses.

Immunohistochemistry

The 4 μm thick paraffin-embedded formalin-fixed tissue sections were de-paraffinized, and heat-based antigen retrieval was performed in 0.1 M citrate buffer (pH 6.0). Endogenous peroxidase activity was inhibited using hydrogen peroxide. The primary antibodies for CD137 (ab3169) and CD137L (ab64912) were purchased from Abcam (Cambridge, MA, USA). The detection system was the streptavidin-biotin-peroxidase complex technique (ABC kit; Vector Laboratories, Burlingame, CA, USA) with diaminobenzidine (DAB; Nichirei Bioscience, Tokyo, Japan) as the chromogen. *In situ* hybridization (ISH) of Epstein–Barr virus-encoded mRNA (EBER) was performed for detection of EBV in tissue sections by Epstein-Barr Virus (EBER) PNA Probe/Fluorescein (DAKO, Carpinteria, CA, USA) and second antibody for Fluorescein (Dako, Glostrup, Denmark).

Immune-fluorescent staining

The expression of CD137 protein on EBV-infected cells was examined by immune-fluorescent staining. Cells were fixed on slides by immersing in 4% paraformaldehyde for 10 min, followed by washing three times in PBS and incubation with mouse monoclonal anti-CD137, goat polyclonal anti-EBNA1) antibodies

(Abcam, Cambridge, MA, USA), Cy5-conjugated Affinipure donkey anti-mouse antibody, and FITC-conjugated donkey anti-goat antibody (Jackson ImmunoResearch Laboratories, Inc. PA, USA). Nuclei were counterstained with ProLong Gold and DAPI (Invitrogen, Carlsbad, CA, USA), and the cells were analyzed by confocal microscopy (Fluoview FV10i, Olympus).

Stimulation of CD137 by ligand-expressing cells and detection of cell viability

The PBMCs were isolated from patients of EBV-T/NK-LPDs. Control CHO or CHO-CD137L cells were stained with PKH-26 (PKH-26 Red Fluorescent Cell Linker Kit; Sigma-Aldrich, St. Louis, MO, USA) according to the manufacturer's instructions, and plated on the wells. The PBMCs were then overlaid on pre-seeded control CHO or CHO-CD137L cells, and cultured with or without etoposide in 10% FCS-RPMI containing 175 U/ml of IL-2. After 48 h incubation, the cells were stained with DiOC6 (Invitrogen, Carlsbad, CA, USA) and removed. The cells were analyzed using a FACS Calibur flow cytometer (Becton, Dickinson and Company, Franklin Lakes, NJ USA), with PKH-26–negative and DiOC6-positive cells considered as living EBV-T/NK cells.

Statistical analysis

For statistical analyses of Figure 3A and 3B, Mann-Whitney test was performed using GraphPad Prism 5 (GraphPad Software, La Jolla, CA, USA). Student t test was performed for Figure 6B and 6C.

The study complied with the principles of the Declaration of Helsinki and was approved by the ethical committee of Tokyo Medical and Dental University (TMDU). Written informed consent was obtained from each patient. The experiments with NOG mice are in accordance with the Guidelines for Animal Experimentation of the Japanese Association for Laboratory Animal Science, as well as ARRIVE guidelines [55]. The experiments were approved by the Institutional Animal Care and Use Committee of TMDU (No. 0140087A).

Supporting Information

Figure S1   CD137L expression in EBV-positive cell lines. Surface expression of CD137L was examined by flow cytometry using an antibody to CD137L (open histogram) or isotype-matched control immunoglobulin (gray, shaded histogram). The mean fluorescent intensity of CD137 was normalized by that of isotype-matched control and expressed as MFIR (mean fluorescence intensity rate) in arbitrary units. CHO-CD137L cells were used as positive control.

Figure S2   CD137 expression in PBMCs from EBV-positive T-NK-lymphoproliferative patients and those from healthy donors (HD). After collection, the cells were cultured with IL-2 for 3 days. The expression was analyzed by flow cytometry using an antibody to CD137 and to surface protein expressed on EBV-positive cells.

Figure S3   Immune-fluorescent staining with anti-LMP1 antibody of cells isolated from the lesions. Mononuclear cells were obtained from the tissue lesions of a model mouse, stained with the antibody. The cells were analyzed by confocal microscopy.

Figure S4   LCL that we used in the study was established as previously described [26]. The infection was confirmed by

RT-PCR for EBNA. We also examined and detected the expression of the lytic protein, BZLF1 [56]. Akata cells [57] stimulated with IgG were used as a positive control for BZLF1 expression. Since BZLF1 was not expressed in them, we concluded that the infection was latent.

Acknowledgments

We are grateful to Dr. Klemens Pichler for providing PGL3-4-1BB. We are also grateful to Dr. Kohei Yamamoto, Ms. Yukana Nakaima, Ms. Kaori Okada, and Ms. Kazumi Fujimoto for excellent technical assistance.

Author Contributions

Conceived and designed the experiments: MY KII SY SF OM AA. Performed the experiments: MY KII LW HK YS TF MK TK NS AA. Analyzed the data: MY KII LW HK YS TF MK TK NS SF OM AA. Contributed reagents/materials/analysis tools: MY KII YS SY TF TK SF OM AA. Wrote the paper: MY KII SY TK SF OM AA. Contributed to the modification of the draft and approved the final submission: MY KII HK LW YS SY TF MK TK NS SF OM AA.

References

1. Chan JKC, Quintanilla-Martinez L, Ferry JA, Peh S-C (2008) Extranodal NK/T-cell lymphoma, nasal type. In: Jaffe E, Harris N, Stein H, editors. World Health Organization Classification of Tumors Pathology and Genetics of Tumours of Haematopoietic and Lymphoid Tissues. Lyon IARC Press. pp. 285–289.

2. Chan JKC, Jaffe ES, Ralfkiaer E, Ko Y-H (2008) Aggressive NK-cell leukemia. In: ES J, NL H, H S, editors. World Health Organization Classification of Tumors Pathology and Genetics of Tumours of Haematopoietic and Lymphoid Tissues. Lyon: IARC Press. pp. 276–277.

3. Quintanilla-Martinez L, Kimura H, Jaffe ES (2008) EBV-positive T-cell lymphoproliferative disorders of childhood. In: Jaffe E, Harris N, Stein H, editors. World Health Organization Classification of Tumors Pathology and Genetics of Tumours of Haematopoietic and Lymphoid Tissues. Lyon IARC Press. pp. 278–280.

4. Kimura H, Ito Y, Kawabe S, Gotoh K, Takahashi Y, et al. (2012) EBV-associated T/NK-cell lymphoproliferative diseases in nonimmunocompromised hosts: prospective analysis of 108 cases. Blood 119: 673–686.

5. Kimura H, Hoshino Y, Kanegane H, Tsuge I, Okamura T, et al. (2001) Clinical and virologic characteristics of chronic active Epstein-Barr virus infection. Blood 98: 280–286.

6. Arai A, Imadome K, Watanabe Y, Yoshimori M, Koyama T, et al. (2011) Clinical features of adult-onset chronic active Epstein-Barr virus infection: a retrospective analysis. Int J Hematol 93: 602–609.

7. Kawa K, Sawada A, Sato M, Okamura T, Sakata N, et al. (2011) Excellent outcome of allogeneic hematopoietic SCT with reduced-intensity conditioning for the treatment of chronic active EBV infection. Bone Marrow Transplant 46: 77–83.

8. Yamaguchi M, Kwong YL, Kim WS, Maeda Y, Hashimoto C, et al. (2011) Phase II study of SMILE chemotherapy for newly diagnosed stage IV, relapsed, or refractory extranodal natural killer (NK)/T-cell lymphoma, nasal type: the NK-Cell Tumor Study Group study. J Clin Oncol 29: 4410–4416.

9. Yamaguchi M, Tobinai K, Oguchi M, Ishizuka N, Kobayashi Y, et al. (2012) Concurrent Chemoradiotherapy for Localized Nasal Natural Killer/T-Cell Lymphoma: An Updated Analysis of the Japan Clinical Oncology Group Study JCOG0211. J Clin Oncol.

10. Croft M (2009) The role of TNF superfamily members in T-cell function and diseases. Nat Rev Immunol 9: 271–285.

11. Pollok KE, Kim YJ, Zhou Z, Hurtado J, Kim KK, et al. (1993) Inducible T cell antigen 4-1BB. Analysis of expression and function. J Immunol 150: 771–781.

12. Pichler K, Kattan T, Gentzsch J, Kress AK, Taylor GP, et al. (2008) Strong induction of 4-1BB, a growth and survival promoting costimulatory receptor, in HTLV-1-infected cultured and patients' T cells by the viral Tax oncoprotein. Blood 111: 4741–4751.

13. Anderson MW, Zhao S, Freud AG, Czerwinski DK, Kohrt H, et al. (2012) CD137 is expressed in follicular dendritic cell tumors and in classical Hodgkin and T-cell lymphomas: diagnostic and therapeutic implications. Am J Pathol 181: 795–803.

14. Zhang Y, Nagata H, Ikeuchi T, Mukai H, Oyoshi MK, et al. (2003) Common cytological and cytogenetic features of Epstein-Barr virus (EBV)-positive natural killer (NK) cells and cell lines derived from patients with nasal T/NK-cell lymphomas, chronic active EBV infection and hydroa vacciniforme-like eruptions. Br J Haematol 121: 805–814.

15. Imadome K, Yajima M, Arai A, Nakazawa A, Kawano F, et al. (2011) Novel Mouse Xenograft Models Reveal a Critical Role of CD4 T Cells in the Proliferation of EBV-Infected T and NK Cells. PLoS Pathog 7: e1002326.

16. Tan JT, Ha J, Cho HR, Tucker-Burden C, Hendrix RC, et al. (2000) Analysis of expression and function of the costimulatory molecule 4-1BB in alloimmune responses. Transplantation 70: 175–183.

17. Lee HW, Park SJ, Choi BK, Kim HH, Nam KO, et al. (2002) 4-1BB promotes the survival of CD8+ T lymphocytes by increasing expression of Bcl-xL and Bfl-1. J Immunol 169: 4882–4888.

18. Takahara M, Kis LL, Nagy N, Liu A, Harabuchi Y, et al. (2006) Concomitant increase of LMP1 and CD25 (IL-2-receptor alpha) expression induced by IL-10 in the EBV-positive NK lines SNK6 and KAI3. Int J Cancer 119: 2775–2783.

19. Ohga S, Nomura A, Takada H, Ihara K, Kawakami K, et al. (2001) Epstein-Barr virus (EBV) load and cytokine gene expression in activated T cells of chronic active EBV infection. J Infect Dis 183: 1–7.

20. Yamanaka Y, Tagawa H, Takahashi N, Watanabe A, Guo YM, et al. (2009) Aberrant overexpression of microRNAs activate AKT signaling via down-regulation of tumor suppressors in natural killer-cell lymphoma/leukemia. Blood 114: 3265–3275.

21. Kutz H, Reisbach G, Schultheiss U, Kieser A (2008) The c-Jun N-terminal kinase pathway is critical for cell transformation by the latent membrane protein 1 of Epstein-Barr virus. Virology 371: 246–256.

22. Eliopoulos AG, Gallagher NJ, Blake SM, Dawson CW, Young LS (1999) Activation of the p38 mitogen-activated protein kinase pathway by Epstein-Barr virus-encoded latent membrane protein 1 coregulates interleukin-6 and interleukin-8 production. J Biol Chem 274: 16085–16096.

23. Dawson CW, Laverick L, Morris MA, Tramoutanis G, Young LS (2008) Epstein-Barr virus-encoded LMP1 regulates epithelial cell motility and invasion via the ERK-MAPK pathway. J Virol 82: 3654–3664.

24. Kaye KM, Izumi KM, Li H, Johannsen E, Davidson D, et al. (1999) An Epstein-Barr virus that expresses only the first 231 LMP1 amino acids efficiently initiates primary B-lymphocyte growth transformation. J Virol 73: 10525–10530.

25. Kim JO, Kim HW, Baek KM, Kang CY (2003) NF-kappaB and AP-1 regulate activation-dependent CD137 (4-1BB) expression in T cells. FEBS Lett 541: 163–170.

26. Imadome K, Shirakata M, Shimizu N, Nonoyama S, Yamanashi Y (2003) CD40 ligand is a critical effector of Epstein-Barr virus in host cell survival and transformation. Proc Natl Acad Sci U S A 100: 7836–7840.

27. Imadome K, Shimizu N, Arai A, Miura O, Watanabe K, et al. (2005) Coexpression of CD40 and CD40 ligand in Epstein-Barr virus-infected T and NK cells and their role in cell survival. J Infect Dis 192: 1340–1348.

28. Mukundan L, Bishop GA, Head KZ, Zhang L, Wahl LM, et al. (2005) TNF receptor-associated factor 6 is an essential mediator of CD40-activated proinflammatory pathways in monocytes and macrophages. J Immunol 174: 1081–1090.

29. Song Z, Jin R, Yu S, Rivet JJ, Smyth SS, et al. (2011) CD40 is essential in the upregulation of TRAF proteins and NF-kappaB-dependent proinflammatory gene expression after arterial injury. PLoS One 6: e23239.

30. Nakaima Y, Watanabe K, Koyama T, Miura O, Fukuda T (2013) CD137 Is Induced by the CD40 Signal on Chronic Lymphocytic Leukemia B Cells and Transduces the Survival Signal via NF-κB Activation. PLoS One 8: e64425.

31. Salih HR, Kosowski SG, Haluska VF, Starling GC, Loo DT, et al. (2000) Constitutive expression of functional 4-1BB (CD137) ligand on carcinoma cells. J Immunol 165: 2903–2910.

32. Alderson MR, Smith CA, Tough TW, Davis-Smith T, Armitage RJ, et al. (1994) Molecular and biological characterization of human 4-1BB and its ligand. Eur J Immunol 24: 2219–2227.

33. Pollok KE, Kim YJ, Hurtado J, Zhou Z, Kim KK, et al. (1994) 4-1BB T-cell antigen binds to mature B cells and macrophages, and costimulates anti-mu-primed splenic B cells. Eur J Immunol 24: 367–374.

34. Salih HR, Schmetzer HM, Burke C, Starling GC, Dunn R, et al. (2001) Soluble CD137 (4-1BB) ligand is released following leukocyte activation and is found in sera of patients with hematological malignancies. J Immunol 167: 4059–4066.

35. Jung HW, Choi SW, Choi JI, Kwon BS (2004) Serum concentrations of soluble 4-1BB and 4-1BB ligand correlated with the disease severity in rheumatoid arthritis. Exp Mol Med 36: 13–22.

36. Hentschel N, Krusch M, Kiener PA, Kolb HJ, Salih HR, et al. (2006) Serum levels of sCD137 (4-1BB) ligand are prognostic factors for progression in acute myeloid leukemia but not in non-Hodgkin's lymphoma. Eur J Haematol 77: 91–101.

37. Kimura H (2006) Pathogenesis of chronic active Epstein-Barr virus infection: is this an infectious disease, lymphoproliferative disorder, or immunodeficiency? Rev Med Virol 16: 251–261.

38. Kasahara Y, Yachie A, Takei K, Kanegane C, Okada K, et al. (2001) Differential cellular targets of Epstein-Barr virus (EBV) infection between acute EBV-associated hemophagocytic lymphohistiocytosis and chronic active EBV infection. Blood 98: 1882–1888.

39. Fox CP, Shannon-Lowe C, Gothard P, Kishore B, Neilson J, et al. (2010) Epstein-Barr virus-associated hemophagocytic lymphohistiocytosis in adults characterized by high viral genome load within circulating natural killer cells. Clin Infect Dis 51: 66–69.

40. Shao Z, Schwarz H (2011) CD137 ligand, a member of the tumor necrosis factor family, regulates immune responses via reverse signal transduction. J Leukoc Biol 89: 21–29.

41. Lee SW, Park Y, So T, Kwon BS, Cheroutre H, et al. (2008) Identification of regulatory functions for 4-1BB and 4-1BBL in myelopoiesis and the development of dendritic cells. Nat Immunol 9: 917–926.

42. Laderach D, Wesa A, Galy A (2003) 4-1BB-ligand is regulated on human dendritic cells and induces the production of IL-12. Cell Immunol 226: 37–44.

43. Pauly S, Broll K, Wittmann M, Giegerich G, Schwarz H (2002) CD137 is expressed by follicular dendritic cells and costimulates B lymphocyte activation in germinal centers. J Leukoc Biol 72: 35–42.

44. Middendorp S, Xiao Y, Song JY, Peperzak V, Krijger PH, et al. (2009) Mice deficient for CD137 ligand are predisposed to develop germinal center-derived B-cell lymphoma. Blood 114: 2280–2289.

45. Melero I, Shuford WW, Newby SA, Aruffo A, Ledbetter JA, et al. (1997) Monoclonal antibodies against the 4-1BB T-cell activation molecule eradicate established tumors. Nat Med 3: 682–685.

46. Narazaki H, Zhu Y, Luo L, Zhu G, Chen L (2010) CD137 agonist antibody prevents cancer recurrence: contribution of CD137 on both hematopoietic and nonhematopoietic cells. Blood 115: 1941–1948.

47. Seo SK, Choi JH, Kim YH, Kang WJ, Park HY, et al. (2004) 4-1BB-mediated immunotherapy of rheumatoid arthritis. Nat Med 10: 1088–1094.

48. Miki T, Kawamata N, Arai A, Ohashi K, Nakamura Y, et al. (1994) Molecular cloning of the breakpoint for 3q27 translocation in B-cell lymphomas and leukemias. Blood 83: 217–222.

49. Okano M, Kawa K, Kimura H, Yachie A, Wakiguchi H, et al. (2005) Proposed guidelines for diagnosing chronic active Epstein-Barr virus infection. Am J Hematol 80: 64–69.

50. Kimura H, Morita M, Yabuta Y, Kuzushima K, Kato K, et al. (1999) Quantitative analysis of Epstein-Barr virus load by using a real-time PCR assay. J Clin Microbiol 37: 132–136.

51. Sinclair AJ, Palmero I, Peters G, Farrell PJ (1994) EBNA-2 and EBNA-LP cooperate to cause G0 to G1 transition during immortalization of resting human B lymphocytes by Epstein-Barr virus. EMBO J 13: 3321–3328.

52. Reedman BM, Klein G (1973) Cellular localization of an Epstein-Barr virus (EBV)-associated complement-fixing antigen in producer and non-producer lymphoblastoid cell lines. Int J Cancer 11: 499–520.

53. Shirakata M, Imadome KI, Okazaki K, Hirai K (2001) Activation of TRAF5 and TRAF6 signal cascades negatively regulates the latent replication origin of Epstein-Barr virus through p38 mitogen-activated protein kinase. J Virol 75: 5059–5068.

54. Nosaka Y, Arai A, Miyasaka N, Miura O (1999) CrkL mediates Ras-dependent activation of the Raf/ERK pathway through the guanine nucleotide exchange factor C3G in hematopoietic cells stimulated with erythropoietin or interleukin-3. J Biol Chem 274: 30154–30162.

55. MacCallum CJ (2010) Reporting animal studies: good science and a duty of care. PLoS Biol 8: e1000413.

56. Iwasaki Y, Chong JM, Hayashi Y, Ikeno R, Arai K, et al. (1998) Establishment and characterization of a human Epstein-Barr virus-associated gastric carcinoma in SCID mice. J Virol 72: 8321–8326.

57. Takada K, Horinouchi K, Ono Y, Aya T, Osato T, et al. (1991) An Epstein-Barr virus-producer line Akata: establishment of the cell line and analysis of viral DNA. Virus Genes 5: 147–156.

8

Reduction of T Cell Receptor Diversity in NOD Mice Prevents Development of Type 1 Diabetes but Not Sjögren's Syndrome

Joanna Kern, Robert Drutel[¤], Silvia Leanhart, Marek Bogacz, Rafal Pacholczyk*

Center for Biotechnology and Genomic Medicine, Georgia Regents University, Augusta, Georgia, United States of America

Abstract

Non-obese diabetic (NOD) mice are well-established models of independently developing spontaneous autoimmune diseases, Sjögren's syndrome (SS) and type 1 diabetes (T1D). The key determining factor for T1D is the strong association with particular MHCII molecule and recognition by diabetogenic T cell receptor (TCR) of an insulin peptide presented in the context of I-A^{g7} molecule. For SS the association with MHCII polymorphism is weaker and TCR diversity involved in the onset of the autoimmune phase of SS remains poorly understood. To compare the impact of TCR diversity reduction on the development of both diseases we generated two lines of TCR transgenic NOD mice. One line expresses transgenic TCRβ chain originated from a pathogenically irrelevant TCR, and the second line additionally expresses transgenic TCRα^{mini} locus. Analysis of TCR sequences on NOD background reveals lower TCR diversity on Treg cells not only in the thymus, but also in the periphery. This reduction in diversity does not affect conventional CD4$^+$ T cells, as compared to the TCR^{mini} repertoire on B6 background. Interestingly, neither transgenic TCRβ nor TCR^{mini} mice develop diabetes, which we show is due to lack of insulin B:9–23 specific T cells in the periphery. Conversely SS develops in both lines, with full glandular infiltration, production of autoantibodies and hyposalivation. It shows that SS development is not as sensitive to limited availability of TCR specificities as T1D, which suggests wider range of possible TCR/peptide/MHC interactions driving autoimmunity in SS.

Editor: John A. Chiorini, National Institute of Dental and Craniofacial Research, United States of America

Funding: This research was supported by grants from National Institute of Allergy and Infectious Diseases of the National Institutes of Health (R01AI081798) and Juvenile Diabetes Research Foundation (RP). The funders had no role in study design, data collection and analysis, decision to publish, or preparation of the manuscript.

Competing Interests: The authors have declared that no competing interests exist.

* Email: rpacholczyk@gru du

¤ Current address: Medical University of South Carolina, College of Medicine, Charleston, South Carolina, United States of America

Introduction

NOD mice serve as well-established models of independently developing autoimmune diseases, Type 1 Diabetes (T1D) and Sjögren's syndrome (SS) [1,2]. T1D is characterized by autoimmune attacks against the pancreatic beta-cells with T cells playing an essential role in the initiation and progression of the disease, leading to hyperglycemia and vascular complications [3,4]. SS is an autoimmune disease with local and systemic manifestations, characterized by mononuclear infiltrates into salivary and lacrimal glands leading to clinical symptoms of dry mouth and dry eyes [5,6]. Glandular infiltrates consist mostly of CD4$^+$ T cells with lesser amounts of CD8$^+$ T cells and B cells. Although factors like viral or bacterial infections, aberrant glandular development or cytokine production are important in the initial phase of the pathogenesis of SS, CD4$^+$ T cells are important players in the onset of autoimmunity and disease progression.

Autoimmunity in NOD mice is attributed to several different events occurring in the thymus and in the periphery. Studies in these mice showed a defect in negative selection [7], perturbed αβ/γδ lineage decision leading to a shift in selection niches [8], reduced relative diversity of thymic Treg cells [9], peripheral

hyper-responsiveness of effector CD4$^+$ T cells [10], multiple binding registers of insulin B:9–23 peptide resulting in poor negative selection in the thymus [11,12], or peripheral post-translational modification of self-peptides/neo-antigens [13]. Despite genetic predispositions, the key component in the development of autoimmune diseases is the recognition of a particular antigen in the context of MHC Class II molecule by CD4$^+$ T cells. The development of diabetes in NOD mice is associated with the key I-A^{g7} molecule (HLA-DQ8 in humans) in the absence of a functional I-E molecule [14,15]. Co-expression of other MHC molecules with I-A^{g7} can prevent development of diabetes in a dominant fashion [14,15]. Replacement of I-A^{g7} with other MHC molecules, like I-A^b, I-A^p or I-A^q, does not promote the development of diabetes yet mice continue to develop autoimmune exocrinopathy and the severity of the SS and the profile of antibodies' specificities vary between congenic mice [16]. In large-scale association study of SS in humans, HLA was found to have the strongest linkage to the disease [17].

The strict dependence of T1D on the particular MHC allele correlates with its primary antigen requirement where insulin B:9–23 peptide has been identified as the epitope necessary for onset of the disease in NOD mice [18]. In SS, no key epitope(s) are identified, although several proteins have been implicated as a source of antigens: Ro/SSA 52 kDa, αFodrin, Muscarinic Acetylcholine 3 Receptor (M3R), α-amylase, islet cell autoantigen-69, kallikrein-13 [19–24]. Recently it has been shown that the transfer of T cells from M3R-immunized M3R$^{-/-}$ mice into Rag$^{-/-}$ mice leads to development of sialadenitis, showing pathogenic potential of M3R specific T cells [25].

Despite the strict requirement of the presence of the insulin B:9–23/I-A^{g7} combination, the development of T1D in NOD mice proceeds even when total TCR diversity and precursor frequency of diabetogenic TCRs is limited. The reduction of TCR diversity by use of TCRβ transgenic mice [26], or great reduction of precursor frequency relying on allelic exclusion escapees on NOD background does not prevent development of T1D [27], although not all endogenous TCRβ chains are permissive for the development of insulin B:9–23 specific TCRs [28]. In SS it is not clear as to what role diversity of interactions between TCRs and different peptide/MHCII complexes play in the onset and development of the disease. Previous studies in patients with SS found that TCR repertoire of infiltrating T cells is to some extent restricted with different dominant clonotypes of Vβ families [29–33]. Despite the lack of dominant Vα/Vβ families or dominant specificity in different patients these studies show clonal expansion of infiltrating T cells, which suggests that the number of epitopes participating in the autoimmunity of the disease is limited [34,35]. However, the weaker dependence of SS on MHC polymorphism suggests broad diversity of possible TCR/peptide/MHCII interactions participating in the pathogenesis of the disease. As the diversity of antigenic specificities and TCR repertoire on T cells involved in SS development is not well understood, we wanted to compare sensitivity of development of SS versus T1D to the diminishing diversities of TCRs in the presence of the same I-A^{g7} molecule in NOD mice. To reduce the diversity of TCRs in NOD mice we generated two types of transgenic strains, in which all T cells express either one transgenic TCRβ chain or additionally co-express TCRα chains from TCRα^{mini} locus [36]. Interestingly, these mice do not develop T1D but still develop SS with glandular infiltrations, autoantibody presence and hyposalivation. We investigated the reasons for the lack of T1D development and the role of reduced diversity on generated repertoires of TCRs on conventional and regulatory T cells in the thymus and periphery of NOD mice.

Materials and Methods

Ethics statement

All mice used in this study were housed in the animal care facility at the Georgia Regents University (GRU). All work involving animals was conducted under protocols approved by the Animal Care and Use Committee at the GRU (#2008−0231). All efforts were made to minimize suffering. Mice were euthanized by CO2 followed by cervical dislocation.

Mice

Production of TCRβ^{Tg} and TCRα^{mini} constructs and generation of transgenic mice on C57BL/6 (B6) background was described previously (Pacholczyk 2006). A similar strategy was used to microinject one or both DNA constructs into zygotes of NOD mice (Transgenic Mice Core Facility, GRU). To eliminate expression of endogenous TCRα chains, NOD.TCRβ^{Tg}.TCRα^{mini} transgenic mice were crossed with NOD.TCRα$^{-/-}$ (NOD.129P2(C)-Tcratm1Mjo/DoiJ) mice purchased from The Jackson Laboratory (Bar Harbor, ME). To facilitate identification

of Treg cells both transgenic lines then were crossed with NOD.FoxP3GFP/cre mice (NOD/ShiLt-Tg(Foxp3-EGFP/cre)1Jbs/J) purchased from The Jackson Laboratory. The B6.Aec1Aec2 (B6.DC) mice were kindly provided by Dr. Ammon Peck [37].

Histology

Organs were removed from each mouse at the time of euthanasia, placed in 10% phosphate-buffered formalin for at least 24 h and then embedded in paraffin. Sections were taken at 5 μm of thickness 200 μm apart. The tissue sections were stained with hematoxylin and eosin (H&E) at the Histology Core Laboratory, GRU. One infiltrate was defined as a cluster of at least 50 nucleated cells, scoring described in figures.

Measurement of saliva flow

Mice were given an i.p. injection of 100 μl of pilocarpine (0.05 mg/ml in PBS) per 20 g of body weight. Saliva was collected for 10 min., starting 1 min. after injection of pilocarpine. The volume of saliva was measured and normalized to the mouse body weight.

Detection of auto-antibodies

Auto-antibodies and total IgG1 were measured using mouse serum with the following ELISA kits: αFodrin (American Research Products), ANA, ssDNA, dsDNA (Immuno-Biological Laboratories) and IgG1 (Immunology Consultants Laboratory). Assays were performed according to manufacturer's protocols with serum dilution 1:100 and 1:50,000 for IgG1. OD$_{450}$ values of negative samples were subtracted from the OD$_{450}$ of experimental samples.

Cell preparation, flow cytometry and cell sorting

Cells were isolated from peripheral lymph nodes (axillary, brachial and inguinal) and thymii by mechanical disruption through nylon mesh. Salivary mandibular and extraorbital lacrimal glands were first cut and digested using collagenase (1 ug/ml) for 30 min in 37°C. Cells were washed and counted (Countess, Invitrogen) and used for staining with monoclonal antibodies: CD4 (clone RM4-5), CD8α (53-6.7), B220 (RA3-6B2), TCRVα2 (B20.1), TCRVβ14 (14-2), TCRβ (H57-597), CD25 (PC61), CD45RB (16A), CD62L (MEL-14), all from BD Biosciences. Stained cells were either analyzed using FACS Canto (BD Biosciences) or sorted on MoFlo Sorter (Cytomation). Dead cells were excluded using forward vs side scatter dot plots and doublets discrimination was accomplished using forward scatter height vs width dot plots. Purities of all sorted populations were above 98%.

Immunization and generation of T cell hybridomas

Mice were immunized at the base of the tail with 50 μg of insulin B:9–23 peptide emulsified in Complete Freund's Adjuvant (Thermo Scientific). One week later lymphocytes were isolated from draining lymph nodes and cultured in vitro for 3–4 days with insulin B:9–23 peptide (50 μg/ml), followed by 3–4 days of expansion with murine recombinant IL-2 (20 U/ml, Peprotech). For generation of allo-specific T cell hybridomas, CD4$^+$ T cells sorted from un-immunized experimental mice were stimulated in vitro by co-culture with splenocytes from B6.TCRα$^{-/-}$ mice, followed by expansion with IL-2. Activated T cells were fused to BW5147 TCRα-β- NFAT-EGFP cells as previously described [38]. BW NFAT-EGFP fusion partner expresses GFP protein under the minimal human IL-2 promoter, which contains NFAT-binding sites [39]. T cell hybridomas were selected using HAT

(Cellgro) selection media by limiting dilution method. For stimulation, cloned T cell hybridomas (10^5 cells) were co-cultured overnight with 5×10^5 splenocytes (from NOD.TCRα−/− or B6.TCRα−/− mice) with or without insulin B:9–23 peptide (50 µg/ml) or anti-CD3 antibody (1 µg/ml). Specific activation of the hybridomas was measured by detection of GFP-positive cells or by detection of IL-2 in culture supernatant using CBA Mouse IL-2 Flex Set (BD Biosciences).

MTT assay

The proliferation of the cells was measured using 3-(4,5-dimethythiazol-2-yl)-2,5-diphenyltetrazolium bromide (MTT; Sigma) assay. On the third day of *in vitro* stimulation 10 µl of MTT (5 mg/ml) was added to each well and incubated for 4 h. After discarding supernatant, the remaining formazan precipitates were dissolved in 150 ul of 70% isopropanol solution (70% isopropanol, 30% water, 0.02N hydrochloric acid) overnight. Absorbance was measured at 570 nm using Microplate Reader (Biotek Synergy HT).

Sequencing

Single cell sorting and sequencing was done as previously described [36]. High-throughput sequencing was done using Ion Torrent platform (Life Technologies) by Genomic Core Facility at GRU. Libraries of the TCRs were prepared according to protocol. Shortly, CDR3α regions were amplified using primers specific for Vα2 and Cα segments with integrated adapters and barcodes, provided by manufacturer. Before sequencing, consistency of samples was checked by 2D-F-SSCP analysis of PCR products from three aliquots of cDNA per each sample [36]. Only samples with three similar/identical profiles were considered without PCR bias and were used for further purification using Agencourt AMPure XP reagent (Beckman Coulter) and used for sequencing. FASTQ files with sequences were processed and analyzed using custom-written program in Pearl (ActivePearl, ActiveState Software Inc.). Sequences with quality score of CDR3α region above 27 were used for analysis. The length of CDR3α region was defined by counting from the third amino acid after the invariant C residue in all Vα regions (Y-L/F-C-A-X-first) to the amino acid immediately preceding common Jα motif (last-F-G-X-F-G-T).

Statistical analysis

The similarity, diversity and richness estimators were calculated using programs designed to measure biodiversity: EstimateS8.2 (Colwell, R. EstimateS: Biodiversity Estimation Software. Program and User's Guide at http://viceroy.eeb.uconn.edu/estimates) and SPADE (Chao, A. and Shen, T.-J. (2010) Program SPADE (Species Prediction And Diversity Estimation). Program and User's Guide published at http://chao.stat.nthu.edu.tw).

Results

Development of T cells in NOD^βTg and NOD^mini mice

We generated TCRβ transgenic mice, in which all T cells use the same TCRβ^Tg chain (Vβ14Dβ2Jβ2.6) and one of the endogenous TCRα chains. The TCRβ transgenic chain originated from I-A^b restricted TCR specific to Ep63 K peptide an analog of Eα 52–68 peptide in which the residue at position 63(I) was substituted with lysine [40]. To further reduce diversity of TCRs we used TCRα^mini transgenic construct, used previously to create TCR^mini mouse on B6 background (B6^mini) [36]. The TCRα^mini transgene allows a single Vα2.9 segment to rearrange to one of the two Jα (Jα26 and Jα2) segments. The generated transgenic mice were further crossed with TCRα^−/− mice to ensure that all

developing T cells use transgenic TCRα^mini locus. To track CD4^+ Foxp3^+ regulatory T (Treg) cells we crossed transgenic mice with NOD.Foxp3.EGFP/cre mice as described in methods. Final characteristics of mice used in this paper were NOD^mini (NOD.TCRα^mini.TCRβ^Tg.TCRα^−/−.Foxp3EGFP/cre), NOD^βTg (TCRβ^Tg.TCRα^+/−.Foxp3EGFP/cre) and NOD (NOD.Foxp3EGFP/cre).

In NOD^mini and NOD^βTg transgenic mice thymic development of T cells proceeds normally, and selection of single positive (SP) thymocytes is very efficient with bias toward CD4^+ T cells in the thymus and in the periphery, similarly to a previously reported bias on B6 background (Fig. 1A, 1B) [36]. TCRβ transgenic mice are characterized by allelic exclusion, resulting in all T cells to express only one transgenic TCRβ chain. It has been proposed that allelic exclusion in NOD mice is less efficient [27]. In our mice all SP thymocytes and peripheral T cells have exclusive expression of transgenic TCRβ^Tg chain (TCRVβ14) in both types of transgenic mice and exclusive expression of TCRα^mini transgene (TCRVα2) in NOD^mini mice (Fig. 1A, 1B). Also we did not observe emergence of the cells bearing TCRs with Vβ segments other than Vβ14 even in older mice. Furthermore, we observed lower percentages of Treg cells in thymii and periphery of transgenic mice as compared to NOD mice and the percentages correlated with diversities of TCRs in analyzed mice (Fig. 1C, 1E). Nevertheless, the total numbers of peripheral Treg cells were similar in all of analyzed mice and reduced percentages of Treg cells were due to more efficient selection of CD4^+ T cells, rather than diversity of TCRs, as we observed this correlation on B6 background and in other types of mice that differ by efficiency of CD4^+ T cells selection (Fig. 1C, 1E) [36,41]. Finally, to check whether this particular TCRVβ14 transgenic chain can impose an unusual restriction on the TCRα repertoire, we evaluated the frequency of individual Vα families. We found no bias in TCR repertoire as the frequency of Vα families usage by CD4^+Vβ14^+ T cells was similar between NOD and NOD^βTg mice (Fig. 1D).

Lack of T cells specific to insulin B:9–23 in NOD transgenic mice

To test development of diabetes we measured blood glucose levels in experimental mice. Surprisingly, neither NOD^βTg nor NOD^mini transgenic mice develop diabetes (Fig. 2A). Evaluation of H&E stained pancreatic sections showed lack of lymphocytic infiltrates in 25 week old transgenic mice, with only insignificant infiltrates found in a few sections of NOD^βTg mice (Fig. 2B). As a control we used non-transgenic littermates of NOD^βTg, NOD.TCRα^+/− mice. These mice developed diabetes and by 30 weeks of age more than 75% of females had high levels of blood glucose (Fig. 2A). One of the possibilities was that the lack of development of diabetes in transgenic mice is due to perturbed proportions of regulatory to effector T cell ratios, which could result in more efficient suppression of potentially diabetogenic T cells. We took advantage of cyclophosphamide treatment, which selectively affects numbers and function of Treg cells and accelerates development of diabetes in NOD mice [42,43]. This treatment however did not cause insulitis nor diabetes in transgenic mice indicating inability of effector T cells to initiate autoimmunity (unpublished data).

The onset of spontaneous diabetes in NOD mice is dependent upon presence of effector T cells specific to insulin B:9–23 antigen and lack of such specificity results in lack of early infiltrates into pancreatic islets [18]. As our mice did not develop islet-infiltrates, we tested their ability to respond to stimulation by insulin B:9–23 peptide (Fig. 3). CD4^+ T cells isolated from NOD^mini, NOD^βTg and NOD mice responded to stimulation by allogeneic spleno-

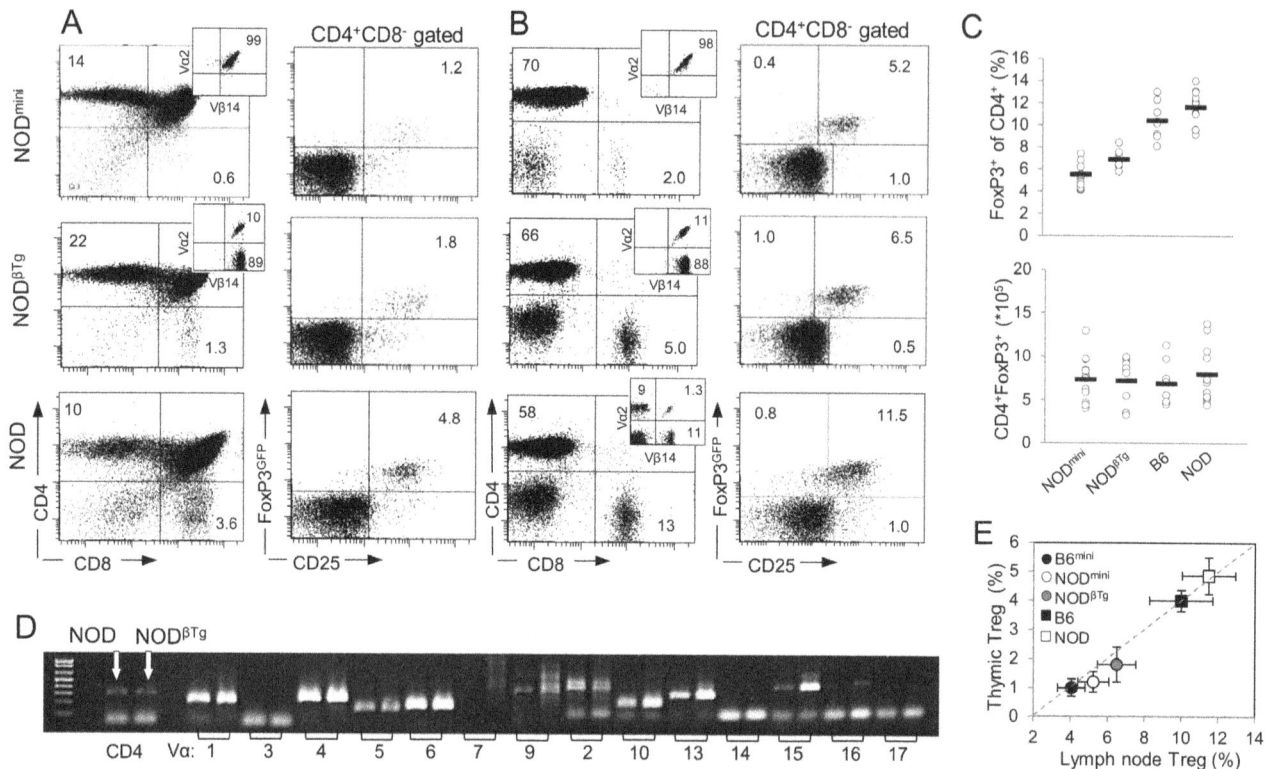

Figure 1. Efficient selection of CD4[+] T lymphocytes in NOD[mini] and NOD[βTg] mice. Lymphocytes isolated from thymii (A) and lymph nodes (B) of indicated mice were stained with monoclonal antibodies and analyzed by flow cytometry. Numbers in quadrants are representative percentages of at least six mice (6 week old) per group. The numbers of thymocytes and lymphocytes ± SD recovered from NOD[mini], NOD[βTg] and NOD mice were: from thymii $78.5 \pm 16.7 \times 10^6$, $72.05 \pm 13.8 \times 10^6$ and $70.1 \pm 14.0 \times 10^6$, and from lymph nodes (axillary, brachial and inguinal) $17.2 \pm 5.8 \times 10^6$, $14.1 \pm 2.5 \times 10^6$, and $13.2 \pm 3.0 \times 10^6$, respectively. (C) Percentages (top) and total numbers (bottom) of CD4[+]Foxp3[+] T cells in peripheral lymph nodes of 6 week old mice; each circle represents individual mouse. (D) Expression of mRNA of TCRVα genes in sorted CD4[+] T cells isolated from NOD and NOD[βTg] mice. Analysis was done by RT-PCR using primers specific to indicated Vα segments and Cα region. (E) Comparison of CD4[+]Foxp3[+] T (Treg) cells from thymii and peripheral lymph nodes of transgenic and wild type B6 and NOD mice. Mean percentage and SD of six young mice per group are shown.

cytes, however only CD4[+] T cells from immunized NOD mice were able to respond to B:9–23 peptide in the presence of syngeneic splenocytes (Fig. 3). As of note, B:9–23 peptide does not bind to I-A[b] molecule and in the presence of B6 splenocytes does not lead to CD4 T cell response [44]. We were also unable to generate B:9–23 specific T cell hybridomas from immunized NOD[mini] and NOD[βTg] mice, however we had no problem generating allo-specific T cell hybridomas from transgenic mice. These results showed that changes introduced by transgenic chains to the TCR repertoire in NOD mice resulted in lack of peripheral specificity to the key antigen required for onset of T1D.

Development of SS in NOD[βTg] and NOD[mini] mice

The lack of T1D in transgenic mice prompted us to test whether reduced TCR diversity will affect development of Sjögren's syndrome – secondary autoimmune disease in NOD mice. It is characterized by lymphocytic infiltrates into salivary and lacrimal glands, production of auto-antibodies and the loss of saliva and tear production by 20 weeks of age [5,45]. Histological evaluation of tissue sections of submandibular salivary and extraorbital lacrimal glands showed focal lymphocytic infiltrates, in both transgenic NOD[mini] and NOD[βTg] and parental NOD mice (Fig. 4). Similarly to the NOD mice, males of both transgenic mice had milder infiltration of salivary glands than females, while the infiltration of lacrimal glands was more prominent in male

NOD[βTg] and NOD[mini] mice. This infiltration is organ specific, as we did not detect infiltrates in lungs, kidney, liver, as well as sublingual and parotid salivary glands and harderian lacrimal glands of 20 week old transgenic mice, similarly to NOD mice (Fig. 4B). Of note, in some of 30 week old NOD[mini] females, but not NOD[βTg] mice, we noticed development of lymphoprolifera-tion, manifested by enlarged lymph nodes and spleen and infiltration into multiple organs (unpublished data). FACS analysis of lymphocytic infiltrates in affected exocrine glands showed that all of the infiltrating CD4[+] T cells expressed transgenic Vβ14 chain in NOD[βTg] mice and Vβ14/Vα2 transgenic chains in NOD[mini] mice (Fig. 4C). This also showed the aforementioned stability of expression of transgenic TCRs in experimental mice.

Development of SS in humans is often correlated with presence of anti-nuclear antibodies (ANA), anti-Ro/SSA, anti-La/SSB, anti-dsDNA, anti-αFodrin and anti-M3R [5,22,46]. In the NOD mouse model of SS, anti-SSA and anti-SSB auto-antibodies are rarely present and they are found at the very low levels [47]. To determine the presence of auto-antibodies in experimental mice, we used ELISA-based assay. For negative control, we used sera from NOD.TCRα[−/−] mice, that do not have T cells. As shown in Fig. 5, transgenic and parental NOD mice from 14–17 week old group had elevated levels of antibodies against αFodrin, ssDNA, dsDNA and ANA. Additionally, we determined the staining pattern of ANA auto-antibodies using immunofluorescent staining of HEp-2 cells (Fig. 5B). The majority (>90%) of NOD[mini] and

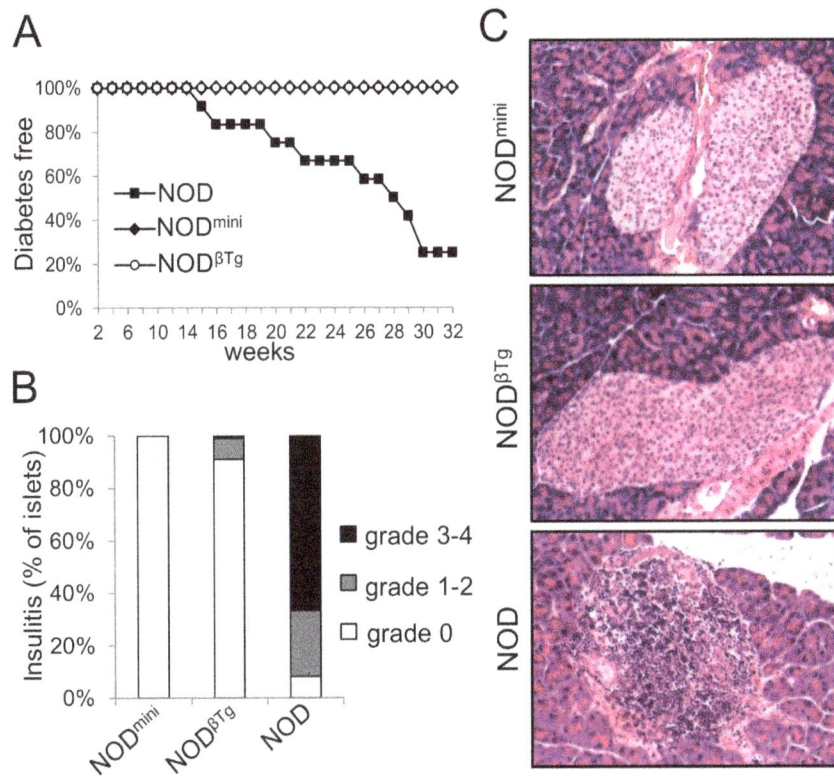

Figure 2. NOD$^{\beta Tg}$ and NOD^{mini} mice do not develop T1D. (A) Incidence of diabetes in mice shown as Kaplan–Meier survival curve. Mice with three consecutive measurements of blood glucose level above 250 mg/dL were considered diabetic. At least twelve mice per group were analyzed; $p<0.05$. (B) H&E staining of pancreatic tissue sections were analyzed for lymphocytic infiltrates and percentages of islets with grade of insulitis were counted. Insulitis was graded based on following criteria: no infiltrates – grade 0; peri-insulitis - grade 1; insulitis $<25\%$ - grade 2; insulitis $<50\%$ - grade 3; insulitis $>50\%$ - grade 4. At least six mice at 20 weeks of age were analyzed with the total number of 140 (NOD^{mini}), 155 (NOD$^{\beta Tg}$) and 160 (NOD) islets. (C) Example of H&E staining of pancreatic tissue sections of indicated mice at 20 weeks of age.

NOD$^{\beta Tg}$ mice tested had a speckled nuclear staining pattern, characteristic for SS development and found in parental NOD mice.

The onset of salivary gland dysfunction and presence of autoantibodies relies on B cells involvement and is dependent on IL-4 mediated IgM to IgG1 class switching [48–50]. Analysis of IgG1 concentration in sera of experimental mice revealed increased levels in older mice with the highest level in NOD^{mini} mice (Fig. 5C). This increase in IgG1 titer correlates with detection of auto-antibodies. Finally, to evaluate glandular dysfunction, we quantified secretion of saliva in 20 wks old mice. Both NOD$^{\beta Tg}$ and NOD^{mini} mice had reduced saliva flow as compared to healthy B6 mice and at the level of the reference parental NOD mice (Fig. 5D). Taken together, glandular infiltration, autoantibody production, and defective salivary secretion is diagnostic of Sjögren's syndrome in transgenic NOD$^{\beta Tg}$ and NOD^{mini} mice, similarly to the parental strain of NOD mice. Interestingly, the timing of infiltrates and levels of autoantibodies and total IgG1 production vary between analyzed mice, which differ only by TCR repertoire diversity.

Diversity of TCR repertoire on CD4$^+$ T cells in NOD^{mini} mice

Lack of certain specificities in NOD^{mini} TCR repertoire and the previously reported lower TCR diversity of thymic Treg cells on NOD background prompted us to take a closer look at the similarity and diversity of TCRα^{mini} repertoires. To determine the

influence of TCR diversity reduction on the selection efficiency of TCRs in NOD mice we started with a single cell analysis to compare to a previously analyzed similar model of TCR^{mini} transgenic mice on "healthy" C57BL/6 background (B6^{mini}) [36]. We compared the similarity between TCR sequences from single cell sorted T$_N$ (CD4$^+$Foxp3$^-$CD45RB$^+$CD62L$^+$) and Treg (CD4$^+$Foxp3$^+$) cells from thymii and peripheral lymph nodes of NOD^{mini} mice. As expected, based on the Morisita-Horn index, the highest similarity was observed between thymic and peripheral subsets of T$_N$ or Treg cells, whereas comparison between populations of T$_N$ and Treg cells showed mostly non-overlapping repertoires with values similar to those observed on B6 background (Fig. 6A and [36]). Previously we've shown that based on abundance coverage estimator (ACE), estimated richness (total unique CDR3α clonotypes in the population) of Treg cells in B6^{mini} mice significantly exceeded estimated richness of T$_N$ cells [36]. Although ACE underestimates true richness at low sample size, it accounts for "unseen sequences" based on low abundance data and is suitable for comparative analyses. We combined thymic and peripheral sequences for each population and calculated the ACE index, based on 578 DNA sequences per subset. The ACE values for T$_N$ and Treg cells were respectively 1187 and 994 for NOD^{mini} mice, and 1184 and 1815 for B6^{mini} mice. Interestingly, estimated ACE value for TCRs on T$_N$ cells from NOD^{mini} mice was comparable to the ACE value for TCRs on T$_N$ cells from B6^{mini} mice. However when we compared the ratio of ACE values for Treg cells between NOD^{mini} and B6^{mini}

A

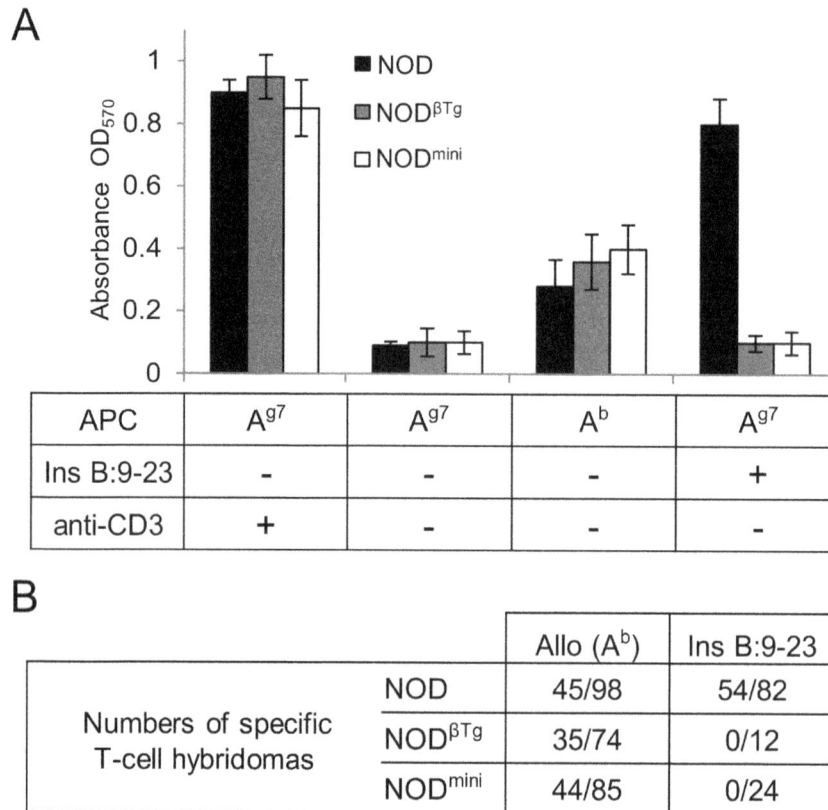

APC	A^{g7}	A^{g7}	A^{b}	A^{g7}
Ins B:9–23	-	-	-	+
anti-CD3	+	-	-	-

B

Numbers of specific T-cell hybridomas		Allo (A^{b})	Ins B:9–23
	NOD	45/98	54/82
	NOD$^{\beta Tg}$	35/74	0/12
	NOD^{mini}	44/85	0/24

Figure 3. Lack of response to insulin B:9–23 peptide in transgenic NOD mice. (A) 5×10^4 of CD4$^+$ T cells sorted from lymph nodes of NOD, NOD$^{\beta Tg}$ and NOD^{mini} mice were cultured in the presence of 5×10^5 splenocytes from NOD.TCR$\alpha^{-/-}$ (A^{g7}) or B6.TCR$\alpha^{-/-}$ (A^{b}) mice and soluble anti-CD3 (1 μg/ml) or insulin B:9–23 peptide (50 μg/ml), as indicated. Proliferation of cells was measured after 3 days by MTT assay [38]. Experiments were done twice with 3 mice per group. (B) T-cell hybridomas specific to allo-antigens or insulin B:9–23 peptide were generated from indicated mice. For generation of B:9–23 specific hybridomas, mice were immunized with the peptide 7 days prior to isolation of lymph nodes for *in vitro* blasts generation [38]. Generated hybridomas were tested for their ability to respond to syngeneic (NOD.TCR$\alpha^{-/-}$) or allogeneic (B6.TCR$\alpha^{-/-}$) splenocytes with or without B:9–23 peptide or anti-CD3. Table shows numbers of identified hybridomas specific to indicated antigens and numbers of hybridomas responding to anti-CD3 stimulation. Table is representative of 3 independent experiments with two mice per group.

mice the number of possible unique TCRs on NOD background was reduced by almost 50% (Fig. 6B).

Previously it has been reported that based on analysis of two selected VJ (TCRα) or one VDJ (TVRβ) rearrangements in wild type mice, TCR repertoire of Treg cells in NOD mice was less diverse as compared to conventional T cells in the thymus, but also less diverse in the thymus of B6 mice [9]. These differences were observed based on calculation of Shannon entropy and normalization to the logarithm of unique sequences [9]. Such transformation is a measure of distribution of frequency of individual species and is a good measure of relative evenness of assemblage [51,52]. Together with richness, evenness is a descriptive measure of diversity not the diversity *per se* [51]. Therefore, as explained by Jost, to put the estimates in perspective, we converted Shannon entropy (diversity index) to "true diversity" by calculating "numbers equivalent" also called "effective number of species" (ENS), to preserve linear scale of comparison [51,53]. The ENS measure represents diversity of a particular sample, and the numeric value represents the theoretical number of equally common unique sequences in the assemblage. Comparison of "true diversity" between B6^{mini} and NOD^{mini} mice showed almost reversal of ratios of diversities between TCRs on T$_N$ and Treg cells, with the differences more profound in the thymus than in the periphery (Fig. 6C). These differences in NOD^{mini} mice were confirmed by high throughput sequencing, and were consistent

regardless of total numbers of sequences analyzed (Fig. 6C, D). Lower diversity of Treg TCR repertoire was visualized empirically by plotting accumulation curves of observed sequences from peripheral T$_N$ and Treg cells (Fig. 6E). These curves show that accumulation of unique CDR3 regions from the first 120 thousands of sequences for each population gives twice as many unique DNA clonotypes in T$_N$ (9757) as compared to Treg cells (4968). This ratio is reversed in comparison to accumulation curves observed in B6^{mini} mice [36]. Collectively our data show that although TCR diversity on Treg cells in NOD^{mini} mice is reduced, conventional T cells retain diverse TCR repertoire at least at the levels found on B6 background.

Discussion

In this study we investigated the impact of the reduction of TCR diversity on the development of two autoimmune diseases in NOD mice; T1D and SS. Previously it has been shown that T1D can develop despite use of transgenic TCRβ chains or reduction of precursor frequency of potentially diabetogenic T cell clones. In our model overall diversity of TCRs was reduced by allelic exclusion caused by use of transgenic TCRβ chain that was not only pathogenically irrelevant, but also was originally selected in B6 mice on I-A^{b} molecule. Despite normal distribution of Vα families in NOD$^{\beta Tg}$ mice, neither insulitis nor diabetes developed.

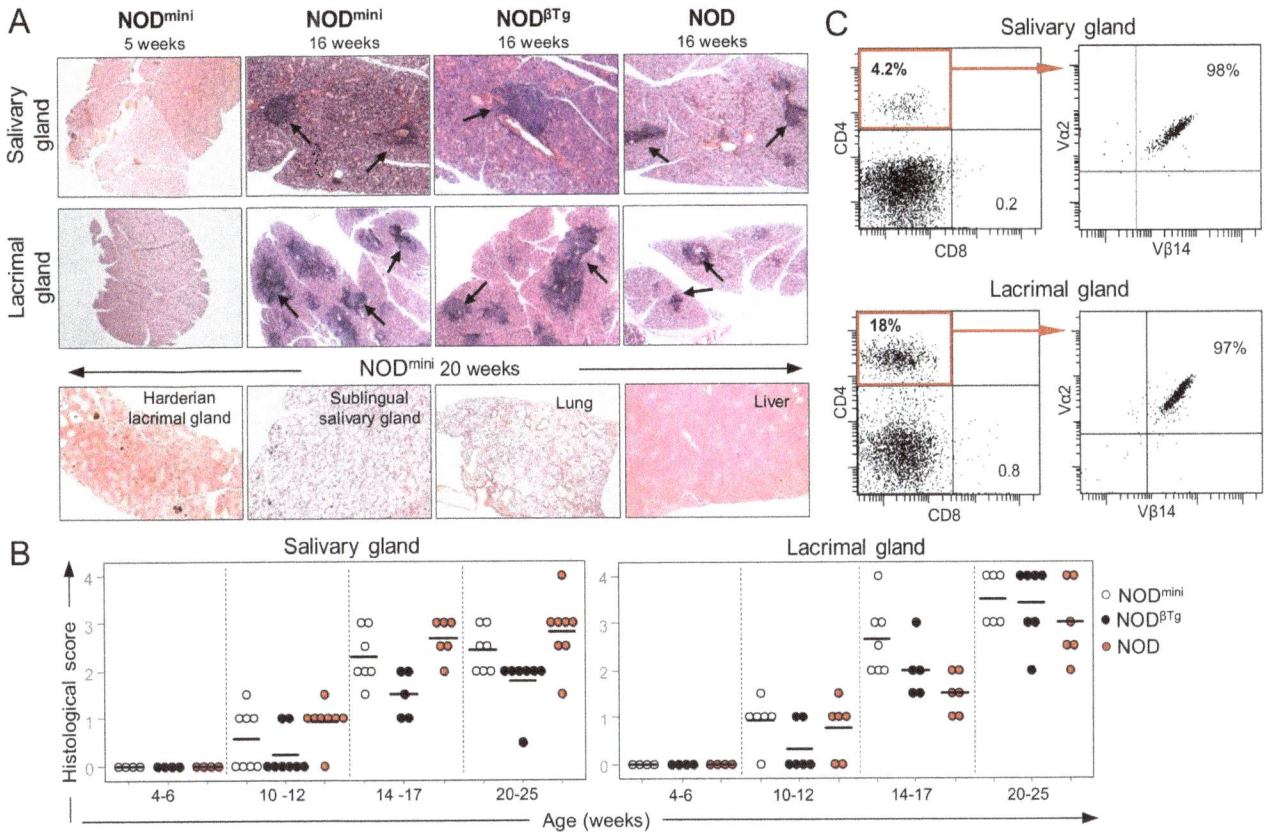

Figure 4. Lymphocytic infiltrates in mandibular salivary and extraorbital lacrimal glands. (A) H&E staining of tissue sections from indicated organs of analyzed mice, showing lymphocytic infiltrates indicated by arrows. (B) Histological score of infiltrated glands in indicated age groups. Scoring criteria: score 0, no infiltrates; score 1–1.5, 1–2 foci per section; score 2–2.5, 3–5 foci per section; score 3, 6–10 foci per section; score 4, more than 10 foci per section. Infiltrate is considered as focus when number of infiltrating cells in continuous space is greater than 50. Three sections at different anatomical locations per organ were analyzed with at least 5 mice per age group. (C) FACS analysis of CD4 T cells infiltrating into salivary and lacrimal glands in 16 week old NOD^{mini} mice. Dot plots on the right show expression of transgenic TCR on CD4$^+$ gated cells.

Conversely, these mice developed infiltrates in salivary and lacrimal glands, leading to autoantibody production and exocrine gland dysfunction. Further reduction of TCR diversity by generation of transgenic mice with TCR^{mini} repertoire, where one Vα segment is allowed to rearrange to only two Jα segments, did not prevent development of SS. Our results indicate that the difference between T1D and SS regarding the dependence on MHC polymorphism is directly correlated to the magnitude of possible TCR/peptide/MHCII interactions participating in the autoimmune phase of the disease.

We show that the lack of development of diabetes or even insulitis in our NOD^{βTg} or NOD^{mini} transgenic mice is due to lack of specificity to the key immunodominant insulin B:9–23 peptide, which is known to be instrumental for the onset of the T1D in NOD mice. The use of transgenic TCRVβ14 chain in our mice did not dramatically influence the ability of its binding to different TCRα chains, as T cells from NOD^{βTg} mice use all Vα families with frequencies found in NOD mice (Fig. 1). This includes efficient amplification of the Vα13 family which contains TRAV5D-4 chain (Vα13s1) that was shown to be sufficient to elicit anti-insulin autoimmunity without bias toward particular Vβ family of TCRβ chain partners [28,54]. Moreover, previous studies show that T cells using Vβ14 family were found on T cells specific to insulin antigen, T cells expanding in pancreatic lymph nodes or in T cells infiltrating pancreatic islets, showing that the Vβ14 family is not negatively influencing the development of

diabetogenic TCRs [55–58]. One cannot exclude the possibility that this particular transgenic TCRVβ14 chain may be unable to pair with appropriate TCRα chain, preventing the ability of the expressed αβTCR to recognize the B:9–23 peptide. This selective requirement for a TCRβ chain would reinforce our observation that development of SS is less dependent than development of T1D on overall TCR diversity and a particular peptide/MHC combination.

Development of T1D relies on different insulin B:9–23 register recognition, allowing escape of specific T cells due to register shifting [11–13]. The lack of peripheral recognition of insulin B:9–23 in our transgenic mice can also be due to the impact of the limited TCR repertoire. Reduction of overall TCR diversity can influence (reduce) the precursor frequency of DP thymocytes bearing potentially autoreactive TCRs, resulting in more efficient negative selection in the thymus of NOD mice. It has been shown that early expression of transgenic αβTCR, due to ERK1/2 defect on NOD background results in greater commitment of the DN thymocytes to αβ lineage "overcrowding" DP compartment [8]. Our TCRα^{mini} transgene has natural timing of expression, similar to B6^{mini} and polyclonal NOD mice, where pre-TCR signaling is not perturbed by early expression of the transgene [36]. As suggested by Mingueneau et. al., in the polyclonal repertoire on the NOD background, the ERK1/2 defect increases the affinity threshold of positive selection, shifting the selection window of thymocytes toward self-reactivity, however not impacting the

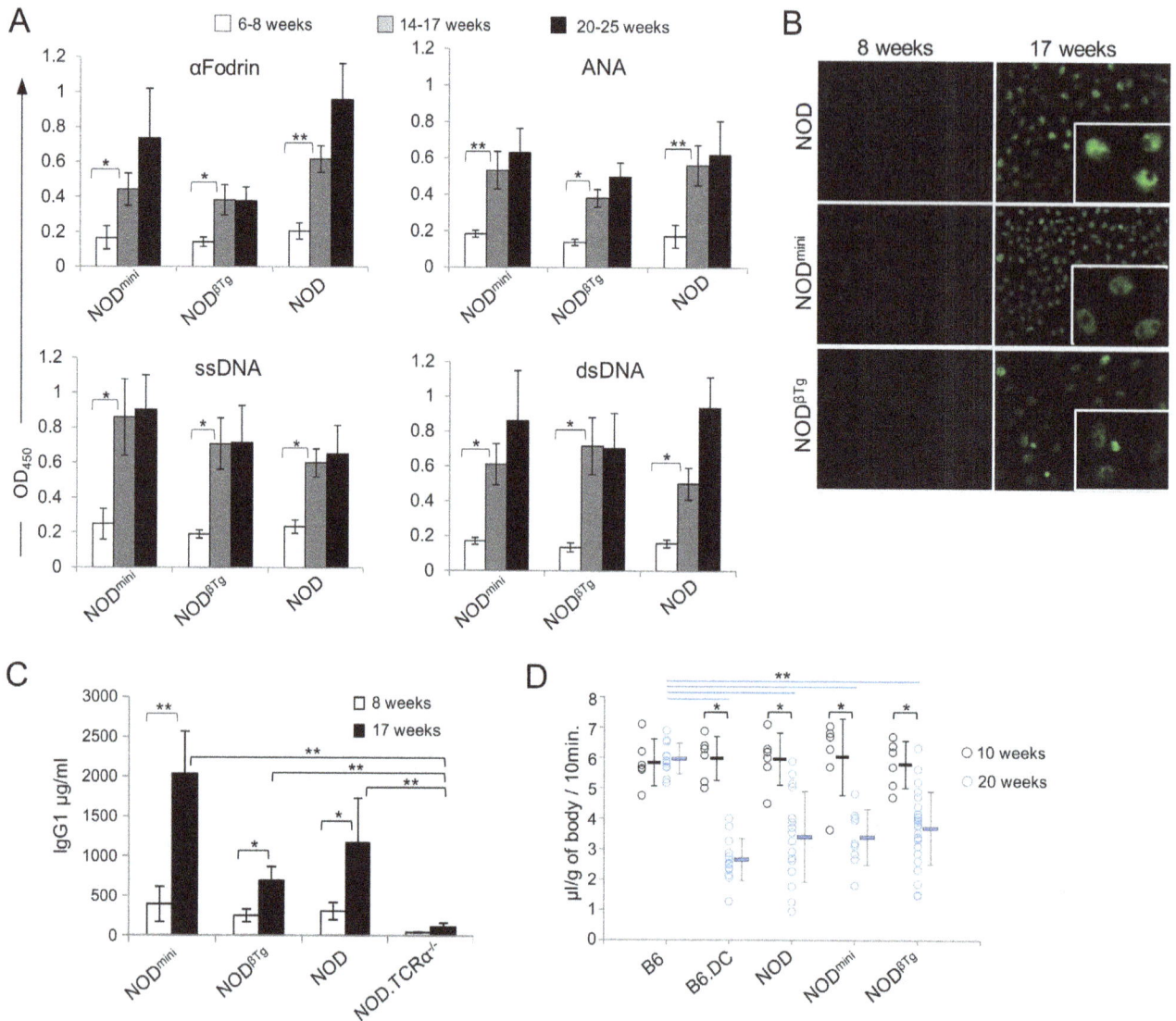

Figure 5. Detection of autoantibodies and hyposalivation in NOD^{mini} and NOD$^{\beta Tg}$ mice. (A) ELISA assay was performed using mouse serum (1:100) from indicated age groups. Each graph represents mean value of OD$_{450}$ and standard deviation for indicated antigens. At least six mice were used per each group. *$p<0.05$, **$p<0.005$. (B) Detection of ANAs pattern using Hep-2 cell line. Sera from mice were diluted 1:40, incubated with HEp-2-fixed slides and evaluated under fluorescent microscope at x20 magnifications. Representative images are shown. (C) Quantitative ELISA analysis of IgG1 levels in sera (1:50,000) from indicated mice. Each bar represents mean value and standard deviation from six mice per experimental groups. (D) Salivary flow rates after pilocarpine injection in indicated mice at 10 and 20 wks of age. Double congenic B6.NODIdd3.NODIdd5 (B6.DC) mice, that develop SS on B6 genetic background, were used as a control. Saliva volume was measured and calculated in mg per mouse body mass. Each circle represents one mouse and horizontal lines indicate mean values of the experimental groups. T-test was used to calculate differences between groups. *$p<0.002$, **$p<0.0002$.

efficiency of negative selection. This results in higher overall self-reactivity of peripheral effector T cells and possibly explains lower diversity of thymic Treg cells on NOD background [8,9]. Considering partial overlap of specificities between Treg and autoreactive T cells, one could suggest similar effect of lower diversity on autoreactive population. However weak and unstable peptide-binding property of I-A^{g7} molecule does not favor the elimination or inactivation of autoreactive T cells [59]. This instability may have additional influence on "a leak" of autoreactive T cells, but also on inefficient generation of Treg population, which may require longer or stronger interactions with self MHC/peptide complexes [60,61]. Therefore the shift in selection window will not impact autoreactive T cells as much as it

will impact Treg cells, after all, Treg development relies on recognition of self-peptide/MHCII complexes in the thymus, whereas thymic escape of autoreactive T cells relies on avoidance of such complexes during negative selection. It is possible that in our model, we reached the threshold of diversity required to generate autoreactive TCR repertoire without "holes" in specificities. Therefore despite reduced TCR diversity of Treg cells mice do not develop diabetes and we were unable to detect insulin B:9–23 specific T cells in the periphery. Similarly, the comparison of TCR^{mini} repertoires between B6 and NOD backgrounds shows minimal impact of the NOD genotype on TCR diversity of conventional CD4$^+$ T cells however it substantially reduces the TCR diversity on Treg cells in NOD mice.

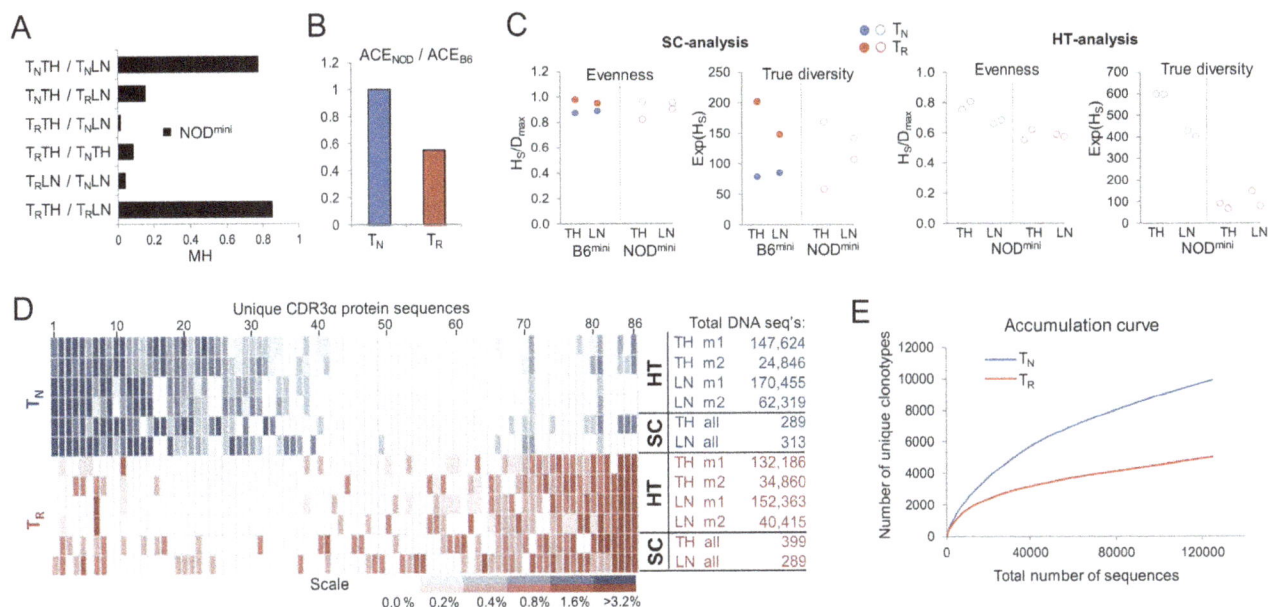

Figure 6. TCR repertoire of naïve and regulatory T cells in NOD^mini mice. (A) Similarity between indicated populations (first 289 single cell sequences per each population) was estimated based on Morisita-Horn index (MH). T_N - naïve CD4+Foxp3−CD45RB+CD62L+ T cells, T_R - regulatory CD4+Foxp3+ T cells, TH - thymus, LN - lymph nodes. (B) Ratio of richness of TCRs on T_N and T_R cells between NOD^mini and B6^mini mice. Abundance coverage estimator (ACE) was calculated based on 578 sequences for each population combined from thymus and peripheral lymph nodes. (C) Evenness and effective number of species (ENS) for analyzed TCR repertoires. Shannon evenness index was calculated as Shannon entropy (H_s) divided by maximum diversity D_{max}, where D_{max} equals natural logarithm of number of unique sequences in analyzed population. ENS (true diversity) was calculated as exponential of Shannon entropy. (D) Comparison of frequency of 20 most dominant unique protein CDR3 clonotypes found in each population indicated on the right of the heat map. Table indicates analyzed populations from lymph nodes and thymii by single cell analysis (SC) and high throughput sequencing (HT). Experimental mouse 1 and 2 are marked as m1 and m2. Numbers next to each population indicate total numbers of DNA sequences analyzed. All 86 unique CDR3α protein sequences in the heat map are shown in Table S1. (E) Accumulation curve of unique DNA clonotypes observed after accumulation of 124,730 sequences for T_N cells and 124,696 for T_R cells. (A–C) All indices were computed based on DNA sequences for each population using software SPADE and EstimateS8.2.

Development of SS in NOD^mini mice is especially interesting, since CD4+ T cells are instrumental in immunopathogenesis and their recognition of self antigens is essential for the onset and progression of the disease [34,62]. It shows that the TCR^mini repertoire is diverse enough not only to drive glandular infiltration and activation of the CD4+ T cells but also the repertoire is still diverse enough to support the full development of the disease with production of Th2-dependent IgG1 pathogenic autoantibodies (Fig. 5C) [50]. Moreover, we noticed differences in timing of infiltrates, levels of autoantibodies and total IgG1 production between transgenic mice and parental NOD mice, which indicates different frequencies of certain TCR specificities between mice. In congenic strains of NOD mice models of SS (NOD.B10-H2^b, NOD.H2^p, NOD.H2^q, NOD.H2^h4) replacement of I-A^g7 with other MHC molecules does not prevent salivary and lacrimal gland infiltration and decreased saliva and tear production [16,48,63]. Interestingly, in NOD.H2^h4, contrary to the parental NOD strain, there is a high frequency of ANA with a high proportion of SSA/Ro and SSB/La observed [63]. Also, NOD.H2^q mice exhibit increased production of lupus-like types of autoantibodies and develop nephritis, as compared to NOD and NOD.H2^p mice [16]. This weak dependence of SS on a particular MHC haplotype in NOD mice correlates with our data that show development of SS despite limited TCR diversity. In human studies it was suggested that production profiles of certain autoantibodies were associated with HLA-DR haplotypes rather than with clinical manifestations [64], however studies of familial inheritance in patients with SS showed a linkage between particular HLA and disease susceptibility [65,66]. The most

recent comprehensive analysis by Sjögren's Genetics Network showed that HLA has the strongest linkage to the SS, although it is not on the level of T1D [17]. Certain HLA haplotypes will influence binding diversity of self or environmental peptides and the nature of antigen presentation to T cells during thymic development or during immune responses in the periphery. Our results from the mouse model emphasize that SS may be less affected by requirement of a unique key antigen/MHCII combination but rather may be more influenced by a wider range of overall TCR/peptide/MHC interactions involved in the onset/progression of the disease. It can be due to a combination of cross-reactivity of the TCR repertoire on SS-specific T cells, wider range of antigens presented by MHCII molecules, higher peripheral self-reactivity of effector T cells, increased tissue expression of MHCII complexes on salivary epithelial cells and de novo expression or post-translational modification of self-antigens [67–69].

Acknowledgments

Cell sorting was performed by Jeanene Pihkala in the GRU FACS Core, the sequencing was performed by John Nechtman in the GRU Genomic Core, and transgenic mice were generated by Gabriela Pacholczyk in the GRU Transgenic Core.

Author Contributions

Conceived and designed the experiments: JK RP. Performed the experiments: JK RD SL MB. Analyzed the data: JK RD SL MB RP. Contributed to the writing of the manuscript: JK RP.

References

1. Chaparro RJ, Dilorenzo TP (2010) An update on the use of NOD mice to study autoimmune (Type 1) diabetes. Expert Rev Clin Immunol 6: 939–955.
2. Lavoie TN, Lee BH, Nguyen CQ (2011) Current concepts: mouse models of Sjogren's syndrome. J Biomed Biotechnol 2011: 549107.
3. Anderson MS, Bluestone JA (2005) The NOD Mouse: A Model of Immune Dysregulation. Annu Rev Immunol 23: 447–485.
4. Mathis D, Vence L, Benoist C (2001) beta-Cell death during progression to diabetes. Nature 414: 792–798.
5. Nguyen CQ, Peck AB (2009) Unraveling the pathophysiology of Sjogren syndrome-associated dry eye disease. Ocul Surf 7: 11–27.
6. Fox RI (2005) Sjogren's syndrome. Lancet 366: 321–331.
7. Kishimoto H, Sprent J (2001) A defect in central tolerance in NOD mice. Nat Immunol 2: 1025–1031.
8. Mingueneau M, Jiang W, Feuerer M, Mathis D, Benoist C (2012) Thymic negative selection is functional in NOD mice. J Exp Med 209: 623–637.
9. Ferreira C, Singh Y, Furmanski AL, Wong FS, Garden OA, et al. (2009) Non-obese diabetic mice select a low-diversity repertoire of natural regulatory T cells. Proc Natl Acad Sci U S A 106: 8320–8325.
10. D'Alise AM, Auyeung V, Feuerer M, Nishio J, Fontenot J, et al. (2008) The defect in T-cell regulation in NOD mice is an effect on the T-cell effectors. Proceedings of the National Academy of Sciences 105: 19857–19862.
11. Stadinski BD, Zhang L, Crawford F, Marrack P, Eisenbarth GS, et al. (2010) Diabetogenic T cells recognize insulin bound to IAg7 in an unexpected, weakly binding register. Proceedings of the National Academy of Sciences 107: 10978–10983.
12. Mohan JF, Petzold SJ, Unanue ER (2011) Register shifting of an insulin peptide–MHC complex allows diabetogenic T cells to escape thymic deletion. J Exp Med 208: 2375–2383.
13. Marrack P, Kappler JW (2012) Do MHCII-Presented Neoantigens Drive Type 1 Diabetes and Other Autoimmune Diseases? Cold Spring Harbor Perspectives in Medicine 2.
14. Wicker LS, Appel MC, Dotta F, Pressey A, Miller BJ, et al. (1992) Autoimmune syndromes in major histocompatibility complex (MHC) congenic strains of nonobese diabetic (NOD) mice. The NOD MHC is dominant for insulitis and cyclophosphamide-induced diabetes. J Exp Med 176: 67–77.
15. Li X, Golden J, Faustman DL (1993) Faulty major histocompatibility complex class II I-E expression is associated with autoimmunity in diverse strains of mice. Autoantibodies, insulitis, and sialadenitis. Diabetes 42: 1166–1172.
16. Lindqvist AKB, Nakken B, Sundler M, Kjellen P, Jonsson R, et al. (2005) Influence on Spontaneous Tissue Inflammation by the Major Histocompatibility Complex Region in the Nonobese Diabetic Mouse. Scand J Immunol 61: 119–127.
17. Lessard CJ, Li H, Adrianto I, Ice JA, Rasmussen A, et al. (2013) Variants at multiple loci implicated in both innate and adaptive immune responses are associated with Sjogren's syndrome. Nat Genet 45: 1284–1292.
18. Nakayama M, Abiru N, Moriyama H, Babaya N, Liu E, et al. (2005) Prime role for an insulin epitope in the development of type[thinsp]1 diabetes in NOD mice. Nature 435: 220–223.
19. Arakaki R, Ishimaru N, Saito I, Kobayashi M, Yasui N, et al. (2003) Development of autoimmune exocrinopathy resembling Sjögren's syndrome in adoptively transferred mice with autoreactive CD4+ T cells. Arthritis Rheum 48: 3603–3609.
20. Takada K, Takiguchi M, Konno A, Inaba M (2005) Autoimmunity against a tissue kallikrein in IQI/Jic Mice: a model for Sjogren's syndrome. J Biol Chem 280: 3982–3988.
21. Winer S, Astsaturov I, Cheung R, Tsui H, Song A, et al. (2002) Primary Sjögren's syndrome and deficiency of ICA69. Lancet 360: 1063–1069.
22. Haneji N, Nakamura T, Takio K, Yanagi K, Higashiyama H, et al. (1997) Identification of alpha-fodrin as a candidate autoantigen in primary Sjogren's syndrome. Science 276: 604–607.
23. Naito Y, Matsumoto I, Wakamatsu E, Goto D, Ito S, et al. (2006) Altered peptide ligands regulate muscarinic acetylcholine receptor reactive T cells of patients with Sjogren's syndrome. Ann Rheum Dis 65: 269–271.
24. Matsumoto I, Maeda T, Takemoto Y, Hashimoto Y, Kimura F, et al. (1999) Alpha-amylase functions as a salivary gland-specific self T cell epitope in patients with Sjogren's syndrome. Int J Mol Med 3: 485–490.
25. Iizuka M, Wakamatsu E, Tsuboi H, Nakamura Y, Hayashi T, et al. (2010) Pathogenic role of immune response to M3 muscarinic acetylcholine receptor in Sjogren's syndrome-like sialoadenitis. J Autoimmun 35: 383–389.
26. Lipes MA, Rosenzweig A, Tan KN, Tanigawa G, Ladd D, et al. (1993) Progression to diabetes in nonobese diabetic (NOD) mice with transgenic T cell receptors. Science 259: 1165–1169.
27. Serreze DV, Johnson EA, Chapman HD, Graser RT, Marron MP, et al. (2001) Autoreactive diabetogenic T-cells in NOD mice can efficiently expand from a greatly reduced precursor pool. Diabetes 50: 1992–2000.
28. Zhang L, Jasinski JM, Kobayashi M, Davenport B, Johnson K, et al. (2009) Analysis of T cell receptor beta chains that combine with dominant conserved TRAV5D-4*04 anti-insulin B: 9–23 alpha chains. J Autoimmun 33: 42–49.
29. Dwyer E, Itescu S, Winchester R (1993) Characterization of the primary structure of T cell receptor beta chains in cells infiltrating the salivary gland in the sicca syndrome of HIV-1 infection. Evidence of antigen-driven clonal selection suggested by restricted combinations of V beta J beta gene segment usage and shared somatically encoded amino acid residues. J Clin Invest 92: 495–502.
30. Matsumoto I, Okada S, Kuroda K, Iwamoto I, Saito Y, et al. (1999) Single cell analysis of T cells infiltrating labial salivary glands from patients with Sjogren's syndrome. Int J Mol Med 4: 519–527.
31. Pivetta B, De Vita S, Ferraccioli G, De RV, Gloghini A, et al. (1999) T cell receptor repertoire in B cell lymphoproliferative lesions in primary Sjogren's syndrome. J Rheumatol 26: 1101–1109.
32. Sumida T, Yonaha F, Maeda T, Tanabe E, Koike T, et al. (1992) T cell receptor repertoire of infiltrating T cells in lips of Sjogren's syndrome patients. J Clin Invest 89: 681–685.
33. Yonaha F, Sumida T, Maeda T, Tomioka H, Koike T, et al. (1992) Restricted junctional usage of T cell receptor V beta 2 and V beta 13 genes, which are overrepresented on infiltrating T cells in the lips of patients with Sjogren's syndrome. Arthritis Rheum 35: 1362–1367.
34. Singh N, Cohen PL (2012) The T cell in Sjogren's syndrome: Force majeure, not spectateur. J Autoimmun 39: 229–233.
35. Sumida T, Tsuboi H, Iizuka M, Hirota T, Asashima H, et al. (2014) The role of M3 muscarinic acetylcholine receptor reactive T cells in Sjögren's syndrome: A critical review. J Autoimmun.
36. Pacholczyk R, Ignatowicz H, Kraj P, Ignatowicz L (2006) Origin and T cell receptor diversity of Foxp3+CD4+CD25+ T cells. Immunity 25: 249–259.
37. Cha S, Nagashima H, Brown VB, Peck AB, Humphreys-Beher MG (2002) Two NOD Idd-associated intervals contribute synergistically to the development of autoimmune exocrinopathy (Sjogren's syndrome) on a healthy murine background. Arthritis Rheum 46: 1390–1398.
38. Pacholczyk R, Kern J, Singh N, Iwashima M, Kraj P, et al. (2007) Nonself-antigens are the cognate specificities of Foxp3+ regulatory T cells. Immunity 27: 493–504.
39. Kisielow J, Tortola L, Weber J, Karjalainen K, Kopf M (2011) Evidence for the divergence of innate and adaptive T-cell precursors before commitment to the alphabeta and gammadelta lineages. Blood 118: 6591–6600.
40. Kraj P, Pacholczyk R, Ignatowicz L (2001) Alpha beta TCRs differ in the degree of their specificity for the positively selecting MHC/peptide ligand. J Immunol 166: 2251–2259.
41. Pacholczyk R, Kraj P, Ignatowicz L (2002) Peptide specificity of thymic selection of CD4+CD25+ T cells. J Immunol 168: 613–620.
42. Lutsiak MEC, Semnani RT, De Pascalis R, Kashmiri SVS, Schlom J, et al. (2005) Inhibition of CD4+25+ T regulatory cell function implicated in enhanced immune response by low-dose cyclophosphamide. Blood 105: 2862–2868.
43. Harada M, Makino S (1984) Promotion of spontaneous diabetes in non-obese diabetes-prone mice by cyclophosphamide. Diabetologia 27: 604–606.
44. Michels AW, Ostrov DA, Zhang L, Nakayama M, Fuse M, et al. (2011) Structure-Based Selection of Small Molecules To Alter Allele-Specific MHC Class II Antigen Presentation. The Journal of Immunology 187: 5921–5930.
45. Cha S, Peck AB, Humphreys-Beher MG (2002) Progress in understanding autoimmune exocrinopathy using the non-obese diabetic mouse: an update. Crit Rev Oral Biol Med 13: 5–16.
46. Atkinson JC, Travis WD, Slocum L, Ebbs WL, Fox PC (1992) Serum anti-SS-B/La and IgA rheumatoid factor are markers of salivary gland disease activity in primary Sjogren's syndrome. Arthritis Rheum 35: 1368–1372.
47. Skarstein K, Wahren M, Zaura E, Hattori M, Jonsson R (1995) Characterization of T cell receptor repertoire and anti-Ro/SSA autoantibodies in relation to sialadenitis of NOD mice. Autoimmunity 22: 9–16.
48. Robinson CP, Yamachika S, Bounous DI, Brayer J, Jonsson R, et al. (1998) A novel NOD-derived murine model of primary Sjogren's syndrome. Arthritis Rheum 41: 150–156.
49. Brayer JB, Cha S, Nagashima H, Yasunari U, Lindberg A, et al. (2001) IL-4-dependent effector phase in autoimmune exocrinopathy as defined by the NOD.IL-4-gene knockout mouse model of Sjogren's syndrome. Scand J Immunol 54: 133–140.
50. Gao J, Killedar S, Cornelius JG, Nguyen C, Cha S, et al. (2006) Sjogren's syndrome in the NOD mouse model is an interleukin-4 time-dependent, antibody isotype-specific autoimmune disease. J Autoimmun 26: 90–103.
51. Jost L (2010) The Relation between Evenness and Diversity. Diversity 2: 207–232.
52. Pielou EC (1966) The measurement of diversity in different types of biological collections. J Theor Biol 13: 131–144.

53. Adelman MA (1969) Comment on the H Concentration Measure as a Numbers-Equivalent. The Review of Economics and Statistics 51: 99–101.

54. Nakayama M, Castoe T, Sosinowski T, He X, Johnson K, et al. (2012) Germline TRAV5D-4 T-Cell Receptor Sequence Targets a Primary Insulin Peptide of NOD Mice. Diabetes 61: 857–865.

55. Simone E, Daniel D, Schloot N, Gottlieb P, Babu S, et al. (1997) T cell receptor restriction of diabetogenic autoimmune NOD T cells. Proceedings of the National Academy of Sciences 94: 2518–2521.

56. Baker FJ, Lee M, Chien Y-h, Davis MM (2002) Restricted islet-cell reactive T cell repertoire of early pancreatic islet infiltrates in NOD mice. Proceedings of the National Academy of Sciences 99: 9374–9379.

57. Marrero I, Hamm DE, Davies JD (2013) High-Throughput Sequencing of Islet-Infiltrating Memory CD4$^+$ T Cells Reveals a Similar Pattern of TCR Vβ Usage in Prediabetic and Diabetic NOD Mice. PLoS ONE 8: e76546.

58. Petrovc Berglund J, Mariotti-Ferrandiz E, Rosmaraki E, Hall H, Cazenave P-A, et al. (2008) TCR repertoire dynamics in the pancreatic lymph nodes of non-obese diabetic (NOD) mice at the time of disease initiation. Mol Immunol 45: 3059–3064.

59. Carrasco-Marin E, Shimizu J, Kanagawa O, Unanue ER (1996) The class II MHC I-Ag7 molecules from non-obese diabetic mice are poor peptide binders. J Immunol 156: 450–458.

60. Aschenbrenner K, D'Cruz LM, Vollmann EH, Hinterberger M, Emmerich J, et al. (2007) Selection of Foxp3+ regulatory T cells specific for self antigen expressed and presented by Aire+ medullary thymic epithelial cells. Nat Immunol 8: 351–358.

61. Fontenot JD, Rasmussen JP, Williams LM, Dooley JL, Farr AG, et al. (2005) Regulatory T cell lineage specification by the forkhead transcription factor foxp3. Immunity 22: 329–341.

62. Sumida T, Tsuboi H, Iizuka M, Nakamura Y, Matsumoto I (2010) Functional role of M3 muscarinic acetylcholine receptor (M3R) reactive T cells and anti-M3R autoantibodies in patients with Sjögren's syndrome. Autoimmunity Reviews 9: 615–617.

63. Burek CL, Talor MV, Sharma RB, Rose NR (2007) The NOD.H2h4 mouse shows characteristics of human Sjögren's Syndrome. J Immunol 178: S232–S223d.

64. Gottenberg JE, Busson M, Loiseau P, Cohen-Solal J, Lepage V, et al. (2003) In primary Sjögren's syndrome, HLA class II is associated exclusively with autoantibody production and spreading of the autoimmune response. Arthritis Rheum 48: 2240–2245.

65. Fox RI, Kang HI (1992) Pathogenesis of Sjögren's syndrome. RheumDisClinNorth Am 18: 517–538.

66. Manoussakis MN, Georgopoulou C, Zintzaras E, Spyropoulou M, Stavropoulou A, et al. (2004) Sjögren's syndrome associated with systemic lupus erythematosus: clinical and laboratory profiles and comparison with primary Sjogren's syndrome. Arthritis Rheum 50: 882–891.

67. Anderton SM (2004) Post-translational modifications of self antigens: implications for autoimmunity. Curr Opin Immunol 16: 753–758.

68. Engelhard VH, Altrich-Vanlith M, Ostankovitch M, Zarling AL (2006) Post-translational modifications of naturally processed MHC-binding epitopes. Curr Opin Immunol 18: 92–97.

69. Moutsopoulos HM, Hooks JJ, Chan CC, Dalavanga YA, Skopouli FN, et al. (1986) HLA-DR expression by labial minor salivary gland tissues in Sjögren's syndrome. Ann Rheum Dis 45: 677–683.

9

Vaccine-Induced Protection of Rhesus Macaques against Plasma Viremia after Intradermal Infection with a European Lineage 1 Strain of West Nile Virus

Babs E. Verstrepen[1], Herman Oostermeijer[1], Zahra Fagrouch[1], Melanie van Heteren[1], Henk Niphuis[1], Tom Haaksma[2], Ivanela Kondova[2], Willy M. Bogers[1], Marina de Filette[3], Niek Sanders[3], Linda Stertman[4], Sofia Magnusson[4], Orsolya Lőrincz[5¤], Julianna Lisziewicz[5¤], Luisa Barzon[6], Giorgio Palù[6], Michael S. Diamond[7], Stefan Chabierski[8], Sebastian Ulbert[8], Ernst J. Verschoor[1]*

1 Department of Virology, Biomedical Primate Research Centre (BPRC), Rijswijk, The Netherlands, 2 Animal Science Department, Division of Pathology and Microbiology, BPRC Rijswijk, The Netherlands, 3 Laboratory of Gene Therapy, Faculty of Veterinary Sciences, Ghent University, Merelbeke, Belgium, 4 Novavax AB, Uppsala, Sweden, 5 eMMUNITY, Inc., Budapest, Hungary, 6 Department of Molecular Medicine, University of Padova, Padova, Italy, 7 Departments of Medicine, Molecular Microbiology and Pathology and Immunology, Washington University School of Medicine, St. Louis, Missouri, United States of America, 8 Department of Immunology, Fraunhofer Institute for Cell Therapy and Immunology, Leipzig, Germany

Abstract

The mosquito-borne West Nile virus (WNV) causes human and animal disease with outbreaks in several parts of the world including North America, the Mediterranean countries, Central and East Europe, the Middle East, and Africa. Particularly in elderly people and individuals with an impaired immune system, infection with WNV can progress into a serious neuroinvasive disease. Currently, no treatment or vaccine is available to protect humans against infection or disease. The goal of this study was to develop a WNV-vaccine that is safe to use in these high-risk human target populations. We performed a vaccine efficacy study in non-human primates using the contemporary, pathogenic European WNV genotype 1a challenge strain, WNV-Ita09. Two vaccine strategies were evaluated in rhesus macaques (*Macaca mulatta*) using recombinant soluble WNV envelope (E) ectodomain adjuvanted with Matrix-M, either with or without DNA priming. The DNA priming immunization was performed with WNV-DermaVir nanoparticles. Both vaccination strategies successfully induced humoral and cellular immune responses that completely protected the macaques against the development of viremia. In addition, the vaccine was well tolerated by all animals. Overall, The WNV E protein adjuvanted with Matrix-M is a promising vaccine candidate for a non-infectious WNV vaccine for use in humans, including at-risk populations.

Editor: Bradley S. Schneider, Metabiota, United States of America

Funding: The project was funded by the European Community FP7 project WINGS (grant no. 261426). The funders had no role in study design, data collection and analysis, decision to publish, or preparation of the manuscript.

Competing Interests: The authors have read the journal's policy and have the following conflicts: SEM and LS are employees of Novavax AB and minority shareholders of Novavax Inc. JL and OL are shareholders of eMMUNITY Inc.

* Email: verschoor@bprc.nl

¤ Current address: eMMUNITY Inc, Bethesda, United States of America

Background

West Nile virus (WNV) is a mosquito-borne flavivirus that is maintained in an enzootic transmission cycle between avian hosts and mosquito vectors, but WNV can also be transmitted to humans and other mammals [1]. Infection in humans is asymptomatic in most cases, but in about 20% of infections it presents as West Nile fever (WNF), and in less than 1% of cases, mainly in elderly and immunosuppressed individuals, as West Nile neuroinvasive disease (WNND) [1].

In recent years, WNV infection has become a public health concern in Europe because of the increasing number of human outbreaks with severe neurological consequences and mortality [2–7]. In addition, WNV has continued to cause large epidemics in

North America, such as those that occurred in Dallas, Texas, in 2012 [8].

Seven different phylogenetic lineages of WNV have been described so far [9,10], but only WNV lineages 1 and 2 have been associated with disease in humans. The different WNV lineages are genetically related, and show 75% to 95% nucleotide identity. In particular, WNV lineage 1 and lineage 2 viruses demonstrate about 75% nucleotide identity and 94% amino acid sequence identity [10,11]. Lineage 1 has a worldwide geographic distribution, and in Europe lineage 1 viruses have been responsible for human cases of WNND in the Mediterranean countries and Eastern Europe since the 1950s [10]. Lineage 2 viruses were originally found only in sub-Saharan Africa and Madagascar, but in 2004 this lineage emerged in Europe, and has spread across the continent [12]. In 1999, a highly virulent WNV lineage 1 strain was introduced into the United States, and rapidly became endemic throughout the continent, affecting wild birds and mammals [13]. Moreover, this strain named NY99, caused a high number of cases of WNF and WNND, leading to considerable morbidity and mortality in humans.

The increasing number of outbreaks, as well as emergence of novel strains belonging to both major lineages, emphasizes the necessity to develop a WNV vaccine [4,5,14,15]. Several WNV vaccines have been licensed for use in horses, but no vaccine for human use has been approved yet [16]. A number of WNV vaccine candidates are currently at different stages of development, and make use of recombinant proteins, plasmid DNA vectors, or chimeric live-attenuated virus approaches [17]. The majority of these vaccines are based on the WNV envelope (E) protein. Either E protein in its native form, a truncated subunit protein 80E, the WNV E immunodominant domain III, or combinations of these compounds are used as immunogens. Most vaccine candidates have been evaluated in rodents [18–21], but such studies may have limited prognostic value for its efficacy in humans given the significant differences in B and T-cell repertoire between both species.

Because of their genetic relatedness to humans, and their relative susceptibility to WNV infection, rhesus macaques may provide a better animal model for the evaluation of the immunogenicity and efficacy of prototype human WNV vaccines. Candidate WNV vaccines that have been tested in non-human primates include recombinant chimeric yellow fever virus or dengue virus as backbone expressing WNV structural genes [22–27], or adjuvanted recombinant E protein [24]. Because of the high impact on human health after its introduction in North America, all WNV vaccines that have been tested in nonhuman primates were based on WNV-NY99, and no data are available of vaccine efficacy to more distantly related European WNV isolates.

We recently performed an experimental infection study in rhesus macaques and common marmosets using the European WNV genotype 1a strain, WNV-Ita09 [28]. Infection in rhesus macaques resulted in a transient viremia with a peak viral load at 2–3 days post-infection, and the emergence of IgM and IgG antibodies within 15 days of infection. After clearance of the viremic phase, WNV was still detectable in tissues like spleen, axillary and inguinal lymph nodes, which resembles the situation observed in human infections [29]. Therefore, rhesus macaques were used in this study to assess vaccine efficacy against the European WNV-Ita09 strain.

Neutralizing antibodies are associated with protection against WNV infection [30,31], whereas T-cells contribute to clearance of infection [32,33]. Because the E protein of WNV is a primary target for CD8 T-cells [34] and neutralizing antibodies [35], we selected it for use in a human WNV subunit vaccine. The immunogens used in our study were derived from the WNV-NY99 strain, and were either the ectodomain of the WNV E protein that was expressed in *E. coli* [36], or a DNA vector expressing the WNV E ectodomain [37].

To increase vaccine induced T-cell responses we formulated the E protein in Matrix-M (Novavax AB). The adjuvant Matrix-M is composed of a specific purified saponin fraction obtained from the tree *Quillaja saponaria* Molina, phosphatidyl choline and cholesterol, and has been shown to increase the migration of the antigen towards the draining lymph nodes [38,39]. An additional strategy to boost the T-cell responses is to prime the immune system with a DNA vaccine [40]. Here, we used a DNA vector expressing the WNV E protein in combination with a mannose-conjugated linear polyethylenimine delivery reagent; WNV-DermaVir [41,42]. The mannose ligand enhances the delivery of DNA to cells expressing mannose-receptors, such as macrophages and dendritic cells, and thus, promotes antigen presentation to T-cells [43].

Two different WNV vaccine strategies were evaluated for immunogenicity and efficacy against WNV-Ita09 challenge. The first strategy consisted of three immunizations with recombinant E protein adjuvanted with Matrix-M. The second strategy entailed a priming immunization with WNV-DermaVir, followed by two booster immunizations with recombinant E protein and Matrix-M. Nine weeks after the last immunization the animals were challenged with the European WNV-Ita09 strain. Both strategies had been evaluated previously in mice, and in that model induced neutralizing antibodies and WNV-specific cellular immune responses [42,44]. Here, in macaques, we observed robust humoral and cellular responses in both vaccination groups although the responses were higher in the protein-only immunization group. Animals in both groups showed consistent vaccine-induced IFNγ responses prior to WNV exposure. After challenge, all vaccinated macaques were completely protected against the development of viremia.

Methods

Ethics statement

This protocol was approved by the Institutional Animal Care and Use Committee (BPRC Dier Experimenten Commissie, BPRC-DEC; DEC advice #724). The qualification of the members of this committee, including their independence from a research institute, is requested in the Dutch law on animal Experiments (Wet op de Dierproeven, 1996). At the BPRC, all animal handling is performed within the Department of Animal Science (ASD) according to Dutch law. A large experienced staff is available, including full-time veterinarians and a pathologist. ASD is regularly inspected by the responsible authority (Voedsel en Waren Autoriteit, VWA), and by an independent Animal Welfare Officer.

The Council of the Association for Assessment and Accreditation of Laboratory Animal Care (AAALAC International) has awarded full accreditation to the BPRC. The BPRC is fully compliant with international demands on animal studies and welfare as set out by the European Convention for the Protection of Vertebrate Animals used for Experimental and other Scientific Purposes, Council of Europe (ETS 123 including the revised Appendix A), Dutch implementing legislation, and the Guide for Care and Use of Laboratory Animals.

The rhesus macaques (*Macaca mulatta*) used in this study were captive-bred for research purposes and housed socially at the Biomedical Primate Research Centre (BPRC) in Rijswijk, The Netherlands. BPRC facilities comply with Dutch law on animal experiments (Wet op de Dierproeven, and its adaptations as published in the Staatscourant), the European Council Directive 86/609/EEC, as well as with the 'Standard for humane care and use of Laboratory Animals by Foreign institutions' identification number A5539-01, provided by the Department of Health and Human Services of the United States of America's National Institutes of Health (NIH).

During the experiment, the animals were pair-housed in a BSL3-facility with spacious cages and were provided with commercial food pellets supplemented with appropriate treats. Drinking water was provided *ad libitum*. Enrichment was provided in the form of pieces of wood, mirrors, food puzzles, a variety of other home-made or commercially available enrichment products. Animals were monitored daily for health and discomfort.

All steps were taken to ameliorate the welfare and to avoid any suffering of the animals. All experimental interventions (immunizations, intradermal injection of WNV, blood samplings) were performed under anesthesia using ketamine. Before euthanasia, animals were first sedated deeply with ketamine, and subsequently euthanized by intracardiac injection of an overdose of pentobarbital.

Animals

Eighteen rhesus macaques (*Macaca mulatta*) were used in this study. All monkeys were adult animals, ranging in age from 5 to 12 years. The animals were in good physical health with normal baseline biochemical and hematological values. At the start of the study, the animals tested negative for antibodies to WNV. To prevent sex, age and weight bias, the animals were assigned randomly to different treatment groups.

Vaccines

The ectodomain of the E protein (amino acid residues 1 to 404) of WNV-NY99 was cloned into the bacterial expression plasmid the pET21a, expressed in *E. coli* and purified as described previously [36]. This antigen was formulated Matrix-M, a mixture of 40 nm particles formed by two separate saponin fractions, i.e. Matrix-A and Matrix-C (Novavax AB, Uppsala, Sweden) [38]. WNV-DermaVir nanoparticles, containing a WNV DNA vaccine that expresses the ectodomain of WNV E protein, were prepared as previously described [42,45].

Experimental set up

A schematic outline of the study is given in **Figure 1**. The animals in group 1 were immunized via three consecutive intramuscular (IM) injections of 20 µg WNV-E mixed with 25 µg Matrix-M at weeks 0, 3 and 6. The animals in group 2 received 100 µg WNV-DermaVir at week 0, given as 8 intradermal injections of 100 µl each in the upper back. Subsequently, the animals were boosted twice at weeks 3 and 6 with 20 µg WNV-E mixed with 25 µg Matrix-M. Nine weeks after the last immunization, all animals, including those in the infection control group (group 3), were challenged by an intradermal injection in the upper back of 2×10^5 TCID$_{50}$ of WNV lineage 1a strain Ita09 [46] in 100 µl saline. This dose was found previously to productively infect rhesus macaques [28]. After WNV infection,

the animals were observed daily for general condition, appetite, and stool until the end of the study, i.e. 14 days post-challenge.

During the immunization period, blood was collected using standard aseptic methods from the femoral vein at the start of the study, two weeks after each immunization, 5 weeks after the last booster immunization, and at challenge (week 15) for determination of biochemical and hematological parameters, and for the analysis of vaccine-induced humoral and cellular immune responses. After challenge, 0.5 ml blood samples were collected on a daily basis until euthanasia for viral load determination using real-time RT-PCR. Additional, larger blood volumes were collected at days 3, 7, and 14 post challenge for hematological and biochemical analysis, and for the evaluation of WNV-specific humoral and cellular immune responses.

Biochemistry and hematology

A panel of hematological parameters, i.e. white blood cell count (WBC), red blood cell count (RBC), hemoglobin, hematocrit, mean cellular volume (MCV), mean corpuscular hemoglobin (MCH), platelets, neutrophils, lymphocytes, monocytes, eosinophils and basophils, was analyzed in peripheral blood using a Sysmex XT-2000iV Automated Hematology Analyzer (Sysmex Nederland B.V., Etten-Leur, The Netherlands). Biochemical analysis, i.e. creatinine, urea, bilirubin, gamma-glutamyltransferase (γGT), aspartate aminotransferase (AST), alanine aminotransferase (ALT), alkaline phosphatase, lactate dehydrogenase (LDH), iron, albumin, total protein, cholesterol and glucose, was assessed using a COBAS Integra 400 plus system (Roche Diagnostics Nederland B.V., Almere, The Netherlands).

Characterization of humoral immune responses

WNV-specific antibodies in EDTA-plasma were detected by ELISA. Briefly, 96-well microtiter plates were coated overnight with 400 ng of the ectodomain of the WNV-NY99 E protein [36], or with 500 ng of hydrogen-peroxide-inactivated WNV-NY99 [47]. The coated plates were incubated for 2 h with 1:50 diluted EDTA plasma, followed by 1 hr incubation with HRP-conjugated goat-anti-human IgG (Thermo Fisher Scientific, Schwerte, Germany). After washing, TMB-substrate (BioLegend, Fell, Germany) was added to the wells and the plate was incubated for 30 min at room temperature in the dark. Then, 1 M H$_2$SO$_4$ was added to stop the reaction and plates were measured at

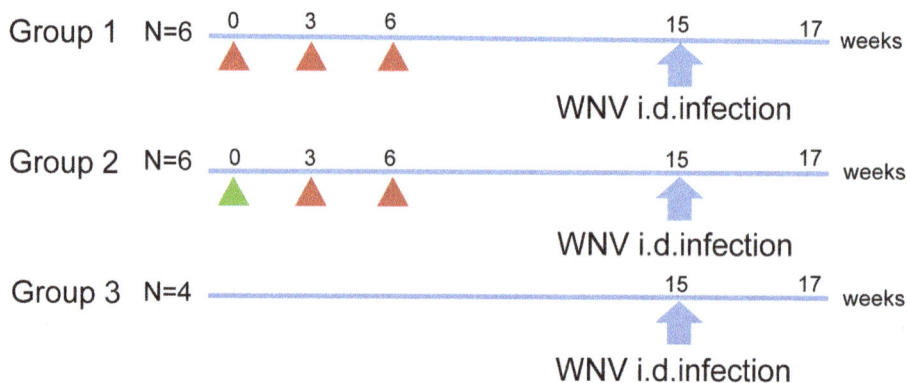

Figure 1. Study outline. Schematic representation of the study with two West Nile virus vaccine strategies. Group 1 received three immunizations with recombinant E protein adjuvanted with Matrix-M (red triangles) at indicated study weeks. Group 2 received one immunization of WNV-DermaVir (green triangle), followed by two immunizations with recombinant E protein adjuvanted with Matrix-M (red triangles). Nine weeks after the last immunization, all animals (including controls) were challenged intradermally with 2×10^5 TCID$_{50}$ of WNV-Ita09. All animals were euthanized 14 days post-challenge (study week 17).

450 nm and 520 nm (reference wavelength) in an ELISA Reader (Infiniti M200, Tecan, The Netherlands).

To determine the *in vitro* neutralizing capacity of sera from vaccinated macaques, plaque-reduction neutralization tests (PRNT50) were performed essentially as described in the Guidelines for plaque reduction neutralization testing of human antibodies to dengue virus (World Health Organization, 2007). Heat-inactivated EDTA plasma samples taken at various time points were serially diluted and mixed with 25 $TCID_{50}$ of WNV-Ita09 (lineage 1), or WNV-AUT08 (lineage 2), before addition to adherent Vero cells. Cytopathic effect (CPE) was visualized using a standard microscope, and the $TCID_{50}$ was calculated using the Karber formula [48].

Determination of cell-mediated immune responses

Cell-mediated immune responses were determined in peripheral blood mononuclear cells (PBMCs) isolated from EDTA-treated blood. PBMCs were tested for WNV-specific secretion using WNV-E protein in ELIspot assays according to the manufacturers' guidelines (U-CyTech, Utrecht, The Netherlands). ELIspot assays were performed on freshly isolated cells at weeks 0, 2, 5, 8, and 11.

To obtain more detailed information on the quality of WNV-specific responses, intracellular cytokine staining (ICS) was performed. Frozen PBMCs, isolated at weeks 0 and 15 were thawed, and intracellular staining was performed as described previously [49] using a panel of monoclonal antibodies; LIVE/DEAD-Aqua (Life Technologies, Grand Island, NY), CD3-AF700, CD8-V500, CD4-PE-Cy7 and IFNγ-PE (all Becton, Dickinson B.V., Breda, The Netherlands). Fluorescence was measured using a FACS LSR2 (Becton, Dickinson and Company, Breda, The Netherlands). Data were analyzed with FlowJo software, version 9.6.4 (Tree Star, Stanford University, USA).

Virus detection in blood and tissue

Viral loads were determined in EDTA-plasma by quantitative real-time RT-PCR as previously described [28,50]. To determine the presence of WNV in tissue samples, 1 mg of snap frozen tissue was added to 1 ml RPMI and was dissociated using a gentleMACS dissociator (Miltenyi Biotec B.V., Leiden, The Netherlands). The homogenate was centrifuged for 10 min at 820× g at room temperature, and the supernatant was filtered through a 40 µm filter. Viral RNA was isolated from 140 µl of filtered homogenate with the QIAamp Viral RNA Mini Kit (QIAGEN Benelux BV, Venlo, the Netherlands), and was subsequently analyzed by PCR, as described previously [28].

Necropsy

Monkeys were euthanized by infusion of pentobarbital (Apharma, Duiven, The Netherlands), and full necropsy was performed. Based on the dissemination data of WNV obtained from an earlier experimental infection study [28], samples were collected from the following organs for PCR analysis; axillary lymph nodes (ln), inguinal ln, mesenteric ln, spleen, urinary bladder, kidney, cerebellum and hippocampus. All samples were snap frozen for WNV-RNA determination.

Statistical analysis

Data obtained with the two vaccine strategies were analyzed and compared using an unpaired t-test in GraphPad Prism version 6.0.

Results

Induction of antibody responses against WNV by both vaccine strategies

Both vaccines were well tolerated by the animals and no local reactions were observed after immunization.

Induction of WNV-specific IgG was measured two weeks after each immunization, and 4 weeks before WNV challenge (**Figure 1**). After the first immunization, very low levels of anti-WNV E IgG were detected (sample:negative ratio (S/N) <40) in only one macaque of the protein-only group (group 1) (**Figure 2A**). After the second protein immunization, 5 of 6 animals from group 1 showed high IgG titers directed against the ectodomain of E, although one animal failed to develop a response that exceeded background levels. In all group 1 animals the IgG response was boosted after the third protein immunization, and remained stable until at least week 11 (one animal was not tested at this time point). In animals of group 2, which first received a DNA vaccine prime followed by two protein booster immunizations, no detectable antibody responses were observed at two weeks after the DNA immunization. After the first E protein boost the levels of E-specific IgG were significantly higher in comparison to the group 1 animals after a single protein immunization, which indicates a priming effect of the DNA vaccine. After the second protein boost the antibody titers in DNA-protein group reached levels that were comparable to those measured in the protein-only group. As expected, no E-specific IgG levels were detected in the control animals prior to WNV challenge. The specificity of the WNV-E protein-specific IgG responses was confirmed by using inactivated whole virus as capture antigen in ELISA (**Figure 2B**).

Vaccine-induced neutralizing antibodies (VN) against WNV were measured using a plaque reduction assay on Vero cells in plasma samples collected at week 0 and week 11. No VN were detectable at the start of the immunization period, but plasma samples collected 5 weeks after the third immunization (week 11) inhibited the infectivity WNV-Ita09, with individual VN titers ranging from 1/3,698 to 1/48,000 (mean value 17,805) in group 1, and from 1/1,567 to 1/21,657 (mean value 12,534) in group 2 (**Figure 2C**). Vaccine-induced neutralizing antibodies cross-neutralized the lineage 2 WNV strain AUT08 with titers ranging from 1/2,828 to 1/160,00 (mean value 6,822) in group 1 animals, and ranging from 1/1,414 to 1/16,000 (mean value 5,771) in group 2 animals (**Figure 2C**). None of the animals in the control group showed neutralizing capacity against the lineage 1 or lineage 2 WNV isolates tested.

CD8 T-cell responses in macaques elicited by WNV vaccines

To determine the cellular immunogenicity of the two WNV vaccine strategies, IFNγ ELIspot assays were performed on isolated peripheral blood mononuclear cells (PBMCs) (**Figure 3A**). Two weeks after the first immunization, a significant difference was observed between the number of spot-forming units (SFU) observed in PBMC from animals that received a protein immunization (70 to 82 SFU per million PBMC) or a DNA immunization (28 to 77 SFU per million PBMC) (p = 0.001). Two weeks after the second immunization, WNV-specific IFNγ responses in both groups were boosted to 155 to 487 SFU in macaques of group 1, and 47 to 117 SFU in the group 2 animals (p = 0.023). The final immunization further augmented the number IFNγ secreting cells in peripheral blood in both vaccine groups, with a more robust response in group 1 animals compared to group 2 (median values of 400 and 274 SFU, respectively, p = 0.0008). Three weeks later, minor changes were observed in

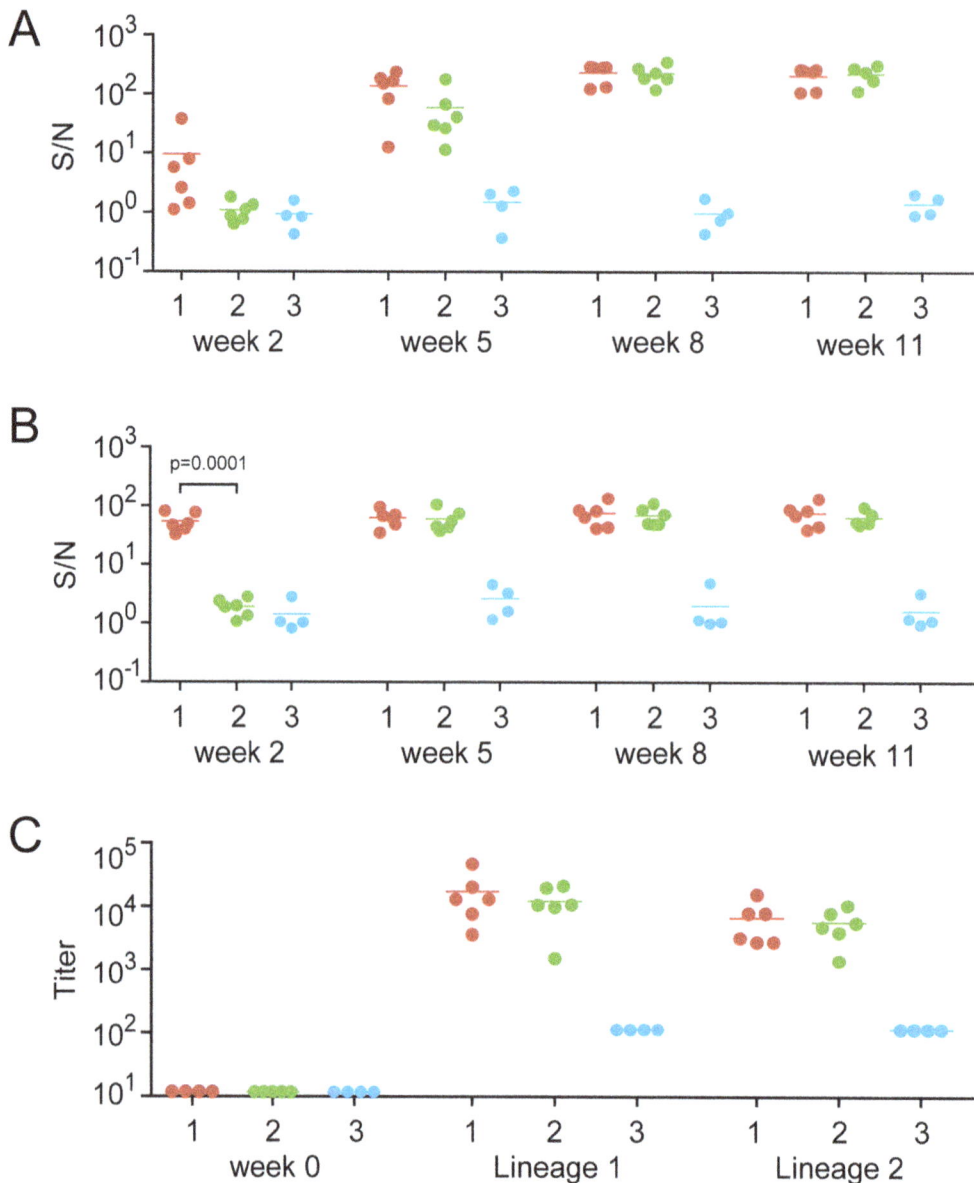

Figure 2. Vaccine-induced antibody responses. Antibodies reactive against (A) the ecto-domain of the WNV E protein, and (B) inactivated WNV were measured in the individual animals at indicated time points. Humoral responses were quantified as sample:negative ratio (S/N). Vaccine-induced neutralizing capacity (PRNT50) of macaque sera was determined using the plaque reduction neutralization test (C). Individual animals are depicted as dots: group 1 (red), group 2 (green), and group 3 (blue). The median value is indicated for each group. Unpaired t-test was used to compare the responses between the groups. Statistical significant differences were defined as p<0.05 and are indicated with arches in the figure.

the number of IFNγ-secreting cells in the different groups. Macaques of group 1 still showed significantly higher number of IFNγ-secreting cells compared to animals belonging to the DNA-protein group (p = 0.0001).

To determine if IFNγ was produced by CD4 T-cells, or by CD8 T-cells, ICS was performed on cells collected at weeks 0 and 15. Cells within the lymphocyte gate were selected based on the expression of CD3 (**Figure S1**). Next, CD4 T-cells and CD8 T-cells were analyzed for their intracellular expression of IFNγ. At week 15, the day of WNV challenge, IFNγ was produced by both CD4 (**Figure 3B**), and CD8 (**Figure 3C**) T-cells in all animals of group 1. This was not observed in the macaques that received the WNV-DermaVir priming immunization, followed by two protein immunizations (group 2). In this group, 2 of 6 animals had IFNγ-

producing CD4 T-cells, and only one animal had IFNγ producing CD8 T-cells.

Determination of WNV vaccine efficacy in rhesus macaques

At week 15, all of the animals were challenged intradermally with 2×10^5 TCID$_{50}$ of WNV lineage 1a strain Ita09. During the 14-day observation period, none of the macaques showed any behavioral changes or health complications. In addition, no changes in rectal body temperature (**Figure S2**), hematological and biochemical parameters were seen, suggesting that all animals remained clinically healthy during the 2-weeks post-challenge follow-up.

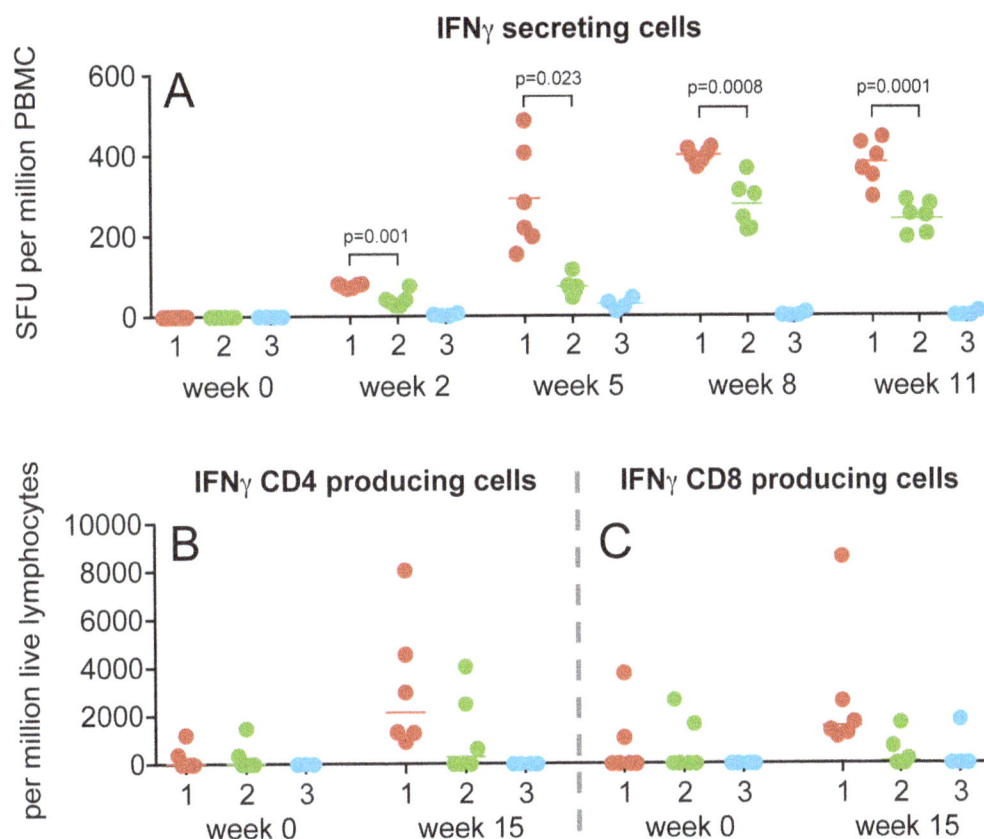

Figure 3. Vaccine-induced T-cell responses. A. IFNγ-secreting cells in blood of the individual animals measured in ELISpot. The responses are presented in spot-forming units (SFU) per million PBMCs. The WNV-specific T-cell responses were calculated by subtraction of the background responses (mean value of triplicate assays plus two times the standard deviation, minus medium alone). Intracellular staining of IFNγ produced by CD4 T-cells (panel B), and CD8 T-cells (panel C). Background IFNγ-responses (number of IFNγ-producing cells with medium alone) were subtracted. Individual animals are depicted as dots: group 1 (red), group 2 (green), and group 3 (blue). The median value is indicated for each group. Unpaired t-test was used to compare the responses between the groups. Statistical significant differences were defined as p<0.05.

The protective capacity of both WNV vaccine strategies was assessed by measuring WNV RNA levels in plasma from the macaques by real-time RT-PCR, and in solid tissues by diagnostic PCR. All vaccinated macaques remained negative for WNV in plasma during the entire follow-up period. In contrast, one day after intradermal infection with WNV, 4 of 6 non-vaccinated controls had become positive for WNV (7.700 to 58.000 RNA copies/ml plasma) (**Table 1**). Two days post-challenge, 5 of 6 control animals were positive for WNV RNA. By day 6 after infection, none of macaques had measurable levels of WNV RNA in peripheral blood. In animal R08058, one of the macaques in the non-vaccinated control group, viral RNA was not detected in peripheral blood at any of the time points tested.

In addition to quantifying WNV by real-time PCR, we tested the plasma taken at 1 to 5 days after WNV exposure for the presence of infectious WNV particles. Plasma of EDTA-treated blood samples was serially diluted, and cultured for 7 days on Vero cells. Only plasma from R03027 (a non-vaccinated control) collected 3 days after WNV exposure caused CPE in Vero cells. Based on a standard curve analysis, the virus titer in this sample was calculated 144 infectious particles per ml of plasma. Sequence analysis confirmed that the CPE in Vero cells was caused by WNV-Ita09 infection.

WNV tissue distribution in vaccinated and non-vaccinated rhesus macaques

In contrast to the control animals, the vaccinated animals did not show plasma viremia despite exposure to WNV. To assess if the vaccine strategies employed in this study conferred sterilizing immunity, we performed PCR analysis on solid tissues that were collected at euthanasia, 14 days post-challenge. **Figure 4** shows the data obtained by qualitative real-time PCR and a nested PCR assay performed on selected tissue samples. WNV RNA was detected in the peripheral lymph nodes (axillary, inguinal or mesenteric ln) from 5 out of 6 non-vaccinated controls. Notably, WNV RNA was also present in the peripheral lymph nodes of animal R08058, the only control that did not show WNV RNA in plasma. In the unvaccinated macaque R03027, although WNV RNA was present in plasma, we did not find WNV RNA in peripheral lymph nodes. In the spleen of this animal, however, the nested PCR assay did detect WNV RNA. The spleen tested positive for WNV RNA in all 6 control animals in at least one of the two PCR assays used. In contrast, WNV RNA was detected in the spleen of 2 out of 12 vaccinated rhesus macaques, including one animal from each of the groups (R06024 and R07121).

The kidney and urinary system have been suggested as potential target organs for WNV infection in humans [2,51]. Here, only two control animals tested positive for WNV RNA in the urinary bladder (R01034) or kidney (R02085). Because WNV disease is

Table 1. Detection of West Nile virus load in plasma of vaccinated and control rhesus macaques.

	Days post-exposure										
	0	1	2	3	4	5	6	8	10	12	14
Group 1: protein only											
R08032	–	–	–	–	–	–	–	–	–	–	–
R08101	–	–	–	–	–	–	–	–	–	–	–
R06024	–	–	–	–	–	–	–	–	–	–	–
R06078	–	–	–	–	–	–	–	–	–	–	–
R03008	–	–	–	–	–	–	–	–	–	–	–
R01080	–	–	–	–	–	–	–	–	–	–	–
Group 2: DNA prime, protein boost											
R08106	–	–	–	–	–	–	–	–	–	–	–
R07121	–	–	–	–	–	–	–	–	–	–	–
R06111	–	–	–	–	–	–	–	–	–	–	–
R06070	–	–	–	–	–	–	–	–	–	–	–
R03020	–	–	–	–	–	–	–	–	–	–	–
R02073	–	–	–	–	–	–	–	–	–	–	–
Group 3: control animals											
R08058	–	–	–	–	–	–	–	–	–	–	–
R06047	–	–	2900	**18000**	1900	–	–	–	–	–	–
R03027	–	**58000**	43000	16800	19000	–	–	–	–	–	–
R02085	–	7700	2800	5500	**61000**	–	–	–	–	–	–
R01034	–	27000	770	**63000**	16000	–	–	–	–	–	–
R05066	–	46000	86000	**110000**	71000	194	–	–	–	–	–

Real time RT-PCR was used to quantify WNV RNA load in plasma at indicated time points after challenge. Virus loads are presented in copies per ml. Peak virus loads are given in bold.

	Group 1 3 x protein						Group 1 1 x DNA, 2 x protein						Group 1 controls					
Real-time PCR / **Diagnostic nested PCR**	R08032	R08101	R06024	R06078	R03008	R01080	R08106	R07121	R06111	R06070	R03020	R02073	R08058	R06047	R03027	R02085	R01034	R05066
Axillary ln								●					●	●		○	●	○
Inguinal ln					○			●					●	○			●	
Mesenteric ln													●					
Spleen			●					●					○	○		○	●	●
Urinary bladder																●		
Thyroid																		
Kidney (L+R)																○		
Adrenal gland																		
Cerebellum																		●
Hippocampus																○		○
Brain stem																		
Parietal cortex																		

Figure 4. Detection of West Nile virus in tissue samples. Tissue samples were analyzed for the presence of WNV RNA by qualitative real-time PCR (red) or a nested PCR assay (orange).

associated with neuroinvasion, different parts of the brain [29], the cerebellum, the hippocampus, the brain stem, and the parietal cortex, were tested. WNV RNA was observed in cerebellum of control animal R05066, and in the hippocampus of 2 control monkeys, i.e. R02085 and R05066.

Discussion

Since its introduction in 1999 into the USA, and the subsequent spread into the New World, WNV has emerged as a serious threat to public health. This opinion is confirmed by an increasing incidence of WNV infections in South-East Europe caused by lineage 1 and 2 WNV strains. Currently, no antiviral treatment or vaccine is available to protect humans from WNV infection. In our study, two WNV vaccine strategies (protein prime + protein boost and DNA prime + protein boost) fully protected monkeys against the development of viremia. Although sterilizing immunity was not achieved, only 3 of 12 vaccinated macaques were positive for WNV RNA in one or more solid tissues compared to 6 out of 6 challenge controls.

This project aimed to develop a vaccine against WNV that is safe for use in the high-risk human target populations, elderly individuals and those having a compromised immune system. Our prototype WNV vaccines were composed of antigens that are safe to use, as they are well-characterized recombinant components (proteins, DNA) that lack the ability to replicate. In preparation of the monkey study, the individual antigens, in combination with DermaVir and Matrix-M, showed safety, immunogenicity, and efficacy in rodents [42,44].

Protein-based vaccines can efficiently protect against a number of viruses by eliciting antibodies, while priming the immune system with a DNA vaccine has been shown to induce CD8 T-cell-

mediated immunity [40]. The correlate of protection against WNV infection has not been fully elucidated although CD8 T-cell and WNV-specific antibody responses are associated with protection from disease or infection [31,32]. The ectodomain of the E protein is highly immunogenic and contains multiple CD8 and CD4 T-cell epitopes [52–54], and was consequently the immunogen of choice in our study. The combination of WNV-E adjuvanted with Matrix-M potently induced WNV-specific IgG antibodies in the macaques, even after the first immunization. In contrast, anti-WNV IgG was not observed after the priming immunization with the WNV-DermaVir nanoparticles. However, when WNV-DermaVir was combined with protein/Matrix-M booster immunizations, a priming effect on the humoral immune responses was seen. In mice, De Filette *et al.* [42] also demonstrated that WNV-DermaVir immunization failed to induce a measurable humoral immune response by itself, but upon protein boosting, DNA-vaccinated mice showed a marked increase in IgG and neutralizing antibody titers against WNV. In addition, mice that were given a WNV-DermaVir priming, followed by a protein boost had a higher amount of IL-4 and IFNγ-producing cells than mice that were given protein immunizations alone. This contrasts with our findings in the rhesus macaques. No evidence was found for an improved CD8 T-cell response due to the WNV-DermaVir priming. However, though the numbers were modest, a CD8 T-cell response was induced in the animals that received the WNV-DermaVir prime while a clear IFNγ producing CD8 T-cell population was shown in all animals from group 1 prior to the challenge. It is conceivable that the limited effect of the DNA priming immunization was caused by use of a too low dose. Others, using 5 to 10 times more DNA than the 100 μg DNA used in this study, did detect a strong priming effect on the immune system of rhesus macaques that resulted in higher and broader T-cell responses [55,56].

We observed cross-protection between North American and European lineage 1 strains, as the vaccine components were based on WNV-NY99, and the challenge strain used in the monkeys was WNV-Ita09 (>99% sequence identity). In mice, E protein/ Matrix-M immunizations also afforded protection against lethal challenge with a lineage 2 strain of WNV [44]. This was not evaluated *in vivo* in macaques, but *in vitro* assays for detection of virus neutralizing IgG showed cross-neutralization of the lineage 2 WNV-AUT08 strain. This is likely because of the conservation of dominant neutralizing epitopes in different regions of WNV E protein between lineage 1 and 2 strains [57].

At present, our results do not tell us which WNV vaccination strategy is best. Both induced complete protection against viremia, but failed to induce sterilizing immunity against intradermal challenge. Although it is speculative, the vaccine may have failed to achieve sterilizing immunity because of the relatively high challenge dose used. Depending on the mosquito species, the dose of WNV inoculated by one mosquito during blood feeding varies between 10^4 and 10^5 PFU [58], and thus the 2.10^5 TCID$_{50}$ challenge dose may have been relatively high.

Several WNV vaccines have been clinically evaluated [59]. Chimeric virus approaches, based of the yellow fever vaccine strain YFV-17D or using dengue virus as viral backbone, showed good immunogenicity in healthy volunteers, but may be unacceptable for vaccine-licensing because of the risk of residual pathogenicity, or reversal to pathogenicity in the human immune-compromised target populations. Safer vaccines that were based on naked DNA or protein subunits also showed good immuno-genicity and induction of neutralizing antibodies in clinical phase I trials, and may therefore be better alternatives. In our pre-clinical macaque model we used a similar subunit and/or DNA vaccine approach, but instead used a European WNV challenge virus. Both the protein only and DNA-protein immunization strategies induced strong humoral and cellular immune responses, and protected healthy rhesus macaques from WNV infection. In recent years, human cases on WNF and WNND in Europe were also caused by WNV lineage 2 viruses, viruses previously thought to be less pathogenic to humans [60]. It is thus of major importance that

our vaccines also elicited neutralizing antibodies that cross-reacted *in vitro* with a WNV lineage 2 strain. It can therefore be concluded that the vaccines described here are promising candidates for the further development of WNV vaccines for at-risk human populations.

Supporting Information

Figure S1   Gating strategy for intracellular IFNγ staining in CD4 and CD8 T-cells. Representative gating strategy to define intracellular IFNγ-staining in CD4 and CD8+ T-cells of vaccinated rhesus macaques. Cytokine-producing T-cells were defined as LIVE/DEAD negative and CD3 positive cells. Next, CD4 positive cells and CD8 positive T-cells were analyzed for IFNγ production.

Figure S2   Rectal body temperatures of rhesus monkeys during the immunization period and after WNV challenge. Rectal body temperature (°C) measured at indicated time points in animals from group 1 (panel A; red), group 2 (panel B; green), and group 3 (panel C; blue). Median rectal body temperature (D) per group at indicated days after experimental WNV infection. Statistically significant differences were defined as $p<0.05$ and are indicated with arches in the figure.

Acknowledgments

We thank Amanda van Geest, Chantal Rongen, Harrypersad Khoen-Khoen, Con Regeer, and Mariska van Etten for the excellent animal care, and Jaco Bakker and Robin van der Schilt for veterinary assistance. We thank Henk van Westbroek for graphics.

Author Contributions

Conceived and designed the experiments: BEV EJV. Performed the experiments: BEV HO ZF MvH HN TH IK WMB MdeF SC. Analyzed the data: BEV EJV. Contributed reagents/materials/analysis tools: MdeF NS LS SM OL JL LB GP MSD. Contributed to the writing of the manuscript: BEV NS SM JL LB MSD SU EJV.

References

1. Petersen LR, Brault AC, Nasci RS (2013) West Nile virus: review of the literature. JAMA 310: 308–315.
2. Murray K, Walker C, Herrington E, Lewis JA, McCormick J, et al. (2010) Persistent infection with West Nile virus years after initial infection. J Infect Dis 201: 2–4.
3. Danis K, Papa A, Theocharopoulos G, Dougas G, Athanasiou M, et al. (2011) Outbreak of West Nile virus infection in Greece, 2010. Emerg Infect Dis 17: 1868–1872.
4. Barzon L, Pacenti M, Franchin E, Lavezzo E, Martello T, et al. (2012) New endemic West Nile virus lineage 1a in northern Italy, July 2012. Euro Surveill 17.
5. Barzon L, Pacenti M, Franchin E, Lavezzo E, Masi G, et al. (2013) Whole genome sequencing and phylogenetic analysis of West Nile virus lineage 1 and lineage 2 from human cases of infection, Italy, August 2013. Euro Surveill 18.
6. Popovic N, Milosevic B, Urosevic A, Poluga J, Lavadinovic L, et al. (2013) Outbreak of West Nile virus infection among humans in Serbia, August to October 2012. Euro Surveill 18.
7. Pervanidou D, Detsis M, Danis K, Mellou K, Papanikolaou E, et al. (2014) West Nile virus outbreak in humans, Greece, 2012: third consecutive year of local transmission. Euro Surveill 19.
8. Chung WM, Buseman CM, Joyner SN, Hughes SM, Fomby TB, et al. (2013) The 2012 West Nile encephalitis epidemic in Dallas, Texas. JAMA 310: 297–307.
9. Vazquez A, Sanchez-Seco MP, Ruiz S, Molero F, Hernandez L, et al. (2010) Putative new lineage of west nile virus, Spain. Emerg Infect Dis 16: 549–552.
10. Pesko KN, Ebel GD (2012) West Nile virus population genetics and evolution. Infect Genet Evol 12: 181–190.
11. Lanciotti RS, Ebel GD, Deubel V, Kerst AJ, Murri S, et al. (2002) Complete genome sequences and phylogenetic analysis of West Nile virus strains isolated from the United States, Europe, and the Middle East. Virology 298: 96–105.
12. Bakonyi T, Ferenczi E, Erdelyi K, Kutasi O, Csorgo T, et al. (2013) Explosive spread of a neuroinvasive lineage 2 West Nile virus in Central Europe, 2008/ 2009. Vet Microbiol 165: 61–70.
13. Murray KO, Mertens E, Despres P (2010) West Nile virus and its emergence in the United States of America. Vet Res 41: 67.
14. ECDC (2012) Epidemiological situation of West Nile virus infection in the European Union.
15. Papa A (2012) West Nile virus infections in Greece: an update. Expert Rev Anti Infect Ther 10: 743–750.
16. De Filette M, Ulbert S, Diamond M, Sanders NN (2012) Recent progress in West Nile virus diagnosis and vaccination. Vet Res 43: 16.
17. Brandler S, Tangy F (2013) Vaccines in development against West Nile virus. Viruses 5: 2384–2409.
18. Wang T, Anderson JF, Magnarelli LA, Wong SJ, Koski RA, et al. (2001) Immunization of mice against West Nile virus with recombinant envelope protein. J Immunol 167: 5273–5277.
19. Pinto AK, Richner JM, Poore EA, Patil, Amanna IJ, et al. (2013) A Hydrogen Peroxide-Inactivated Virus Vaccine Elicits Humoral and Cellular Immunity and Protects against Lethal West Nile Virus Infection in Aged Mice. J Virol 87: 1926–1936.
20. Widman DG, Ishikawa T, Winkelmann ER, Infante E, Bourne N, et al. (2009) RepliVAX WN, a single-cycle flavivirus vaccine to prevent West Nile disease, elicits durable protective hematumity in hamsters. Vaccine 27: 5550–5553.

21. Spohn G, Jennings GT, Martina BE, Keller I, Beck M, et al. (2010) A VLP-based vaccine targeting domain III of the West Nile virus E protein protects from lethal infection in mice. Virol J 7: 146.

22. Arroyo J, Miller C, Catalan J, Myers GA, Ratterree MS, et al. (2004) ChimeriVax-West Nile virus live-attenuated vaccine: preclinical evaluation of safety, immunogenicity, and efficacy. J Virol 78: 12497–12507.

23. Monath TP, Liu J, Kanesa-Thasan N, Myers GA, Nichols R, et al. (2006) A live, attenuated recombinant West Nile virus vaccine. Proc Natl Acad Sci U S A 103: 6694–6699.

24. Lieberman MM, Nerurkar VR, Luo H, Cropp B, Carrion R Jr, et al. (2009) Immunogenicity and protective efficacy of a recombinant subunit West Nile virus vaccine in rhesus monkeys. Clin Vaccine Immunol 16: 1332–1337.

25. Pletnev AG, Swayne DE, Speicher J, Rumyantsev AA, Murphy BR (2006) Chimeric West Nile/dengue virus vaccine candidate: preclinical evaluation in mice, geese and monkeys for safety and immunogenicity. Vaccine 24: 6392–6404.

26. Widman DG, Ishikawa T, Giavedoni LD, Hodara VL, Garza Mde L, et al. (2010) Evaluation of RepliVAX WN, a single-cycle flavivirus vaccine, in a non-human primate model of West Nile virus infection. Am J Trop Med Hyg 82: 1160–1167.

27. Whiteman MC, Li L, Wicker JA, Kinney RM, Huang C, et al. (2010) Development and characterization of non-glycosylated E and NS1 mutant viruses as a potential candidate vaccine for West Nile virus. Vaccine 28: 1075–1083.

28. Verstrepen BE, Fagrouch Z, van Heteren M, Buitendijk H, Haaksma T, et al. (2014) Experimental infection of rhesus macaques and common marmosets with a European strain of West Nile virus. PLoS Negl Trop Dis 8: e2797.

29. Busch MP, Kleinman SH, Tobler LH, Kamel HT, Norris PJ, et al. (2008) Virus and antibody dynamics in acute west nile virus infection. J Infect Dis 198: 984–993.

30. Diamond MS, Shrestha B, Mehlhop E, Sitati E, Engle M (2003) Innate and adaptive immune responses determine protection against disseminated infection by West Nile encephalitis virus. Viral Immunol 16: 259–278.

31. Diamond MS, Shrestha B, Marri A, Mahan D, Engle M (2003) B cells and antibody play critical roles in the immediate defense of disseminated infection by West Nile encephalitis virus. J Virol 77: 2578–2586.

32. Shrestha B, Diamond MS (2004) Role of CD8+ T cells in control of West Nile virus infection. J Virol 78: 8312–8321.

33. Brien JD, Uhrlaub JL, Nikolich-Zugich J (2007) Protective capacity and epitope specificity of CD8(+) T cells responding to lethal West Nile virus infection. Eur J Immunol 37: 1855–1863.

34. Purtha WE, Myers N, Mitaksov V, Sitati E, Connolly J, et al. (2007) Antigen-specific cytotoxic T lymphocytes protect against lethal West Nile virus encephalitis. Eur J Immunol 37: 1845–1854.

35. Throsby M, Ter Meulen J, Geuijen C, Goudsmit J, de Kruif J (2007) Mapping and analysis of West Nile virus-specific monoclonal antibodies: prospects for vaccine development. Expert Rev Vaccines 6: 183–191.

36. Oliphant T, Nybakken GE, Austin SK, Xu Q, Bramson J, et al. (2007) Induction of epitope-specific neutralizing antibodies against West Nile virus. J Virol 81: 11828–11839.

37. Schneeweiss A, Chabierski S, Salomo M, Delaroque N, Al-Robaiy S, et al. (2011) A DNA vaccine encoding the E protein of West Nile virus is protective and can be boosted by recombinant domain DIII. Vaccine 29: 6352–6357.

38. Bengtsson KL, Karlsson KH, Magnusson SE, Reimer JM, Stertman L (2013) Matrix-M adjuvant: enhancing immune responses by 'setting the stage' for the antigen. Expert Rev Vaccines 12: 821–823.

39. Magnusson SE, Reimer JM, Karlsson KH, Lilja L, Bengtsson KL, et al. (2013) Immune enhancing properties of the novel Matrix-M adjuvant leads to potentiated immune responses to an influenza vaccine in mice. Vaccine 31: 1725–1733.

40. Koup RA, Graham BS, Douek DC (2011) The quest for a T cell-based immune correlate of protection against HIV: a story of trials and errors. Nat Rev Immunol 11: 65–70.

41. Lorincz O, Toke ER, Somogyi E, Horkay F, Chandran PL, et al. (2012) Structure and biological activity of pathogen-like synthetic nanomedicines. Nanomedicine 8: 497–506.

42. De Filette M, Soehle S, Ulbert S, Richner J, Diamond MS, et al. (2014) Vaccination of mice using the West Nile virus E-protein in a DNA prime-protein boost strategy stimulates cell-mediated immunity and protects mice against a lethal challenge. PLoS One 9: e87837.

43. Diebold SS, Kursa M, Wagner E, Cotten M, Zenke M (1999) Mannose polyethylenimine conjugates for targeted DNA delivery into dendritic cells. J Biol Chem 274: 19087–19094.

44. Magnusson SE, Karlsson KH, Reimer JM, Corbach-Sohle S, Patel S, et al. (2014) Matrix-M adjuvanted envelope protein vaccine protects against lethal lineage 1 and 2 West Nile virus infection in mice. Vaccine 32: 800–808.

45. Toke ER, Lorincz O, Somogyi E, Lisziewicz J (2010) Rational development of a stable liquid formulation for nanomedicine products. Int J Pharm 392: 261–267.

46. Barzon L, Franchin E, Squarzon L, Lavezzo E, Toppo S, et al. (2009) Genome sequence analysis of the first human West Nile virus isolated in Italy in 2009. Euro Surveill 14.

47. Amanna IJ, Raue HP, Slifka MK (2012) Development of a new hydrogen peroxide-based vaccine platform. Nat Med 18: 974–979.

48. Karber G (1931) 50% end-point calculation Arch Exp Pathol Pharmakol 162: 480–483.

49. Donaldson MM, Kao SF, Eslamizar L, Gee C, Koopman G, et al. (2012) Optimization and qualification of an 8-color intracellular cytokine staining assay for quantifying T cell responses in rhesus macaques for pre-clinical vaccine studies. J Immunol Methods 386: 10–21.

50. Lanciotti RS, Kerst AJ, Nasci RS, Godsey MS, Mitchell CJ, et al. (2000) Rapid detection of west nile virus from human clinical specimens, field-collected mosquitoes, and avian samples by a TaqMan reverse transcriptase-PCR assay. J Clin Microbiol 38: 4066–4071.

51. Nolan MS, Podoll AS, Hause AM, Akers KM, Finkel KW, et al. (2012) Prevalence of chronic kidney disease and progression of disease over time among patients enrolled in the Houston West Nile virus cohort. PLoS One 7: e40374.

52. Hughes HR, Crill WD, Davis BS, Chang GJ (2012) A West Nile virus CD4 T cell epitope improves the immunogenicity of dengue virus serotype 2 vaccines. Virology 424: 129–137.

53. Netland J, Bevan MJ (2013) CD8 and CD4 T cells in west nile virus immunity and pathogenesis. Viruses 5: 2573–2584.

54. Larsen MV, Lelic A, Parsons R, Nielsen M, Hoof I, et al. (2010) Identification of CD8+ T cell epitopes in the West Nile virus polyprotein by reverse-immunology using NetCTL. PLoS One 5: e12697.

55. Mooij P, Nieuwenhuis IG, Knoop CJ, Doms RW, Bogers WM, et al. (2004) Qualitative T-helper responses to multiple viral antigens correlate with vaccine-induced immunity to simian/human immunodeficiency virus infection. J Virol 78: 3333–3342.

56. Rollier C, Verschoor EJ, Paranhos-Baccala G, Drexhage JA, Verstrepen BE, et al. (2005) Modulation of vaccine-induced immune responses to hepatitis C virus in rhesus macaques by altering priming before adenovirus boosting. J Infect Dis 192: 920–929.

57. Oliphant T, Engle M, Nybakken GE, Doane C, Johnson S, et al. (2005) Development of a humanized monoclonal antibody with therapeutic potential against West Nile virus. Nat Med 11: 522–530.

58. Styer LM, Kent KA, Albright RG, Bennett CJ, Kramer LD, et al. (2007) Mosquitoes inoculate high doses of West Nile virus as they probe and feed on live hosts. PLoS Pathog 3: 1262–1270.

59. Ishikawa T, Yamanaka A, Konishi E (2014) A review of successful flavivirus vaccines and the problems with those flaviviruses for which vaccines are not yet available. Vaccine 32: 1326–1337.

60. Sambri V, Capobianchi M, Charrel R, Fyodorova M, Gaibani P, et al. (2013) West Nile virus in Europe: emergence, epidemiology, diagnosis, treatment, and prevention. Clin Microbiol Infect 19: 699–704.

10

Replication Rates of *Mycobacterium tuberculosis* in Human Macrophages Do Not Correlate with Mycobacterial Antibiotic Susceptibility

Johanna Raffetseder[9], **Elsje Pienaar**[9¤a], **Robert Blomgran, Daniel Eklund, Veronika Patcha Brodin, Henrik Andersson, Amanda Welin**[¤b], **Maria Lerm***

Division of Microbiology and Molecular Medicine, Department of Clinical and Experimental Medicine, Faculty of Health Sciences, Linköping University, Linköping, SE-58185, Sweden

Abstract

The standard treatment of tuberculosis (TB) takes six to nine months to complete and this lengthy therapy contributes to the emergence of drug-resistant TB. TB is caused by *Mycobacterium tuberculosis* (Mtb) and the ability of this bacterium to switch to a dormant phenotype has been suggested to be responsible for the slow clearance during treatment. A recent study showed that the replication rate of a non-virulent mycobacterium, *Mycobacterium smegmatis,* did not correlate with antibiotic susceptibility. However, the question whether this observation also holds true for Mtb remains unanswered. Here, in order to mimic physiological conditions of TB infection, we established a protocol based on long-term infection of primary human macrophages, featuring Mtb replicating at different rates inside the cells. During conditions that restricted Mtb replication, the bacterial phenotype was associated with reduced acid-fastness. However, these phenotypically altered bacteria were as sensitive to isoniazid, pyrazinamide and ethambutol as intracellularly replicating Mtb. In support of the recent findings with *M. smegmatis,* we conclude that replication rates of Mtb do not correlate with antibiotic tolerance.

Editor: Jordi B. Torrelles, The Ohio State University, United States of America

Funding: The project was funded by the Bill & Melinda Gates Foundation (www.gatesfoundation.org), the Swedish Research Council (grant numbers 2009-3821 and 2012-3349, www.vr.se), the Swedish International Development Cooperation Agency (www.sida.se), the Swedish Heart-Lung Foundation (www.hjart-lungfonden.se), King Oscar II Foundation, Carl Trygger Foundation (www.carltryggersstiftelse.se), and the Clas Groschinsky Foundation (www.groschinsky.org). The funders had no role in study design, data collection and analysis, decision to publish, or preparation of the manuscript.

Competing Interests: The authors have declared that no competing interests exist.

* Email: maria.lerm@liu.se

¤a Current address: Department of Microbiology and Immunology, Department of Chemical Engineering, University of Michigan, Ann Arbor, Michigan, 48109-2136, United States of America
¤b Current address: Phagocyte Research Laboratory, Department of Rheumatology and Inflammation Research, Sahlgrenska Academy, University of Gothenburg, Gothenburg, SE-41346, Sweden

[9] These authors contributed equally to this work.

Introduction

Tuberculosis (TB) is caused by *Mycobacterium tuberculosis* (Mtb), which primarily infects alveolar macrophages. Depending on the host immune status, the infection has different outcomes. In immunocompetent hosts, the bacterium may be controlled through innate immune mechanisms and/or by adaptive immunity [1,2]. In some individuals, the immune system fails to control the infection and the disease progresses to active TB. Factors that contribute to disease progression include HIV co-infection, malnutrition and predisposing genetic variations [1].

Treatment of TB requires administration of several drugs for at least 6 to 9 months, leading to high costs, side-effects and the emergence of drug-resistant strains associated with patient non-compliance. Therefore, one of the key elements in improved global TB control is a more effective treatment regimen to shorten the time of sterilizing antibiotic therapy by several months. Altered bacterial phenotypes have been suggested to be responsible for

tolerance of Mtb against antibiotics, and the prevailing view is that slow- or non-replicating bacteria in hypoxic granulomas are phenotypically tolerant towards antibiotics and thus responsible for the long time required for TB treatment. The hypoxic conditions in the granuloma have been mimicked *in vitro* by progressive oxygen depletion of cultures, rendering Mtb tolerant to isoniazid (INH) [3]. Although the absence of oxygen could directly affect the efficacy of INH [4,5,6], the tolerance has been attributed to the absence of replication [3].

In the human lung, Mtb can persist without the presence of granuloma [7], or in replicating and non-replicating states in subclinical lesions [8]. In the mouse model, Mtb can persist [9] although mice do not form hypoxic granulomas [10,11,12], and before the onset of adaptive immunity, substantial killing occurs [13]. Altogether, this speaks for a major role for innate immunity, at least during the early phase of infection and raises the question of tolerant Mtb being located outside of granulomas. Macrophages, constituting the primary target of infection and the first line of host defense, exert a range of pressures on the bacilli, forcing them to adapt to the harsh intracellular conditions and to shift phenotype, as shown earlier in different macrophage-based models [14,15,16] and mimicked in broth models [17]. We have shown that primary human macrophages are able to control bacterial net growth through mechanisms dependent on phagolysosomal functionality [18]. So far, Mtb replication and death rates have been difficult to determine and often neglected, although considerable evidence exists for divergent numbers of live and dead (or non-culturable) bacteria *in vivo* and *in vitro* [13,19,20,21]. The link between mycobacterial replication and drug tolerance is still not clear, and a recent study in a non-virulent mycobacterium, *Mycobacterium smegmatis*, elegantly showed that tolerance correlates with expression fluctuations of katG (a mycobacterial catalase-peroxidase which protects Mtb from oxidative stress but also transforms INH into its active form [22]) and is independent of replication rate [23]. Furthermore, asymmetrical division of *M. smegmatis* resulting in phenotypically heterogeneous siblings growing at different rates did not cause any differences in antibiotic susceptibilities [24].

With this study, we take these findings into a more physiological setting and evaluate drug susceptibility of phenotypically different, virulent Mtb inside human monocyte-derived macrophages (hMDM). We observed that hMDMs are able to restrict intracellular Mtb net growth for at least 10 days, provided that the initial bacterial burden was low. During growth restriction, Mtb displayed a phenotype that was rich in lipid bodies, but negative for acid-fast staining, both of which are features that have been linked to persistent Mtb. A higher bacterial burden, on the other hand, promoted an actively replicating phenotype that was positive for acid-fast staining. Finally, we tested whether the susceptibility towards first- and second-line TB drugs was different in the characterized phenotypes. Consistently with the findings obtained with *M. smegmatis*, we demonstrate that an altered replication rate of Mtb did not influence the susceptibility of the bacterium to antibiotics.

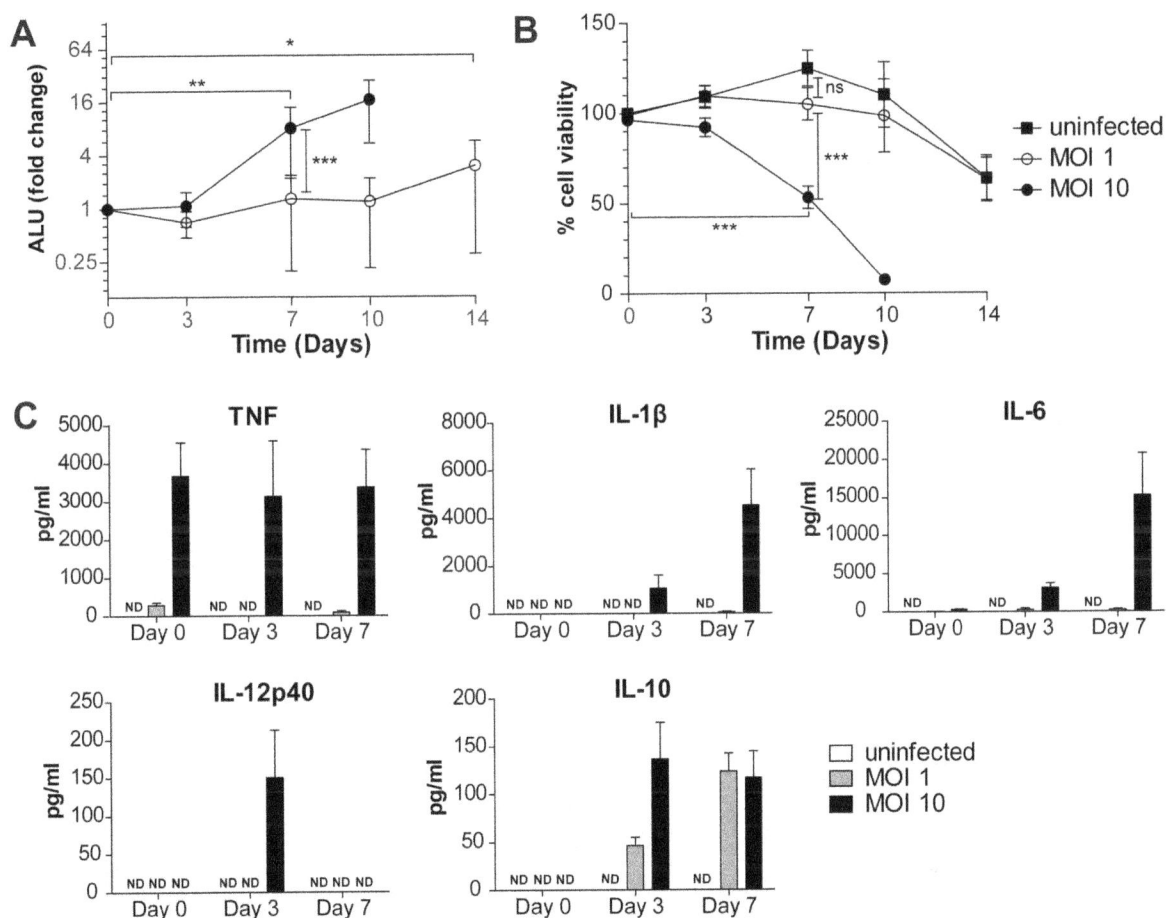

Figure 1. Kinetics of Mtb growth, macrophage cell death and cytokine secretion. Bacterial fold change (A; normalized to day 0 values of the respective MOI) and percentage of macrophage survival (B; normalized to uninfected controls on day 0) were measured during 14 days of H37Rv infection using luminometry for bacterial numbers and calcein-AM for macrophage viability. Arbitrary luminescence units (ALU) for medium supernatant and lysate (Figure S1) measurements were added to give totals (A). n = 7–32 and symbols and error bars represent means and 95% confidence intervals. Comparisons between MOI 1 and MOI 10 (and uninfected controls for (B)) at different time points were done using unmatched 2-way ANOVA of normalized values and Bonferroni post-hoc test for multiple comparisons. Significant changes compared to day 0 were determined using 1-way ANOVA of normalized values and Dunnett's test, and only the first time point significantly different from day 0 is indicated with asterisks (A and B). *p<0.05, **p<0.01, ***p<0.001. (C) For cytokine analysis, medium supernatants were saved on the respective days of infection and analyzed by cytokine bead array for the indicated cytokines. n = 5–7 and bars and error bars depict means and SEMs, respectively. ND: Not detected.

Results

Macrophages control Mtb net growth during a low burden infection

In order to establish whether unstimulated hMDMs were able to restrict growth of virulent Mtb for an extended period of time, we performed infection experiments through 14 days of infection. We found that infection of hMDMs with Mtb H37Rv at a multiplicity of infection (MOI) of 1 did not result in any significant net increase in bacterial numbers for at least 10 days, a period during which cell viability of infected cells was similar to uninfected cells (Figure 1A and B). On the contrary, infection with a higher MOI (MOI 10) resulted in significant bacterial growth by day 7 (Figure 1A), coinciding with extensive cell death (Figure 1B) and release of Mtb from dying cells causing an increase in the extracellular fraction, but not in the cell-associated fraction (Figure S1).

The different outcomes of MOI 1 and MOI 10 infection prompted us to map the inflammatory response of the cells to the different bacterial loads. Cells infected with MOI 10 released high amounts of TNF at day 0, and of IL-1β, IL-6, IL-12p40 and IL-10 starting from day 3. Cells infected with MOI 1 initially secreted TNF at levels corresponding to approximately 10% of the amount secreted from the MOI 10-infected cells. However, at day 3, there was no detectible TNF secretion from MOI 1-infected cells, followed by a slight increase by day 7. The other investigated pro-inflammatory cytokines were low (IL-6 on day 3 and IL-1β and IL-6 on day 7) or undetectable (IL-1β and IL-12p40 on day 3) during MOI 1 infection. On the other hand, the levels of the anti-inflammatory cytokine IL-10 increased by day 3 and were equal for both MOIs by day 7. Uninfected cells did not release any of the cytokines measured (Figure 1C), and hMDMs exhibited a heterogeneous phenotype at the time of infection, expressing both M1 and M2 macrophage makers (Figure S2 and Table S1), corresponding to a more dynamic classification of macrophages, as proposed by Mosser and Edwards [25], rather than the conventional IFNγ-/IL-4-induced M1/M2 phenotypes.

During the course of infection, bacterial numbers were measured using a H37Rv strain carrying a luciferase-encoding plasmid with a hygromycin resistance marker (pSMT1). To rule out the possibility of changes in luciferase expression after infection, we routinely correlated arbitrary luminescence units (ALU) to bacterial CFU. During extended macrophage infection,

ALU and CFU correlated well and most importantly, bacterial numbers were not underestimated when using luminometry (Figure S3A). Furthermore, the luminescent signal did not diminish when hygromycin is absent indicating that plasmid loss does not occur during a time period of at least 14 days (Figure S3B). This is further supported by earlier publications on the same plasmid showing that CFU and ALU correlate well for at least 60 days in a murine infection model [26].

Bacterial replication rates are dependent on the initial bacterial burden

To investigate whether the absence of intracellular net growth during MOI 1 infection reflects bona fide non-replicating bacteria or a dynamic equilibrium (growth balanced by killing by macrophages), we used the replication clock plasmid [13]. Briefly, this low copy plasmid is lost from each generation at a constant rate, and together with the proportion of plasmid-containing Mtb, this rate can be used to derive the replication (r) and death (d) rates of the bacteria in a given population at a given time point.

Analysis of plasmid loss from intracellular bacteria revealed that during the initial phase of MOI 1 infection, there was no significant loss of plasmid (Figure 2A, estimated generation time of 6.5 days or 158 h). Between day 7 and 14 of MOI 1 infection, a shorter generation time of 1.5 days (38 h) was accompanied by an increase in bacterial death rate (r = 0.43 and d = 0.40, Figure 2B), suggesting growth balanced by killing during the later phase of infection. Both phases are consistent with the absence of net growth as observed in Figure 1A. For the time span between day 0 and day 7 during MOI 10 infection, Mtb was estimated to replicate once every 3 days (76 h, r = 0.22, d = 0.07, Figure 2B). The larger difference between r and d during MOI 10 compared to MOI 1 infection is reflected in the observed net growth during MOI 10 infection (Figure 1A). The method likely underestimates the replication rate (and hence overestimates the generation time) of the MOI 10 infection, since dying macrophages release replicating bacteria into the supernatant. For comparison, we determined the generation time in broth for H37Rv to be 37 hours.

Intracellular bacterial phenotype

Next, we characterized whether the slow-growing Mtb during MOI 1 infection displayed an altered phenotype, as compared to the actively growing Mtb during MOI 10 infection. Persistent Mtb

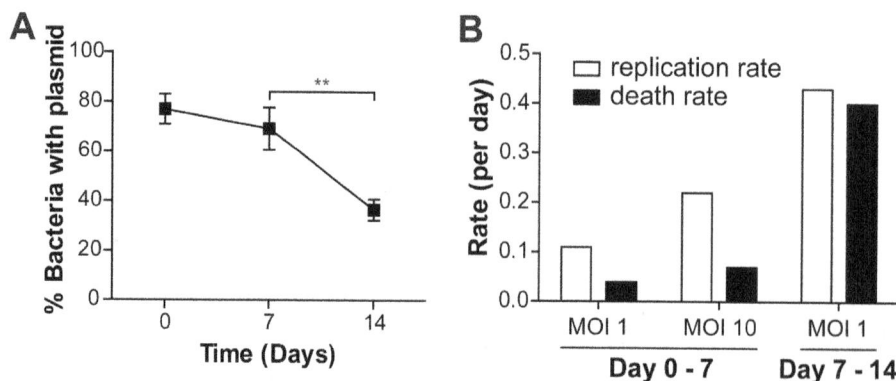

Figure 2. Loss of clock plasmid in the intracellular fraction and estimated mycobacterial replication and death rates. (A) CFU counts from cell lysates during MOI 1 infection on kanamycin-containing plates normalized to total CFU counts on plates without kanamycin. Differences in percentage of bacteria containing the clock plasmid was analyzed using 1-way ANOVA and Tukey's post-hoc test. n = 8–11. **p<0.01. (B) Estimated replication and death rates (per day) for intracellular Mtb were calculated from clock plasmid CFU data. Rates for MOI 10 infection between day 7 and 14 could not be determined due to extensive cell death.

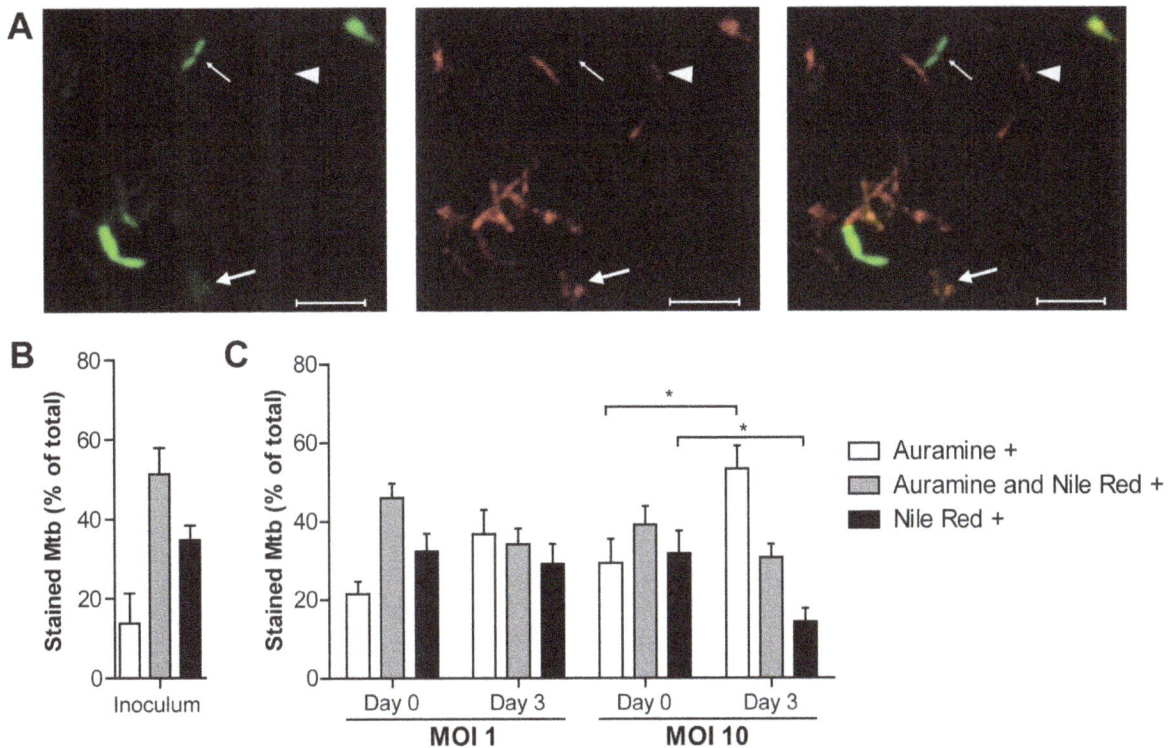

Figure 3. Phenotypic characteristics of Mtb inoculum and during macrophage infection. (A) Representative image of intracellular Mtb stained with Auramine O and Nile Red, counted as either Auramine O-positive (thin arrow), Nile Red-positive (arrowhead) or as positive for both stainings (thick arrow). Scale bar: 5 μm. (B) Percentage of bacteria stained with Auramine O, Nile Red or both in the inoculum. n = 3. (C) Percentage of Auramine O/Nile Red-positive intracellular bacteria, using hMDMs from 20 different donors. Significant changes were determined using 1-way ANOVA comparison followed by Bonferroni's multiple comparison test. *$p < 0.05$. Bars and error bars represent means and SEMs respectively.

are characterized by reduced acid-fastness and intrabacterial accumulation of lipid bodies, as observed *in vivo* in the lungs of latently infected individuals, in sputum from TB patients and in an *in vitro* multiple-stress dormancy model [17,27,28]. In order to determine the phenotype of intracellular Mtb, we implemented a combined acid-fast (Auramine O) and lipid body (Nile Red) staining technique [17]. Representative images of stained intracellular Mtb are shown in Figure 3A. The inoculum displayed a mixed phenotype, with 14% of bacteria being positive for Auramine O only, 51% positive for both Auramine and Nile Red, and 35% positive for Nile Red only (Figure 3B).

One hour after infection (Day 0) with either MOI 1 or MOI 10, the staining pattern of intracellular Mtb resembled the inoculum (Figure 3B and C), indicating that no phenotypic shift occurred during the first hour of infection. This phenotype was not altered during MOI 1 infection by day 3 (Figure 3C), suggesting that the macrophages were able to maintain the initial bacterial phenotype. In contrast, there was a shift in the staining pattern of Mtb infecting the macrophages at the MOI 10 ratio, with a significant increase in Auramine-positive and a significant decrease in Nile Red-positive bacteria (Figure 3C). This phenotypic shift coincided with the bacterial replication observed during MOI 10 infection.

Antibiotic susceptibility of different Mtb phenotypes

Having established that our primary human macrophages were able to maintain an altered, slow-growing and lipid-rich phenotype of Mtb, we tested whether the sensitivity of these bacteria towards some first- and second-line antimycobacterial drugs was different

from the sensitivity of actively replicating, acid-fast bacteria in the same system.

To this end, antibiotics at concentrations based on human peak serum levels were added 1 hour after infection with either MOI 1 or MOI 10 and the number of intracellular bacteria was measured 4 days later. At this time point, no replication had taken place in the MOI 1 situation, whereas one replication had occurred in the MOI 10 situation (as determined by the clock plasmid experiment), thus reflecting situations with non-replicating and replicating bacteria, respectively (schematically outlined in Figure 4A). Significant reduction of bacterial numbers was seen after treatment with three of the first-line drugs ethambutol (EMB), INH and pyrazinamide (PZA) (Figure 4B), but there was no difference between the two MOIs. One possible interpretation of this result may be that the bacteria need time to shift to a different phenotype in the MOI 10 situation. To test this, we performed an additional experiment, in which the antibiotics were added 3 days after infection. Again, bacterial numbers were determined 4 days after addition of antibiotics, and INH was found to significantly kill intracellular bacteria (Figure 4C), but without any difference in antibiotic susceptibility between MOI 1 and MOI 10 infection. The same set of experiments was carried out with second-line drugs (amikacin, capreomycin, kanamycin, metronidazole and streptomycin), but none of the tested drugs caused any significant reduction in bacterial numbers as compared to untreated controls. As observed with the first-line drugs, there was no difference between the two MOIs (Figure S4), and none of the tested first- and second-line drugs rescued cell viability as compared to the untreated controls (Figure S5).

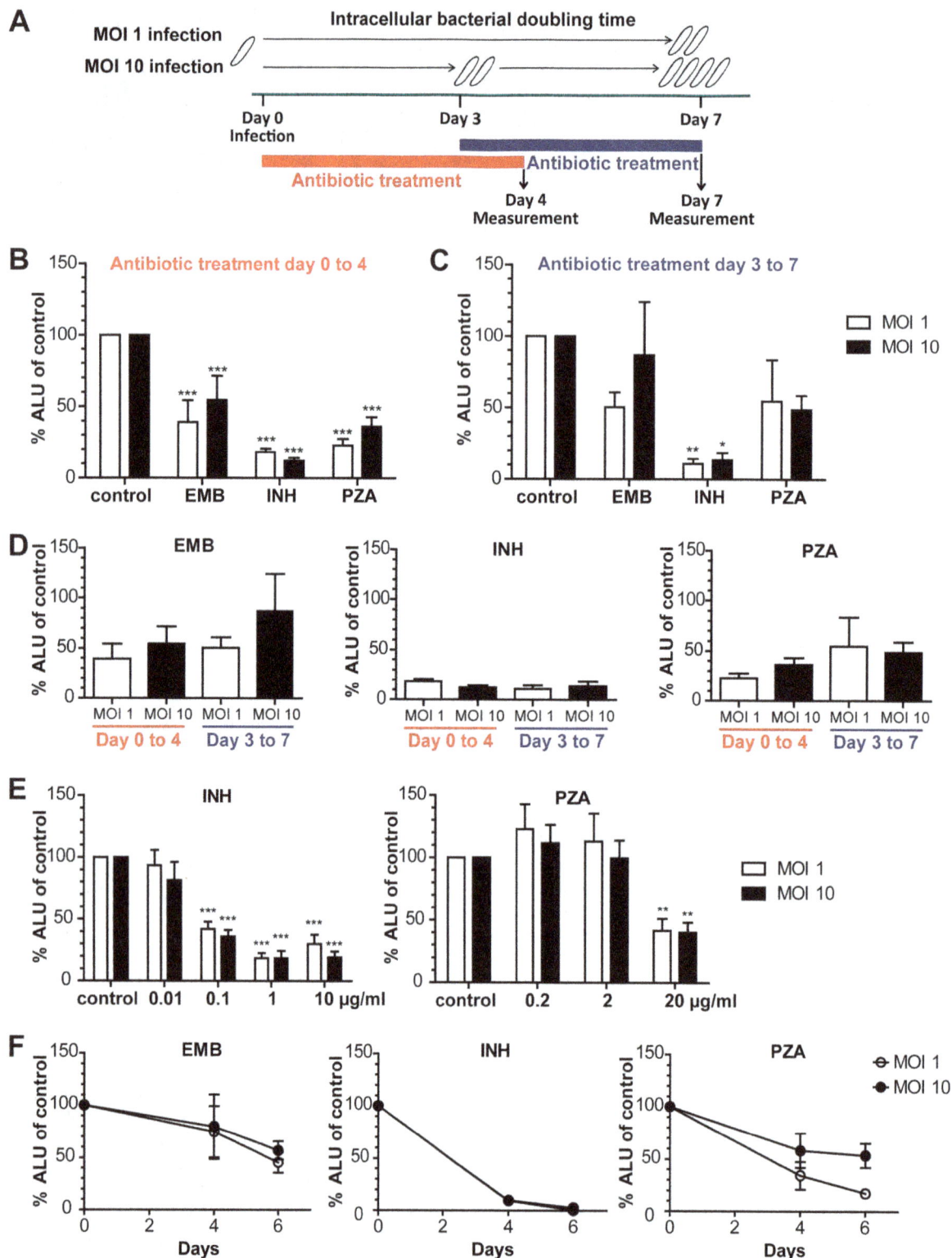

Figure 4. Antibiotic susceptibility of intracellular Mtb. (A) Schematic outline of the experiments, with antibiotics being added either 1 h (B) after infection or after 3 days (C) when Mtb in MOI 10-infected cells already had replicated once. Intracellular bacteria were quantified 4 days later on day 4 or 7, respectively. Antibiotics were used at the following concentrations derived from human peak serum levels: 1 μg/ml ethambutol (EMB), 10 μg/ml isoniazid (INH) and 20 μg/ml pyrazinamide (PZA). ALU as a measure of bacterial numbers were normalized against untreated controls of the same donor. Significant changes were determined using 2-way ANOVA followed by Bonferroni's post-hoc test comparing treated samples to untreated control. Differences between MOIs were not significant. (D) contains the data from (B) and (C). Groups were compared using 1-way ANOVA and Tukey's post-hoc test. No significant differences were found. (E) Lower concentrations of INH and PZA were added than in B–D (0.01, 0.1 and 1 μg/ml INH and 0.2 and 2 μg/ml PZA), and intracellular bacteria were measured on day 4. Significant differences between treated samples and untreated control were determined using 2-way ANOVA followed by Bonferroni's post-hoc test (indicated with asterisks). No significant difference

between MOIs was found. (F) Antibiotics were added 1 h after infection as in (B) and (E), but infection was extended beyond day 4 with another measurement on day 6. n = 5–10 in (B–D), n = 3 in (E) and n = 3 in (F). Bars and error bars represent means and SEMs, respectively. *p<0.05, **p<0.01 and ***p<0.001.

Using the data presented in Figure 4B and 4C, we made a statistical comparison of the percentage of bacteria remaining after 4 days of antibiotics treatment independently of whether the antibiotics were added at day 0 or day 3. The efficacy of EMB, INH and PZA did not differ between MOIs and time points (Figure 4D), indicating that the antibiotic susceptibility was not dependent on the replicative state of the bacteria. In order to rule out that the concentrations of drugs are too high to discriminate between tolerant and susceptible bacteria, we tested lower concentrations of the drugs with the best intracellular effect, INH and PZA, but again, no significant differences between MOIs could be observed (Figure 4E). Treatment with antibiotics was also extended beyond 4 days, showing that bacterial numbers can be further diminished (Figure 4F), which speaks against a residual tolerant population.

The antibiotics were demonstrated to be effective against H37Rv in 7H9 broth cultures (Figure S6), with the exception of PZA that requires acidic pH for activity and was not expected to have any effect in broth, as well as metronidazole which requires anaerobic conditions [3,29]. All the other first and second line drugs effectively killed bacteria in broth, indicating that the bacteria used are genotypically susceptible to those antibiotics.

We also assessed whether treatment with INH, PZA and EMB affected the two studied phenotypes differently using the Auramine O/Nile Red staining protocol on intracellular Mtb after 4 days of infection. The activities of the studied drugs did not affect a certain phenotype more than the other, however, the reliability of the method could have been influenced by the fact that also antibiotic-killed bacteria were stained as indicated by the fragmented appearance of many bacteria (not shown).

Discussion

Aiming to understand how Mtb phenotypes relate to the lengthy treatment required for TB, we investigated antibiotic susceptibility of Mtb inside macrophages. Two major findings guided the investigation: first, evidence has accumulated that not only necrotic granulomas but also macrophages can harbor altered phenotypes of Mtb [14,15,16,30,31,32], and second, that antibiotic susceptibility might not necessarily be coupled to mycobacterial replication rate [23].

We found that unstimulated primary human macrophages harbored an altered phenotype of Mtb during low-burden infection, characterized by slow replication, lipid bodies and reduced acid-fast staining and that this phenotype exhibited similar antibiotic susceptibility as did actively replicating, acid-fast Mtb. The control of bacterial net growth in human macrophages infected with a low bacterial burden was earlier shown to depend on effective phagosomal acidification [18], while macrophages infected with Mtb at higher MOIs undergo necrotic cell death coinciding with intracellular replication [33]. In the present study, long-term infection experiments showed that the balance between macrophages and Mtb at the low MOI could be maintained for at least 10 days. While restriction of mycobacterial growth has been described in other macrophage-based systems, this was dependent on manipulation of the macrophages via factors such as IFN-γ, TNF, GM-CSF or hypoxic conditions [14,15,16]. These studies only describe the absolute numbers of intracellular bacteria and do not provide information about bacterial replication and killing

rates. We included the clock plasmid replication rate analysis [13] in order to distinguish lack of replication from coincident replication and death, both of which would result in unchanged bacterial numbers over time. During low MOI infection, an early phase of slow replication was followed by a phase of faster replication and compensatory killing. The fact that a period of bacterial turnover follows the initial phase suggests that Mtb dynamically cycles between actively replicating and non- or slow-replicating states. A possible explanation for the low bacterial death rate during the early stage of MOI 1 infection is that macrophage effector functions are ineffective against this phenotype of Mtb, which would provide a rationale for its existence. Our observation of an initial stage of slow-replicating bacteria is contrary to previous findings with Mtb CDC1551 infection of murine bone marrow-derived macrophages [19], which showed higher replication (and death) rates associated with a net decrease in bacterial load in the initial phase of the infection, followed by lower replication (and death) rates coincident with a net increase in bacterial numbers. The divergent results may be explained by differential inherent ability of murine and human macrophages to control Mtb infection, by strain variability and possibly also by factors affecting the phenotype(s) of the Mtb inoculum.

The absence of cytokine release from uninfected cells confirms that the cells were not pre-activated and suggests that factors acting inside the cells rather than mediators acting via auto- or paracrine routes contribute to the restriction of intracellular Mtb growth. Analyzing the Mtb inoculum, we found that both replicating (acid-fast-positive) and persister-like (lipid-rich/acid-fast-negative) bacteria were present, probably due to our unagitated Mtb culture conditions. This inoculum phenotypically resembles Mtb found in sputum from TB patients [28], thus constituting a physiologically relevant source of Mtb. Characterization of intracellular Mtb at the higher MOI revealed a significant shift towards the acid-fast-positive, lipid body-negative phenotype, which correlated with a higher replication rate. In contrast, the mixed Mtb phenotypes observed during initial infection were maintained throughout the experiment at the low MOI. Cell wall alterations leading to decreased acid-fastness are features of Mtb persistence in vivo [27,34], and both lost acid-fastness and accumulation of lipid bodies can be induced in a multiple-stress dormancy model [17], and in hypoxic macrophages [14]. In contrast, we show that unstimulated macrophages can harbor an altered Mtb phenotype under normal oxygen pressure. We were unable to quantify whether simultaneous bacterial replication and persistence occurs within the same cell since we could not distinguish the borders of individual cells using this staining protocol. However, the frequent appearance of Auramine O-positive bacteria in the vicinity of Nile Red-positive bacilli suggests that both phenotypes can exist in the same cell. Since the inoculum used in this study contained a mixture of Mtb phenotypes, we cannot make conclusions regarding the ability of the macrophages to induce a phenotypic shift from actively replicating to a lipid-body-rich and acid-fast-negative phenotype. Although this question needs further attention, previous studies have reported induction of stress-regulated genes in Mtb upon uptake into macrophages [19,35], suggesting that the pathogen alters its phenotype to endure the stressful intracellular environment.

Phenotypic drug tolerance has been attributed to the absence of replication, e.g. in *E. coli* [36] and recently also in intracellular *Salmonella* [37]. We found that EMB, INH and PZA efficiently killed intracellular bacilli, and the extent of killing was independent of the MOI, i.e. of the bacterial replication rate. Regardless of MOI and of the time point of addition of antibiotics, the susceptibility pattern was similar, suggesting that antibiotic tolerance of intracellular bacteria does not correlate with bacterial replication rates. Our results provide two possible explanations to the enigmatic fact that INH, which has been traditionally viewed as a drug that is ineffective against non-replicating Mtb [3], is successfully used to treat latent TB [38]. First, we show that it is possible that a macrophage population can balance growth by killing, housing actively replicating bacteria without a net increase of bacterial load, which has been shown to be the case in a mouse model for chronic TB [13]. More importantly, we show that independently of replication rates, INH is as effective in killing Mtb. Our data are supported by the recent study by Wakamoto et al. [23], in which INH tolerance of *Mycobacterium smegmatis* correlates with fluctuations in *katG* expression rather than replication rate. Another study led to a different conclusion and showed THP1 macrophage-induced tolerance to INH in replicating *Mycobacterium marinum* bacteria [30]. In the present study, we cannot exclude the possibility that activated or immunosuppressed macrophages would have rendered Mtb tolerant to INH or the other drugs tested here. We did not measure KatG fluctuations, and to our knowledge, this has not been studied inside macrophages. Furthermore, our model does not necessarily account for the Mtb phenotype found in the hypoxic core of granulomas, where Mtb might undergo a truly non-replicating state (Wayne) or be tolerant to INH due to other factors like oxygen inavailability [4,5]. The absence of activity of second-line drugs in our study is most likely explained by limited intracellular activity of these drugs [39]. Other studies, showing good intracellular effect of these antibiotics, did not investigate macrophage viability [40].

Although first-line drugs effectively killed the bacteria in MOI 10-infected cells in the present study, the treatment did not significantly rescue macrophage viability. The finding suggests that the initial bacterial load rather than the absolute numbers of bacteria determines cell death, however, the reason for this needs further investigation.

To conclude, unstimulated human macrophages were able to maintain phenotypically altered Mtb exhibiting some characteristics of persisters, which supports a role for innate immune cells in latent TB. Being based on infected primary human macrophages as opposed to broth cultures, our model provides a physiological environment in which altered Mtb phenotypes can be studied. Furthermore, we challenge the view that Mtb replication rates determine antibiotic susceptibility inside macrophages.

Materials and Methods

Ethics statement

Blood, collected at the blood bank at Linköping University Hospital, was obtained from healthy donors, who had given written consent for research use of the donated blood in accordance with the Declaration of Helsinki. Since blood donation is classified as a negligible risk to the donors and since only de-identified samples were delivered to the researchers, this study did not require a specific ethical approval according to paragraph 4 of the Swedish law (2003:460) on Ethical Conduct in Human Research.

Bacteria

Mtb H37Rv (ATCC) carrying the luciferase-encoding pSMT1 plasmid [26] or both the pSMT1 and the "clock plasmid" pBP10 [13] were grown in Middlebrook 7H9 broth (Difco, Becton Dickinson) supplemented with glycerol, Tween-80 and albumin-dextrose-catalase (ADC, Becton Dickinson) as described earlier [41], and reseeded into fresh medium 7 days before infection. Bacteria carrying the plasmids were selected with 100 µg/ml hygromycin (Sigma) for pSMT1 and 75 µg/ml kanamycin (Sigma) for pBP10.

Human monocyte-derived macrophages

For the preparation of hMDMs from heparinized whole blood or buffy coats, isolation of the mononuclear cell fraction using LymphoPrep (Axis Shield) and differentiation of monocytes were performed as described [18,33]. Monocytes were allowed to differentiate into hMDMs for 5–8 days in Dulbecco's Modified Eagle Medium (DMEM, Gibco) containing 80 µM L-Glutamine (Gibco) and 10% non-heat inactivated human serum (from blood bank at Linköping University Hospital) pooled from 5 donors. The day before infection, cells were trypsinized and re-seeded in serum-containing medium: 1×10^5 cells/well in triplicates in black 96-well plates (Greiner) for determination of bacterial growth and cell viability, and 2.5×10^5 cells/coverslip for staining.

Macrophage characterization

For staining of intracellular macrophage markers, cells were treated with Cytofix/Cytoperm™ (BD Pharmingen) before staining with antibodies. Antibody manufacturers and concentrations used are given in Table S2. Samples stained with fluorophore-conjugated secondary antibodies only served as background controls for intracellularly stained samples. Isotype antibody-treated cells were used as background controls and single- and non-stained cells for color compensation. 10,000 events/sample were acquired using a Gallios Flow Cytometer (Beckman Coulter) and data was analyzed using Kaluza or Flowjo.

Experimental infection

For infection, bacteria were passaged through a 27 gauge needle to remove aggregates and diluted in serum-free medium as described earlier [41], then added to the macrophages at an MOI of 1 or 10. After 1 hour of incubation, the medium was replaced by fresh DMEM containing human serum. For long-term infections, medium was changed on day 3, 7 and 10. For antibiotic susceptibility experiments, antibiotics (all from Sigma Aldrich) were added 1 hour or 3 days after infection. Intracellular bacterial numbers and cell viability were evaluated 4 days after addition of antibiotics as described below. Uninfected and untreated controls were included for all time points. Day 0 measurements were done 2 to 4 hours after infection.

Antibiotic susceptibility in broth

Mtb H37Rv expressing luciferase from the pSMT1 plasmid were prepared from the same culture as used for infection and diluted in Middlebrook 7H9 broth supplemented with Tween 80 and ADC, with or without antibiotics, to a concentration of 10^5 CFU/ml. Antibiotic concentrations used were the same as in the macrophage experiments. After 4 days of incubation, bacterial numbers were determined using the luminescence-based method described below.

Measurement of bacterial numbers and cell viability

Bacterial numbers were determined by a luminescence-based method published previously [41]. Aliquots of medium supernatants and lysates containing luciferase-expressing bacteria were transferred to white 96-well plates (Greiner), and flash luminescence after injection of the luciferase substrate (1% decanal, Sigma Aldrich) was measured in a plate reader (GloMax-Multi+ Detection System with Instinct Software, Promega). The remaining supernatants were pooled, spun down and frozen at −80°C for cytokine analysis, and cell viability was determined as described below prior to subjecting the cells to hypotonic lysis. Arbitrary luminescence units (ALU) obtained from supernatant and lysate measurements were corrected for background luminescence using ALU values from uninfected cells. In order to calculate the total values for each well (intracellular and extracellular bacteria), the ALUs of the supernatant and lysates were standardized for dilutions and summed up. For bacterial growth, the median value of each triplicate of all time points was normalized to the day 0 median of the same experiment (fold change) or normalized to medians of untreated controls of the same day in the antibiotics experiments.

To determine cell viability, cells were washed three times with PBS, followed by 30 min incubation with 4 µM calcein-AM (Molecular Probes). Fluorescence was measured in a plate reader. Arbitrary fluorescence units of infected samples were normalized to those of uninfected cells measured on day 0.

Correlating arbitrary luminescence units to CFU

In order to ensure the stable expression of the luciferase-encoding pSMT1 plasmid in Mtb H37Rv after macrophage infection and to exclude the possibility of underestimating the actual bacterial load due to plasmid loss, ALU measured in medium supernatants and lysates were repeatedly correlated to CFU obtained by traditional plating of the same samples. To do so, supernatant and lysate samples from triplicate wells were pooled, serially diluted and plated in triplicates on Middlebrook 7H10 agar supplemented with ADC. CFUs were counted after two and three weeks of incubation at 37°C, ALU und CFU calculated per well and the median CFU value was correlated to the mean ALU value (since triplicates had been pooled). In order to check for plasmid loss when bacteria are maintained without hygromycin, H37Rv expressing luciferase were grown in 7H9 broth supplemented with ADC in the presence and absence of the selecting antibiotic hygromycin. Every few days, ALUs were measured.

Cytokine analysis

Cytokine analysis was performed using the human flex sets for TNF, IL-1β, IL-6, IL-10 and IL-12p40 for Cytokine Bead Array (Becton Dickinson), according to the manufacturer's instructions followed by an additional fixation step (4% paraformaldehyde for 30 min). Samples were measured using a Gallios Flow Cytometer (Beckman Coulter) and data were analyzed using Kaluza software (Beckman Coulter).

Evaluation of replication rates

The loss of the clock plasmid from intracellularly replicating bacteria was determined by CFU plating of cell lysates on Middlebrook 7H10 plates supplemented with ADC with and without 75 µg/ml kanamycin. Bacteria containing the plasmid grow on both plates, whereas CFUs of bacteria without the plasmid appear only on kanamycin-free plates. The rate of plasmid loss (segregation rate) was determined in logarithmic

phase cultures to be 0.2. Bacterial replication and death rates can be calculated from the segregation rate, total CFU and plasmid containing fractions as outlined elsewhere [13].

Staining of Mtb

Staining of the inoculum and intracellular Mtb was adapted from Garton et al. [42]. Inoculum was streaked on microscope slides, dried and heat-fixed. hMDMs infected on glass coverslips were fixed with 4% paraformaldehyde either 1 hour or 3 days after infection. Microscope slides and coverslips were treated with Auramine O solution (TB Auramine M by Becton Dickinson), acid alcohol and Nile Red (Sigma Aldrich). Between all steps, slides were washed with water. Samples were mounted with fluorescence mounting medium (DAKO). Microscopy was performed using a Zeiss LSM 700 confocal microscope, taking Z-stacks and using the Zen software (Zeiss) for image projection. Bacteria were evaluated for staining with Auramine O and Nile Red.

Supporting Information

Figure S1 Kinetics of Mtb growth in the extracellular and cell-associated fraction. Bacterial fold-change in the macrophage supernatant (A) and lysate (B) during the long-term infection experiments shown in Figure 1A and 1B. Bacterial numbers were measured using luminometry and expressed ALU normalized to Day 0 values. n = 7–32 and symbols and error bars represent means and 95% confidence intervals. Comparisons between MOI 1 and MOI 10 at different time points were done using unmatched 2-way ANOVA of normalized values and Bonferroni post-hoc test for multiple comparisons. Significant changes compared to day 0 were determined using 1-way ANOVA of normalized values and Dunnett's test, and only the first time point significantly different from day 0 is indicated with asterisks. **p<0.01, ***p<0.001.

Figure S2 Macrophage characterization. Surface (CD206, CD 163, DC-SIGN, CD86 and CD14) and intracellular (iNOS2, arginase I, and CD119) staining of hMDMs differentiated for 8 days. Plots show representative expression in one of six donors. Dashed lines show background fluorescence.

Figure S3 Correlation of arbitrary luminescence units to CFU, and plasmid stability. (A) ALUs from Mtb expressing luciferase were measured in aliquots of the cell lysates, and aliquots of the same samples were used for CFU plating. ALU/well and CFU/well are shown over time from one representative donor of four. (B) Mtb expressing luciferase were grown in the presence and absence of the selecting antibiotic hygromycin and bacterial numbers were quantified by luminometry. One representative experiment of two is shown.

Figure S4 Intracellular susceptibility of Mtb to second-line TB drugs. Antibiotics were added either 1 h after infection (A) or on day 3 (B) after infection. Intracellular bacterial numbers were measured 4 days later, on day 3 or day 7, respectively. Antibiotics were used at the following concentrations: 1 µg/ml amikacin (AMI), 30 µg/ml capreomycin (CAP), 10 µg/ml kanamycin (KAN), 10 µg/ml metronidazole (MTZ) and 10 µg/ml streptomycin (STR). Bacterial numbers were normalized against untreated controls of the same donor. Significant differences were determined using 2-way ANOVA followed by Bonferroni's multiple comparison test comparing treated samples to untreated control. n = 3–6 and bars and error bars represent means and SEMs, respectively.

Figure S5 Cell viability of infected macrophages treated with first- and second-line TB drugs. First-line drug treatments in (A) and (B) correspond to the bacterial growth data shown in Figure 4B and 4C, and second-line drug treatments in (C) and (D) correspond to Figure S4. Antibiotics were added 1 h after infection (A) and (C) or on day 3 (B) and (D), and cell viability was measured at the same time point as intracellular bacterial numbers were determined, on day 4 or 7, respectively and normalized against the cell viability of uninfected cells from the same day. Significant differences were determined using 2-way ANOVA followed by Bonferroni's multiple comparison test comparing treated samples to untreated but infected control. Bars and error bars represent means and SEMs, respectively. *p<0.05, **p<0.01 and ***p<0.001.
(EPS)

Figure S6 Antibiotic susceptibility of H37Rv in 7H9 broth. Luciferase-expressing Mtb H37Rv were inoculated in 7H9 broth and exposed to first- and second-line drugs or left untreated (Control) for 4 days. The antibiotic concentrations used were the same as in Figure 4 and Figure S4. The number of bacteria in the samples was then assessed using luminometry and normalized to untreated controls. Bars depict means from four (EMB, INH, PZA) or two (AMI, CAP, KAN, MTZ, STR) independent experiments and error bars represent SEM.
(EPS)

Table S1 Macrophage markers on hMDMs from cells from six independent donors.
(DOC)

Table S2 Antibodies used for macrophage characterization.
(DOC)

Acknowledgments

We are grateful to Professor David Sherman for providing us with the replication clock plasmid, and to Professor Jan Ernerudh and Judit Svensson for advice on macrophage characterization.

Author Contributions

Conceived and designed the experiments: JR EP RB DE VPB AW ML. Performed the experiments: JR EP RB DE VPB AW. Analyzed the data: JR EP RB DE HA VPB AW. Contributed reagents/materials/analysis tools: HA. Contributed to the writing of the manuscript: JR EP RB DE AW ML.

References

1. Lawn SD, Zumla AI (2011) Tuberculosis. Lancet 378: 57–72.
2. Schon T, Lerm M, Stendahl O (2013) Shortening the 'short-course' therapy-insights into host immunity may contribute to new treatment strategies for tuberculosis. J Intern Med 273: 368–382.
3. Wayne LG, Hayes LG (1996) An in vitro model for sequential study of shiftdown of Mycobacterium tuberculosis through two stages of nonreplicating persistence. Infect Immun 64: 2062–2069.
4. Youatt J (1960) The uptake of isoniazid and related compounds by Mycobacteria. Aust J Exp Biol Med Sci 38: 331–337.
5. Zabinski RF, Blanchard JS (1997) The Requirement for Manganese and Oxygen in the Isoniazid-Dependent Inactivation of Mycobacterium tuberculosis Enoyl Reductase. J Am Chem Soc 119: 2331–2332.
6. Magliozzo RS, Marcinkeviciene JA (1996) Evidence for Isoniazid Oxidation by Oxyferrous Mycobacterial Catalase−Peroxidase. J Am Chem Soc 118.
7. Hernandez-Pando R, Jeyanathan M, Mengistu G, Aguilar D, Orozco H, et al. (2000) Persistence of DNA from Mycobacterium tuberculosis in superficially normal lung tissue during latent infection. Lancet 356: 2133–2138.
8. Young DB, Gideon HP, Wilkinson RJ (2009) Eliminating latent tuberculosis. Trends Microbiol 17: 183–188.
9. McCune RM Jr, McDermott W, Tompsett R (1956) The fate of Mycobacterium tuberculosis in mouse tissues as determined by the microbial enumeration technique. II. The conversion of tuberculous infection to the latent state by the administration of pyrazinamide and a companion drug. J Exp Med 104: 763–802.
10. Via LE, Lin PL, Ray SM, Carrillo J, Allen SS, et al. (2008) Tuberculous granulomas are hypoxic in guinea pigs, rabbits, and nonhuman primates. Infect Immun 76: 2333–2340.
11. Aly S, Wagner K, Keller C, Malm S, Malzan A, et al. (2006) Oxygen status of lung granulomas in Mycobacterium tuberculosis-infected mice. J Pathol 210: 298–305.
12. Tsai MC, Chakravarty S, Zhu G, Xu J, Tanaka K, et al. (2006) Characterization of the tuberculous granuloma in murine and human lungs: cellular composition and relative tissue oxygen tension. Cell Microbiol 8: 218–232.
13. Gill WP, Harik N, Whiddon MR, Liao RP, Mittler JE, et al. (2009) A replication clock for Mycobacterium tuberculosis. Nat Med 15: 211–214.
14. Daniel J, Maamar H, Deb C, Sirakova TD, Kolattukudy PE (2011) Mycobacterium tuberculosis Uses Host Triacylglycerol to Accumulate Lipid Droplets and Acquires a Dormancy-Like Phenotype in Lipid-Loaded Macrophages. PLoS Pathog 7: e1002093.
15. Estrella JL, Kan-Sutton C, Gong X, Rajagopalan M, Lewis DE, et al. (2011) A Novel in vitro Human Macrophage Model to Study the Persistence of Mycobacterium tuberculosis Using Vitamin D(3) and Retinoic Acid Activated THP-1 Macrophages. Front Microbiol 2: 67.
16. Vogt G, Nathan C (2011) In vitro differentiation of human macrophages with enhanced antimycobacterial activity. J Clin Invest 121: 3889–3901.
17. Deb C, Lee CM, Dubey VS, Daniel J, Abomoelak B, et al. (2009) A novel in vitro multiple-stress dormancy model for Mycobacterium tuberculosis generates a lipid-loaded, drug-tolerant, dormant pathogen. PLoS One 4: e6077.
18. Welin A, Raffetseder J, Eklund D, Stendahl O, Lerm M (2011) Importance of phagosomal functionality for growth restriction of Mycobacterium tuberculosis in primary human macrophages J Innate Immun 3: 508–518.
19. Rohde KH, Veiga DF, Caldwell S, Balazsi G, Russell DG (2012) Linking the transcriptional profiles and the physiological states of Mycobacterium tuberculosis during an extended intracellular infection. PLoS Pathog 8: e1002769.
20. Muñoz-Elías E, Timm J, Botha T, Chan W-T, Gomez J, et al. (2005) Replication dynamics of Mycobacterium tuberculosis in chronically infected mice. Infect Immun 73: 546–551.
21. Lin P, Ford C, Coleman M, Myers A, Gawande R, et al. (2014) Sterilization of granulomas is common in active and latent tuberculosis despite within-host variability in bacterial killing. Nature Med 20: 75–79.
22. Sherman DR, Sabo PJ, Hickey MJ, Arain TM, Mahairas GG, et al. (1995) Disparate responses to oxidative stress in saprophytic and pathogenic mycobacteria. Proc Natl Acad Sci U S A 92: 6625–6629.
23. Wakamoto Y, Dhar N, Chait R, Schneider K, Signorino-Gelo F, et al. (2013) Dynamic persistence of antibiotic-stressed mycobacteria. Science 339: 91–95.
24. Santi I, Dhar N, Bousbaine D, Wakamoto Y, McKinney JD (2013) Single-cell dynamics of the chromosome replication and cell division cycles in mycobacteria. Nat Commun 4: 2470.
25. Mosser DM, Edwards JP (2008) Exploring the full spectrum of macrophage activation. Nat Rev Immunol 8: 958–969.
26. Snewin VA, Gares MP, Gaora PO, Hasan Z, Brown IN, et al. (1999) Assessment of immunity to mycobacterial infection with luciferase reporter constructs. Infect Immun 67: 4586–4593.
27. Seiler P, Ulrichs T, Bandermann S, Pradl L, Jorg S, et al. (2003) Cell-wall alterations as an attribute of Mycobacterium tuberculosis in latent infection. J Infect Dis 188: 1326–1331.
28. Garton NJ, Waddell SJ, Sherratt AL, Lee SM, Smith RJ, et al. (2008) Cytological and transcript analyses reveal fat and lazy persister-like bacilli in tuberculous sputum. PLoS Med 5: e75.
29. Zhang Y, Scorpio A, Nikaido H, Sun Z (1999) Role of acid pH and deficient efflux of pyrazinoic acid in unique susceptibility of Mycobacterium tuberculosis to pyrazinamide. J Bacteriol 181: 2044–2049.
30. Adams KN, Takaki K, Connolly LE, Wiedenhoft H, Winglee K, et al. (2011) Drug tolerance in replicating mycobacteria mediated by a macrophage-induced efflux mechanism. Cell 145: 39–53.
31. Peyron P, Vaubourgeix J, Poquet Y, Levillain F, Botanch C, et al. (2008) Foamy macrophages from tuberculous patients' granulomas constitute a nutrient-rich reservoir for M. tuberculosis persistence. PLoS Pathog 4: e1000204.
32. Caceres N, Tapia G, Ojanguren I, Altare F, Gil O, et al. (2009) Evolution of foamy macrophages in the pulmonary granulomas of experimental tuberculosis models. Tuberculosis (Edinb) 89: 175–182.
33. Welin A, Eklund D, Stendahl O, Lerm M (2011) Human Macrophages Infected with a High Burden of ESAT-6-Expressing M. tuberculosis Undergo Caspase-1- and Cathepsin B-Independent Necrosis. PLoS One 6: e20302.
34. Bhatt A, Fujiwara N, Bhatt K, Gurcha SS, Kremer L, et al. (2007) Deletion of kasB in Mycobacterium tuberculosis causes loss of acid-fastness and subclinical latent tuberculosis in immunocompetent mice. Proc Natl Acad Sci U S A 104: 5157–5162.
35. Tailleux L, Waddell SJ, Pelizzola M, Mortellaro A, Withers M, et al. (2008) Probing host pathogen cross-talk by transcriptional profiling of both Mycobacterium tuberculosis and infected human dendritic cells and macrophages. PLoS One 3: e1403.

36. Balaban NQ, Merrin J, Chait R, Kowalik L, Leibler S (2004) Bacterial persistence as a phenotypic switch. Science 305: 1622–1625.

37. Helaine S, Cheverton A, Watson K, Faure L, Matthews S, et al. (2014) Internalization of *Salmonella* by macrophages induces formation of nonreplicating persisters. Science 343: 204–208.

38. Zumla A, Atun R, Maeurer M, Mwaba P, Ma Z, et al. (2011) Viewpoint: Scientific dogmas, paradoxes and mysteries of latent *Mycobacterium tuberculosis* infection. Trop Med Int Health TM & IH 16: 79–83.

39. Dhillon J, Mitchison DA (1989) Activity and penetration of antituberculosis drugs in mouse peritoneal macrophages infected with *Mycobacterium microti* OV254. Antimicrob Agents Chemother 33: 1255–1259.

40. Rastogi N, Labrousse V, Goh KS (1996) *In vitro* activities of fourteen antimicrobial agents against drug susceptible and resistant clinical isolates of *Mycobacterium tuberculosis* and comparative intracellular activities against the virulent H37Rv strain in human macrophages. Curr Microbiol 33: 167–175.

41. Eklund D, Welin A, Schon T, Stendahl O, Huygen K, et al. (2010) Validation of a medium-throughput method for evaluation of intracellular growth of *Mycobacterium tuberculosis*. Clin Vaccine Immunol 17: 513–517.

42. Garton NJ, Christensen H, Minnikin DE, Adegbola RA, Barer MR (2002) Intracellular lipophilic inclusions of mycobacteria *in vitro* and in sputum. Microbiology 148: 2951–2958.

11

Hyaluronidase Modulates Inflammatory Response and Accelerates the Cutaneous Wound Healing

Marcio Fronza[1,4], Guilherme F. Caetano[2], Marcel N. Leite[2], Claudia S. Bitencourt[1], Francisco W. G. Paula-Silva[1], Thiago A. M. Andrade[2], Marco A. C. Frade[2], Irmgard Merfort[3], Lúcia H. Faccioli[1]*

1 Departamento de Análises Clínicas, Toxicológicas e Bromatológicas, Faculdade de Ciências Farmacêuticas de Ribeirão Preto, Universidade de São Paulo, Ribeirão Preto, São Paulo, Brazil, 2 Departamento de Clínica Médica, Divisão de Dermatologia, Faculdade de Medicina de Ribeirão Preto, Universidade de São Paulo, Ribeirão Preto, São Paulo, Brazil, 3 Department of Pharmaceutical Biology and Biotechnology, University of Freiburg, Freiburg, Germany, 4 Departamento de Farmácia, Universidade de Vila Velha, Vila Velha, Espirito Santo, Brazil

Abstract

Hyaluronidases are enzymes that degrade hyaluronan an important constituent of the extracellular matrix. They have been used as a spreading agent, improving the absorption of drugs and facilitating the subcutaneous infusion of fluids. Here, we investigated the influence of bovine testes hyaluronidase (HYAL) during cutaneous wound healing in *in vitro* and *in vivo* assays. We demonstrated in the wound scratch assay that HYAL increased the migration and proliferation of fibroblasts *in vitro* at low concentration, e.g. 0.1 U HYAL enhanced the cell number by 20%. HYAL presented faster and higher reepithelialization in *in vivo* full-thickness excisional wounds generated on adult Wistar rats back skin already in the early phase at 2nd day post operatory compared to vehicle-control group. Wound closured area observed in the 16 U and 32 U HYAL treated rats reached 38% and 46% compared to 19% in the controls, respectively. Histological and biochemical analyses supported the clinical observations and showed that HYAL treated wounds exhibited increased granulation tissue, diminished edema formation and regulated the inflammatory response by modulating the release of pro and anti-inflammatory cytokines, growth factor and eicosanoids mediators. Moreover, HYAL increased gene expression of peroxisome proliferator-activated receptors (PPAR) γ and PPAR β/δ, the collagen content in the early stages of healing processes as well as angiogenesis. Altogether these data revealed that HYAL accelerates wound healing processes and might be beneficial for treating wound disorders.

Editor: Masaya Yamamoto, Institute for Frontier Medical Sciences, Kyoto University, Japan

Funding: The authors are grateful to the São Paulo Research Foundation (FAPESP, grant # 2011/23992-3 and grant # 2009/07169-5) and Conselho Nacional de Desenvolvimento Científico e Tecnológico (CNPq) for financial support. The funders had no role in study design, data collection and analysis, decision to publish, or preparation of the manuscript.

Competing Interests: The authors have declared that no competing interests exist.

* Email: faccioli@fcfrp.usp.br

Introduction

A wound can be defined as a disruption of the anatomical, normal cellular and functional continuity of a structure. Thus, wound healing is a succession of complicated biochemical and cellular events that aims to restore the structural and functional integrity of the wounded tissue. The healing of cutaneous wounds is a multifaceted biological process that can be divided in three overlapping phases: inflammation, tissue formation, and tissue remodeling. The extracellular matrix synthesis and remodeling occurs during the entire processes [1,2]. Immediately after the skin injury, a rapid and coordinated response of several cell types is triggered, including circulating platelets, leukocytes, keratinocytes, fibroblasts and endothelial cells. The release of cytokines, eicosanoids, growth factors and activation of transcriptional regulation genes are required to mediate the communication between different cell types aiming the proper healing of full-thickness wounds [3–5]. Defects or imbalance in this process might destroy the delicate equilibrium of cells and soluble factors necessary for complete wound repair, resulting in fibrotic scar

[6,7]. These complex interaction processes responsible for the homeostasis of mature skin is tightly regulated through different molecular targets. Among such targets are transcription factors that control various pathways in cellular repair. In particular, the involvement of peroxisome proliferator-activated receptors (PPARs) has received special attention for their protective and healing attributes in tissue injury and wound repair [8,9].

Hyaluronic acid (HA) is a structural component of the extracellular matrix (ECM), but can also be located intracellular and increased following trauma. In the earliest phase of wound healing, there is a strict increase in HA in the site of injury, as a result of a combination of increased synthesis and impaired clearance [10,11]. The role of HA during wound repair is not well understood. HA displays antioxidant properties and can modulate wound healing by promoting cell migration and proliferation, facilitating leukocytes infiltration and improving tissue hydration [12,13]. However, elevated HA levels are often observed in hyperproliferative epidermis in the setting of acute inflammation, so-called inflammatory hyperplasia [14]. Degradation of HA mostly results from the enzymatic action of HYAL [15] which was recognized as a "spreading factor" by hydrolyzing the dermal barrier. HYAL has been therapeutically used for many years based on their properties in facilitating the subcutaneous infusion and dispersion of fluids thus improving absorption of drugs [16–19], besides its ability to reduce bleomycin-induced lung injury and fibrosis [20–22].

Although HYAL is involved in wound healing the exact mode of action is still unknown. Therefore, this study propose to investigate the mechanisms of action of the bovine testes HYAL in different stages of cutaneous wound healing using *in vitro* and *in vivo* models. Our results demonstrated that HYAL accelerated the wound healing process and might be beneficial for treating wound disorders.

Materials and Methods

Cell lines, chemicals and biochemicals

Swiss 3T3 albino mouse fibroblasts (Cell Line Service, Rio de Janeiro, Brazil - ATCC CCL-92) were maintained in Dulbecco's modified Eagle's medium (DMEM) supplemented with 10% fetal bovine serum (FBS), 100 IU/ml penicillin and 100 µg/ml streptomycin, at 37°C in a containing 5% CO_2 humidified atmosphere (all Gibco-BRL, Netherlands). HYAL from bovine testes (H3884), collagen solution, type I from rat tail and platelet derived growth factor-BB (PDGF) were from Sigma Chemical Co, MO, USA, Mitomycin C (Bristol-Myers) from a local pharmacy shop, enzyme-linked immunosorbent assays (ELISAs) for TNF-α, IFN-γ, IL-6, IL1-α, IL1-β, IL-10, IL-4, IL-5, TGF-β1 and VEGF from R & D Systems (Minneapolis, USA) and for the eicosanoids (PGE_2, PGD_2 and LTB_4) from Cayman Chemical (An Arbor, USA). Coomassie protein assay reagent from Thermo Scientific (Rockford, USA). Illustra RNAspin Mini Isolation Kit from GE Healthcare, (UK). Reverse transcription (High Quality cDNA Reverse Transcriptase Kit) and TaqMan primers were from Applied Biosystems (CA, USA).

Animals

48 adult male Wistar rats (*Rattus norvegicus*) (180–230 g), aged 6 to 7 weeks were obtained from the central Bioterium of the Medical School, Ribeirão Preto, University of São Paulo (FMRP-USP). In order to prevent skin lesions from fighting males, which may interfere with wound repair, animals were housed singly (1 week pre- and for the entire period post wounding). Animals were maintained under standard laboratory conditions with a 12 h light-dark cycle and a free access to food and water. All mouse experiments were conducted in accordance with the Brazilian Committee for animal care and use (COBEA) guidelines and approved by the University Animal Care Committee at USP-RP (process 2012.1.397.53.2).

In vitro cell migration assay

The proliferation and migration abilities of fibroblasts exposed to hyaluronidase were assessed using a scratch wound assay, which measures the expansion of a cell population on surfaces. The assay was performed as previously described [23] and in the Protocol S1.

In vivo wound-healing experiments

The animals were randomly divided in three groups (n = 16) and subdivided in four subgroups (n = 4). The groups were evaluated for 21 days in defined post-operatory periods according to standards protocols [24,25]. The following groups were used: in the vehicle-control group (control) the animals were only treated with 0.2 g/wound of 2% hydroxyethylcellulose gel base; in the hyaluronidase 16 U (HYAL 16 U) and hyaluronidase 32 U

(HYAL 32 U) groups the wounds were treated with hydroxyethyl-cellulose gel in a way that 0.2 g contained 16 and/or 32 U of active drug/wound, respectively. The pH value in the gels was monitored to be around 6.0 confirming optimal conditions for bovine testis HYAL activity [26]. The enzymatic activity of the HYAL used in the current study was turbidimetrically determined before and after the gel preparations using the methodology described by Pessini et al. (2001) [27]. Hydrolytic activity of hyaluronidase was preserved in the gel preparation (Table S1). Detailed information is given in the Protocol S1. The choice of hydroxyethylcellulose gel delivery system was based on its wide spread application in the pharmaceutical industry and its high biocompatibility [28]. As a comparator arm, a vehicle control containing the same formulation as the study product without the active agent was used [29]. Prior to the excisional wound induction, the animals were weight and deeply anesthetized by intraperitoneal (i.p.) administration of an association between ketamin (80 mg/Kg) and xylazine (15 mg/Kg). After shaving and cleaning with 70% ethanol two full thickness excision wounds were made on the dorsum cervical region of each rat with sterile 150 mm punch biopsy (Stiefel Laboratories, Offenbach, Germany). Immediately after the surgery and daily afterwards on the same hour, the control group and the HYAL treated groups received their respective treatments. The animals were euthanatized at 2nd, 7th, 14th and 21st post-operatory days and the wounds and their surrounding areas were cut with a sterile biopsy punch. One wound of each animal was snap frozen in liquid nitrogen and stored at −70°C. The other wound was used to perform histological analysis.

Rate of wound closure determination – morphometric evaluation

The morphometric analysis of the wounds was performed using images of the wounds at days zero, 2, 5, 7, 10, 14 and day 21 post-operatory to determine the remained wound area using Image J software (NIH, USA) [30]. The rate of wound closure that represents the percentage of wound reduction from the original wound size was calculated using the following formula: wound area day 0 – wound area (day 2, 5, 7, 10, 14 and 21)/wound area day 0×100. Values expressed as percentage of the healed wounds.

Histological analysis

The wound specimens were fixed in 4% phosphate-buffered formaldehyde at days 0, 2, 7, 14 and 21 post-wounding and processed according to the standard routine light microscope tissue protocols. The processed tissues were embedded in paraffin and serial sections of 5 µm-thick were mounted on glass slides, dewaxed, rehydrated to distilled water, and stained with hematoxylin and eosin (H&E) as well as with the solution of Sirius Red F3BA saturated in aqueous picric acid [20]. The slides were examined and photomicrographed in a blinded fashion using digital camera (LEICA DFC 280, Germany) attached to a light microscope (LEICA DM 4000B, Germany). Quantitative analysis of inflammatory infiltrate and angiogenesis by image analysis was determined as previously described [24,31] and in the Protocol S1. Photographs taken from the Picrosirius red-stained sections were used for quantifying the collagen content in the wound tissue [24]. The morphometric analysis corresponding to the area occupied by the fibers were determined by digital densitometry recognition and expressed as percentage of the total area of the field using Image J software (NIH, USA). Detailed information is given in the Protocol S1.

Cytokines and lipid mediators measurements

Tissue sections of wound biopsies treated with vehicle-control or HYAL 16 U were homogenized (Mixer Homogenizer, Labortechnik, Germany), centrifuged at 1500 g and stored at $-70°C$ until assayed. The homogenate fluid obtained were used to measure TNF-α, IFN-γ, IL-6, IL1-α, IL1-β, IL-10, IL-4, IL-5, TGF-β1 and VEGF by Enzyme-Linked Immunosorbent Assay (ELISA) techniques using specific antibodies (purified and biotinylated) and cytokine standards, according to the manufacturer's instructions (R&D Systems, Minneapolis, USA). Optical densities were measured at 450 nm in a microplate reader (μQuant, Biotek Instruments Inc.). Cytokine levels were expressed in pg, sensitivities were >10 pg/ml.

PGE$_2$, PGD$_2$ and LTB$_4$ were measured using ELISA according to the manufacturer's instructions (BD Biosciences and Cayman Chemical). The optical density of samples was determined at 420 nm in a microplate reader (μQuant, Biotek Instruments Inc.), and concentrations of eicosanoids were calculated based on the standard curve. The detection limit was 7.8 pg/ml for PGE$_2$, 19.5 pg/ml for PGD$_2$ and 3.9 pg/ml for LTB$_4$.

Total protein quantification

Total proteins were quantified in a homogenate fluid obtained from tissue sections of wounds treated with vehicle-control or 16 U HYAL by Coomassie protein assay reagent (Rockford, USA), according to the manufacturer's instructions.

Measurement of myeloperoxidase (MPO)

To determine the accumulation of neutrophils, MPO activity was assayed in wounds lysate according previous reports [24,32] with minor modifications as described in the Protocol S1.

Measurement of hydroxyproline

The amount of hydroxyproline present in the biopsies, which represents the collagen content in the wounds, was determined as previously described [33] with minor modifications as described in the Protocol S1.

Total RNA Extraction and qRT-PCR

To verify the expression of mRNA for PPAR α, PPAR γ and PPAR δ, the RNA was extracted from wounds biopsies after 16 U HYAL treatment and were analyzed by qRT-PCR. Relative quantification was performed using the $\Delta\Delta$Ct method according to the Protocol S1.

Statistical analysis

Statistical analyses were performed using GraphPad software (San Diego, CA, 176 USA). Data were expressed as mean $\pm$ standard error of mean (SEM). Statistical variations among groups were determined using one way analysis of variance (ANOVA) followed by Dunnett's post-test or two-way- ANOVA when appropriated. Values of $p < 0.05$ were considered significant.

Results

HYAL increased migration and proliferation of fibroblasts *in vitro* in a dose-dependent manner

The activity of HYAL (0.1 to 32 U) and its influence on proliferation and/or migration of 3T3 mouse fibroblasts were investigated using the scratch assay. HYAL dose-dependently enhanced the cell number in the gap with values ranging from $20 \pm 3.8\%$ (0.1 U) to $92 \pm 6.3\%$ (16 U). PDGF was used as positive control and exhibited a stimulatory effect of $52 \pm 4.7\%$ (2 ng/ml)

(Figure S1). Increased cell numbers can be due to immigration and/or proliferation of the migrated cells. To better distinguish between these two effects, mitomycin C (5 μg/ml) was added to the "wounded" monolayer cultures of fibroblasts together with either PDGF (2 ng/ml) or HYAL (0.1 U to 32 U). As addition of mitomycin C prevents mitosis and thereby proliferation, the remaining increase in the cell number is only due to migration [34,35]. The total cell numbers slightly decreased using mitomycin C and either PDGF or HYAL for all tested concentrations (see Figure S1) indicating that the observed effect in the *in vitro* scratch assay may be mainly due to migration and only marginally to proliferation.

HYAL accelerates wound closure *in vivo*

As showed in Figure 1, the wounds treated with 16 U or 32 U HYAL presented faster and higher reepithelialization compared to vehicle-control group. Selected doses of 16 U and 32 U were based on the *in vitro* scratch assay, in which these concentrations exhibited the maximum stimulatory effects on fibroblasts proliferation and migration, as well as on our previous *in vivo* studies using HYAL [20]. Wound closure area observed in the 16 U and 32 U HYAL reached 38% and 46% compared to only 19% in the controls already in the early stage (2nd day), respectively. After 5 and 7 days the closure wound in the 16 U and 32 U HYAL reached 67% and 68% (at day 5) and 85% and 89% (at day 7) as compare to 40% and 69% observed in control group, respectively. Interesting, by day 14 the wounds of HYAL-treated rats were completely closed, whereas the wounds of control rats had not yet completely healed. This observation suggests that HYAL positively influenced the wound healing process and that 16 U or 32 U HYAL treatments healed the full thickness wound in a similar speed. Therefore, the following experiments were performed using only 16 U HYAL.

HYAL affects cellular recruitment and edema formation

Histological analysis from the skin revealed significantly increased cellularity in the wounds of 16 U HYAL treated rats at days 2 and 7 compared to controls (Figure 2A, B). The density of cells 14 and 21 days post wounding were similar between treated and control groups and gradually decreased to physiological levels at 21st day. To evaluate whether neutrophils may have accumulated or have been activated, the activity of myeloperoxidase (MPO) was studied. As expected, MPO activity was very low in the intact skin (day zero) (Figure 2C). However, at day 2 post-wounding, MPO levels markedly increased in the animals treated with 16 U HYAL. At day 7, MPO activity in treated rats declined to similar levels as in the controls and both gradually declined thereafter to normal concentration at day 14 as observed in the day zero. To study if the decrease in MPO activity may have an influence on the edema we analyzed the total protein content in homogenate skin biopsies. We observed that HYAL significantly reduced the edema formation evidenced by lower amount of protein at day 2 and at day 7 after excision wounds being daily treated with 16 U HYAL and compared to vehicle-control group (Figure 2D). After 14 and 21 days no difference was observed between experimental groups, and the amount of protein declined to similar concentrations detected in unwound control tissue.

HYAL induces cytokine release and eicosanoid generation, and temporarily increases TGF-β in the skin wound biopsies

Neutrophils were proven to be attracted to the wounded sites which may be induced by various cytokines. However, neutrophils

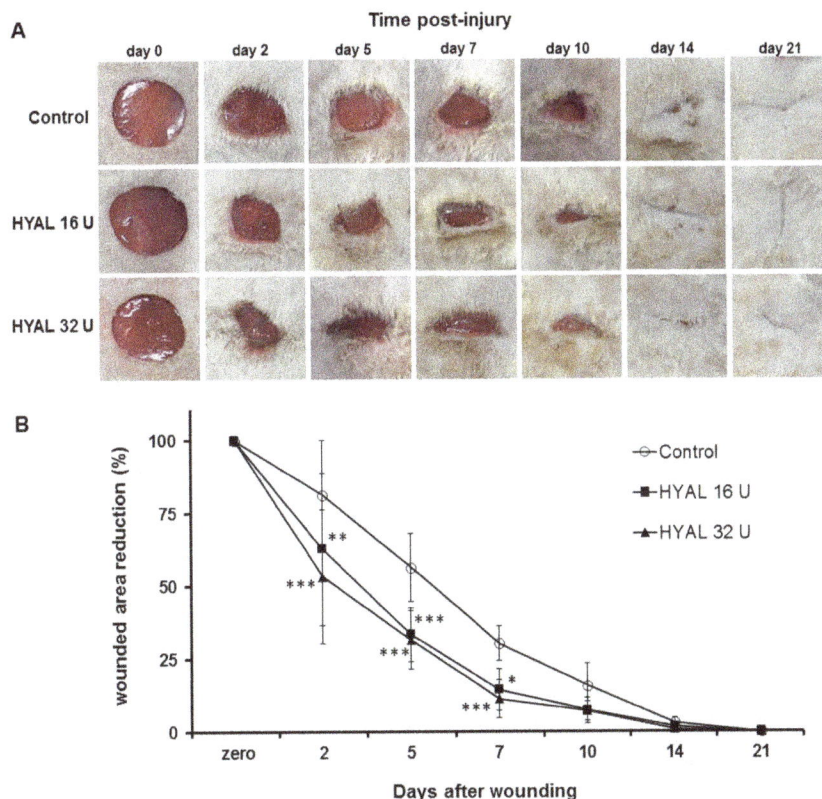

Figure 1. Topical application of HYAL accelerates wound closure in full-thickness excisional wounds. (A) Representative photographs taken from the 150 mm diameter full-thickness wounds of the Wistar rats. Macroscopic changes in skin wound sites induced by topical application of vehicle, HYAL 16 U and HYAL 32 U at day 0 (picture taken immediately after injury) 2, 5, 7, 10, 14 and day 21 are shown. (B) Rate of wound closure induced by topical application of vehicle (control group), HYAL 16 U and HYAL 32 U at day 2, 5, 7, 10, 14 and day 21 are given. Data are expressed as percentage of reduction area from the original wound size (day zero). Values are mean $\pm$ SEM (n = 8 to 16 wounds/group), $*P<0.05$, $**P<0.01$, $***P<0.001$ compared to control group by two-way-ANOVA.

themselves can also be activated releasing cytokines which have an impact on further steps in the wound healing process. Therefore, we evaluated the impact of HYAL on different cytokines. In fact, 16 U HYAL altered the release of pro- and anti-inflammatory cytokines in a time-dependent manner (Figure 3). Enhanced production of IL1-α, TNF-α, IL-4 and IL-10 at day 2 was observed compared to vehicle-control group (Figure 3A, B, C e D). Except of IL1-α all other cytokines declined at day 7 and this continuously. Only TNF-α was still slightly, but significantly increased at day 7 compared to the controls. After 14 days, there were no significant changes in the levels of the studied cytokines, while at day 21, a significant decrease in the IL1-α and TNF-α amount could be observed. TGF-β production was increased after 2 days, peaked at day 7 and then decreased after 14 and 21 days to control level in the wound biopsies (Figure 3E). Levels of IL-6, IL1-β, IFN-γ and IL-5 were not detected after HYAL treatment during the time-course of this experiment. Eicosanoids were also altered by HYAL treatment. Compared to controls, we observed a significant peak in the production of PGE$_2$ and LTB$_4$ after 2 days of HYAL treatment (Figure 3F, G). Subsequently, both lipid mediators decreased to baseline levels, after 14 days for LTB$_4$ and 21 days for PGE$_2$ post-wounding, respectively. Low concentrations of PGD$_2$ where observed in the first days of HYAL treatment, however a significant increase in the production of PGD$_2$ was observed at day 7 (Figure 3H).

HYAL temporarily affects collagen accumulation

Collagen deposition is an important event in the development of granulation tissue. We could observe that HYAL treated wounds revealed a marked and robust increase in the organization of collagen fibers, detected after staining with Picrosirius red in the wound biopsy, bridging the gaps in the skin compared to the vehicle-treated animals (Figure 4A). At days 2 and 7, the collagen content in the 16 U HYAL treated group was significantly higher than in the vehicle-control group, whereas after 14 and 21 days the collagen amount was similar between the groups with a slight decrease in the HYAL treated group at day 21 post wounding (Figure 4B). To confirm these histological findings, the collagen content was also measured by calculating the amount of hydroxyproline in the homogenate tissue of the wounds after 2, 7, 14 and 21 days post-wounding. The results of the hydroxyproline content in the skin after 2 days and 7 days by daily 16 U HYAL treatment showed a significant higher concentration compared to the controls (Figure 4C). Interestingly, after 21 days of 16 U HYAL wound treatment, the collagen content was significantly reduced compared to the control group.

HYAL affects neovascularization

The number of blood vessels in the HYAL treated wound was determined using different techniques. Figure 5A exemplarily illustrates photomicrographs of blood vessels in tissue sections from the wounds. The number of blood vessels in the 16 U HYAL

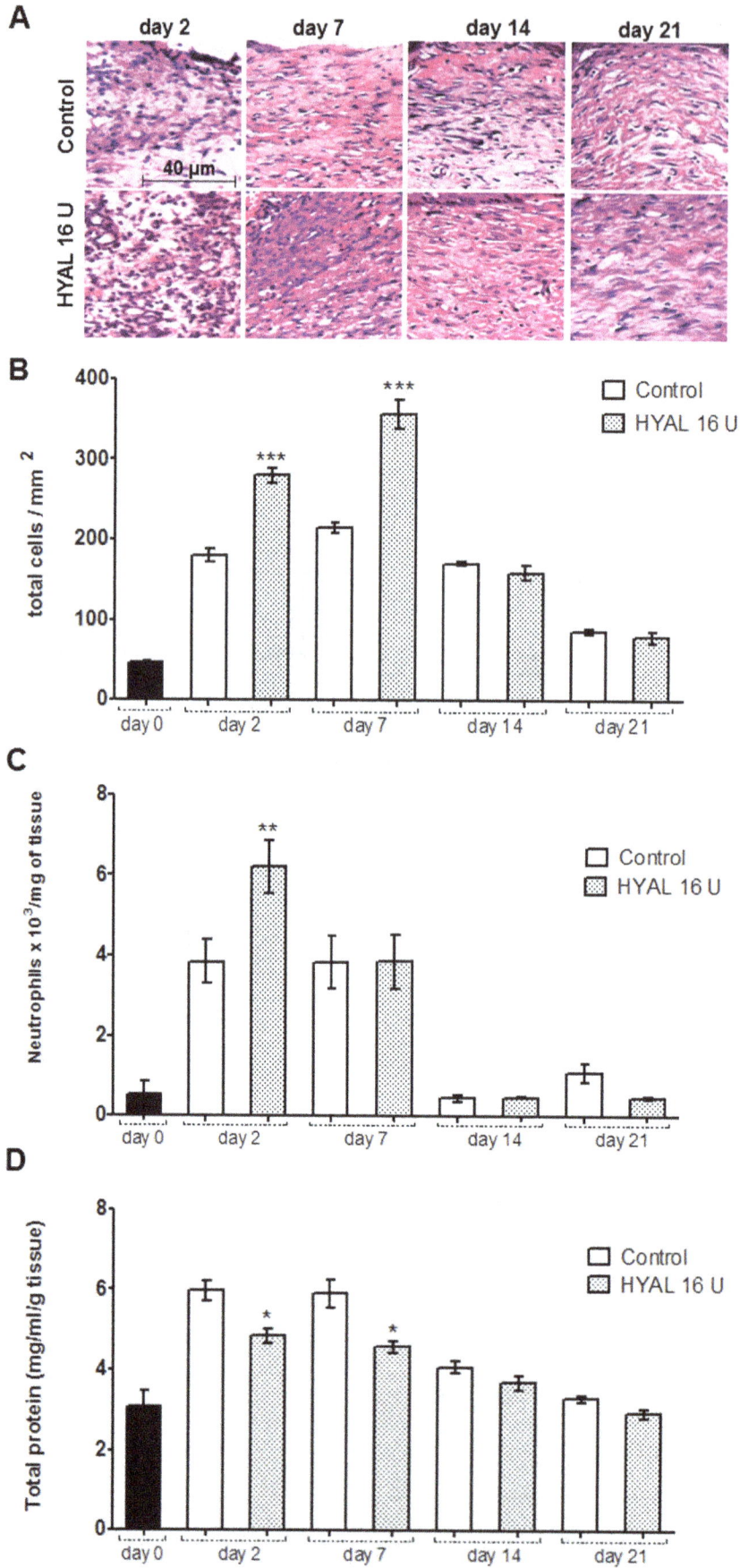

Figure 2. HYAL affects cellular recruitment and edema formation. Animals were topically treated either with vehicle (control group) or HYAL 16 U daily. Paraffin-wound sections were stained with HE to evaluate the inflammatory infiltrate response by image analysis. (A) The sections were photographed at 400x. The ImageJ software was used to count the inflammatory cells in wound tissue specimens at day 2, 7, 14 and 21 post wounding in at least ten random optic fields per group. (B) Histogram of a quantitative analysis of inflammatory infiltrate counted. (C) Tissue neutrophil accumulation determined by MPO levels in wound biopsies. (D) The total protein content was measured according to Coomassie assay. Values represent mean ± SEM (n = 8 wounds/group), *$P<0.05$, **$P<0.01$, ***$P<0.001$ compared to control group by one-way-ANOVA.

treated wounds determined by morphometric analyses was increased after 7, 14 and 21 days (Figure 5B). Levels of VEGF, a signal protein that stimulates angiogenesis, measured by ELISA in the wound tissue homogenate was enhanced in 16 U HYAL treated wounds at day 2 post wounding (Figure 5C).

HYAL differently influenced PPAR gene expression in the wound tissue

PPAR α and δ (also called β) have been shown to be important for the rapid epithelialization of wound skin and PPAR γ during the resolution phase of wound repair. To study the impact of HYAL on PPAR gene expression (*Ppara*, *Pparg* and *Ppard*), the skin extracts dissected from the cutaneous wounds were analyzed by qRT-PCR. The three PPAR isotypes were expressed in the skin at all-time points, but in a different manner (Figure 6). mRNA for PPAR α (*Ppara*) was inhibited in the cutaneous wound, compared to unwounded skin (day 0). Interestingly, a time-dependent increased expression of *Ppara* was observed after daily treatment of 16 U HYAL until day 21, reaching finally a similar expression level as the physiological one (Figure 6A). Levels of PPAR δ mRNA were only increased at day 2 (fold increase 1.62), but returned to levels measured in the unwounded tissue (Figure 6B). mRNA of PPAR γ showed the highest fold increase at day 2 (fold increase 5.3) and decreased to levels in the range of the controls (Figure 6C).

Discussion

Wounds cause discomfort and are prone to infection and other complications. Moreover, diseases like diabetes, immunosuppression diseases, ischemia and ageing lead to a delay in wound healing. Therefore, agents that accelerate healing are important and research to find potent agents are a challenging task. Our aim was to evaluate whether HYAL is not only a spreading agent to improve the bioavailability of drugs as known from the literature [17,18] but has also a wound healing potential.

The *in vitro* scratch assay performed with HYAL and 3T3 mouse fibroblasts provided first preliminary insights that HYAL mainly influence the migration of the fibroblasts. It can be assumed that then also the rebuilding of new granulation tissue may be positively influenced [3]. This *in vitro* assay has been demonstrated to be a convenient and suitable in vitro test that gives robust and reproducible results for the migration of fibroblasts in an artificial wounded area [23,36,37]. However, it has to be taken into account that the 3T3 fibroblast cell line may be behave differently from primary fibroblasts and most important, this *in vitro* assay cannot replace *in vivo* studies. Therefore, we studied the wound healing activity of HYAL in the *in vivo* model of the skin excisional wound in rats. Macroscopic examination showed that the healing rate of HYAL treated wounds was significantly higher already in the early phase at day 2 compared to the controls (Figure 1A). The wound closure involves a complex orchestrated interaction of different cell types including neutrophils, macrophages, keratinocytes, fibroblasts and endothelial [6]. It is well known that recruitment of neutrophils within the first hours and days and macrophages in the later phase of

inflammation that occurs in site of the skin injury is crucial. These cells have the competence to remove cellular debris and dead cells and therefore supporting the wound healing processes [4,5]. We demonstrate that HYAL increased myeloperoxidase activity in the neutrophils at day 2 which is probably related to an enhanced recruitment of mononuclear cells as reported in the literature [32]. Moreover, at 2nd and 7th day post-wounding cellularity and release of cytokines, growth factors and lipid mediators is increased according to our data (Figure 2 and 3). Pro-inflammatory cytokines, including IL1-α, IL1-β, IL6, and TNF-α, play an important role in wound repair. They influence various processes at the wound site, such as stimulation of keratinocyte and fibroblast proliferation, synthesis and breakdown of extracellular matrix proteins, fibroblast chemotaxis, and regulation of the immune response [6]. In addition, IL-10 plays a major role in the limitation and termination of the inflammatory response, regulating the growth and differentiation of various immune cells, keratinocytes and endothelial cells [5]. The observed effect suggested that HYAL has a different impact on the release of the cytokines depending on the stage of the inflammatory process and could therefore control the degree and duration of the inflammatory response. Beside cytokines, lipid mediators such as prostaglandins (PGs) and leukotrienes (LTs) can also be released during different stages of the healing phases. They are reported to play a crucial role in the initiating and resolution of acute inflammation during wound healing [38–40]. Our findings (Figure 3F, G, H) corroborate with previous data [41,42], demonstrating that during the wound repair, a gradual shift in the metabolism of arachidonic acid from the pro-inflammatory PGE_2 to anti-inflammatory PGD_2 occurs and that this shift in the metabolism of arachidonic acid may be responsible for initiating endogenous mechanism resulting in wound healing.

We could also demonstrate that HYAL differently affects the expression of transcription factors peroxisome proliferator-activated receptors (PPARs), which have received attention because of their protective and healing properties in tissue injury and wound repair [9,43,44]. Our results showed increased levels of PPAR δ and PPAR γ mRNA, but decreased levels of PPAR α mRNA after HYAL treatment in the first stage (day 2) compared to the unwounded tissue and the vehicle-control in the wounded tissue (Figure 6). The increased gene expression corroborated with previous reports where PPAR δ was demonstrated to be activated by the stress-associated protein kinase pathway in response to inflammatory cytokines, such as TNF-α and IL1, and down-regulated by TGF-β1 after a skin injury, playing an important role for new tissue development [8,45,46]. mRNA increased expression of PPAR γ accompanied with increased levels of PGD_2 is in agreement with the literature [41]. It is reported that upregulation of PPAR γ during the resolution phase of wound repair concomitant with PGD_2 expression is responsible for initiating the endogenous mechanism which results in healing/resolution.

Collagen is the major component of the connective tissue. Hence, the healing processes depend on its regulatory production, deposition and subsequent maturation. As the ECM can have positive or negative effects, the right balance and shifts in synthesis versus catabolism of collagen during the healing process are

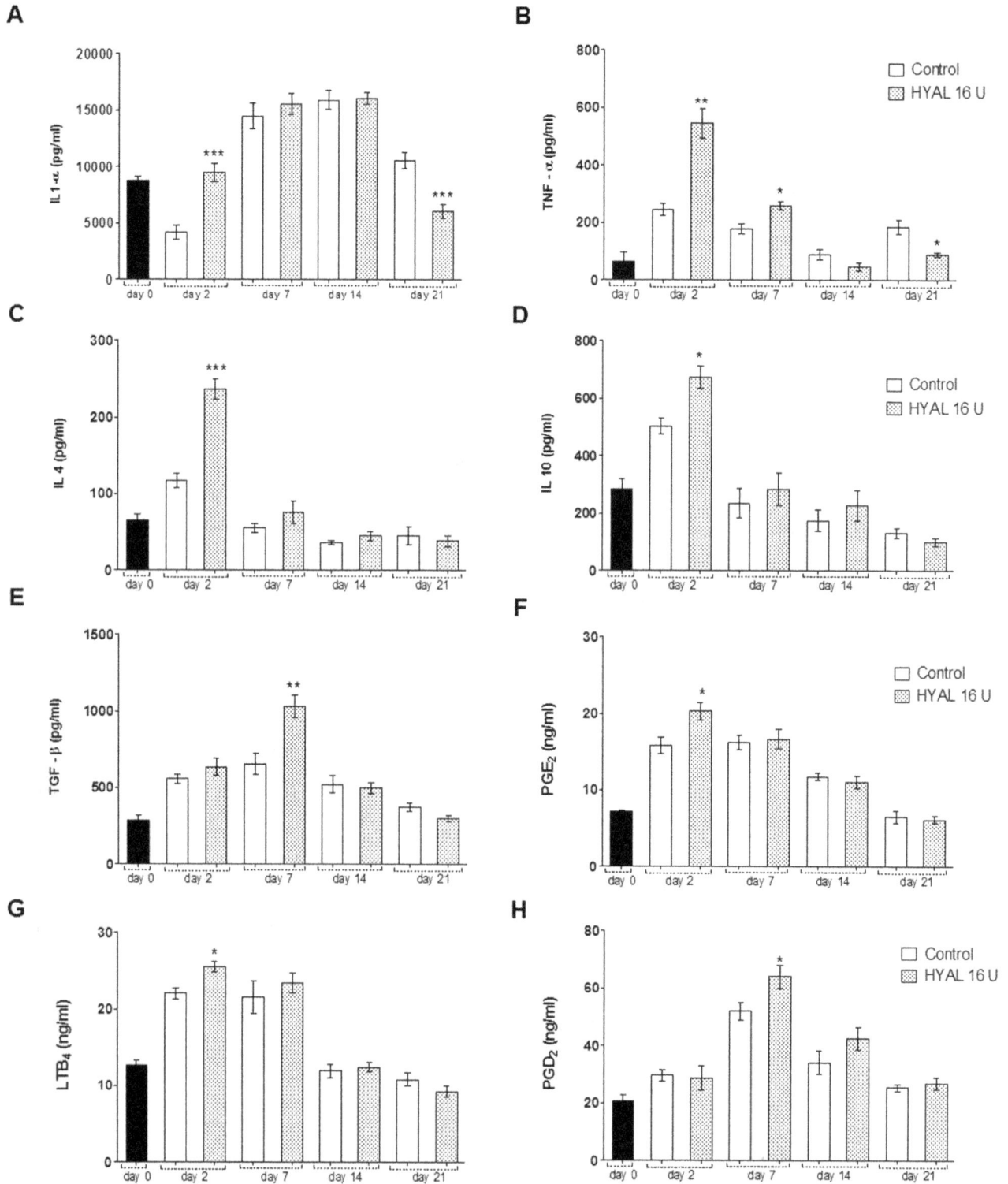

Figure 3. HYAL modulates cytokines and induces eicosanoid generation in the skin wound biopsies. Homogenates were prepared from the wound biopsies obtained from animals at day 0, 2, 7, 14 and 21 treated with 16 U HYAL or with vehicle-control. (A) IL1-α, (B) TNF-α, (C) IL-4, (D) IL-10, (E) TGF-β, (F) PGE$_2$, (G) LTB$_4$ and (H) PGD$_2$ were assayed by ELISA. Data are means $\pm$ SEM (n = 8 wounds/group), *$P<0.05$, **$P<0.01$, ***$P<0.001$ compared to control group by one-way-ANOVA.

important to prevent and avoid keloid scarring. Keloid is often considered to be the result of a prolonged proliferative and a delayed remodeling phase which contain disorganized and large collagen fibers, whereas hypertrophic scars exhibit thin fibers which are organized into nodules [7,47,48]. The enhanced collagen in skin wounds of HYAL treated rats in the first stages

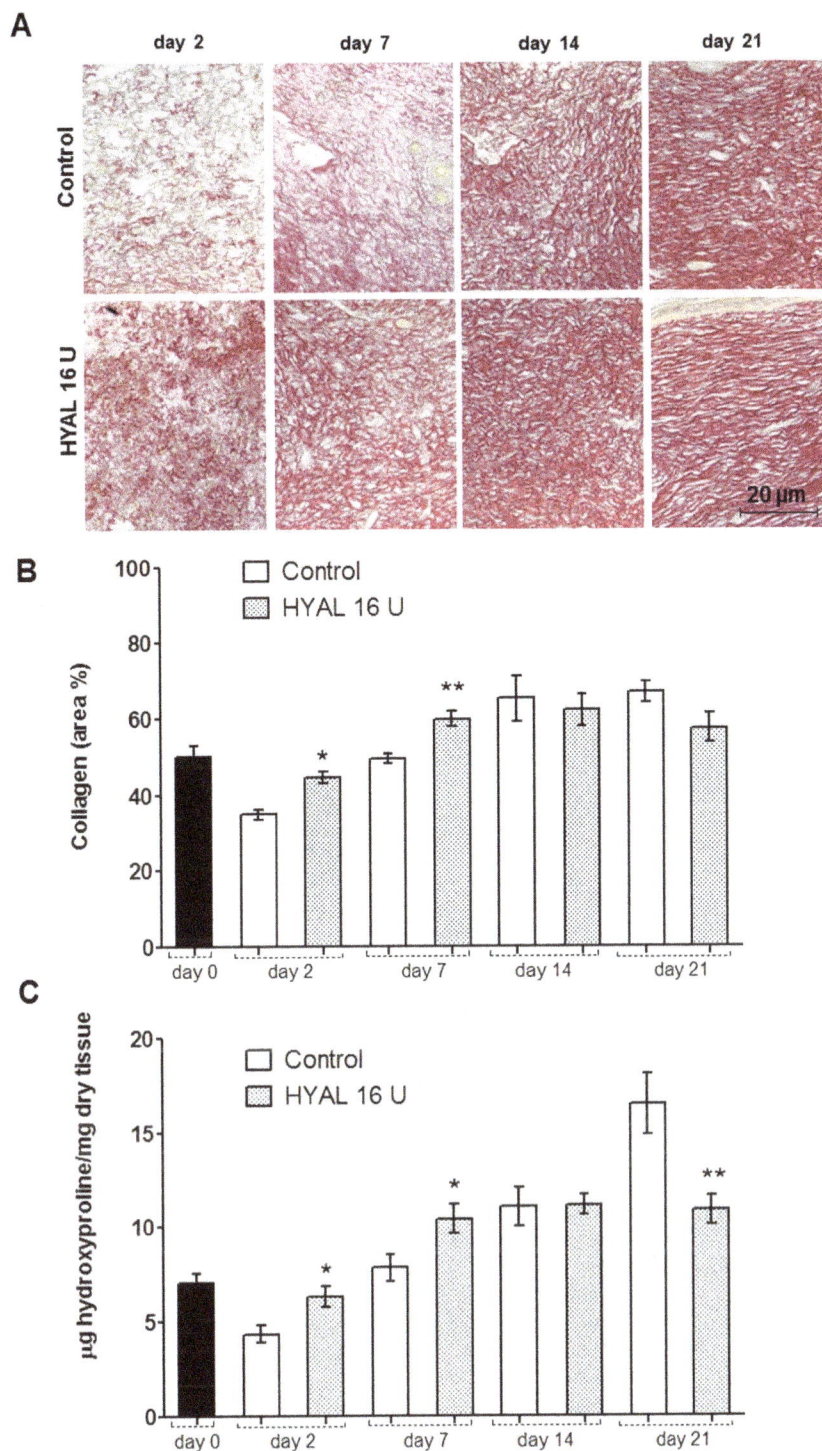

Figure 4. Collagen accumulation in wound areas of HYAL and vehicle-control treated rats at day 2, 7, 14 and 21 after wounding. (A) Representative photomicrograph of wounds tissue sections stained with picrosirius red staining (200x), note the collagen intensity and disposition of fibers (red). (B) Collagen content measured by digital densitometry is shown as a result of collagen content in each specimen in percentage. (C) Determination of wound hydroxyproline content as an indicator of collagen levels. μg of hydroxyproline/mg of dry wound specimen content was measured at day zero, 2, 7, 14 and 21 after injury. Data represent means ± SEM (n = 8 wounds/group), *$P < 0.05$, **$P < 0.01$ compared to control group by one-way-ANOVA.

stabilizes the new granulation tissue formation and may consequently accelerate the rate of wound closure. Importantly, collagen amount was diminished at day 21 post-wounding which may contribute to anti-fibrotic scar formation and a better distribution and organization of collagen fibers (Figure 4). During the entire process of healing, modulation of the ECM metabolism has been

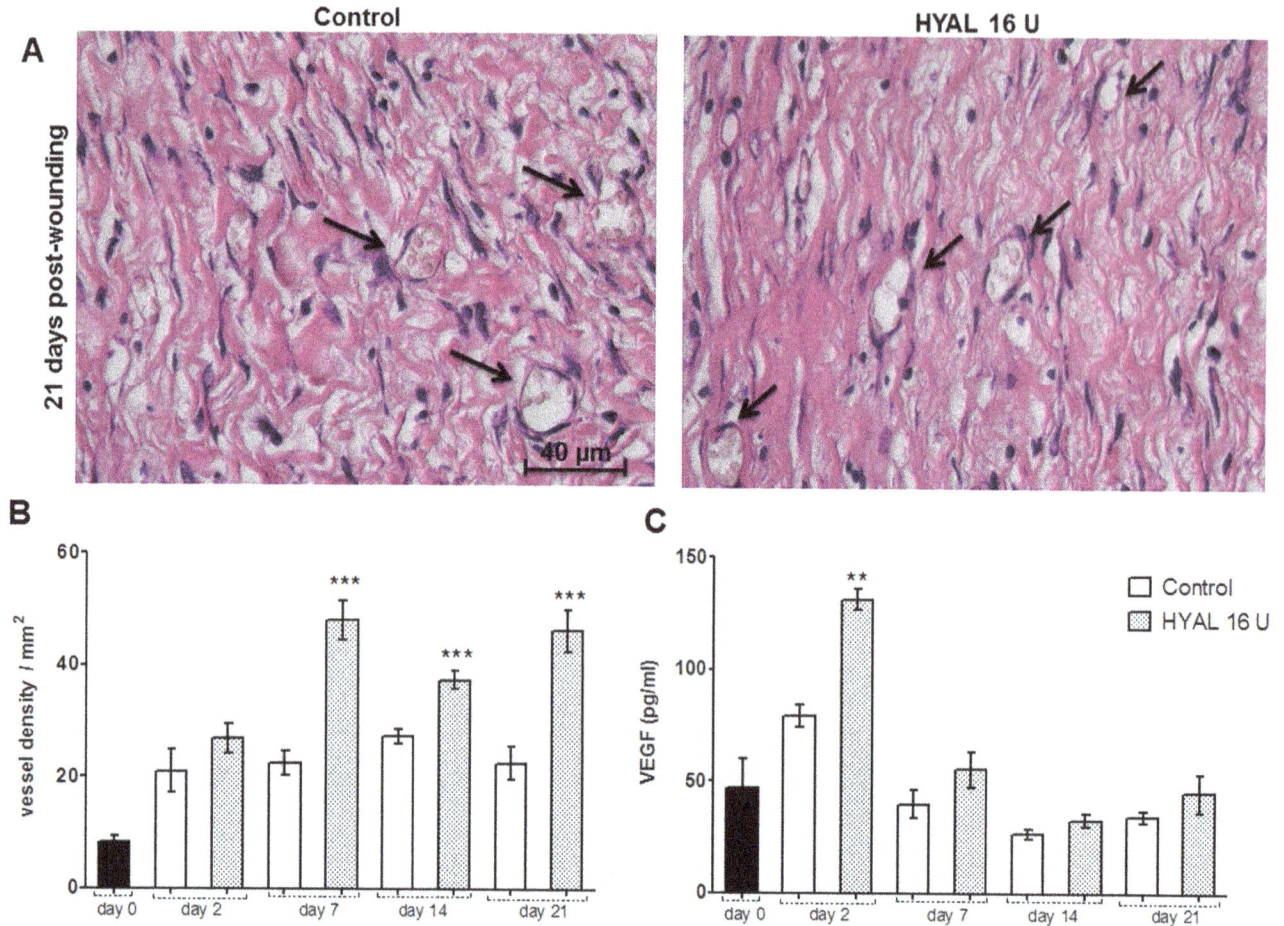

Figure 5. Neovascularization induced by HYAL. Animals were topically treated either with vehicle (control group) or HYAL 16 U daily. Paraffin-wound sections were stained with HE to evaluate the angiogenic response by image analysis. The sections were photographed at 400x. The ImageJ software was used to count the blood vessels in wound tissue specimens at day 2, 7, 14 and 21 post wounding in at least ten random optic fields per group. (A) Representative photomicrograph of blood vessels (black arrow) in wound tissue specimens at day 21 post-wounding. (B) Histogram of a quantitative analysis of vascular density counted. (C) Vascular endothelial growth factor (VEGF) expression measured in the supernatant of wound tissue homogenate by ELISA. Data represent means ± SEM (n = 8 wounds/group), **$P<0.01$, ***$P<0.001$ compared to control group by one-way-ANOVA.

extensively demonstrated to be mainly regulated by adequate temporal secretion of TGF-β1 [49]. At early stages the synthesis and deposition of collagen are essential and treatment of wounds with anti TGF-β antibodies resulted in delayed wound healing, demonstrating the importance of collagen content at this stage for proper healing [50]. Therefore, the observed increased TGF-β1 secretion at day 7 after HYAL treatment (Figure 3E) is in agreement with this previous report. Altogether, these observed effects of HYAL on collagen content and maturation process in rat skin may be beneficial for clinical use helping to prevent exacerbated wound healing processes such as hypertrophic and contracted scars.

Another important fact during wound healing is the angiogenesis that exerts dual function by providing the essential nutrients required and the oxygen to the wounded site, thus promoting granulation tissue formation [1,2]. HYAL treatment was found to increase the angiogenesis as evidenced histologically by the increased blood vessel density in the wound (Figure 5) and the expression of VEGF, which might be responsible to trigger the angiogenesis. The observed decrease in the VEGF protein expression after 2 days is in agreement with the previous studies

showing that transcription and secretion are elevated in the acute wounds. Expression of VEGF proteins during healing of cutaneous wounds was demonstrated to be induced within 24 h of skin injury, was maximal at 2–3 days and declined to basal level after 7 days of skin injury [51,52]. Moreover, it has been suggested that low molecular weight HA stimulates formation on new blood vessels and contributes to wound healing [53–55]. Therefore the angiogenic activity may be attributed to degradation products of hyaluronic acid of a specific size by HYAL, which has yet to be proven experimentally.

Conclusions

Taken together, under *in vivo* conditions we could show that HYAL accelerates the wound closure in the full-thickness excisional model in Wistar rats and give further insights how this wound healing properties can be explained on the molecular level. HYAL regulates the inflammatory response by mediating pro and anti-inflammatory cytokines like TNFα, IL-1α, IL-10 and IL-4,

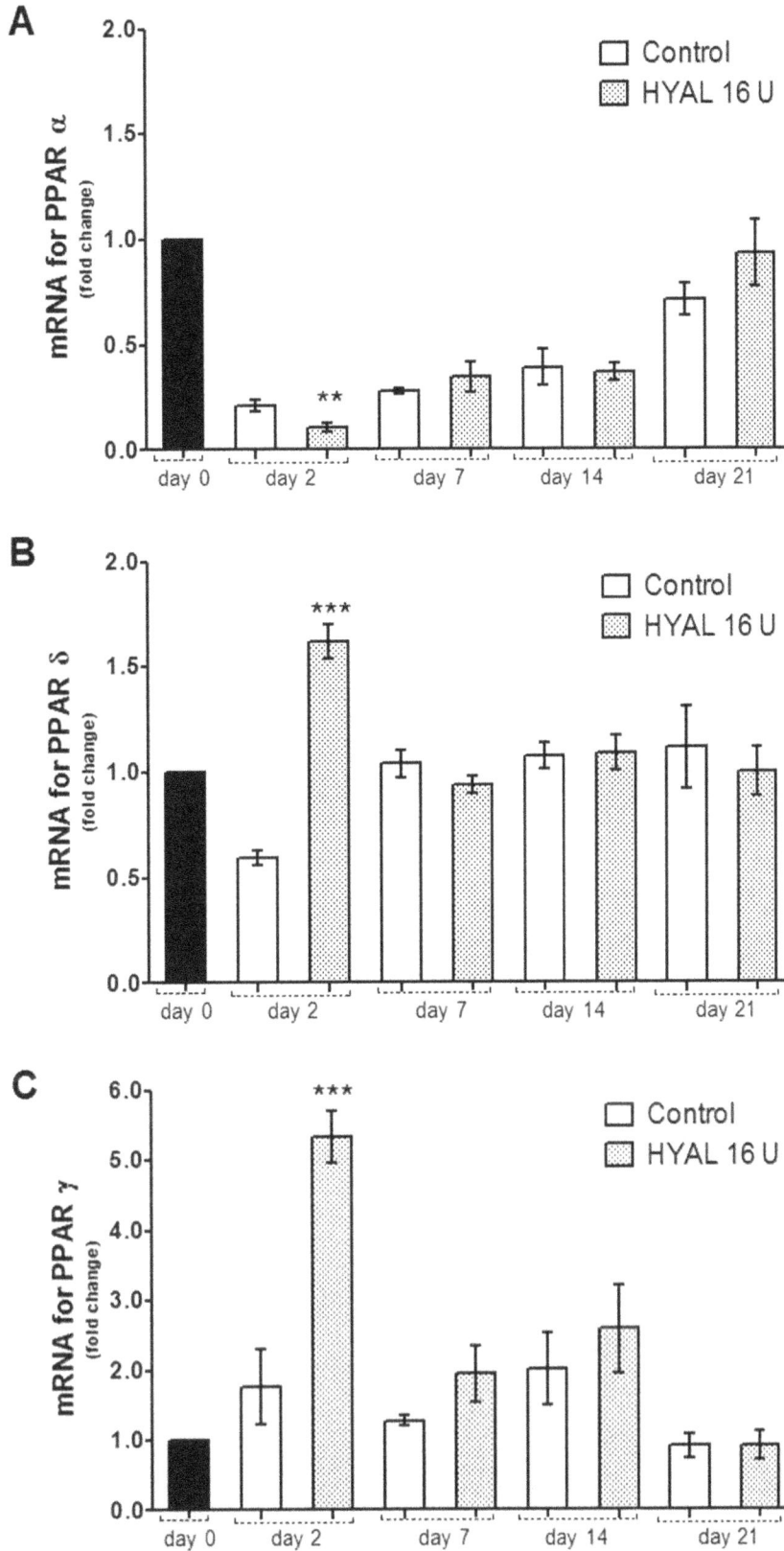

Figure 6. PPARs gene expression in skin biopsies dissected from the cutaneous wounds after HYAL treatment analyzed by qRT-PCR. A) mRNA for PPAR α, B) PPAR δ and C) PPAR γ determined by qRT-PCR. *Ppar* expression was normalized by *Gapdh* and *beta-actin*. Animals were topically treated with the vehicle (control group) or 16 U HYAL daily for 2, 7, 14 and 21 days, respectively. Data represent means ± SEM (n = 8 wounds/group), **$P<0.01$, ***$P<0.001$ compared to control group by one-way-ANOVA.

lipid mediators like PGE_2, LTB_4 and PGD_2, and the transcription factors PPARs δ, α and γ. Moreover, the enzyme contributes to the balance between synthesis and deposition of collagen and promotes angiogenesis. Therefore, HYAL may have a potential as a healing promoting agent for cutaneous injuries.

Supporting Information

Figure S1 Effect of HYAL on the migratory and proliferative activities of 3T3 mouse fibroblasts in the scratch assay. The experiments were performed in the absence (open bars) or presence (filled bars) of 5 µg/ml of antimitotic mitomycin C after 14 h incubation (37°C, 5% CO_2) in DMEM medium supplemented with 10% fetal bovine serum. HYAL was tested at concentration ranging from 0.1 U to 32 U. PDGF-BB was used as positive control at 2 ng/ml concentration. Data are expressed as percentage of cell numbers in the injured area, compared to the control group (DMEM medium only). Bars represent the mean ± SEM of three independent experiments, **$P < 0.01$, ***$P < 0.001$ compared to control group by two-way-ANOVA.

Table S1 Comparison of hyaluronidase enzyme activity in solution with in the gel preparations.

Acknowledgments

The authors wish to thank Dra. Karla de Castro Figueiredo Bordon for the determination of enzymatic activity of hyaluronidase from the Departamento de Física e Química da Faculdade de Ciências Farmacêuticas de Ribeirão Preto, Universidade de São Paulo, Brazil and Tina Wardecki, Department of Pharmaceutical Biology and Biotechnology, University of Freiburg, Freiburg, Germany, for revised and controlled the statistical analysis.

Author Contributions

Conceived and designed the experiments: MF LHF MACF IM. Performed the experiments: MF GFC MNL TAMA CSB FWGPS. Analyzed the data: MF CSB FWGPS LHF MACF IM. Wrote the paper: MF LHF MACF IM.

References

1. Schreml S, Szeimies RM, Prantl L, Landthaler M, Babilas P (2010) Wound healing in the 21st century. Journal of the American Academy of Dermatology 63: 866–881.
2. Singer AJ, Clark RAF (1999) Mechanisms of disease - Cutaneous wound healing. New England Journal of Medicine 341: 738–746.
3. Gurtner GC, Werner S, Barrandon Y, Longaker MT (2008) Wound repair and regeneration. Nature 453: 314–321.
4. Martin P, Leibovich SJ (2005) Inflammatory cells during wound, repair: the good, the bad and the ugly. Trends in Cell Biology 15: 599–607.
5. Werner S, Grose R (2003) Regulation of wound healing by growth factors and cytokines. Physiological Reviews 83: 835–870.
6. Barrientos S, Stojadinovic O, Golinko MS, Brem H, Tomic-Canic M (2008) Growth factors and cytokines in wound healing. Wound Repair and Regeneration 16: 585–601.
7. Shih B, Garside E, McGrouther DA, Bayat A (2010) Molecular dissection of abnormal wound healing processes resulting in keloid disease. Wound repair and regeneration 18: 139–153.
8. Icre G, Wahli W, Michalik L (2006) Functions of the peroxisome proliferator-activated receptor (PPAR) alpha and beta on skin homeostasis, epithelial repair, and morphogenesis. Journal of Investigative Dermatology Symposium Proceedings 11: 30–35.
9. Montagner A, Philippe V, Tan NS, Wahli W, Michalik L (2011) The nuclear hormone receptor PPAR beta as a regulator of skin healing and carcinogenesis. Journal of Investigative Dermatology 131: 2154–2154.
10. Dechert TA, Ducale AE, Ward SI, Yager DR (2006) Hyaluronan in human acute and chronic dermal wounds. Wound Repair and Regeneration 14: 252–258.
11. Toole BP (2004) Hyaluronan: From extracellular glue to pericellular cue. Nature Reviews Cancer 4: 528–539.
12. Chen WY, Abatangelo G (1999) Functions of hyaluronan in wound repair. Wound repair and regeneration: official publication of the Wound Healing Society [and] the European Tissue Repair Society 7: 79–89.
13. Ghazi K, Deng-Pichon U, Warnet JM, Rat P (2012) Hyaluronan fragments improve wound healing on in vitro cutaneous model through P2X7 purinoreceptor basal activation: role of molecular weight. PloS one 7: e48351.
14. Jameson JM, Cauvi G, Sharp LL, Witherden DA, Havran WL (2005) gamma delta T cell-induced hyaluronan production by epithelial cells regulates inflammation. Journal of Experimental Medicine 201: 1269–1279.
15. El-Safory NS, Fazary AE, Lee CK (2010) Hyaluronidases, a group of glycosidases: Current and future perspectives. Carbohydrate Polymers 81: 165–181.
16. Lee A, Grummer SE, Kriegel D, Marmur E (2010) Hyaluronidase. Dermatologic Surgery 36: 1071–1077.
17. Dunn AL, Heavner JE, Racz G, Day M (2010) Hyaluronidase: a review of approved formulations, indications and off-label use in chronic pain management. Expert Opinion on Biological Therapy 10: 127–131.
18. Adams L (2011) Adjuvants to local anaesthesia in ophthalmic surgery. The British journal of ophthalmology 95: 1345–1349.
19. Knight E, Carne E, Novak B, El-Shanawany T, Williams P, et al. (2010) Self-administered hyaluronidase-facilitated subcutaneous immunoglobulin home therapy in a patient with primary immunodeficiency. Journal of clinical pathology 63: 846–847.
20. Bitencourt CS, Pereira PA, Ramos SG, Sampaio SV, Arantes EC, et al. (2011) Hyaluronidase recruits mesenchymal-like cells to the lung and ameliorates fibrosis. Fibrogenesis & tissue repair 4: 3.
21. Dygai AM, Skurikhin EG, Ermakova NN, Pershina OV, Krupin VA, et al. (2013) Antifibrotic activity of hyaluronidase immobilized on polyethylenoxide under conditions of bleomycin-induced pneumofibrosis. Bulletin of experimental biology and medicine 154: 388–392.
22. Dygai AM, Skurikhin EG, Ermakova NN, Pershina OV, Krupin VA, et al. (2013) Antifibrotic effect of combined treatment with neuroleptic drug and immobilized hyaluronidase in pulmonary fibrosis. Bulletin of experimental biology and medicine 154: 329–333.
23. Fronza M, Heinzmann B, Hamburger M, Laufer S, Merfort I (2009) Determination of the wound healing effect of Calendula extracts using the scratch assay with 3T3 fibroblasts. Journal of Ethnopharmacology 126: 463–467.
24. Andrade TA, Iyer A, Das PK, Foss NT, Garcia SB, et al. (2011) The inflammatory stimulus of a natural latex biomembrane improves healing in mice. Brazilian journal of medical and biological research 44: 1036–1047.
25. Birch M, Tomlinson A, Ferguson MW (2005) Animal models for adult dermal wound healing. Methods in molecular medicine 117: 223–235.
26. Kemparaju K, Girish KS (2006) Snake venom hyaluronidase: a therapeutic target. Cell Biochemistry and Function 24: 7–12.
27. Pessini AC, Takao TT, Cavalheiro EC, Vichnewski W, Sampaio SV, et al. (2001) A hyaluronidase from Tityus serrulatus scorpion venom: isolation, characterization and inhibition by flavonoids. Toxicon: official journal of the International Society on Toxinology 39: 1495–1504.
28. Hoare TR, Kohane DS (2008) Hydrogels in drug delivery: Progress and challenges. Polymer 49: 1993–2007.
29. FDA (2006) Guidance for industry: chronic cutaneous ulcer and burn wounds-developing products for treatment. Official publication of the US Department of Health and Human Services - Food and Drug Administration (FDA) - Center for Drug Evaluation and Research (CDER) - Center for Biologics Evaluation and Research (CBER) - Center for Devices and Radiological Health (CDRH) 18p.
30. Minatel DG, Frade MA, Franca SC, Enwemeka CS (2009) Phototherapy promotes healing of chronic diabetic leg ulcers that failed to respond to other therapies. Lasers in surgery and medicine 41: 433–441.
31. Noursadeghi M, Tsang J, Haustein T, Miller RF, Chain BM, et al. (2008) Quantitative imaging assay for NF-kappaB nuclear translocation in primary human macrophages. Journal of immunological methods 329: 194–200.
32. Souza DG, Cassali GD, Poole S, Teixeira MM (2001) Effects of inhibition of PDE4 and TNF-alpha on local and remote injuries following ischaemia and reperfusion injury. British Journal of Pharmacology 134: 985–994.
33. Reddy GK, Enwemeka CS (1996) A simplified method for the analysis of hydroxyproline in biological tissues. Clinical biochemistry 29: 225–229.
34. Wong CM, Yam JW, Ching YP, Yau TO, Leung TH, et al. (2005) Rho GTPase-activating protein deleted in liver cancer suppresses cell proliferation and invasion in hepatocellular carcinoma. Cancer research 65: 8861–8868.
35. Buonomo R, Giacco F, Vasaturo A, Caserta S, Guido S, et al. (2012) PED/PEA-15 controls fibroblast motility and wound closure by ERK1/2-dependent mechanisms. Journal of cellular physiology 227: 2106–2116.

36. Liang CC, Park AY, Guan JL (2007) In vitro scratch assay: a convenient and inexpensive method for analysis of cell migration in vitro. Nature Protocols 2: 329–333.

37. van Horssen R, Galjart N, Rens JA, Eggermont AM, ten Hagen TL (2006) Differential effects of matrix and growth factors on endothelial and fibroblast motility: application of a modified cell migration assay. Journal of cellular biochemistry 99: 1536–1552.

38. Aoki T, Narumiya S (2012) Prostaglandins and chronic inflammation. Trends in Pharmacological Sciences 33: 304–311.

39. Futagami A, Ishizaki M, Fukuda Y, Kawana S, Yamanaka N (2002) Wound healing involves induction of cyclooxygenase-2 expression in rat skin. Laboratory Investigation 82: 1503–1513.

40. Green JA, Stockton RA, Johnson C, Jacobson BS (2004) 5-Lipoxygenase and cyclooxygenase regulate wound closure in NIH/3T3 fibroblast monolayers. American Journal of Physiology-Cell Physiology 287: C373–C383.

41. Kapoor M, Kojima F, Yang LH, Crofford LJ (2007) Sequential induction of pro- and anti-inflammatory prostaglandins and peroxisome proliferators-activated receptor-gamma during normal wound healing: A time course study. Prostaglandins Leukotrienes and Essential Fatty Acids 76: 103–112.

42. Nelson AM, Loy DE, Lawson JA, Katseff AS, Fitzgerald GA, et al. (2013) Prostaglandin D2 inhibits wound-induced hair follicle neogenesis through the receptor, Gpr44. The Journal of investigative dermatology 133: 881–889.

43. Michalik L, Desvergne B, Tan NS, Basu-Modak S, Escher P, et al. (2001) Impaired skin wound healing in peroxisome proliferator-activated receptor (PPAR)alpha and PPAR beta mutant mice. Journal of Cell Biology 154: 799–814.

44. Michalik L, Wahli W (2006) Involvement of PPAR nuclear receptors in tissue injury and wound repair. Journal of Clinical Investigation 116: 598–606.

45. Chong HC, Tan MJ, Philippe V, Tan SH, Tan CK, et al. (2009) Regulation of epithelial-mesenchymal IL-1 signaling by PPAR beta/delta is essential for skin homeostasis and wound healing. Journal of Cell Biology 184: 817–831.

46. Tan NS, Michalik L, Noy N, Yasmin R, Pacot C, et al. (2001) Critical roles of PPAR beta/delta in keratinocyte response to inflammation. Genes & Development 15: 3263–3277.

47. Santibanez JF, Quintanilla M, Bernabeu C (2011) TGF-beta/TGF-beta receptor system and its role in physiological and pathological conditions. Clinical Science 121: 233–251.

48. Wynn TA (2008) Cellular and molecular mechanisms of fibrosis. The Journal of pathology 214: 199–210.

49. Siebert N, Xu WG, Grambow E, Zechner D, Vollmar B (2011) Erythropoietin improves skin wound healing and activates the TGF-beta signaling pathway. Laboratory Investigation 91: 1753–1765.

50. Lu L, Saulis AS, Liu WR, Roy NK, Chao JD, et al. (2005) The temporal effects of anti-TGF-beta 1, 2, and 3 monoclonal antibody on wound healing and hypertrophic scar formation. Journal of the American College of Surgeons 201: 391–397.

51. Brown LF, Yeo KT, Berse B, Yeo TK, Senger DR, et al. (1992) Expression of vascular permeability factor (vascular endothelial growth factor) by epidermal keratinocytes during wound healing. The Journal of experimental medicine 176: 1375–1379.

52. Shukla A, Dubey MP, Srivastava R, Srivastava BS (1998) Differential expression of proteins during healing of cutaneous wounds in experimental normal and chronic models. Biochemical and biophysical research communications 244: 434–439.

53. Sattar A, Rooney P, Kumar S, Pye D, West DC, et al. (1994) Application of angiogenic oligosaccharides of hyaluronan increases blood vessel numbers in rat skin. The Journal of investigative dermatology 103: 576–579.

54. Slevin M, Kumar S, Gaffney J (2002) Angiogenic oligosaccharides of hyaluronan induce multiple signaling pathways affecting vascular endothelial cell mitogenic and wound healing responses. The Journal of biological chemistry 277: 41046–41059.

55. West DC, Hampson IN, Arnold F, Kumar S (1985) Angiogenesis induced by degradation products of hyaluronic acid. Science 228: 1324–1326.

12

Erythrocyte Stiffness during Morphological Remodeling Induced by Carbon Ion Radiation

Baoping Zhang[1,2,3], Bin Liu[3,4], Hong Zhang[4], Jizeng Wang[1,2,3]*

1 School of Civil Engineering and Mechanics, Lanzhou University, Lanzhou, 730000, PR China, 2 Key Laboratory of Mechanics on Disaster and Environment in Western China, The Ministry of Education of China, Lanzhou University, 730000, PR China, 3 Institute of Biomechanics and Medical Engineering, Lanzhou University, Lanzhou, 730000, PR China, 4 Department of Heavy Ion Radiation Medicine, Institute of Modern Physics, Chinese Academy of Sciences, Lanzhou 730000, PR China

Abstract

The adverse effect induced by carbon ion radiation (CIR) is still an unavoidable hazard to the treatment object. Thus, evaluation of its adverse effects on the body is a critical problem with respect to radiation therapy. We aimed to investigate the change between the configuration and mechanical properties of erythrocytes induced by radiation and found differences in both the configuration and the mechanical properties with involving in morphological remodeling process. Syrian hamsters were subjected to whole-body irradiation with carbon ion beams (1, 2, 4, and 6 Gy) or X-rays (2, 4, 6, and 12 Gy) for 3, 14 and 28 days. Erythrocytes in peripheral blood and bone marrow were collected for cytomorphological analysis. The mechanical properties of the erythrocytes were determined using atomic force microscopy, and the expression of the cytoskeletal protein spectrin-α1 was analyzed via western blotting. The results showed that dynamic changes were evident in erythrocytes exposed to different doses of carbon ion beams compared with X-rays and the control (0 Gy). The magnitude of impairment of the cell number and cellular morphology manifested the subtle variation according to the irradiation dose. In particular, the differences in the size, shape and mechanical properties of the erythrocytes were well exhibited. Furthermore, immunoblot data showed that the expression of the cytoskeletal protein spectrin-α1 was changed after irradiation, and there was a common pattern among its substantive characteristics in the irradiated group. Based on these findings, the present study concluded that CIR could induce a change in mechanical properties during morphological remodeling of erythrocytes. According to the unique characteristics of the biomechanical categories, we deduce that changes in cytomorphology and mechanical properties can be measured to evaluate the adverse effects generated by tumor radiotherapy. Additionally, for the first time, the current study provides a new strategy for enhancing the assessment of the curative effects and safety of clinical radiotherapy, as well as reducing adverse effects.

Editor: Juan Carlos del Alamo, University of California San Diego, United States of America

Funding: This work was supported by grants from the National Natural Science Foundation of China (grants No. 11032006, No. 11072094, and No. 11121202), the PhD Program Foundation of the Ministry of Education of China (grant No. 20100211110022), and New Century Excellent Talents in University (program No. NCET-10-0445). The funders had no role in study design, data collection and analysis, decision to publish, or preparation of the manuscript.

Competing Interests: The authors have declared that no competing interests exist.

* Email: jizengwangibme@gmail.com

Introduction

Ionizing radiation and radiotherapy commonly encounter problems not only due to the action of the treated tumor but also due to the adverse effects of irradiation on non-target cells or tissues [1]. Over the past decades, due to their high targeting ability and distinct curative effects, radioactive rays and ion beams have been intensively researched. Thus, special charged ion beam-carbon ion beams (CIBs) have great potential for the development of radiation therapy. Because CIBs have a special energy beam path, the so-called Bragg peak characteristic of its occurrence provides a higher relative biological effectiveness (RBE) than low linear energy transfer (LET) radiation (X-rays, γ-rays and electron beams) [2,3]. Thus, heavy ion beams ($^{12}C^{6+}$ ions) can precisely target the nidus and avoid energy loss, leading to improved targeting with greater curative effect and better local control at the tumor site than is possible with conventional X-rays or similar treatments [4,5]. However, although the beams have many advantages in their application, the adverse effects of treatment caused by the rays themselves remain an inevitable problem. Improving the maximum targeting of radiation therapy and reducing its adverse effects on normal cells remain major research focuses for tumor radiotherapy. Previous studies mainly emphasized the direct effects of cellular lethality caused by the irradiation of human organs or tissues [6] or investigated these aspects within the context of chromosomal rearrangement and mutation in the genetic material arising from energy deposition [7–9]. Additionally, whether the therapeutic success that is possible with X-ray treatment can also be achieved with heavy ion radiation is a major question.

The organs of the blood and hematopoietic systems are vulnerable to radiation [10–14]. Indeed, many studies have shown that radiation can cause a decrease in the visible components of blood [15], cell morphology changes, alterations to the electrolyte state in peripheral blood (PB), mild hyperplasia in the bone marrow (BM) [16], serious inhibition or even destruction of the bone marrow [17,18], a reduction in the production of erythrocytes [19], changes in the aggregation state of platelets [20], and induction of the transformation of normal stem cells into tumor stem cells [20–22]. Thus, a hemogram of the blood system is often used initially as an approximate guide to assess the adverse effects caused by radiotherapy to the human body. Indeed, CIR may cause changes of in the hemogram and myelogram. Likewise, biological function and morphology must be in conformity with each other to determine the occurrence of disease. However, several investigations have indicated that radiation induces a series of complex and dynamic changes in cell shape as well as membrane damage and that a close relationship exists among the membrane skeleton components [23] and the function and antioxidant effects of electrolytes [9], [24]–such as changes in cell membrane permeability and alterations of the membrane and cytoskeleton–which can cause changes in the membrane, including organizational and metabolic changes [25], eventually leading to cell dysfunction.

Some considerable insights have already been obtained concerning the physiological or pathological processes of cell movement, invasion and migration through cell biomechanics research. Presently, cell mechanics are favored for understanding the problem. Additionally, not only is the cell membrane considered a very important factor in the response to damage; the cytoskeleton also plays a key role, being the most direct embodiment of cell morphology changes. For instance, the role of cytoskeletal morphological remodeling in tumor development is a crucial problem. Thus far, very few studies have assessed the biomechanical principles underlying the cytoskeletal morphological remodeling induced by radiation to evaluate the safety of ion radiotherapy in the human body through using morphological remodeling mechanics at the cellular level to understand how heavy ion radiation affects organs and tissues of the body from the perspective of biomechanics. This study investigates the mechanical properties of the membrane surface, cytoskeletal morphological remodeling and cytoskeletal protein levels to clarify the morphological remodeling process of the cytoskeleton. Normal erythrocytes have good mechanical properties that depend on an equilibrium state between two parameters–morphological motion and deformations–in particular, the geometric shape and biophysical characteristics of the spherical surface area, the viscosity of the cytoplasm, and the elasticity of the membrane. Alteration of any of these factors can lead to the differences in the cell membrane and the cytoskeletal structure. Previous studies have shown that some erythrocyte-related diseases are associated with the following three significant characteristics: the typical biconcave disc shape, the phospholipid bilayer membrane and the cytoskeleton meshwork. If these shape-changing agents cause area differences between the change in membrane morphology and mechanical properties of the cell, the process of the disease is altered [26]. Therefore, the size and shape, the phospholipid bilayer membrane and the cytoskeletal network govern the deformation and damage of erythrocytes and are widely considered to represent changes in biological behavior or function [27–29]. Typical illnesses related to erythrocyte dysfunction include malaria [30–34], sickle cell anemia [35,36], hemolytic anemia [37,38], cancer [39], spherocytosis and elliptocytosis [30], [40], and diabetes mellitus [41]. Thus, it has been vital to study the pathophysiology of these diseases [27], [42,43].

Biological-type atomic force microscopy (BT-AFM) can allow the direct visualization of cell morphology changes in erythrocytes at the micro-nano level using an inverted microscope and measurement of the mechanical properties of biological specimens [44,45]. However, measurement of the dynamic properties of cells

as a characteristic feature can provide important information regarding their physical state [46,47]. Current literature has suggested that altering the physical properties of the cytoplasm and membrane-cytoskeleton in erythrocytes can result in morphologically distinct signals [46], [48]. Thus, the remarkable changes in erythrocyte morphology result from a coupled dynamic response of the phospholipid bilayer membrane and an elastic spectrin molecular meshwork on the cytoplasmic face [27], [31], [42], [49–51]. Generally, erythrocyte damage depends on the phospholipid bilayer membrane of an adult red cell (mainly including membrane proteins or enzymatic erythrocyte defects), which is supported on its inner surface by a complex arrangement of spectrin-spectrin molecular interactions of cytoskeletal proteins (membrane skeleton). A major component of cytoskeletal proteins is the neofunctionalized protein spectrin, called an erythrocyte "ghost", that was first reported to be isolated from human erythrocytes in 1968 by Marchesi and Steers [52,53]. Studies have demonstrated that some examples of unhealthy cell morphology changes produce adverse outcomes, and these changes were focused on the interactions between the cell membrane and the cytoskeleton [50], [54,55]. Additionally, previous theoretical research has contributed to a reliance on numerical modeling for the analysis of the membrane shape and surface free energy [48], [56–60], partly revealing the time-dependent relationship between the shape changes and deformability of erythrocytes [61], as well as displaying the elastic response of erythrocytes to small and large deformations [62–65]. Therefore, through quantitative measurement of the inherent behavior of erythrocytes, such as the elasticity of the cell membrane (cell stiffness), cell membrane contributions to the local or nonlocal bending deformation in the process of damage, changes in tension in the membrane-skeleton system, and the membrane surface area and size of erythrocytes [66], the degree of erythrocyte damage can be further assessed.

Herein, this paper will provide further insight into the adverse effects in erythrocytes related to radiation by examining the changes in microstructure and mechanical properties that have been used to analyze the functional relationship of erythrocytes before and after irradiation. We investigated whether subtle changes in the morphology and mechanical properties of cells can be used to assess the effects of radiation and to better depict the correlations among signal molecules involved in the configuration of the cytoskeleton, cell morphology changes, and the dynamic mechanical properties of cells in the process of damage. Based on these attempts, we focused on a new method of explaining the deformation or damage via the mechanical mechanism of erythrocyte morphological remodeling in different irradiated groups. Thus, according to the established parameters and these insights, we hypothesized the quantitation of the degree of erythrocyte damage to better explain cytoskeleton signaling dominated by biochemical molecules involved in the erythrocyte cytoskeleton morphological remodeling process, the biomechanical mechanism underlying erythrocyte induction by irradiation, and the relationship between the erythrocyte shape and injury rate to provide a theoretical base. In the present article, cell stiffness was chosen to meticulously estimate biological and adverse effects in erythrocytes during irradiation. Finally, this new perspective should be exploited to develop biomechanics to better assess the onset or progression of damage caused by ionizing radiation and to identify novel potential biomechanical targets or characteristics for therapeutic interventions.

Materials and Methods

Animals

SPF-class female Syrian golden hamsters (6–8 weeks old and weighing 80–100 g) provided by the Lanzhou Institute of Biological Products (Lanzhou, China) were used in the current study. All of the animals were maintained under standardized conditions (temperature, $22\pm2°C$; humidity, $40\pm10\%$; light/dark cycle, 12 h:12 h) and given standard food and water ad libitum. The animal experimental protocols were approved by the Animal Experiment Medicine Center of Lanzhou University. A total of 156 hamsters were randomly divided into three groups: a carbon ion irradiation group (1 Gy, 2 Gy, 4 Gy, or 6 Gy; six hamsters per group), an X-ray irradiation group (2 Gy, 4 Gy, 6 Gy, or 12 Gy; six hamsters per group), and a control non-irradiated group (0 Gy; twelve hamsters per group).

Irradiation procedure

Each hamster was positioned in a chamber attached to the irradiation equipment at the Heavy Ion Research Facility in Lanzhou (HIRFL, Institute of Modern Physics, Chinese Academy of Sciences, Lanzhou, China). The whole body of the hamster was irradiated with $^{12}C^{6+}$ ion beams at an energy of 270 MeV/u and LET of 10 keV/m, with a dose rate of 0.3 Gy/min. When $^{12}C^{6+}$ ion beams at 200 MeV/u and 31.3 keV/m of the beam entered the chamber, the $^{12}C^{6+}$ ion dose of 0.5 Gy corresponded to a fluence of 3.0×10^7 particles/cm^2. The carbon ions were equipped with a passive beam delivery system. The data were controlled automatically by a microcomputer during irradiation. Particle fluences were determined from an air-ionization chamber signal according to the calibration of the detector (PTW-UNIDOS; PTW-Freiburg Co., Wiesbaden, Germany). Similarly, animals exposed to X-rays were given whole-body radiation using an X-ray therapy machine (Elekta BMEI Medical Equipment Co. Ltd, Beijing, China) at a source-to-surface distance (SSD) of 100 cm and a dose rate of 2 Gy/min [67].

Preparation of erythrocytes in peripheral blood and bone marrow

The experiments complied with the laboratory animal disposal regulations of the Animal Ethics Committee at Lanzhou University. Animals were sacrificed at different time points to collect peripheral blood (PB) and bone marrow (BM) following treatment with different doses of radiation. Briefly, fresh peripheral blood and bone marrow were retrieved from the hamsters. First, the animals were anesthetized with 0.3% pentobarbital sodium at the injection concentration range of 30–35 mg/kg body weight. After adequate anesthetization, dissection was performed, the abdominal vein was exposed, and then the blood from the abdominal vein was retrieved using an anti-coagulated tube containing EDTA. After the plasma and buffy coat were removed, the erythrocytes were washed three times in an iso-osmotic HEPES-Ringer's buffer [68] (centrifugation at $1000\times g$ for 10 min at room temperature (RT)). Following the final wash, the erythrocytes were resuspended in HEPES-Ringer's buffer (100 mM NaCl, 10 mM HEPES, 4 mM KCl, 1 mM CaCl$_2$, 0.7 mM NaH$_2$PO$_4$, 0.6 mM MgSO$_4$, and 5 mM glucose) with 1 mg/mL of bovine serum albumin (BSA). The final dilution of the erythrocyte pellet ranged from 1:10,000 to 1:50,000, which was sufficient to separate individual erythrocytes by several cell diameters on a microscope slide. Erythrocyte ghosts were prepared from these samples by hemolysis using a standard procedure [69] and phosphate-buffered saline (PBS, 151.2 mmol/L NaCl, 5.6 mmol/L KCl, 5.48 mmol/L Na$_2$HPO$_4$, 0.32 mmol/L NaH$_2$PO$_4$, pH 7.4, osmotic pressure 300 mosmol/kg). First, one drop of the suspension was placed on a glass substrate treated with poly-L-lysine (P4832; Sigma) and was then incubated for 1 hour at 37°C. Next, one drop of 0.5% glutaraldehyde was added for 1.5 min to fix the erythrocyte membrane to the substrate. Finally, the pretreated cells were washed with phosphate buffer solution to remove the unbound cells and glutaraldehyde. The samples were immediately subjected to AFM.

The whole femurs of hamsters were dissected, and then the bone was cut from the knee to the hip buttock to better expose the bone marrow (BM). With a pointed tip, the area around the bone marrow was mixed evenly. The bone marrow was removed (approximately 0.5 mm^3) with the tips of a pair of tweezers, and its color and status were then recorded to prior loading into 1.5–2.0 mL of serum in vitro. The bone marrow-serum mixture was mixed by aspiration with a glass dropper tip approximately 20 times until the mixture was evenly dispersed, carefully avoiding the production of bubbles. Finally, using a trace sample gun, 50 μl of the bone marrow fluid (depending on the amount of bone marrow retrieved) was removed to be applied to a centrifugal smear machine small funnel at 600–800 r/min using a 10-min medium speed centrifuge. The pre-coated glass slide with the cells was removed, and the follow-up test was completed.

Cytological analysis of the proportion of irradiated erythrocytes in the bone marrow

BM smear samples were prepared on different of substrates using three glass slides: one slide was used for Swiss-Giemsa staining, another was used to determine the number of nucleated cells in the BM, and the third was counted at low magnification. The BM cytological report contained four grades of activity: hyperactive, active, reduced and significantly reduced. Additionally, the erythroid cells in the BM smear were classified into four clinical types–pronormoblasts, basophilic erythroblasts, polychromatophilic erythroblasts and normoblasts–and then the proportion of the total number of nucleated cells was determined under oil. According to cell counting principles, the samples were divided into three types–low, medium and high cell count. Additionally, each slide was observed no fewer than 30 times, and each observation involved the selection of several fields for statistical processing parameters.

Atomic force microscopy analysis of the changes in morphology and mechanical properties in erythrocytes induced by CIR or X-rays

A NanoWizard III AFM (JPK Instruments, Germany) mounted on an inverted optical microscope (Axiovert 200; Carl Zeiss Microimaging) was used for cell imaging and force spectroscopy. Silicon nitride cantilevers (PNP-DB; NanoWorld) with a nominal spring constant of 0.06 N/m (f$_0$: 17 kHz) were used in all of the experiments. For each cantilever, the spring constant was determined using the thermal noise constant calibration method. To ensure reproducibility in force application, the cantilever sensitivity and spring constant were calibrated before each experiment using JPK Instruments software 4.2.61. The optical microscope was used to select the desired cell and position the AFM tip. All of the AFM images and measurements were obtained in contact mode in air.

AFM imaging and measurement

Erythrocyte imaging was performed on glass slides at RT. The AFM had a maximum scanning range from 50×50 μm bar (Fast × Slow) to 5×5 μm bar (Fast × Slow) and a vertical range (Z-direction) of 15 μm. Pretreated cells were imaged using a pixel resolution of 512 pixels at a line rate of 0.10–0.30 Hz. The imaging parameters were carefully monitored to achieve good contrast with scanning forces as determined from force distance curves in the experiment. Elastic modulus (cell stiffness) determination is detailed in Section 2.5.2 below. Regarding radiation dose changes, a series of 50–100 curves of elastic modulus measurements in the erythrocytes was performed for each specimen in which the probe was placed over the sample surface and then pushed against the sample. The force acting between the tip and the sample caused a deflection of the cantilever that was recorded as a function of the relative sample position as a force curve. **Figure 1** shows two curves, one obtained from a soft erythrocyte and the other from a hard material. After subtraction of these two curves, the force-versus-indentation curve was obtained. In this experiment, the glass coverslip was taken as a zero-reference hard surface and was used for calibration, and the calibration curve was recorded each time together with a newly prepared erythrocyte sample. Ultimately, all of the AFM data were acquired and analyzed using two proprietary codes–a topographical image analysis code and a code for force curve analysis–using JPK instruments data processing software version 4.2.61.

Elastic modulus determination

Using AFM for nanoindentation is a useful tool to determine elastic properties such as the elastic modulus of biological samples [61], [70–73]. Cantilevers serve as soft nanoindenters that allow local testing of small and inhomogeneous samples such as cells or tissues. To calculate the parameter of interest, various models are used, but most of them are based on the Hertz model, modified to match the experimental conditions concerning the indenter's shape or the thickness of the sample [74–76]. The cell elastic modulus was calculated by applying the modified Hertz model contact theory to the force curves [35], [75], [77,78]. Thus, it is assumed that the surface is continuous, frictionless and incompressible (similar to rubber) at small deformations [79], and also consider the indentation is considered to be negligible compared with the sample thickness, to reflect the real situation of the cells and to ensure that the indentation depth is optimized. The Hertz model is valid for small indentations (5–10% of the height of the

cell, approximately, 200–500 nm) where the substrate does not influence the calculations [45], [78], [80]. There may be additional limitations in the indentation depth if the tip shape model is an approximation.

In the present study, tiny force probes were employed during the entire experimental process, and the probes were modified by attaching 6-μm diameter polystyrene microspheres (Base Line Chromtech Research Centre, Tianjin, China) onto the cantilever with epoxy resin glue (Epoxy F-05 Clear; Alteco, Japan). Additionally, the cell deformation nonlinearity was reduced due to a more homogeneous contact between the cells and probe. Elastic modulus measurements were derived from the force-distance profiles (extended curves) acquired at different locations on the cells, and JPK instruments software was used for this purpose. Microprobes were positioned on the cell membrane under optical control, in accordance with the method described by Ketene [81], and force curves were acquired at a sampling rate of 5 kHz and a constant approach velocity of ~1.0 μm/s. The movement is sufficiently slow that the viscous contributions are small, and force measurements are dominated by elastic behavior [82,83]. A maximum force of 3.5 ± 1.0 nN was implemented for all of the force curves to maintain a basis for comparison among the cells. In light of these claims, the parabolic model is often used if the indenter is a sphere because it is relatively easy to fit and yields a reasonable approximation for small indentations. Because the tip that comes in contact with the cell sample is spherical in shape, the model [84] predicts the relationship between the applied force and the indentation depth of the AFM cantilever into the soft sample by the following equation:

$$F = \frac{4E^*}{3}\sqrt{R}.\delta^{\frac{3}{2}} \qquad (1)$$

where F is the applied force, R is the radius of the sphere, δ is the indentation, and E^* is the relative Young's modulus term:

$$\frac{1}{E^*} = \frac{(1-v_{tip}^2)}{E_{tip}} + \frac{(1-v_{cell}^2)}{E_{cell}} \qquad (2)$$

Here, v is Poisson's ratio, and E_{tip} and E_{cell} represent the Young's

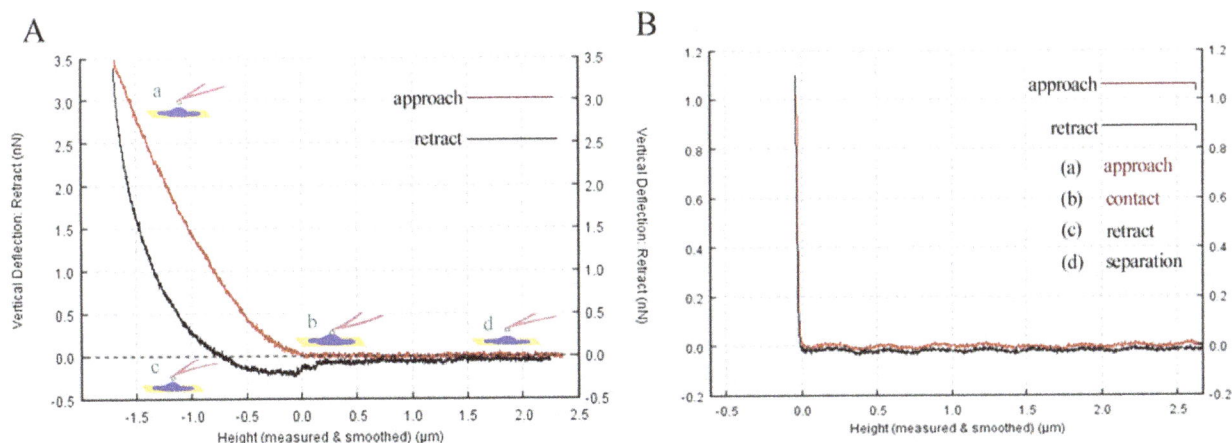

Figure 1. Force distance curve taken on the erythrocyte, Extend (or approach) (dark red) and retract (dark) curve clearly show hysteresis owing to the viscous and plastic behavior of the erythrocyte. (A) Cantilever deflection dependence on the tip sample distance (Z coordinate), and determination of the force-versus-indentation curves for control erythrocytes. **(B)** The straight line corresponds to curves measured on hard, non-deformable surface (glass coverslip) as the calibration curves. Lowercase letters show the marching trajectory of the probe in the whole process, and it consists of four steps, approach, contact, retract and separation (in **A**).

modulus of the tip and the cell, respectively. If the assumption of an infinitely hard needlepoint tip is employed, then $E_{tip} >> E_{cell}$. Thus, equation (2) could be simplified to the following:

$$\frac{1}{E^*} = \frac{(1 \text{-} v_{cell}^2)}{E_{cell}} \qquad (3)$$

where v depends on the material. For soft biological samples (i.e., cells, soft tissue, lipid bilayers and vesicles) [35], Poisson's ratio was assumed to be 0.5 in accordance with the incompressibility assumption usually employed for cells. Finally, the Hertz model equation assumes the following format:

$$F = \left[\frac{4\sqrt{R}}{3(1\text{-}v_{cell}^2)}E_{cell}\right] . \delta^{\frac{3}{2}} \qquad (4)$$

However, regarding equation (4), it is difficult to determine the exact point at which the tip and the cell membrane come into contact, resulting in an inability to judge the most appropriate force curve to which the Hertz model is fitted. As a result, the following equation can be applied:

$$F^{2/3} = \left[\frac{4\sqrt{R}}{3(1\text{-}v_{cell}^2)}E_{cell}\right]^{2/3} . \delta \qquad (5)$$

Additionally, when the dependence of the deformation on the force becomes linear, we use the indentation (δ) described as the difference in the relative changes of the piezo scanner displacement (z) and cantilever deflection (d). We obtain the following equation by replacing δ:

$$\delta = (z - z_0) - (d - d_0) \qquad (6)$$

where z_0 and d_0 are both the x and y coordinates of initial contact between the tip and the cell sample to identify the initial contact point. To attain the use of visual means to approximate the contact point for the fit region range, we adopt a semi-automated, mathematical approximation for the contact point. To better calculate the Young's modulus, we substitute equation (6) into equation (5) to produce the formula below:

$$F^{2/3} = \left[\frac{4\sqrt{R}}{3(1\text{-}v_{cell}^2)}E_{cell}\right]^{2/3}(z - d) \text{-} \left[\frac{4\sqrt{R}}{3(1\text{-}v_{cell}^2)}E_{cell}\right]^{2/3}(z_0 - d_0) \quad (7)$$

Thus, this equation can be analyzed as a line in the ($F^{2/3}$, z–d) plane, from which the Young's modulus (E) can be directly calculated from the linear slope and contact point (z_0-d_0) through the intercept of Eq. (7) [82], [85–87]. In addition, the Hertz model assumes linearity, so it can be further analyzed according to the following formula:

$$y = kx + b \qquad (8)$$

The slope information of the indentation curve (k) was used to calculate the Young's modulus (E):

$$\left[\frac{4\sqrt{R}}{3(1\text{-}v_{cell}^2)}E_{cell}\right]^{2/3} = slope_{indentation} = k \qquad (9)$$

Solving for E_{cell}, we obtain the following:

$$E_{cell} = k^{3/2} \left[\frac{3(1\text{-}v_{cell}^2)}{4\sqrt{R}}\right] \qquad (10)$$

Equation (7) should give a good linear fit line for the indentation data. The Young's modulus of the cell is considered a constant within the range of force applied to it. Presently, the contact point can be approximately represented by the b term in the following equation:

$$b = \text{-}\left[\frac{4\sqrt{R}}{3(1\text{-}v_{cell}^2)}E_{cell}\right]^{2/3}(z_0 - d_0) \qquad (11)$$

However, z_0 and d_0 are both the x and y coordinates of the initial point of contact. d_0 refers to the deflection offset that is experienced during force curve acquisition and can be determined conveniently by simply observing the raw deflection $vs.$ piezo position data. We solve for z_0 as follows:

$$z_0 = \text{-}\frac{b}{k} + d_0 \qquad (12)$$

Ultimately, we will acquire a more accurate fitting region (z_0, d_0) for the Hertz model. All of the data analysis and curve fitting of the Hertz model to the collected force-indentation data were performed using JPK IP software, which offered automatic fitting for all of the indenter shapes. Finally, the elastic modulus (E) calculations were performed using the JPK IP software.

Extraction and purification of scaffolding protein in irradiated erythrocytes, and western blot analysis of the expression of spectrin-α1

First, the erythrocytes were purified within 48 hours from hamster whole blood and were then isolated by centrifugation at $600 \times g$ for 20 min at 4°C. After removing the plasma and buffy coat by careful aspiration, the erythrocyte pellet was resuspended in cold isotonic buffer (145 mM NaCl, 5 mM KCl, 5 mM HEPES, pH 7.4) and then centrifuged again at $2,000 \times g$ for 10 min at 4°C. Thereafter, the erythrocyte suspension was washed with isotonic buffer four times to completely remove the plasma and buffy layers. Next, to remove white blood cells from the erythrocyte suspensions, the samples were passed through white blood cell filters (Leukotrap RC; Pall Corporation, East Hills, NY) twice. In each step of the purification process, the upper layer was removed. The erythrocytes were finally resuspended in cold isotonic buffer at pH 7.4, made up to a hematocrit of approximately 50%, and stored at 4°C until further analysis.

Erythrocyte samples were purified as described above and were incubated for 10 min at 4°C in buffer containing 1% Triton X-100, 100 mg/mL PMSF, and 1 mM EDTA. The cell lysates were then centrifuged at $30,000 \times g$ at 4°C. The obtained supernatants and pellets, as well as the control (intact cell suspension in PBS), were treated with sample buffer (125 mmol/L Tris-HCl, pH 6.8, 2% sodium dodecyl sulfate (SDS), 10% β-mercaptoethanol, 10% glycerol, and 0.01% bromophenol blue) and heated at 100°C for 8 min. Standard immunoblot procedures were used for all of the samples using the indicated antibody combinations. The protein samples were subjected to 6% SDS-PAGE gel electrophoresis followed by electrotransfer onto PVDF membranes in 0.2 M glycine-NaOH transfer buffer with 0.01% SDS. Filters were blocked for 2 h at RT with blocking buffer (10% FSC, 0.1% Tween-20, and PBS) and subsequently incubated for 2 h at RT in blocking buffer containing monoclonal spectrin-α1 primary antibody (sc-15371; Santa Cruz Biotechnology) at a dilution of 1:1,000. Membranes were washed and incubated for 2 h at RT in blocking buffer containing 1:10,000 affinity-purified goat anti-rabbit IgG (H&L) antibody (7074; Cell Signaling Technology) secondary antibody and then were extensively washed. Next, the antibody conjugate was decanted and washed for 30 min with agitation in wash buffer (TBS with 0.1% Tween-20), changing the wash buffer every 5 min. Protein visualization was performed using ECL reagents (Super Signal West Pico Chemiluminescent Substrate; 34077; Pierce) followed by photography. Normal untreated cells with extraction buffer were used as controls. Western blot analysis was performed using a color scanner by densitometry (HP Scan jet Enterprise 7000n) and analyzed using the Image J software (NIH).

Statistical analysis

Except where noted, data are reported as the mean ± standard error, and statistical comparisons were performed using one-way ANOVA followed by the Tukey-Kramer HSD test for pair-wise comparisons. p values less than 0.05 were considered significant. All statistical analyses were performed using SPSS 11.5 (Statistical Product and Service Solutions) (Stanford University, USA).

Results

3.1 Radiation-induced morphological changes of erythrocytes in hamster peripheral blood via optical microscope observation

Morphological changes were observed in normal and irradiated erythrocytes by optical microscopy. Non-irradiated erythrocytes in peripheral blood were typically biconcave discs, resembling round cakes that were thinner at the center and thicker at the edges. However, after irradiation with CIR for 3 days, these cells appeared to have undergone shrinkage and were irregular, and the edges of some cells exhibited abnormal spines or ruffles. As shown in **Figure 2**, these changes were associated with decreased erythrocyte levels, and the number of abnormally shaped cells increased gradually. Moreover, quantitative analysis was performed on the inherent physicochemical parameters of the erythrocytes, such as the size, shape, effective area of the membrane, and average volume of the cells after irradiation by CIR and X-rays. The results showed that these morphological changes were closely correlated with ionizing irradiation, and a dose-time effect relationship was observed in the irradiated group of erythrocytes with respect to the different radiation doses (**Table 1**).

3.2 Influence of the proportion of erythroid cells in bone marrow exposed to radiation

Changes in the BM erythrocytes after irradiation were analyzed using a tangible cell-counting method. The purpose of our observations was to compare the characteristics among the different cell population types in the total number of BM cells and to understand the distribution characteristics of erythroid cells in BM caused by irradiation. The results revealed a mild myeloproliferative effect with small doses of radiation. Additionally, given the priority of the early development of erythroid cells, the pronormoblasts and basophilic erythroblasts seemed to demonstrate a tendency to increase with increasing absorbed doses of CIR; however, this change in the X-ray radiation group was not obvious. When the radiation dose increased, an obvious inhibitory effect was shown on BM. However, the proportions of polychromatophilic erythroblasts and normoblasts decreased significantly following both types of irradiation. In addition, the data indicated the presence of the myeloid maturation stage in a significantly higher proportion of granulocytes. Furthermore, the annular core, class changes and lack of particles were easily observed via the additive pleochroism of the erythrocytes (**Figure 3** and **Figure 4**).

3.3 Alterations of erythrocyte morphology and mechanical properties triggered by radiation evaluated using atomic force microscopy

3.3.1 AFM topographic imaging. AFM experiments were performed on erythrocytes that were spin-coated onto glass slides, representing the surface effects of the measurement period. Image acquisition was performed in contact mode, and the mechanical properties of the erythrocytes were measured using the force spectrum of the AFM. The AFM probe not only senses the differences in the surface and local mechanical properties in the cell, it also leads to differential surface deformation and contributes to image contrast. During AFM raster scanning, the AFM tip presses against the soft cell membrane into the cytosol until the membrane is resisted by the underlying stiffer structures, resulting in the sub-membrane structures appearing elevated and being detected in deflection images. Thus, through the analysis of AFM topographic images, including height-measured images, deflection images and 3D images, the imaging results can connect the membranous structure and function to reveal the variations in the microstructure of erythrocytes exposed to radiation. Unaffected erythrocytes are typically smooth, biconcave discs; when the cells were irradiated, a series of changes, ranging from minute to major, was captured throughout the whole process using BT-AFM, as detailed below (**Figure 5**).

3.3.2 AFM measurement of the elastic modulus (cell stiffness) of irradiated erythrocytes. The elastic modulus is often used to describe the mechanical properties of cells and other biological samples. The modified Hertz model fit well to the experimental data obtained by AFM measurement, and the calculated value of the elastic modulus was obtained using JPK Instruments data processing software. Stiffness measurements for the erythrocytes treated with different radiation doses were recorded relative to the reference hard material at 3, 14 and 28 days. The results are shown as histograms in **Figure 6** (including, carbon ion beams and X-rays), with the bin size reflecting the confidence interval of the measurements. The average values of the elastic modulus were obtained by fitting the Gaussian distribution to the histograms. Justification for using a normal distribution function for the analysis of the experimental data was provided by performing the Shapiro–Wilk normality test. This procedure indicated that all of the distributions from **Figure 6** were normal at the level of $\alpha = 0.05$. Furthermore, the equality of variance was successfully verified using Levene's test, and the statistical evaluation of the differences among the distributions was performed using analysis of variance (ANOVA). The ANOVA results showed that the means were different at the

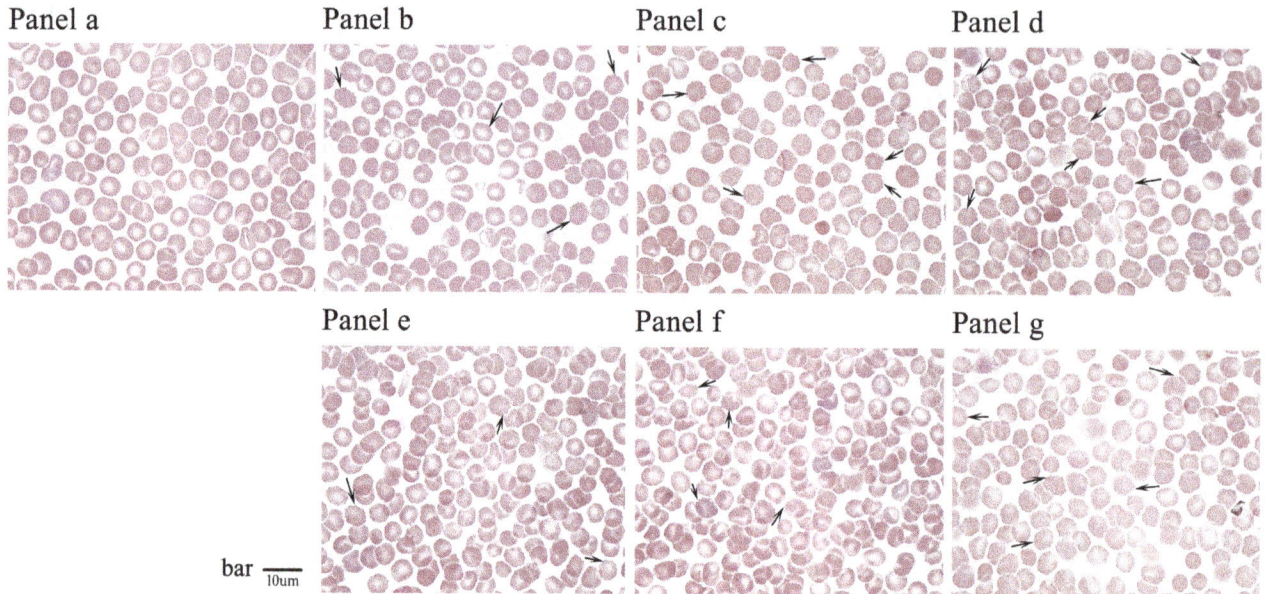

Figure 2. Photographs of analysis the changes of gross morphology of erythrocytes in blood smear at 3d after whole-body exposure to $^{12}C^{6+}$ ions or X-rays (by 100×oil immersion observation). Panel **a**: Non-irradiated control group erythrocytes (0 Gy); Panel **b–d**: erythrocytes of carbon ions radiation groups (Radiation dose: 2 Gy, 4 Gy and 6 Gy); and Panel **e–g**: erythrocytes of X-rays radiation groups (Radiation dose: 4 Gy, 6 Gy and 12 Gy). Black arrows indicate the morphological changes of erythrocytes. The scale bar is 10 μm.

level of $\alpha = 0.01$. The time dependence of the average elastic modulus is shown in **Figure 7**. The error bars in this figure represent half-widths of the normal distributions from **Figure 7**. It could be concluded that the elastic modulus of the phospholipid bilayer membrane in erythrocytes decreases slightly over time with exposure to large doses of radiation. Additionally, an interesting phenomenon is evident in the figure: with the increasing radiation doses, the elastic modulus also decreased. In the experiment, the changes in the elastic modulus were due to different radiation doses with CIR or X-rays, triggering injury to the membrane-cytoskeleton system.

Figure 8 shows scatter plots of the elastic modulus values of the irradiated and non-irradiated groups over 3, 14, and 28 days calculated from the average of the approach force curves, and the results are shown as box-plots in which the scattered dots represent the effective sample point number. The data indicate that there were similar trends in variations of the elastic modulus according to the different doses of radiation in the erythrocyte samples, possibly indicating that the elastic modulus was proportional to the radiation dose.

3.4 Spectrin-α1 specifically participates in the morphological remodeling of irradiated erythrocytes

After exposure to CIR, the expression of spectrin-α1 protein significantly decreased in erythrocytes. With increasing radiation doses, spectrin-α1 protein expression was reduced. From 3 to 28 days after exposure to CIR, spectrin-α1 expression steadily decreased with increasing radiation doses. However, for X-rays, when small doses (<4 Gy) of radiation were utilized, spectrin-α1 expression was slightly augmented for a short time (approximately 14 days); with larger doses of radiation, spectrin-α1 expression appeared to be inhibited. As shown in **Figure 9**, the changes in erythrocyte morphology at the micro-nano scale level illustrate the integrity of the cell membrane and the stability of the cytoskeleton, which are dependent on protein conformation.

3.5 Comparison of the variation between the average of the elastic modulus and the mean density levels of spectrin-α1 caused by radiation

As indicated in **Table 2**, noticeable differences were observed for all of the data before and after irradiation. The mean density values of spectrin-α1 protein expression were significantly lower in the irradiated samples than in the non-irradiated samples ($p < 0.05$), and the difference in the elastic modulus of both groups is clearly shown in **Table 2**. In particular, after exposure to CIR for 3 days, with increasing radiation dose from 2 Gy to 6 Gy, the mean density values of spectrin-α1 protein expression ranged from 0.99 ± 0.16 to 0.75 ± 0.15, which was significantly different from those of the control non-irradiated group ($p<0.05$). However, at 14 days, the radiation-exposed cells showed mean density values of spectrin-α1 protein expression between 1.03 ± 0.19 to and 0.71 ± 0.17 with increasing radiation dose. At 28 days, the mean density values of spectrin-α1 protein expression ranged from 1.39 ± 0.12 to 0.57 ± 0.13. Furthermore, the mean elasticity modulus values of the irradiated group were reduced with increasing radiation dose from 10.62 ± 1.57 kPa to 5.08 ± 0.59 kPa after irradiation for 3 days; at 14 and 28 days, the average value of the Young's modulus ranged from 9.42 ± 0.66 kPa to 4.98 ± 0.76 kPa and from 8.22 ± 1.33 kPa to 4.72 ± 0.74 kPa, respectively. For X-ray radiation, results similar to those obtained with CIR were observed (**Table 2**). Thus, in summary, the results indicate that when the micromorphology and microstructure of an erythrocyte change from a typically smooth, biconcave disc to a cell surface with corrugated, irregular, and rolling regional topography, changes in the elastic modulus and morphology occur in parallel with the irradiation process. Additionally, the fact is the elastic modulus values always increase when young cells become old cells in process, the form of change coexist in the process of erythrocyte changes by CIR induced, but the radiation induce the cell apoptosis that is a programmed cell death process along with the evolution of time, the activation of

Table 1. Measurement of the changes of erythrocytes shape by induced of $^{12}C^{6+}$ ions and X-rays radiation in *Mesocricetus auratus*.

Group	Cells No.	Length(μm)	Width(μm)	Perimeter(μm)	Thickness(μm)	ROI area(μm²)	Volume(μm³)
Control 0Gy	1500	7.25±0.13	6.12±0.10	584.14±36.78	2.0	20517.44±3651.02	41.03±7.30
$^{12}C^{6+}$ions 2Gy	410	6.85±0.15▲	5.96±0.20	563.95±57.72▲	2.0	19019.15±3120.58	38.04±6.24▲
4Gy	376	6.72±0.16▲	5.85±0.11▲	547.98±47.86▲	2.0	18178.41±2933.45	36.36±5.87▲
6Gy	373	5.96±0.24▲	5.55±0.15▲	529.38±40.77▲	2.0	17317.20±2419.97	34.63±4.84▲
X-rays 4Gy	652	7.0±0.11▲▲	5.8±0.16▲▲	570.7±57.43▲▲	2.0	19496.54±2975.36	38.99±5.95▲▲
6Gy	325	6.8±0.15▲▲	5.6±0.12▲▲	535.6±37.50▲▲	2.0	18659.76±2260.22	37.32±4.52▲▲
12Gy	554	6.1±0.18▲▲	5.4±0.10▲▲	519.0±45.65▲▲	2.0	17734.23±2747.42	35.47±5.49▲▲

Note. Measurement of the morphological differences of erythrocytes had indicated the obvious impact of $^{12}C^{6+}$ ions or X-rays radiation with Image J software. And these general varies mainly includes the physical and chemical parameters of the erythrocyte, such as length, width, perimeter, thickness, ROI area and volume (of average value). Because of the average thickness of erythrocytes in mammals is around in the range of 1.0–2.5 μm, and using an optical microscope in the experiment, so as to calculate the volume, we taken the average thickness value of 2.0 μm to obtain the relative size of erythrocytes. And in the list of **Tab.**, ▲ Black triangle symbols significant statistical significance compared with the control group in carbon ion radiation ($p<0.05$), but ▲▲ double triangle line represent the differences results by inducing X-rays ($p<0.05$). (In detail, for length, Control vs C ions-2Gy, p=0.000, $p<$ 0.05; Control vs C ions-4Gy, p=0.000, $p<0.05$; Control vs C ions-6Gy, p=0.000, $p<0.05$; Control vs X rays-6Gy, p=0.000, $p<0.05$; for width, Control vs C ions-4Gy, p=0.479, p>0.05; Control vs C ions-2Gy, p=0.000, $p<0.05$; Control vs X rays-6Gy, p=0.000, $p<0.05$; Control vs X rays-12Gy, p=0.000, $p<0.05$; for perimeter, Control vs C ions-2Gy, p=0.002, $p<0.05$; Control vs C ions-4Gy, p=0.000, $p<0.05$; Control vs X rays-4Gy, p=0.027, $p<0.05$; Control vs X rays-6Gy, p=0.000, $p<0.05$; Control vs X rays-12Gy, p=0.000, $p<0.05$; for volume, Control vs C ions-2Gy, p=0.000, $p<0.05$; Control vs C ions-4Gy, p=0.000, $p<0.05$; Control vs X rays-4Gy, p=0.000, $p<0.05$; Control vs X rays-6Gy, p=0.000, $p<0.05$; Control vs X rays-12Gy, p=0.000, $p<0.05$).)

signaling molecules, then the series of cascading effects of transduction pathway [88,89]. Specific mechanisms with age may be different from the mechanism of apoptosis, maybe there are some commonness, and also differences. Clearly, age-related changes have showed a transitions from physiological to pathological state, and the change of age relative to the apoptosis process is negligible. Therefore, the elastic modulus may function as a "biomarker" in the process and can be used to assess the harmful effects to erythrocytes or other cell types/tissues triggered by irradiation. The assessment of a single cell or group of cells may be sufficient to connect the biomechanical properties of cells and the protein molecular signaling cascade.

3.6 Spatial correlation of the expression of cytoskeletal protein spectrin-α1 and the elastic modulus in irradiated erythrocytes

After the experimental groups were exposed to CIR or X-rays, the spatial relationships between spectrin-α1 protein expression and the elastic modulus in erythrocytes were examined. We correlated the value measured for the elastic modulus of the erythrocyte membrane using BT-AFM with the expression of the cytoskeletal protein spectrin-α1. Qualitatively, the elastic modulus appeared to be positively correlated with the relative expression of spectrin-α1 (i.e., a high modulus was observed in regions with higher protein expression in the context of irradiation) and was also correlated with radiation dose (low modulus in regions with lower protein level in the context of irradiation). Additionally, there was a special dose-response relationship between the elastic modulus and the radiation dose: when the irradiation dose increased, the elastic modulus increased as well (**Figure 10**). Based on these findings, Pearson's correlation coefficient (r) was calculated between the elastic modulus and the relative level of cytoskeletal protein spectrin-α1. In control erythrocyte samples, there appeared to be no correlation among high-modulus regions, low-modulus regions and spectrin-α1 protein expression. After treatment with radiation, the average modulus was reduced, and the area of the cell membrane appeared to be more correlated with the modulus. Reflecting these findings, after exposure to CIR for 3 days, Pearson's correlation coefficient (r) between the modulus and spectrin-α1 protein expression was relatively strong and significant ($r_{3c}=0.678$, $p<0.01$) compared with the other time points. At 14 days of irradiation with CIR, Pearson's correlation coefficient showed a positive correlation ($r_{14c}=0.639$, $p<0.01$); at 28 days of irradiation by CIR, the correlation coefficient was also positive ($r_{28c}=0.438$, $p<0.01$). For X-rays, there were radiation effects similar to those of CIR among the different groups: at 3, 14 and 28 days, the correlation coefficients were ($r_{3x}=0.390$, $p<0.05$), ($r_{14x}=0.301$, $p<0.01$) and ($r_{28x}=0.353$, $p<0.01$), respectively.

Discussion

The inherent mechanical characteristics of cells are an important manifestation of their physical state under external perturbation

The mechanical properties of individual cells have been regarded as unique indicators that can constantly reflect the changes in their states caused by cellular events and pathological conditions. Simply put, alterations in biological activity or transformation of cell states can also trigger changes in the mechanical properties of cells. In particular, alterations in cell stiffness or the elastic modulus have been used as biological markers for cellular phenotypic events and diseases [90]. The

Panel a   Panel b   Panel c   Panel d

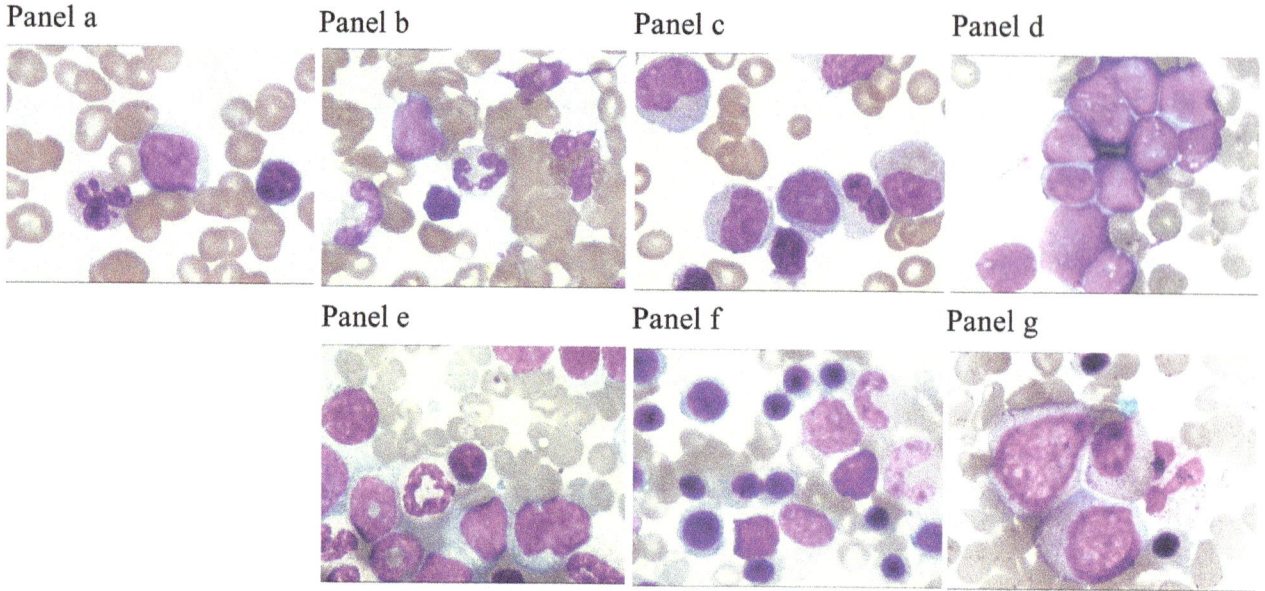

Panel e   Panel f   Panel g

Figure 3. The distribution characteristics of erythrocytes in BM at 3d after exposed by different doses of $^{12}C^{6+}$ ions or X-rays. Cytology analysis the distribution of erythrocytes in BM. In detailed, Panel **a**: Non-irradiated control group erythrocytes (0Gy); Panel **b–d**: erythrocytes of carbon ions radiation groups (Radiation dose: 2Gy, 4Gy and 6Gy); panel **e–g**: erythrocytes of X-rays radiation groups (Radiation dose: 4Gy, 6Gy and 12Gy). And BM aspirate smear from irradiated golden hamster showing abnormal erythroblasts indicative of a cell-division defect, or dysplasia. The cytology image was observed with 100×oil immersion, in the picture, pink represents the erythrocytes.

mechanical properties of cells are largely attributable to the cytoskeleton components and the cytoskeletal architecture, which maintain the basic form of cells. Thus, for the abovementioned changes in a cell's life cycle, visualizing the changes in the mechanical properties of cells exposed to some type of stimulus and the association of these changes with the biomechanics of

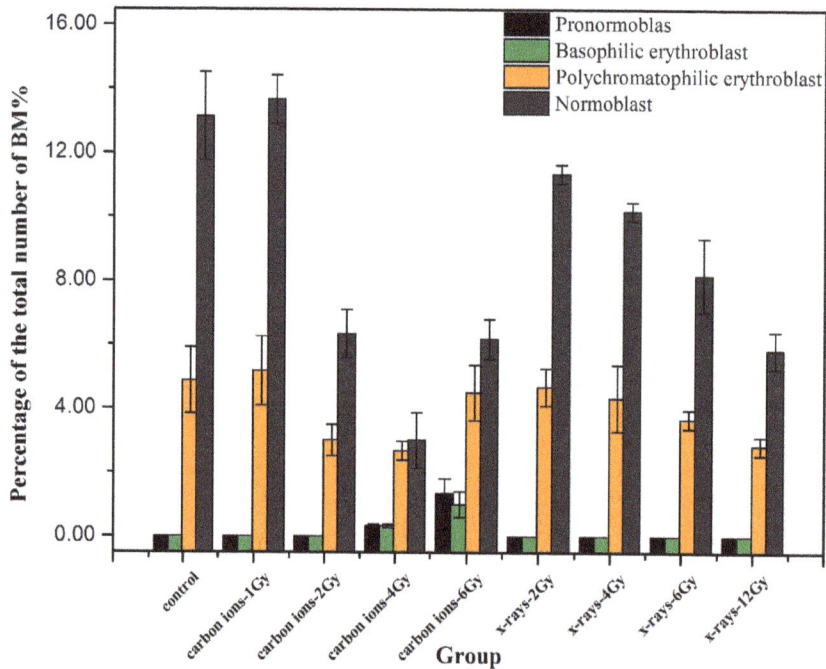

Figure 4. The number of erythroid cells in BM accounted for the relative percentage of the total of BM cells after exposed carbon ion beams or X-rays. From the column chart showed that the pronormoblast and basophilic erythroblast seemed upward tendency with the increasing of absorbed dose in carbon ions radiation, but the change in X-rays radiation groups seemed to be not obvious, as for the polychromatophilic erythroblast and normoblast, the percentage of cells number had decreased significantly in two types of irradiation, and the differences between groups had significant statistical significance ($p<0.05$).

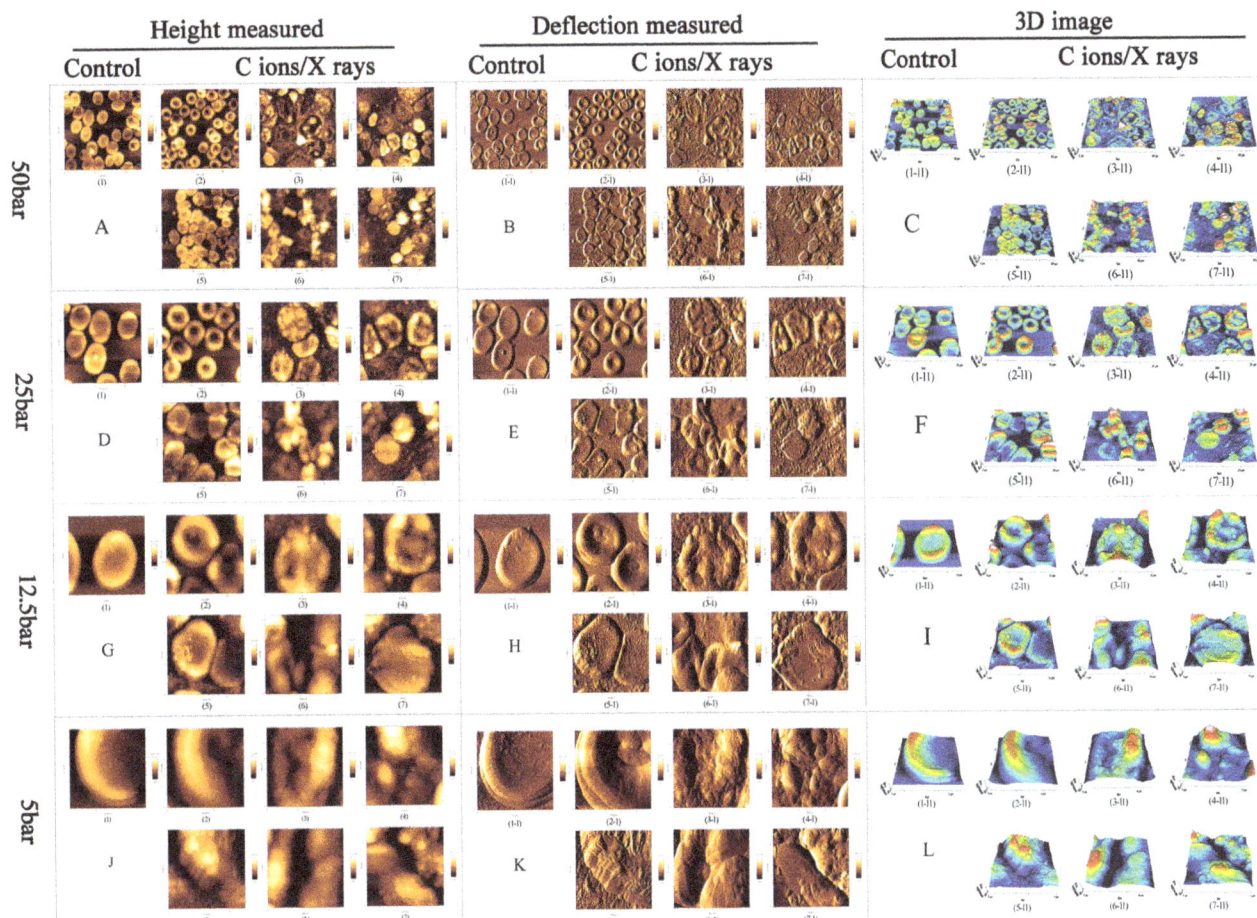

Figure 5. Effects of radiation on micromorphology in erythrocytes membrane. (**A–L**) Surface imaging of erythrocytes induced by carbon ion beams and X-rays radiation using biological type atomic force microscopy; and the graph **A**, **B** and **C** showed respectively for the Height measured image, Deflection image and 3D image at scan scale of 50 μm (Fast)×50 μm bar (Slow), [for **A**:(1) Control; (2) C ions 2Gy; (3) C ions 4Gy; (4) C ions 6Gy; (5) X-rays 4Gy; (6) X-rays 6Gy; (7) X-rays 12Gy; for **B**: (1–1) Control; (2–1) C ions 2Gy; (3–1) C ions 4Gy; (4–1) C ions 6Gy; (5–1) X-rays 4Gy; (6–1) X-rays 6Gy; (7–1) X-rays 12Gy; for **C**: (1–11) Control; (2–11) C ions 2Gy; (3–11) C ions 4Gy; (4–11) C ions 6Gy; (5–11) X-rays 4Gy; (6–11) X-rays 6Gy; (7–11) X-rays 12Gy]. But the graph **D–F** showed respectively for the Height measured image, Deflection image and 3D image at scan scale of 25 μm (Fast) ×25 μm bar (Slow); the graph **G–I** showed respectively for the Height measured image, Deflection image and 3D image at scan scale of 12.5 μm (Fast) ×12.5 μm bar (Slow); the graph **J–L** showed respectively for the Height measured image, Deflection image and 3D image at scan scale of 5 μm (Fast) × 5 μm bar (Slow). In addition, for a smaller scan scale was the same grouping as 50 μm (Fast) × 50 μm bar (Slow) bar. Here, the schematic showed different doses and type radiation for the influence of micromorphology of erythrocytes, and this fine change was captured by AFM.

cellular events have very important significance. Previously, the spectrin skeleton of erythrocytes was studied as a model tethered membrane [91], and many results have suggested that spectrin is a vital scaffold protein involved in signaling pathway organization, influencing changes in cytoskeletal structure and controlling membrane function.

Radiation induces changes in erythrocyte stiffness during morphological remodeling

In the present study, the mechanical properties of erythrocytes were assessed by combining the use of biological-type AFM, cytological analysis of samples of peripheral blood and optical microscopy of bone marrow after irradiation by CIR or X-rays. The experimental results suggested that there was a clear relationship between changes in cell morphology and variations in mechanical properties; this relationship was mainly manifested in the following respects. First, in terms of morphology, a normal erythrocyte is a biconcave disc resembling a round cake, has a

uniform size, has no nucleus, appears as a bilaterally indented sphere of approximately 4–8 μm in diameter (in mammals; in humans, 6–9 μm), has a thickness of approximately 1.0–2.5 μm, and has a relatively uniform, flat, and smooth membrane surface that is structured and maintains some continuity. However, after 3 days of irradiation with CIR, these cells underwent shrinkage and became irregular, and some exhibited abnormal spines or ruffles on the edges; additionally, the membrane area exhibited discontinuities and an undulating surface (**Figure 1**). Furthermore, the cytological smear method was used and analyzed with the NIH Image J software to reveal changes in the cell form in peripheral blood samples and in the proportions of different cell types in the marrow. The inherent parameters, such as the length, width, perimeter, thickness, ROI area and volume were quantitatively analyzed. Measurement of the results showed that the average value of the length was reduced from approximately 7.25 ± 0.13 μm to 5.96 ± 0.24 μm, the average value of the width was reduced from approximately 6.12 ± 0.10 μm to

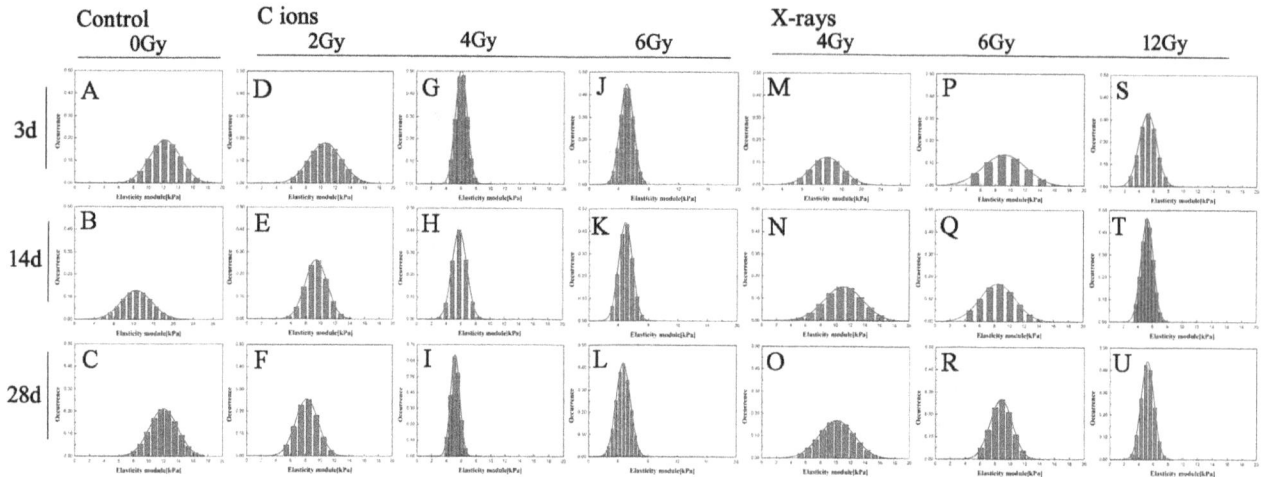

Figure 6. Histograms of erythrocytes elasticity modulus distributions induced by C ions or X-rays exposed for 3, 14 and 28 days.
The bar graph (**A**), (**B**) and (**C**) represented control erythrocytes (0 Gy), 3d, 14d and 28d, respectively; the bar graph (**D**), (**E**) and (**F**) represented carbon ions 2 Gy, 3d, 14d and 28d, respectively; the bar graph (**G**), (**H**) and (**I**) represented carbon ions 4 Gy, 3d, 14d and 28d, respectively; the bar graph (**J**), (**K**) and (**L**) represented carbon ions 6 Gy, 3d, 14d and 28d, respectively. But the bar graph (**M**), (**N**) and (**O**) showed X-rays 4 Gy, 3d, 14d and 28d, respectively; the bar graph (**P**), (**Q**) and (**R**) showed X-rays 6 Gy, 3d, 14d and 28d; the bar graph (**S**), (**T**) and (**U**) showed X-rays 12 Gy, 3d, 14d and 28d, respectively.

5.40±0.10 µm, the average value of the perimeter was reduced from approximately 584.14±36.78 µm to 519.0±45.65 µm, the ROI area was reduced from approximately 20517.44±3651.02 µm^2 to 17317.20±2419.97 µm^2, and the average volume was reduced from approximately 41.03±7.30 µm^3 to 34.63±4.84 µm^3. Additionally, the average thickness of erythrocytes in mammals is in the range of approximately 1.0–2.5 µm. Using an optical microscope, an average thickness value of 2.0 µm was found and used to calculate the relative volume of the erythrocytes. Additionally, using the tangible cell counting method to analyze the proportion of erythroid cells in BM, there was a mild myeloproliferative effect of small doses of radiation. Furthermore, given the priority of the early development of erythroid cells, the pronormoblasts and basophilic erythroblasts seemed to demonstrate a tendency to increase with increasing absorbed CIR doses; however, this change was not obvious in the X-ray radiation group. Taken together, these results indicated that when the radiation dose increased, there was an obvious inhibitory effect on BM; thus, the proportions of polychromatophilic erythroblasts and normoblasts decreased significantly with both types of irradiation (**Figure 2** and **Figure 3**).

Most importantly, BT-AFM was employed in this study as a powerful and versatile tool to study the mechanical properties at the micro-nano scale for the analysis of fine surface structure changes on erythrocytes, emphasizing the role of the cell membrane and the integrity of the membrane in cell mechanical stability following radiation exposure. This study investigated the microstructural and mechanical properties of erythrocytes and quantified the deformation and damage to the membrane skeleton. In particular, as shown in **Figure 5**, AFM topographic images reveal the fine variations induced by radiation, and the images were obtained of shrunken, irregular, ruffled-edge shapes and progressively discontinuous membrane structures. Next, a conclusion can be drawn based on the relative elastic modulus or stiffness, which depends on the precise measurement of the mechanical properties of the cell membrane. The mean elastic modulus of erythrocytes irradiated with increasing CIR doses was decreased to between 10.62±1.57 (kPa) and 5.08±0.59 (kPa) at

3 days after irradiation; at 14 and 28 days, the average values of the elastic modulus ranged from 9.42±0.66 (kPa) to 4.98±0.76 (kPa) and 8.22±1.33 (kPa) to 4.72±0.74 (kPa), respectively. For X-ray radiation, similar results were observed to those obtained with CIR. Thus, fundamental alterations in erythrocyte stiffness were triggered by the different radiation types, at different times and with different doses. Furthermore, the combination, the distribution, and the changes in stiffness were also different, as shown in **Figures 6, 7** and **8**. This strategy allowed us to perform nanobiological analysis of the erythrocytes after irradiation, further improving our knowledge of the aspects and dynamics of the mechanical properties of erythrocytes.

Spectrin-α1, a neofunctionalized cytoskeletal protein of erythrocytes, is involved in mediating changes in erythrocyte stiffness during the morphological remodeling process induced by radiation

The membrane skeleton, a dense proteinaceous network, is thought to be responsible for the remarkable morphological changes and mechanical properties of erythrocytes [92], allowing them to withstand and respond to different mechanical stresses and tension caused by external perturbations experienced throughout their 120-day lifespan [93]. The basic shape of an erythrocyte can be visualized by observing the spectrin-containing sub-membranous cytoskeleton because this structure preserves the outline of the cell. The spectrin molecules form pentagonal or hexagonal arrangements, which are composed of tetramers of spectrin subunits associating with short actin filaments at either end of the tetramer. These short actin filaments act as junctional complexes, allowing the formation of a hexagonal mesh and scaffolding. This assembly configuration not only plays an important role in the maintenance of plasma membrane shape, integrity, and cytoskeletal structure, influence influencing deformability or resulting in damage [90], [94,95] and finally determining biological behavior and functional aspects [96–99]; it can also produce a rapid response and break the tetramers [100]. A dysfunctional underlying membrane skeleton results in the erythrocyte membrane being partially devoid of a spectrin-actin

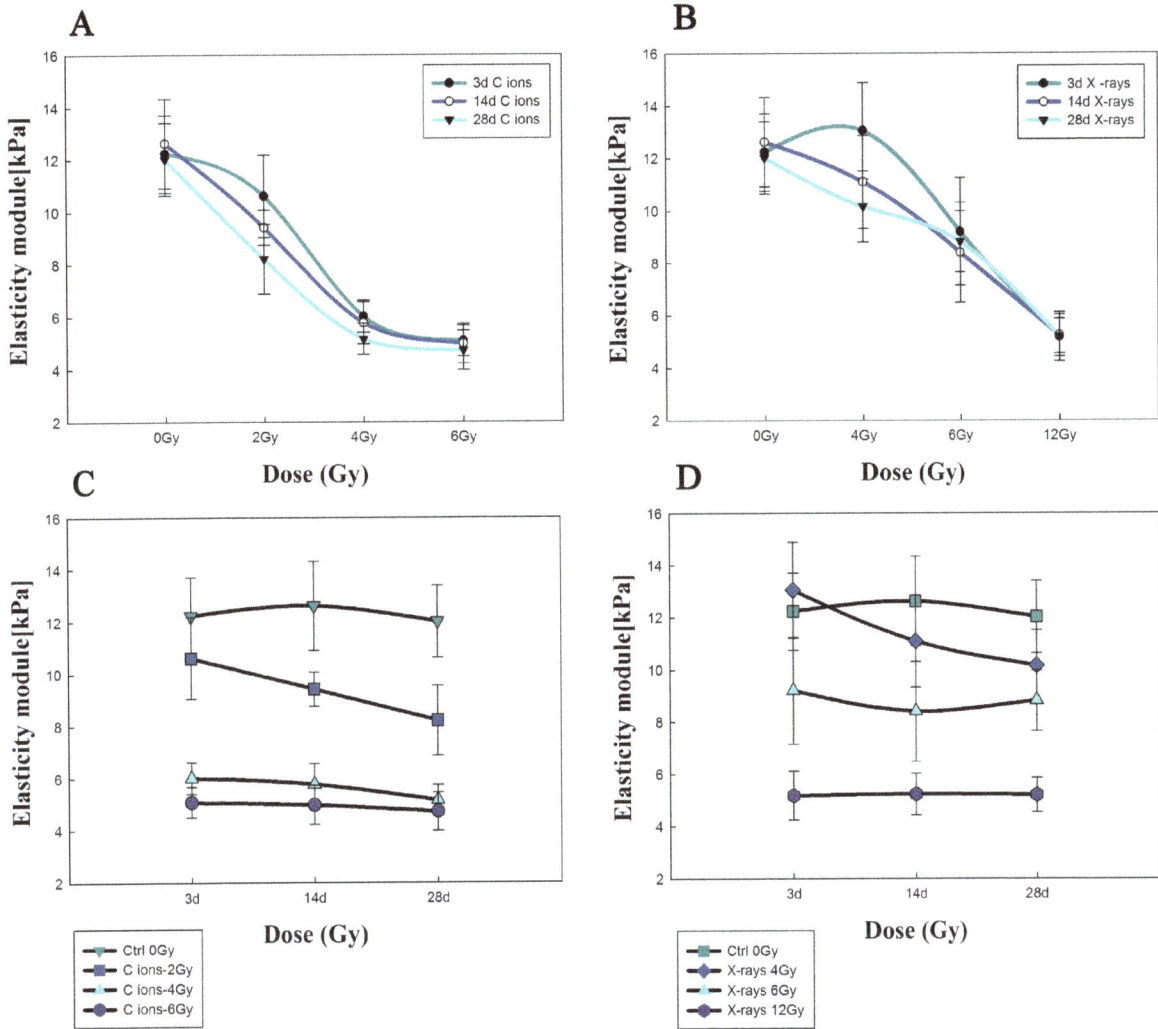

Figure 7. The change of elasticity modules of erythrocytes induced by C ions or X-rays radiation. And the groups displayed as a function of the dependent manner on dosage (**A** and **B**) and time (**C** and **D**). Error bars represent half-widths of the normal distributions fitted to the respective histograms.

network, no longer existing as a ghost, and causing disruption of the unique arrangement of spectrin, F-actin, protein 4.1 and ankyrin, with direct and indirect connections to the membrane bilayer with its immersed integral proteins [101] (**Figure 11**). Consequently, the distribution of membrane tension is regulated by signaling molecules through the activated complex signaling transduction pathway to mediate the biochemical reaction between target proteins or molecules [102–104] and triggering exquisite changes in cell shape or membrane damage [105]. Similarly, it was reported that the skeleton began to fragment and became a small, approximately 50-nm inverted vesicle [52], producing changes in cell shape and stability regarding the filamentous network. Consequently, the importance of this structure is highlighted by the above discussion noting that spectrin is a structural platform for the stabilization and activation of membrane channels, receptors and transporters in mammals; however, it is also closely related to cell physiology and pathology [106,107].

Many studies have shown that the measurement of mechanical properties in biological samples can explain the biomechanical mechanism of organism units in various physiological and

pathological states. Recent evidence suggests that shear can induce the unfolding of spectrin within erythrocytes [108], forcing changes in protein structure by the unfolding of specific regions, and that the spectrin repeat unit can be subjected to reversible unfolding and refolding using 20-pN forces [109]. Regarding the erythrocyte cytoskeleton, spectrin comprises a tetrameric or higher oligomeric protein arranged as antiparallel filamentous heterodimers of α and β subunits [52], [110], which is easy to open or fold; moreover, spectrin is organized in a scaffold located at the intracellular side of the plasma membrane in eukaryotic cells, and is linked to several integral membrane proteins through a helical repeating unit. Additionally, spectrin and a few other proteins assemble into a building block and share a common structural fold with all of the spectrin repeat units [52]. Ultimately, the crystal structure of the assembled protein shows that it maintains an uninterrupted helical structure [111], creating a steady state for the cytoskeleton meshwork and maintaining the native cell shape. In the present study, the expression of the cytoskeletal protein spectrin-α1 was analyzed using a quantitative immunoblot technique after irradiation, and the results showed that CIR or X-rays can cause the expression of spectrin-α1 to decrease

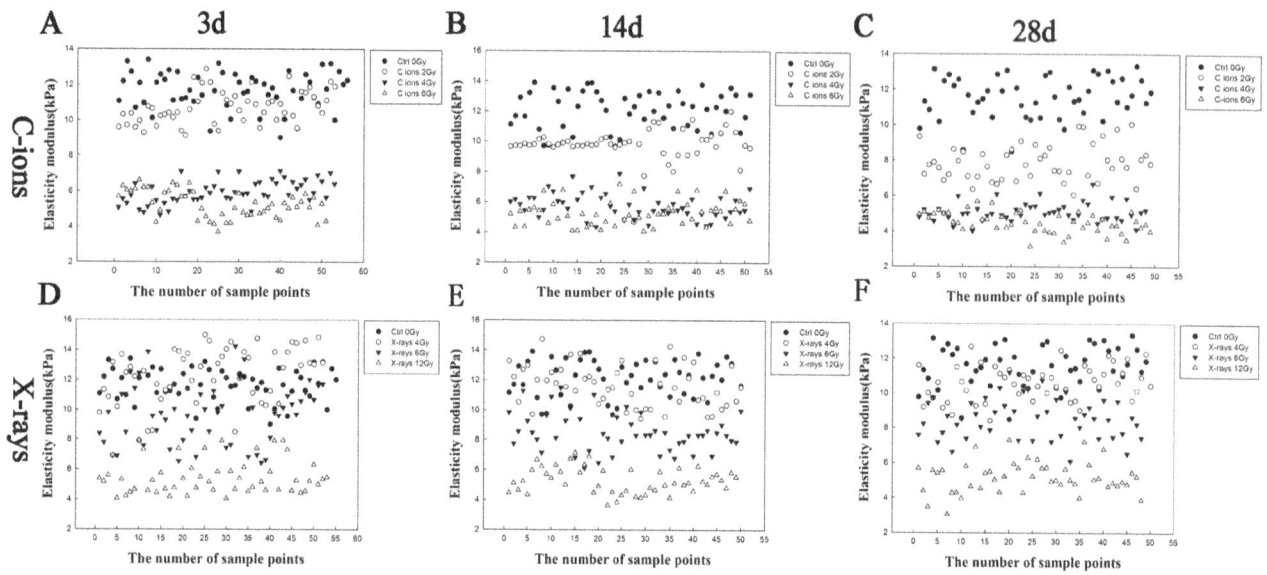

Figure 8. Variations of elasticity modulus for different doses of radiation in erythrocyte samples–control erythrocytes, and after suffering from the irradiation dose, the distribution effect of elasticity modulus was showed by scatters dots (A–F).

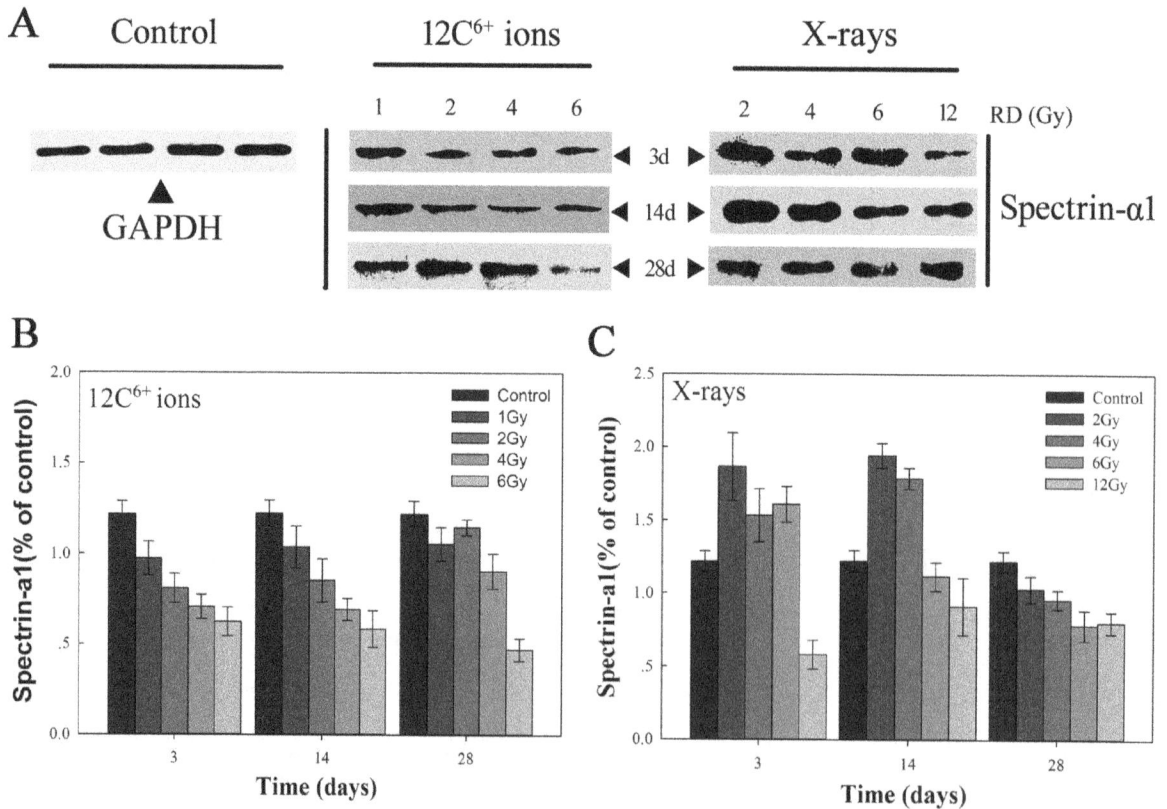

Figure 9. Spectrin-α1 is specifically targeted to drive erythrocyte skeleton impairment by C ions or X-rays radiation induction. Western blotting analyzed of the change of erythrocytes skeleton proteins spectrin-α1 expression after treated with radiation (**A**). (**B**) After C ions exposed at 3, 14 and 28d, the change of skeleton protein expression in different radiation groups. (**C**) After X-rays exposed at 3, 14 and 28d, and skeleton protein expression was also monitored by WB in different radiation groups. Error bars represent standard deviation from more triplicate valid data.

Table 2. Average values of Young's modulus and mean density values of spectrin-α1 expression for the change of RBCs distributions according to different radiation groups.

Group	Spectrin-α1 protein expression (mean density)			Young's modulus (kPa)		
	3d	14d	28d	3d	14d	28d
Control	1.21±0.07	1.22±0.62	1.22±0.64	12.23±1.48	12.62±1.71	12.02±1.38
C ions 2Gy	0.99±0.16▼	1.03±0.19▼	1.39±0.12▼##	10.62±1.57	9.42±0.66	8.22±1.33
4Gy	0.88±0.14▼	0.82±0.13▼	1.10±0.18▼##	6.02±0.60△#	5.77±0.80△#	5.17±0.60△#
6Gy	0.75±0.15▼	0.71±0.17▼	0.57±0.13▼##	5.08±0.59△#	4.98±0.76△#	4.72±0.74△#
X-rays 4Gy	1.86±0.26▼	2.17±0.14	1.16±0.14##	13.05±1.84	11.09±1.77	10.16±1.35
6Gy	1.95±0.20▼	1.36±0.17	0.95±0.17▼##	9.20±2.05△	8.40±1.91△	8.82±1.17△
12Gy	0.67±0.16▼	1.11±0.27▼	0.97±0.14▼	5.18±0.94△#	5.23±0.80△#	5.21±0.66△#

Errors are a standard deviation of the mean (SEM).
Note, △ White triangles represents the statistical significance compared with the control group, #the pound sign shows the plot as time goes on and the difference mean Young's modulus(E) between each dose group (*mean ± SEM*). (for 3d, Control *vs* C ions-2Gy, p = 0.114, *p>0.05*; Control *vs* C ions-4Gy, p = 0.000, *p<0.01*; Control *vs* C ions-6Gy, p = 0.000, *p<0.01*; Control *vs* X rays-4Gy, p = 0.200, *p>0.05*; Control *vs* X rays-6Gy, p = 0.000, *p<0.01*; Control *vs* X rays-12Gy, p = 0.000, *p<0.01*; for 14d, Control *vs* C ions-2Gy, p = 0.000, *p<0.01*; Control *vs* C ions-4Gy, p = 0.000, *p<0.01*; Control *vs* C ions-6Gy, p = 0.000, *p<0.01*; Control *vs* X rays-4Gy, p = 0.243, *p>0.05*; Control *vs* X -rays-6Gy, p = 0.000, *p<0.01*; Control *vs* X rays-12Gy, p = 0.000, *p<0.01*;for 28d, Control *vs* C ions-2Gy, p = 0.095, *p>0.05*; Control *vs* C ions-4Gy, p = 0.000, *p<0.01*; Control *vs* C ions-6Gy, p = 0.000, *p<0.01*; Control *vs* X -rays-4Gy, p = 0.871, *p>0.05*; Control *vs* X rays-6Gy, p = 0.000, *p<0.01*; Control *vs* X rays-12Gy, p = 0.000, *p<0.01*). But ▼ blank triangles standards for the differences of spectrin-α1 protein average level (sp) and mean Young's modulus (E) in different time points (*mean ± SEM*). ##Double pound sign shows the plot as time goes on and the difference of protein between each dose group. (for 3d, Control *vs* C ions-2Gy, p = 0.000, *p<0.01*; Control *vs* C ions-4Gy, p = 0.000, *p<0.01*; Control *vs* C ions-6Gy, p = 0.000, *p<0.01*; Control *vs* X rays-4Gy, p = 0.013, *p<0.05*; Control *vs* X rays-6Gy, p = 0.000, *p<0.01*; Control *vs* X rays-12Gy, p = 0.000, *p<0.01*; for 14d, Control *vs* C ions-2Gy, p = 0.000, *p<0.01*; Control *vs* C -ions-4Gy, p = 0.000, *p<0.01*; Control *vs* C ions-6Gy, p = 0.000, *p<0.01*; Control *vs* X rays-4Gy, p = 0.000, *p<0.01*; Control *vs* X rays-6Gy, p = 0.020, *p<0.05*; Control *vs* X rays-12Gy, p = 0.023, *p<0.05*; for 28d, Control *vs* C -ions-2Gy, p = 0.010, *p<0.05*; Control *vs* C ions-4Gy, p = 0.046, *p<0.05*; Control *vs* C ions-6Gy, p = 0.000, *p<0.01*; Control *vs* X rays-4Gy, p = 0.341, *p>0.05*; Control *vs* X rays-6Gy, p = 0.000, *p<0.01*; Control *vs* X rays-12Gy, p = 0.002, *p<0.01*).

significantly in irradiated erythrocytes. This effect relied on different radiation doses, and the data obtained showed a relationship between the expression of cytoskeletal protein spectrin-α1 and changes in cell stiffness in the irradiated group, as well as a negative correlation regarding changes in erythrocyte stiffness during the morphological remodeling process. Additionally, regarding the AFM experimental data, examination of these changes in mechanical properties by the response to force is one of the most straightforward visual indices to evaluate the membrane damage mechanism caused by radiation, assess the overall performance of protein conformation and the protein grid in the erythrocyte membrane skeleton, and increase the understanding of the radiation-induced morphological remodeling-cytoskeletal remodeling process.

Erythrocyte stiffness during morphological remodeling can be used as a biomarker to estimate the adverse effects induced by ionizing radiation

Based on the established parameters, the present study evaluated the roles of cell morphology and cell stiffness during the erythrocyte morphological remodeling process to determine the adverse effects on erythrocytes following exposure to radiation. The influence of the combination of cell signaling with the interactions of membrane phospholipids in vertical force interactions, horizontal interactions, and lateral network interactions of the spectrin structure were emphasized in the current study. Thus, it is necessary to clarify two basic problems of the mechanics induced by the effects of radiation. The first problem is the relationship between the stability of the membrane-associated cytoskeleton and changes in the mechanical properties (e.g., the stiffness or elastic modulus and the viscosity) of the erythrocytes. Another problem is that the shear stress or tension created by the effects of deformation or damage after radiation might influence

how the radiation alters the cell behavior in various mechano-signaling processes, such as changes in cell shape, cell migration, cell movement and cell apoptosis. Thus, to solve these two problems, a link must be created between the biochemical molecules (proteins) and the response to force (cell stiffness) to improve our understanding of why mechanically induced changes in the protein structure within erythrocytes are likely to be important not only to cell deformability or damage but also to various mechano-signaling processes [35], [112].

When the erythrocytes were subjected to radiation, the cells first responded to the radiation at the cellular level. Next, the effect was further expanded via a signaling cascade starting at the level of proteins and molecules. Similarly to a scaffold protein, spectrin functions as a supporting protein of the erythrocyte membrane skeleton. Spectrin can organize and mediate signaling molecules into particular domains of specific signaling pathways that depend not only on the targeting affinity of proteins of the signaling pathway but also on the circumstances under which the expression of these signaling pathway components were increased and position these components in response to the radiation that activated the signal transduction pathway. Next, using this procedure, membrane proteins (comprising membrane channels, receptors and adhesion molecules) on the erythrocyte surface were activated to recruit target proteins to a specified location, organize them by affinity, and bind them into large biological macromolecular complexes. However, for spectrin proteins, posttranslational protein modifications of phosphorylation and dephosphorylation are involved in positioning and recruiting target proteins [52], resulting in a disturbance of the dynamic balance of the formation and depolymerization of scaffolding proteins [113]. This disturbance leads to the openings in the structure, rotation, and fracture, causing cytoskeleton rearrangement and collapse of the membrane skeleton due to radiation effects, in addition to directly affecting and modulating the mechanical stability of the erythro-

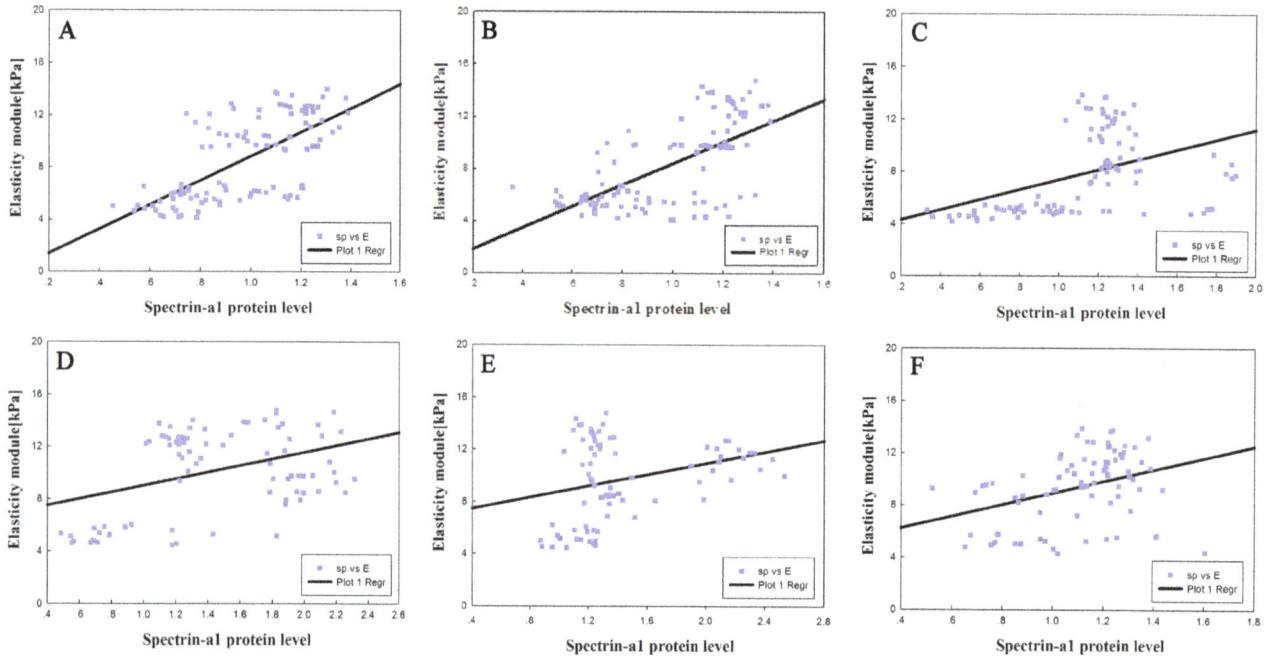

Figure 10. Spatial correlation of nanoscale modulus and spectrin-α1 protein expression with different doses of C ions or X-rays irradiated. With the increasing of radiation dosage, the relative protein expression of spectrin-α1 (sp) seemed more spatially correlated to elastic modulus (E) than low dose radiation (**A–F**). Comparison of correlation of the modulus in the same areas with Pearson's testing. In control erythrocyte samples, there appeared to be non-correlation among the Young's modulus in high-modulus regions, or low-modulus regions and the expression of spectrin-α1 protein. After treated with the radiation, the average elastic modulus was reduced and areas of cell membrane appeared to be more correlated with the modulus. Through the Pearson's correlation coefficient between modulus and spectrin-α1protein level by western blotting detection. Reflective of these findings, after exposure by carbon ion beams at 3 days, Pearson's correlation coefficient (r) between modulus and spectrin-α1 protein expression were relatively strong but significant ($r_{3c} = 0.678$, $p < 0.01$) compared with others time points; At 14 days irradiated by carbon ions, Pearson's correlation coefficient between them showed positive correlation ($r_{14c} = 0.639$, $p < 0.01$); at 28 days irradiated by carbon ions, the correlation coefficient was ($r_{28c} = 0.438$, $p < 0.01$). For X-rays, there were similar radiation effects with carbon ion beams in different groups, respectively, at 3, 14 and 28 days, the correlation coefficient were ($r_{3x} = 0.390$, $p < 0.05$), ($r_{14x} = 0.301$, $p < 0.01$) and ($r_{28x} = 0.353$, $p < 0.01$).

cyte plasma membrane. The direct effects manifest as uneven changes in the regional distribution of tension forces on the cell membrane surface; thus, the deformation or damage to the erythrocyte morphological remodeling process can be assessed.

However, for morphology-cytoskeleton remodeling, tension or stress forces are always involved in this complex coupling process. The cascade effects in the pathway are caused by biological composite macromolecules that can produce changes in the cytoskeleton-associated proteins in the spatial conformation of the erythrocyte–e.g., spectrin. There is a rigorous procedure to facilitate the interaction and fine-tune the activity and crosstalk among the proteins within the entire assembly. This targeted protein expression shows increased biological activity, which influences the activity of downstream proteins under their control, until the dynamic balance of the molecules is again coordinated. Thus, different molecular assemblies in different regions operate on the functions or implement local "microdomains" of the cell. However, the complexity of this response relies on several components of the membrane skeleton, and the stiffness of spectrin upon phosphorylation may permit the formation of many junctions to allow fast, reversible rearrangement of the spectrin network upon large deformations, thus indirectly modulating the mechanical stability of the membrane [114]. Certainly, the membrane stability depends largely on resultant forces in three directions to transfer the spatial effects of deformation or damage to the scaffolding proteins. If the protein chains are to be studied as a geometric unit, some of the mechanical behavior must be evaluated under the stress-induced load bearing of the protein

structural unit (**Figure 11**). Additionally, the surface density of the filaments decreases from the center to the edge of the membrane-skeleton, and the overall thickness of the membrane-skeleton also increases from the edge of the cells (54 nm) to the center (110 nm) [115], suggesting a distribution imbalance between the surface density and the membrane-skeleton thickness, leading to tension of the membrane surface. The stress of the cytoskeleton protein chain as a unit inside the cell is unevenly distributed in partial regions or across the entire cell span. The direction of force is along the three axes; thus, the spectrin tetramers can dissociate transiently into dimers, and some of the repeating units of the spectrin chains can unfold. The dissociation of the spectrin tetramers leads to relatively unimpeded translational diffusion of transmembrane proteins and may be expected to allow them to form irregular clusters [116]. Therefore, in horizontal-plane interactions, including spectrin dimers, tetramers, hexamers and octamers, and even higher oligomeric proteins, the tension generates the interactions between the protein chains. In vertical-force interactions, the direction of the force mainly originates from two complexes, which produce shear force by the junctional complex and the AE1-ankyrin complex. The force of the lateral network interactions is more complex and presents numerous binding sites and binding proteins for a broad diversity of partners. There are mainly F-actin binding sites, actin-binding sites, and tropomyosin-, tropomodulin-, adducin-, and dematin-binding proteins participating in local regions of the network to dynamically change the mechanical properties, thus facilitating reversible deformations that the erythrocyte undergoes in different external environments

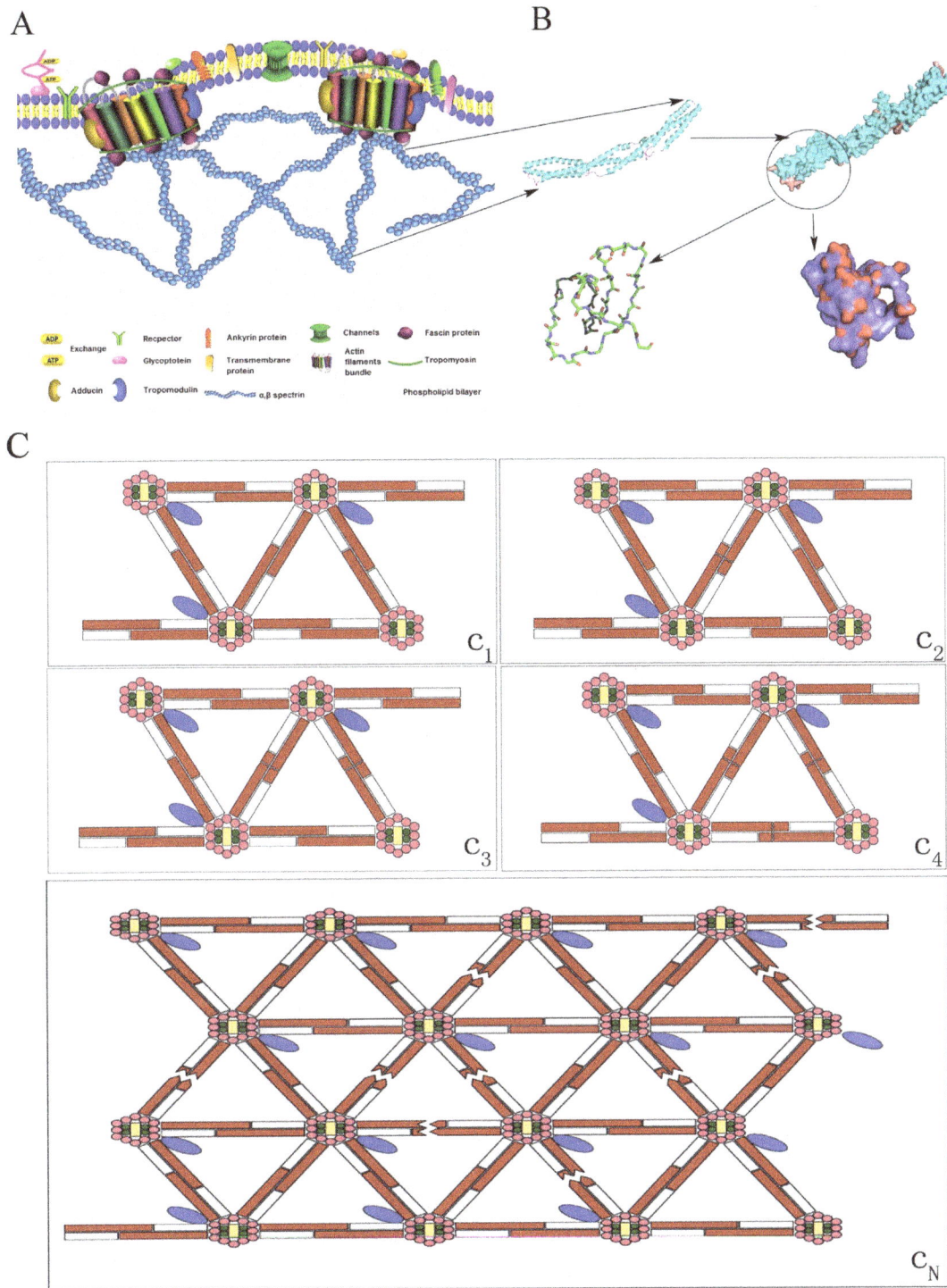

Figure 11. This picture shown the assembly structure of the scaffold protein spectrin and its spatial configuration, and were proposed a deformation hypothesis of our model. (A) The figure was a schematic diagram of spectrin and other cytoskeletal molecules. **(B)** Stereoview ribbon diagram of the overall structure of spectrin protein in all the repeats around the kink region. The first and second repeat (α, β subunit) were shown in light blue, and the linker region between repeats in purple, Residues were numbered according to the SWISS-PROT NP_003117.2 entry, and the residues from 1 to 2149 aa of Homo sapiens. Lastly, the software of the PyMOL Molecular Graphics Systerm was used to simulate the molecular structure, including a complete of the molecular structure and partial structure were displayed. **(C)** A series of random deformation process will be shown. The figure was α-spectrin in dark red band, and β-spectrin with a white band, the shape of saw tooth was rupture boundary. C_1 represented for completely without any deformation, then, C_2, C_3 and C_4 respectively shown that from a set of skeleton to three groups of skeleton were broken. But the case of C_N manifested randomly the fracture of cytoskeletal protein. Thus, this phenomenon could reflect the uninterrupted and dynamic of changes from small deformation to large deformation during the radiation, and more details were explained in the article.

[117,118] (as shown in **Figure 11**). The topographic and mechanical mapping of single components at the cytoplasmic face reveal that, surprisingly, the erythrocyte membrane mechanics are regulated by spectrin phosphorylation related to the metabolic state and the assembly of structural elements in the membrane [111]. Of course, to a certain extent, the local distortion or ratio of damage in cells is mainly determined by the radiation dose. Thus, the spectrins can fully dominate the deformation or damage of the cytoskeletal meshwork in the morphological remodeling process [119]. Considering the current knowledge that spectrin proteins can trigger a biological effect sufficient to change the local or overall cell morphology, as well as the mechanical and structural properties that are changed, few data are available on the interactions of spectrin with several participants in a particular pathway, organizing it into a chain of signaling events. However, according to the present study, the spectrins could be considered docking proteins in the morphological remodeling process induced by radiation.

Conclusion

In summary, our results suggest that CIR could influence the amount of components and reorganize the spectrin-α1 protein of the membrane-skeleton system, as well as affect the distribution of the regional tension or stress (force), resulting in changes in the surface topographical microstructure and mechanical properties (cell stiffness) in the erythrocyte morphological remodeling process. Additionally, we show how spectrin-α1 protein could be used as a biomarker to detect erythrocyte membrane deformation or damage and how this protein promotes the study of the biomechanical properties of signaling domains extending from the cell surface to deeper parts within the erythrocytes. These findings may bridge the gap between numerous interdependent behaviors of biological molecules and their mechanical properties to reveal the effects of deformation or damage or to assess the adverse effects on erythrocytes induced by radiation, thereby providing an inherent force-biochemical coupling analytical approach. The use of heavy ion radiation ($^{12}C^{6+}$ ions) has been proven to possess unique biological advantages in radiation therapy. Incidentally, we also suggest using heavy ion beam radiation pretreatment for the storage of erythrocytes, an application that has not yet been reported in the literature.

Author Contributions

Conceived and designed the experiments: BPZ JZW. Performed the experiments: BPZ BL. Analyzed the data: BPZ JZW. Contributed reagents/materials/analysis tools: BPZ BL. Contributed to the writing of the manuscript: BPZ. Obtained permission for use of Heavy ion radiation: HZ. Reviewed the manuscript: HZ.

References

1. Umegaki K, Sugisawa A, Shin SJ, Yamada K, Sano M (2001) Different onsets of oxidative damage to DNA and lipids in bone marrow and liver in rats given total body irradiation. Free Radic Biol Med 31: 1066–1074. PubMed: 11677039.

2. Matsunaga A, Ueda Y, Yamada S, Harada Y, Shimada H, et al. (2010) Carbon-ion beam treatment induces systemic antitumor immunity against murine squamous cell carcinoma. Cancer 116: 3740–3748. PubMed: 20564091.

3. Suzuki Y, Nakano T, Ohno T, Oka K (2008) Comparison of the radiobiological effect of carbon ion beam therapy and conventional radiation therapy on cervical cancer. J Radiat Res 49: 473–479. PubMed: 18622131.

4. Ghosh S, Narang H, Sarma A, Krishna M (2011) DNA damage response signaling in lung adenocarcinoma A549 cells following gamma and carbon beam irradiation. Mutat Res/Fundamental and Molecular Mechanisms of Mutagenesis 716: 10–19. PubMed: 21839752.

5. Afrin R, Nakaji M, Sekiguchi H, Lee D, Kishimoto K, et al. (2012) Forced extension of delipidated red blood cell cytoskeleton with little indication of spectrin unfolding. Cytoskeleton (Hoboken) 69: 101–112. PubMed: 22213694.

6. Nomura T, Hongyo T, Nakajima H, Li LY, Syaifudin M, et al. (2008) Differential radiation sensitivity to morphological, functional and molecular changes of human thyroid tissues and bone marrow cells maintained in SCID mice. Mutat Res/Genetic Toxicology and Environmental Mutagenesis 657: 68–76. PubMed: 18778792.

7. Coates PJ, Lorimore SA, Wright EG (2004) Damaging and protective cell signalling in the untargeted effects of ionizing radiation. Mutat Res/Fundamental and Molecular Mechanisms of Mutagenesis 568: 5–20. PubMed: 15530535.

8. Gavara N, Chadwick RS (2012) Determination of the elastic moduli of thin samples and adherent cells using conical atomic force microscope tips. Nat Nanotechnol. 7: 733–736. PubMed: 23023646.

9. Wang Y, Liu L, Pazhanisamy SK, Li H, Meng A, et al. (2010) Total body irradiation causes residual bone marrow injury by induction of persistent oxidative stress in murine hematopoietic stem cells. Free Radic Biol Med 48: 348–356. PubMed: 19925862.

10. Bao Y, Chen H, Hu Y, Bai Y, Zhou M, et al. (2012) Combination effects of chronic cadmium exposure and gamma-irradiation on the genotoxicity and cytotoxicity of peripheral blood lymphocytes and bone marrow cells in rats. Mutat Res/Genetic Toxicology and Environmental Mutagenesis 743: 67–74. PubMed: 22245108.

11. Mukherjee D, Coates PJ, Rastogi S, Lorimore SA, Wright EG (2013) Radiation-induced bone marrow apoptosis, inflammatory bystander-type signaling and tissue cytotoxicity. Int J Radiat Biol 89: 139–146. PubMed: 23078404.

12. Li Q, Sun H, Xiao F, Wang X, Yang Y, et al. (2014) Protection against radiation-induced hematopoietic damage in bone marrow by hepatocyte growth factor gene transfer. Int J Radiat Biol 90: 36–44. PubMed: 24059647.

13. Liesveld JL, Rubin P, Constine LS (2014) Hematopoietic System. ALERT• Adverse Late Effects of Cancer Treatment: Springer. pp. 623–655.

14. Wang C, Nakamura S, Oshima M, Mochizuki-Kashio M, Nakajima-Takagi Y, et al. (2013) Compromised hematopoiesis and increased DNA damage following non-lethal ionizing radiation of a human hematopoietic system reconstituted in immunodeficient mice. Int J Radiat Biol 89: 132–137. PubMed: 23020858.

15. Hu S, Cucinotta FA (2011) Characterization of the radiation-damaged precursor cells in bone marrow based on modeling of the peripheral blood granulocytes response. Health Phys 101: 67–78. PubMed: 21617393.

16. Li W, Wang G, Cui J, Xue L, Cai L (2004) Low-dose radiation (LDR) induces hematopoietic hormesis: LDR-induced mobilization of hematopoietic progenitor cells into peripheral blood circulation. Exp Hematol 32: 1088–1096. PubMed: 15539087.

17. Grande T, Bueren JA (2006) The mobilization of hematopoietic progenitors to peripheral blood is predictive of the hematopoietic syndrome after total or partial body irradiation of mice. Int J Radiat Oncol Biol Phys 64: 612–618. PubMed: 16414374.

18. Moroni M, Coolbaugh TV, Lombardini E, Mitchell JM, Moccia KD, et al. (2011) Hematopoietic radiation syndrome in the Gottingen minipig. Radiat Res 176: 89–101. PubMed: 21520996.

19. Peslak SA, Wenger J, Bemis JC, Kingsley PD, Frame JM, et al. (2011) Sublethal radiation injury uncovers a functional transition during erythroid maturation. Exp Hematol 39: 434–445. PubMed: 21291953.

20. Moroni M, Elliott TB, Deutz NE, Olsen CH, Owens R, et al. (2014) Accelerated Hematopoietic Syndrome after Radiation Doses Bridging Hematopoietic (H-ARS) and Gastrointestinal (GI-ARS) Acute Radiation Syndrome: Early Hematological Changes and Systemic Inflammatory Response Syndrome in Minipig. Int J Radiat Biol: 90: 363–372. PubMed: 24524283.

21. Manda K, Kavanagh JN, Buttler D, Prise KM, Hildebrandt G (2014) Low dose effects of ionizing radiation on normal tissue stem cells. Mutat Res Rev Mutat Res pii: S1383–5742(14)00017-9. PubMed: 24566131.

22. Kulkarni S, P Ghosh S, Hauer-Jensen M, Sree Kumar K (2010) Hematological targets of radiation damage. Curr Drug Targets 11: 1375–1385. PubMed: 20583980.

23. Lara PC, López-Peñalver JJ, Farias VdA, Ruiz-Ruiz MC, Oliver FJ, et al. (2013) Direct and bystander radiation effects: A biophysical model and clinical perspectives. Cancer Lett pii: S0304–3835(13)00659-9. PubMed: 24045041.

24. Garaj-Vrhovac V, Gajski G, Pažanin S, Šarolić A, Domijan A-M, et al. (2011) Assessment of cytogenetic damage and oxidative stress in personnel occupationally exposed to the pulsed microwave radiation of marine radar equipment. Int J Hyg Environ Health 214: 59–65. PubMed: 20833106.

25. Park HJ, Griffin RJ, Hui S, Levitt SH, Song CW (2012) Radiation-induced vascular damage in tumors: implications of vascular damage in ablative hypofractionated radiotherapy (SBRT and SRS). Radiat Res 177: 311–327. PubMed: 22229487.

26. Weng H, Guo X, Papoin J, Wang J, Coppel R, et al. (2014) Interaction of Plasmodium falciparum knob-associated histidine-rich protein (KAHRP) with

erythrocyte ankyrin R is required for its attachment to the erythrocyte membrane. Biochim Biophys Acta 1838: 185–192. PubMed: 24090929.

27. Park Y, Best CA, Badizadegan K, Dasari RR, Feld MS, et al. (2010) Measurement of red blood cell mechanics during morphological changes. Proc Natl Acad Sci U S A 107: 6731–6736. PubMed: 20351261.

28. Zou S, Chisholm R, Tauskela JS, Mealing GA, Johnston LJ, et al. (2013) Force Spectroscopy Measurements Show That Cortical Neurons Exposed to Excitotoxic Agonists Stiffen before Showing Evidence of Bleb Damage. PLoS One 8: e73499. PubMed: 24023686.

29. de Oliveira M, Vera C, Valdez P, Sharma Y, Skelton R, et al. (2010) Nanomechanics of multiple units in the erythrocyte membrane skeletal network. Ann Biomed Eng 38: 2956–2967. PubMed: 20490687.

30. Lim CT, Li A (2011) Mechanopathology of red blood cell diseases–Why mechanics matters. Theoretical and Applied Mechanics Letters 1: 014000-014000-014006.

31. Rojas-Aguirre Y, Hernández-Luis F, Mendoza-Martínez C, Sotomayor CP, Aguilar LF, et al. (2012) Effects of an antimalarial quinazoline derivative on human erythrocytes and on cell membrane molecular models. Biochim Biophys Acta 1818: 738–746. PubMed: 22155684.

32. Samanta S, Dutta D, Ghoshal A, Mukhopadhyay S, Saha B, et al. (2011) Glycosylation of Erythrocyte Spectrin and Its Modification in Visceral Leishmaniasis. PLoS One 6: e28169. PubMed: 22164239.

33. Shi H, Liu Z, Li A, Yin J, Chong AG, et al. (2013) Life Cycle-Dependent Cytoskeletal Modifications in Plasmodium falciparum Infected Erythrocytes. PLoS One 8: e61170. PubMed: 23585879.

34. An X, Mohandas N (2010) Red cell membrane and malaria. Transfus Clin Biol 17: 197–199. PubMed: 20674435.

35. Mohandas N, Evans E (1994) Mechanical properties of the red cell membrane in relation to molecular structure and genetic defects. Annu Rev Biophys Biomol Struct 23: 787–818. PubMed: 7919799.

36. Maciaszek JL, Lykotrafitis G (2011) Sickle cell trait human erythrocytes are significantly stiffer than normal. J Biomech 44: 657–661. PubMed: 21111421.

37. Delaunay J (2007) The molecular basis of hereditary red cell membrane disorders. Blood Rev 21: 1–20. PubMed: 16730867.

38. Debaugnies F, Cotton F, Boutique C, Gulbis B (2011) Erythrocyte membrane protein analysis by sodium dodecyl sulphate-capillary gel electrophoresis in the diagnosis of hereditary spherocytosis. Clin Chem Lab Med 49: 485–492. PubMed: 21231903.

39. Katira P, Zaman MH, Bonnecaze RT (2012) How changes in cell mechanical properties induce cancerous behavior. Phys Rev Lett 108: 028103. PubMed: 22324713.

40. Li J, Lykotrafitis G, Dao M, Suresh S (2007) Cytoskeletal dynamics of human erythrocyte. Proc Natl Acad Sci U S A 104: 4937–4942. PubMed: 17360346.

41. Lekka M, Fornal M, Pyka-Fościak G, Lebed K, Wizner B, et al. (2005) Erythrocyte stiffness probed using atomic force microscope. Biorheology 42: 307–317. PubMed: 16227658.

42. Bao G, Suresh S (2003) Cell and molecular mechanics of biological materials. Nat Mater 2: 715–725. PubMed: 14593396.

43. Suresh S, Spatz J, Mills J, Micoulet A, Dao M, et al. (2005) Connections between single-cell biomechanics and human disease states: gastrointestinal cancer and malaria. Acta Biomater 1: 15–30. PubMed: 16701777.

44. Stewart MP, Toyoda Y, Hyman AA, Müller DJ (2012) Tracking mechanics and volume of globular cells with atomic force microscopy using a constant-height clamp. Nat Protoc 7: 143–154. PubMed: 22222789.

45. Zuk A, Targosz-Korecka M, Szymonski M (2011) Effect of selected drugs used in asthma treatment on morphology and elastic properties of red blood cells. Int J Nanomedicine 6: 249–257. PubMed: 21499423.

46. Szarama KB, Gavara N, Petralia RS, Kelley MW, Chadwick RS (2012) Cytoskeletal changes in actin and microtubules underlie the developing surface mechanical properties of sensory and supporting cells in the mouse cochlea. Development 139: 2187–2197. PubMed: 22573615.

47. Li M, Liu L, Xi N, Wang Y, Dong Z, et al. (2012) Atomic force microscopy imaging and mechanical properties measurement of red blood cells and aggressive cancer cells. Sci China Life Sci 55: 968–973. PubMed: 23160828.

48. Heinrich V, Ritchie K, Mohandas N, Evans E (2001) Elastic thickness compressibilty of the red cell membrane. Biophys J 81: 1452–1463. PubMed: 11509359.

49. Park Y, Best CA, Auth T, Gov NS, Safran SA, et al. (2010) Metabolic remodeling of the human red blood cell membrane. Proc Natl Acad Sci U S A 107: 1289–1294. PubMed: 20080583.

50. Peng Z, Li X, Pivkin IV, Dao M, Karniadakis GE, et al. (2013) Lipid bilayer and cytoskeletal interactions in a red blood cell. Proc Natl Acad Sci U S A 110: 13356–13361. PubMed: 23898181.

51. Svetina S, Kuzman D, Waugh RE, Ziherl P, Žekš B (2004) The cooperative role of membrane skeleton and bilayer in the mechanical behaviour of red blood cells. Bioelectrochemistry 62: 107–113. PubMed: 15039011.

52. Machnicka B, Czogalla A, Hryniewicz-Jankowska A, Bogusławska DM, Grochowalska R, et al. (2013) Spectrins: A structural platform for stabilization and activation of membrane channels, receptors and transporters. Biochim Biophys Acta 1838: 620–634. PubMed: 23673272.

53. Marchesi VT, Steers E, Jr. (1968) Selective solubilization of a protein component from red cell membrane. Science 159: 203–204. PubMed: 5634911.

54. Švelc T, Svetina S (2012) Stress-free state of the red blood cell membrane and the deformation of its skeleton. Cell Mol Biol Lett 17: 217–227. PubMed: 22302416.

55. Foretz M, Hébrard S, Guihard S, Leclerc J, Do Cruzeiro M, et al. (2011) The AMPKγ1 subunit plays an essential role in erythrocyte membrane elasticity, and its genetic inactivation induces splenomegaly and anemia. FASEB J 25: 337–347. PubMed: 20881209.

56. Kim Y, Kim M, Shin JH, Kim J (2011) Characterization of cellular elastic modulus using structure based double layer model. Med Biol Eng Comput 49: 453–462. PubMed: 21221828.

57. Strey H, Peterson M, Sackmann E (1995) Measurement of erythrocyte membrane elasticity by flicker eigenmode decomposition. Biophys J 69: 478–488. PubMed: 8527662.

58. Cardamone L, Laio A, Torre V, Shahapure R, DeSimone A (2011) Cytoskeletal actin networks in motile cells are critically self-organized systems synchronized by mechanical interactions. Proc Natl Acad Sci U S A 108: 13978–13983. PubMed: 21825142.

59. Fedosov DA, Caswell B, Karniadakis GE (2010) Systematic coarse-graining of spectrin-level red blood cell models. Comput Methods Appl Mech Eng 199: 1937–1948. PubMed: 24353352.

60. Zhu Q, Vera C, Asaro RJ, Sche P, Sung LA (2007) A hybrid model for erythrocyte membrane: a single unit of protein network coupled with lipid bilayer. Biophys J 93: 386–400. PubMed: 17449663.

61. Kozlova EK, Chernysh AM, Moroz VV, Kuzovlev AN (2012) Analysis of nanostructure of red blood cells membranes by space Fourier transform of AFM images. Micron 44: 218–427. PubMed: 22854216.

62. Li X, Peng Z, Lei H, Dao M, Karniadakis GE (2014) Probing red blood cell mechanics, rheology and dynamics with a two-component multi-scale model. Philos Trans A Math Phys Eng Sci 372: 20130389. PubMed: 24982252.

63. Callan-Jones A, Albarran Arriagada OE, Massiera G, Lorman V, Abkarian M (2012) Red Blood Cell Membrane Dynamics during Malaria Parasite Egress. Biophys J 103: 2475–2483. PubMed: 23260049.

64. Boey SK, Boal DH, Discher DE (1998) Simulations of the Erythrocyte Cytoskeleton at Large Deformation. I. Microscopic Models. Biophys J 75: 1573–1583. PubMed: 9726958.

65. Discher DE, Boal DH, Boey SK (1998) Simulations of the Erythrocyte Cytoskeleton at Large Deformation. II. Micropipette Aspiration. Biophys J 75: 1584–1597. PubMed: 9726959.

66. De Nunzio C, Aronson W, Freedland SJ, Giovannucci E, Parsons JK (2012) The correlation between metabolic syndrome and prostatic diseases. Eur Urol 61: 560–570. PubMed: 22119157.

67. Ma X, Zhang H, Wang Z, Min X, Liu Y, et al. (2011) Chromosomal aberrations in the bone marrow cells of mice induced by accelerated (12) C (6+) ions. Mutat Res/Fundamental and Molecular Mechanisms of Mutagenesis 716: 20–26. PubMed: 21843535.

68. Sheetz MP, Casaly J (1980) 2, 3-Diphosphoglycerate and ATP dissociate erythrocyte membrane skeletons. J Biol Chem 255: 9955–9960. PubMed: 7430109.

69. Lin S, Snyder C (1977) High affinity cytochalasin B binding to red cell membrane proteins which are unrelated to sugar transport. J Biol Chem 252: 5464–5471. PubMed: 407226.

70. Kunda P, Pelling AE, Liu T, Baum B (2008) Moesin controls cortical rigidity, cell rounding, and spindle morphogenesis during mitosis. Curr Biol 18: 91–101. PubMed: 18207738.

71. Ludwig T, Kirmse R, Poole K, Schwarz US (2008) Probing cellular microenvironments and tissue remodeling by atomic force microscopy. Pflugers Arch 456: 29–49. PubMed: 18058123.

72. Takeuchi M, Miyamoto H, Sako Y, Komizu H, Kusumi A (1998) Structure of the erythrocyte membrane skeleton as observed by atomic force microscopy. Biophys J 74: 2171–2183. PubMed: 9591644.

73. Swihart A, Mikrut J, Ketterson J, Macdonald R (2001) Atomic force microscopy of the erythrocyte membrane skeleton. J Microsc 204: 212–225. PubMed: 11903798.

74. Alonso JL, Goldmann WH (2003) Feeling the forces: atomic force microscopy in cell biology. Life Sci 72: 2553–2560. PubMed: 12672501.

75. Sneddon IN (1965) The relation between load and penetration in the axisymmetric Boussinesq problem for a punch of arbitrary profile. Int J Engi Sci 3: 47–57. doi.org/10.1016/0020-7225(65)90019-4.

76. Rico F, Roca-Cusachs P, Gavara N, Farré R, Rotger M, et al. (2005) Probing mechanical properties of living cells by atomic force microscopy with blunted pyramidal cantilever tips. Phys Rev E Stat Nonlin Soft Matter Phys 72: 021914. PubMed: 16196611.

77. Johnson K, Kendall K, Roberts A (1971) Surface energy and the contact of elastic solids. Proc Roya Soci Lond 324: 301–313. doi.jstor.org/stable/78058.

78. Dimitriadis EK, Horkay F, Maresca J, Kachar B, Chadwick RS (2002) Determination of elastic moduli of thin layers of soft material using the atomic force microscope. Biophys J 82: 2798–2810. PubMed: 11964265.

79. Carl P, Schillers H (2008) Elasticity measurement of living cells with an atomic force microscope: data acquisition and processing. Pflugers Arch 457: 551–559. PubMed: 18481081.

80. Li Q, Lee G, Ong C, Lim C (2008) AFM indentation study of breast cancer cells. Biochem Biophys Res Commun 374: 609–613. PubMed: 18656442.

81. Ketene AN (2011) The AFM Study of Ovarian Cell Structural Mechanics in the Progression of Cancer: Virginia Polytechnic Institute and State University. doi.scholar.lib.vt.edu/theses/available/etd-05182011-152552.

82. Ketene AN, Schmelz EM, Roberts PC, Agah M (2012) The effects of cancer progression on the viscoelasticity of ovarian cell cytoskeleton structures. Nanomedicine 8: 93–102. PubMed: 21704191.

83. Lu Y-B, Franze K, Seifert G, Steinhäuser C, Kirchhoff F, et al. (2006) Viscoelastic properties of individual glial cells and neurons in the CNS. Proc Natl Acad Sci U S A 103: 17759–17764. PubMed: 17093050.

84. Strobl JS, Nikkhah M, Agah M (2010) Actions of the anti-cancer drug suberoylanilide hydroxamic acid (SAHA) on human breast cancer cytoarchitecture in silicon microstructures. Biomaterials 31: 7043–7050. PubMed: 20579727.

85. Darling EM, Topel M, Zauscher S, Vail TP, Guilak F (2008) Viscoelastic properties of human mesenchymally-derived stem cells and primary osteoblasts, chondrocytes, and adipocytes. J Biomech 41: 454–464. PubMed: 17825308.

86. Guo S, Akhremitchev BB (2006) Packing density and structural heterogeneity of insulin amyloid fibrils measured by AFM nanoindentation. Biomacromolecules 7: 1630–1636. PubMed: 16677048.

87. Nikkhah M, Strobl JS, De Vita R, Agah M (2010) The cytoskeletal organization of breast carcinoma and fibroblast cells inside three dimensional (3-D) isotropic silicon microstructures. Biomaterials 31: 4552–4561. PubMed: 20207413.

88. Ghorai A, Bhattacharyya NP, Sarma A, Ghosh U (2014) Radiosensitivity and Induction of Apoptosis by High LET Carbon Ion Beam and Low LET Gamma Radiation: A Comparative Study. Scientifica (Cairo) 2014: 438030. PubMed: 25018892.

89. Xu H, Gao L, Che T, Du W, Li Q, et al. (2012) The effects of $^{12}C^{6+}$ irradiation on cell cycle, apoptosis, and expression of caspase-3 in the human lung cancer cell line h1299. Cancer Biother Radiopharm 27: 113–118. PubMed: 22242595.

90. Haghparast SMA, Kihara T, Shimizu Y, Yuba S, Miyake J (2013) Actin-based biomechanical features of suspended normal and cancer cells. J Biosci Bioeng 116: 380–385. PubMed: 23567154.

91. Schmidt CF, Svoboda K, Lei N, Petsche IB, Berman LE, et al. (1993) Existence of a flat phase in red cell membrane skeletons. Science 259: 952–955. PubMed: 8438153.

92. Machnicka B, Grochowalska R, Bogusławska D, Sikorski A, Lecomte M (2012) Spectrin-based skeleton as an actor in cell signaling. Cell Mol Life Sci 69: 191–201. PubMed: 21877118.

93. Franke R, Scharnweber T, Fuhrmann R, Mrowietz C, Jung F (2013) Effect of radiographic contrast media (Iodixanol, Iopromide) on the spectrin/actin-network of the membranous cytoskeleton of erythrocytes. Clin Hemorheol Microcirc 54: 273–285. PubMed: 23666115.

94. Sonmez M, Ince HY, Yalcin O, Ajdžanović V, Spasojević I, et al. (2013) The effect of alcohols on red blood cell mechanical properties and membrane fluidity depends on their molecular size. PloS One 8: e76579. PubMed: 24086751.

95. Kuriakose S, Dimitrakopoulos P (2013) Deformation of an elastic capsule in a rectangular microfluidic channel. Soft Matter. 9: 4284–4296. PubMed: 23585769.

96. Hansen J, Skalak R, Chien S, Hoger A (1996) An elastic network model based on the structure of the red blood cell membrane skeleton. Biophys J 70: 146–166. PubMed: 8770194.

97. Kabaso D, Shlomovitz R, Auth T, Lew VL, Gov NS (2010) Curling and local shape changes of red blood cell membranes driven by cytoskeletal reorganization. Biophys J 99: 808–816. PubMed: 20682258.

98. Afrin R, Nakaji M, Sekiguchi H, Lee D, Kishimoto K, et al. (2012) Forced extension of delipidated red blood cell cytoskeleton with little indication of spectrin unfolding. Cytoskeleton 69: 101–112. PubMed: 22213694.

99. Liu F, Burgess J, Mizukami H, Ostafin A (2003) Sample preparation and imaging of erythrocyte cytoskeleton with the atomic force microscopy. Cell Biochem Biophys 38: 251–270. PubMed: 12794267.

100. Salomao M, An X, Guo X, Gratzer WB, Mohandas N, et al. (2006) Mammalian αI-spectrin is a neofunctionalized polypeptide adapted to small highly deformable erythrocytes. Proc Natl Acad Sci U S A 103: 643–648. PubMed: 16407147.

101. Chan MM, Wooden JM, Tsang M, Gilligan DM, Hirenallur-S DK, et al. (2013) Hematopoietic Protein-1 Regulates the Actin Membrane Skeleton and Membrane Stability in Murine Erythrocytes. PLoS One 8: e54902. PubMed: 23424621.

102. Nambiar R, McConnell RE, Tyska MJ (2009) Control of cell membrane tension by myosin-I. Proc Natl Acad Sci U S A 106: 11972–11977. PubMed: 19574460.

103. Muravyov AV, Tikhomirova IA (2013) Role molecular signaling pathways in changes of red blood cell deformability. Clin Hemorheol Microcirc 53: 45–59. PubMed: 22951624.

104. Corre I, Niaudet C, Paris F (2010) Plasma membrane signaling induced by ionizing radiation. Mutat Res 704: 61–67. PubMed: 20117234.

105. Daniels G (2007) Functions of red cell surface proteins. Vox Sang 93: 331–340. PubMed: 18070278.

106. Buys AV, Van Rooy M-J, Soma P, Van Papendorp D, Lipinski B, et al. (2013) Changes in red blood cell membrane structure in type 2 diabetes: a scanning electron and atomic force microscopy study. Cardiovasc Diabetol 12: 25. PubMed: 23356738.

107. Dubreuil RR (2006) Functional links between membrane transport and the spectrin cytoskeleton. J Membr Biol 211: 151–161. PubMed: 17091212.

108. Johnson CP, Tang H-Y, Carag C, Speicher DW, Discher DE (2007) Forced unfolding of proteins within cells. Science 317: 663–666. PubMed: 17673662.

109. Discher DE, Carl P (2001) New insights into red cell network structure, elasticity, and spectrin unfolding-a current review. Cell Mol Biol Lett 6: 593–606. PubMed: 11598637.

110. Broderick M, Winder S (2005) Spectrin, alpha-actinin, and dystrophin. Adv Protein Chem 70: 203–246. PubMed: 15837517.

111. Kusunoki H, MacDonald RI, Mondragón A (2004) Structural insights into the stability and flexibility of unusual erythroid spectrin repeats. Structure 12: 645–656. PubMed: 15062087.

112. Pan CQ, Sudol M, Sheetz M, Low BC (2012) Modularity and functional plasticity of scaffold proteins as p(l)acemakers in cell signaling. Cell Signal 24: 2143–2165. PubMed: 22743133.

113. Zhu Q, Asaro RJ (2008) Spectrin folding versus unfolding reactions and RBC membrane stiffness. Biophys J 94: 2529–2545. PubMed: 18065469.

114. Picas L, Rico Fl, Deforet M, Scheuring S (2013) Structural and Mechanical Heterogeneity of the Erythrocyte Membrane Reveals Hallmarks of Membrane Stability. ACS Nano 7: 1054–1063. PubMed: 23347043.

115. Nans A, Mohandas N, Stokes DL (2011) Native ultrastructure of the red cell cytoskeleton by cryo-electron tomography. Biophys J 101: 2341–2350. PubMed: 22098732.

116. Blanc L, Salomao M, Guo X, An X, Gratzer W, et al. (2010) Control of erythrocyte membrane-skeletal cohesion by the spectrin-membrane linkage. Biochemistry 49: 4516–4523. PubMed: 20433199.

117. Koshino I, Mohandas N, Takakuwa Y (2012) Identification of a novel role for dematin in regulating red cell membrane function by modulating spectrin-actin interaction. J Biol Chem 287: 35244–35250. PubMed: 22927433.

118. Baines A (2010) Evolution of the spectrin-based membrane skeleton. Transfus Clin Biol 17: 95–103. PubMed: 20688550.

119. Zhang R, Brown FL (2008) Cytoskeleton mediated effective elastic properties of model red blood cell membranes. J Chem Phys 129: 065101. PubMed: 18715105.

13

Poikilocytosis in Rabbits: Prevalence, Type, and Association with Disease

Mary M. Christopher[1]*, **Michelle G. Hawkins**[2], **Andrew G. Burton**[3]

1 Department of Pathology, Immunology and Microbiology, University of California Davis, Davis, CA, 95616, United States of America, 2 Department of Medicine and Epidemiology, University of California Davis, Davis, CA, 95616, United States of America, 3 William R. Pritchard Veterinary Medical Teaching Hospital, University of California Davis, Davis, CA, 95616, United States of America

Abstract

Rabbits (*Oryctolagus cuniculus*) are a popular companion animal, food animal, and animal model of human disease. Abnormal red cell shapes (poikilocytes) have been observed in rabbits, but their significance is unknown. The objective of this study was to investigate the prevalence and type of poikilocytosis in pet rabbits and its association with physiologic factors, clinical disease, and laboratory abnormalities. We retrospectively analyzed blood smears from 482 rabbits presented to the University of California-Davis Veterinary Medical Teaching Hospital from 1990 to 2010. Number and type of poikilocytes per 2000 red blood cells (RBCs) were counted and expressed as a percentage. Acanthocytes ($>$3% of RBCs) were found in 150/482 (31%) rabbits and echinocytes ($>$3% of RBCs) were found in 127/482 (27%) of rabbits, both healthy and diseased. Thirty-three of 482 (7%) rabbits had $>$30% acanthocytes and echinocytes combined. Mild to moderate ($>$0.5% of RBCs) fragmented red cells (schistocytes, microcytes, keratocytes, spherocytes) were found in 25/403 (6%) diseased and 0/79 (0%) healthy rabbits ($P = 0.0240$). Fragmentation and acanthocytosis were more severe in rabbits with inflammatory disease and malignant neoplasia compared with healthy rabbits ($P < 0.01$). The % fragmented cells correlated with % polychromasia, RDW, and heterophil, monocyte, globulins, and fibrinogen concentrations ($P < 0.05$). Echinocytosis was significantly associated with renal failure, azotemia, and acid-base/electrolyte abnormalities ($P < 0.05$). Serum cholesterol concentration correlated significantly with % acanthocytes ($P < 0.0001$), % echinocytes ($P = 0.0069$), and % fragmented cells ($P = 0.0109$), but correlations were weak (Spearman $\rho < 0.02$). These findings provide important insights into underlying pathophysiologic mechanisms that appear to affect the prevalence and type of naturally-occurring poikilocytosis in rabbits. Our findings support the need to carefully document poikilocytes in research investigations and in clinical diagnosis and to determine their diagnostic and prognostic value.

Editor: Jan S. Suchodolski, GI Lab, United States of America

Funding: The authors have no support or funding to report.

Competing Interests: The authors have declared that no competing interests exist.

* Email: mmchristopher@ucdavis.edu

Introduction

Poikilocytosis is the presence of abnormally shaped erythrocytes in peripheral blood. Identification of poikilocytes is an important part of blood smear evaluation because shape changes often are associated with specific diseases, providing clues to underlying pathogenesis and facilitating diagnosis and treatment. Poikilocytes can result from biochemical changes, toxins, or physical damage to erythrocytes; regardless of cause, they can shorten erythrocyte survival and contribute to anemia [1,2]. In healthy pigs and young goats and calves, poikilocytes (acanthocytes, echinocytes, dacryocytes) are found normally in peripheral blood, without apparent pathologic consequence [1].

Rabbits are popular companion animals, are raised for meat, and are used extensively as animal models of human disease, including atherosclerosis, disorders of lipid metabolism, diabetes, and cardiovascular disease [3–5]. Acanthocytes have been observed in blood smears from healthy laboratory rabbits [6]. Described in 1967 as "thorn apple"-shaped red blood cells (RBCs), numerous acanthocytes (or acantho-echinocytes) were observed together with small microcytes about one-fourth the size

of a normal red cell [7]. Sanderson and Phillips [8] later described echinocytes, acanthocytes, and schistocytes in cardiac and arterial blood smears from healthy New Zealand White rabbits; they concluded that the poikilocytes were probably artifact and "indicative of a poorly prepared smear". However, while echinocytes can be the result of artifact (crenation), acanthocytes and schistocytes are pathologic cells that involve splenic remodeling and occur with in vivo fragmentation or membrane lipid abnormalities [1,9,10]. Acanthocytes, echinocytes, and occasionally schistocytes have been associated with liver disease and hypercholesterolemia in humans [2,10,11], dogs [12], and cats [13] and with disseminated intravascular coagulation and some types of neoplasia in dogs [12,14,15]. Red cell shape abnormalities (mainly acanthocytes) also are well described in laboratory rabbits [16,17] and dogs [18] fed atherogenic diets. In our hematology laboratory we have occasionally observed poikilocytes in companion rabbits presented to the University of California-Davis Veterinary Medical Teaching Hospital (VMTH). To the authors' knowledge, no studies have been done to quantify poikilocytes in healthy rabbits or to investigate possible links between poikilocytes and clinical or biochemical variables. A better understanding of red cell morphology in rabbits would be beneficial to researchers and clinicians alike.

The objectives of this study were to retrospectively characterize the prevalence, type, and severity of poikilocytes in a large cohort of rabbits and to investigate associations between poikilocytes and physiologic factors (age, sex, and breed), clinical disease, and CBC and biochemical findings. We hypothesized that poikilocytes in rabbits would be associated with specific diseases or laboratory abnormalities.

Materials and Methods

Study design and data collection

Electronic medical records from the University of California-Davis VMTH were searched retrospectively for rabbit visits between 1990 and 2010 at which a complete blood count (CBC) was done. Cases were excluded if a blood smear was not available or if a clinical diagnosis was not provided. Repeat visits by the same rabbit were excluded. Patient number, date, signalment (age, sex, breed), clinical and pathologic diagnoses, and CBC and biochemistry results were recorded. Age was reported in years and categorized as adult ($\geq$1 year old) or juvenile (<1 year). Clinical diagnoses were those reported in the visit summary by the clinician, and were based on the results of physical examination, laboratory tests, imaging, and occasionally, histopathology. Pathology results (biopsy and necropsy) were recorded if they were obtained within 6 months of the CBC and/or were relevant to the primary clinical disease. Healthy rabbits were those presented for routine physical examination or elective spay or neuter.

Hematology and biochemistry data

From January, 1990 to September, 2001 hematology results were obtained using a Baker Systems 9110 Plus hematology analyzer (BioChem ImmunoSystems Inc., Allentown, PA, USA). From September, 2001 to December, 2010 hematology results were obtained using an ADVIA 120 hematology system (Siemens Healthcare Diagnostics Inc., Tarrytown, NY, USA) with the rabbit setting in MultiSpecies System Software. Differential counts were obtained manually by counting 200 leukocytes in Wright-Giemsa-stained blood smears. Total plasma protein concentration was determined by refractometry and fibrinogen concentration was determined using the heat precipitation method. Hemolysis (pink plasma color) was qualitatively evaluated as mild, moderate, or marked. Biochemical results were obtained on a Roche Hitachi 917 analyzer (Roche Diagnostics Corporation, Indianapolis, IN, USA) from 2006 to 2010, Hitachi 717^c from 1997 to 2005, and Coulter Dacos analyzer (Coulter Electronics Inc, Hialeah, FL, USA) from 1990 to 1996. When instruments were upgraded, results were calibrated to retain consistency in results between analyzers.

Quantitation of poikilocytes

Original blood samples had been collected and processed according to our laboratory's standard operating procedure. Whole blood was placed into tubes containing EDTA and smears were prepared, air-dried, and stained by certified medical technologists within ~1 hour of collection. Poikilocytes were reported semiquantitatively (eg, few, moderate, many) by the technologists. Smears were coverslipped prior to storage in the laboratory slide archive.

On each original stained smear, 2000 RBCs were counted and characterized at 1000X magnification by a senior clinical

pathology resident (AGB) blinded to information about the rabbit. Poikilocytes were defined based on standard morphology and counting was limited to representative monolayer fields in which about half the erythrocytes were touching but did not overlap [1,19,20]. In severely anemic patients, counting was limited to areas where erythrocytes were separated by no more than one cell diameter. The number and type of poikilocytes were recorded and expressed as a percentage of RBCs. Poikilocytosis was subsequently classified as none (0%), rare (0.05–0.5%), mild (>0.5–3%), moderate (>3–10%), or marked (>10%). The number and percentage of polychromatophils were also recorded.

A board-certified clinical pathologist (MMC) independently determined % poikilocytes in a subset of the smears, also in a blinded manner; results from the two observers were averaged for analysis. The subset included a random sample consisting of every 10th slide (according to laboratory accession number) and all samples where the qualitative poikilocyte results in the original hematology report were widely discrepant from the quantitative results.

Statistical methods

Data were compiled in an Excel (Microsoft Corp, Redmond, WA, USA) spreadsheet and examined for aberrant entries. Statistical analyses were done using JMP 10.0.0 (SAS Institute Inc, Cary, NC, USA). Poikilocyte percentages were tested for normality by examination of histograms and Shapiro-Wilk tests. Differences in % poikilocytes between groups were evaluated using Wilcoxon/Kruskal-Wallis rank sums tests. Rabbits with none, rare, and mild (few) poikilocytes were combined and compared with those having moderate to marked poikilocytosis. Differences in age and hematologic and biochemical data were analyzed using Student's t test or ANOVA. Chi square analysis was used to compare nominal data. A multivariate model using Spearman's rank test was used to evaluate correlations among % poikilocytes and CBC and biochemistry variables. Principal component analysis was done using % poikilocytes and selected CBC and biochemistry variables. A P-value of.05 was used to indicate statistical significance.

Results

Nine-hundred-seventy-five rabbit visits with at least partial CBC results were identified during the 20-year period. Of these, 406 samples were excluded as repeat CBCs; 48 were excluded because smears were missing; 25 were excluded because they were native brush rabbits (*Sylvalagus bachmani*); and 14 were excluded because a clinical diagnosis was not reported. In total, 482 rabbits were included in the study.

Rabbits ranged from 3 months to 12 years of age (median 4 years), with 428 adults and 54 juveniles. Rabbits included 205 females (113 intact, 92 spayed) and 277 males (137 intact, 140 castrated). Rabbit breeds included Netherland Dwarf (n = 64), Lop (60), Mini-Lop (30), Mini-Rex (28), Holland Lop (20), New Zealand White (16), Dutch (13), Rex (10), Angora (8), French Lop (8), Flemish Giant (6), English Spot (5), English Lop (4), Dwarf (4), Dwarf Hotot (3), Lionhead (2), Chinchilla Rabbit (2), 1 each Dwarf Lionhead, Finnish Giant, Florida White, Havana, Hottot, Jersey Wooly, Lop-eared Angora, Norwegian Dwarf, and crossbred (21); breed was not specified for 170 rabbits.

Of the 482 rabbits, 79 were healthy and 403 were diseased. The mean ($\pm$ SD) age of healthy rabbits (1.6$\pm$1.9 years) was significantly lower than that of diseased rabbits (4.6$\pm$2.8 years) (P<0.0001, Student's t test). No difference was found in the proportion of females and males or in breed distribution between healthy and diseased rabbits.

Prevalence and type of poikilocytes

A total of 155/482 (32%) smears were quantified by two observers, with good agreement in % poikilocytes (average difference 0.05% ± 5% over a range of 0 to 70%). In the remaining smears, quantitative findings were similar to poikilocytes noted (or not) in the original laboratory report.

A majority of rabbits 251/482 (52%) had none, rare, or mild (<3%) poikilocytosis; 90/482 (19%) rabbits had moderate and 141 (29%) had marked poikilocytosis. Acanthocytes and echinocytes were the most frequently observed poikilocytes, with no significant difference between healthy and diseased rabbits (Figures 1–3). One-hundred-fifty of 482 (31%) rabbits had moderate to marked acanthocytosis and 127/482 (27%) had moderate to marked echinocytosis. Of these, 10 (2%) rabbits (including 1 healthy rabbit) had >30% acanthocytes and 11 (2%) rabbits (including 2 healthy rabbits) had >30% echinocytes. Acanthocytes and echinocytes often were observed together (Spearman $\rho = 0.3896$, P<0.0001) and overlapped in morphology; 33/482 (7%) rabbits had >30% acanthocytes and echinocytes combined. Acanthocyte morphology ranged from cells with one to two elongated blebs to multiple, smooth to sharply spiculated and irregularly-placed projections. Echinocytes had fine- to blunt-tipped, evenly spaced, short projections; those with blunt-tipped projections sometimes occurred together with irregularly-spiculated acanthocytes. No significant difference in the percentage of acanthocytes and echinocytes was observed between healthy and ill rabbits.

Schistocytes, microcytes, keratocytes, and spherocytes (subsequently combined as "fragmented" red cells) were observed in low numbers, with 457/482 (95%) rabbits having none to rare fragmented cells and 25/482 (5%) having mild to moderate fragmentation (Figures 1–3). Only diseased rabbits had mild to moderate fragmentation (P = 0.0024, Chi square), and a higher percentage of fragmented cells was found in diseased compared with healthy rabbits (P = 0.0240, Wilcoxon) (Figure 2). Fragmented red cells usually were found together with acanthocytes, with or without echinocytes. Percent fragmented cells correlated significantly with % acanthocytes (Spearman's $\rho = 0.4400$, P<0.0001) and to a lesser extent with % echinocytes (Spearman's $\rho = 0.2861$, P<0.0001. Microcytes often were very small, less than one-fourth the diameter of a normal red cell. Ovalocytes, dacryocytes, blister cells, and knizocytes were observed in low numbers in a few rabbits, as were occasional stomatocytes, target cells and ghost cells; because of their low frequency, these poikilocytes were not analyzed further.

No significant difference in % poikilocytes was observed between samples with none (n = 374), slight (n = 101), or moderate (n = 7) sample hemolysis. Further, neither moderate to marked acanthocytosis or echinocytosis nor mild to moderate fragmentation were associated with the presence of sample hemolysis. None of the 7 samples with moderate hemolysis had increased fragmentation and only 3/98 samples with mild to moderate fragmentation had slight hemolysis.

Poikilocytes and physiologic factors

Associations between poikilocytes and physiologic factors were evaluated in clinically healthy rabbits (n = 79). Healthy rabbits included 47 adults and 32 juveniles ranging from 3 months to 8 years of age. No significant difference in % poikilocytes or in the proportion of samples with moderate to marked poikilocytosis was found between adult and juvenile rabbits; no correlation was found between age and % poikilocytes.

Healthy rabbits included 32 females (28 intact, 4 spayed) and 47 males (35 intact, 12 castrated). Female rabbits had a slightly higher

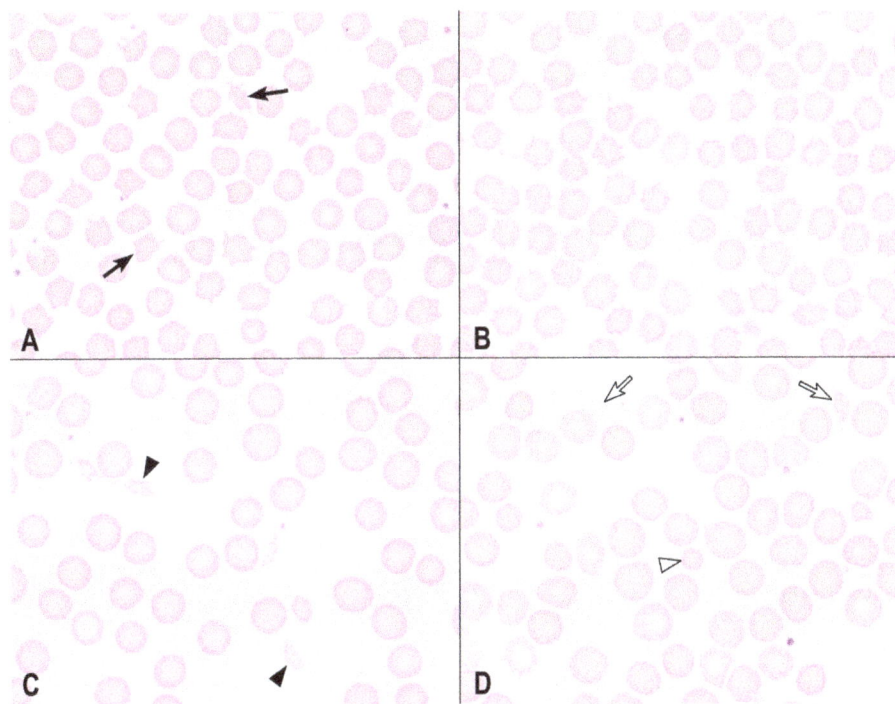

Figure 1. Poikilocytes in blood smears from rabbits. (A) Acanthocytes (arrows) in a healthy rabbit; (B) echinocytes in a rabbit with renal failure; (C) schistocytes (closed arrowheads) in a rabbit with a dental abscess; and (D) spherocytes (open arrowhead) and schistocytes (open arrows) in a rabbit with a mandibular abscess. Wright-Giemsa stain. Scale bar = 10 μm.

HEALTHY RABBITS (n = 79)

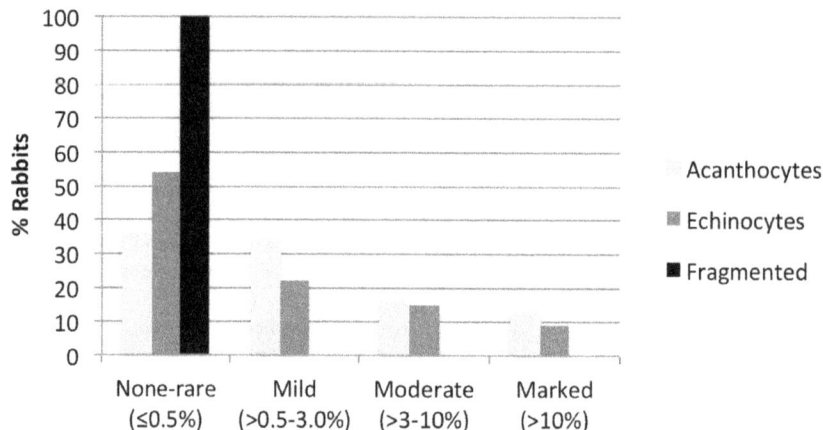

DISEASED RABBITS (n = 403)

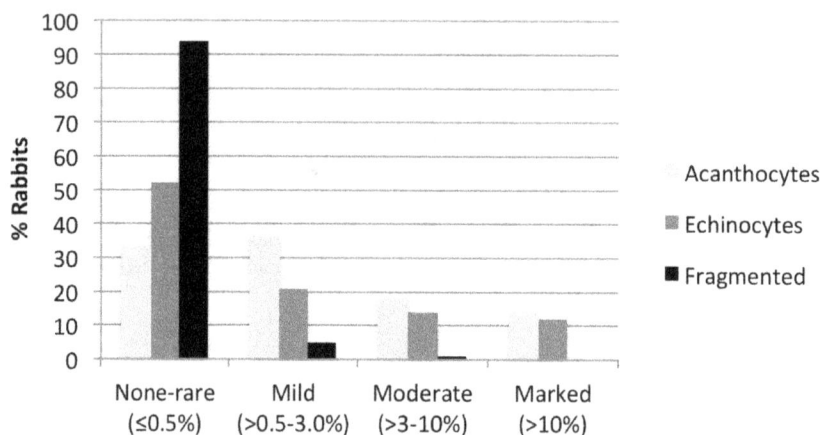

Figure 2. Prevalence of poikilocytes in 492 rabbits. Fragmented cells include schistocytes, keratocytes, microcytes, and spherocytes.

% echinocytes (median 0.8%, range 0–31.0%) than male rabbits (median 0.1%, range 0–28.8%) (P = 0.0309, Wilcoxon). A higher proportion of females than males had moderate to marked acanthocytosis (41/32, 44% vs 9/47, 15%) and echinocytosis (12/32, 84% vs 7/47, 15%) (P<0.05, Chi square).

Healthy rabbits included Netherland Dwarf (14), Mini-Rex (5), Dutch (4), Holland Lop (4), and Lop (4), New Zealand White (2), Mini-Lop (2), Lionhead (2), English Spot (2), 1 each of Angora, Dwarf, Dwarf Lionhead, English Lop, Flemish Giant, Hottot, and Rex; and cross-breed (5), breed was not reported for 28 rabbits. No significant breed difference was found in % poikilocytes or in the proportion of samples with moderate to marked poikilocytes, however samples sizes were small.

Poikilocytes and disease

Diseased rabbits were classified into 12 organ groups based on primary diagnosis (Table 1). Pathology results were available for 101/403 (25%) diseased rabbits, including 70 necropsy (with histopathology), 27 biopsy, and 4 cytology results. Rabbits also were grouped based on the specific disease process; groups with 10

or more rabbits were analyzed statistically for associations with poikilocytosis (Table 2).

No difference in the % or severity of acanthocytes and echinocytes was found on the basis of organ system, but a significantly lower % fragmented cells was found in healthy rabbits and in rabbits with ophthalmic disease compared with other organ systems (P<.05, Wilcoxon). Moderate to marked acanthocytosis and mild to moderate fragmentation were observed significantly more often in rabbits with septic and inflammatory disorders compared with healthy rabbits (Table 2). A significantly higher % of echinocytes (P = 0.0086) and moderate to marked echinocytosis (Table 2) were observed in rabbits with renal failure compared with healthy rabbits.

Poikilocytes and laboratory abnormalities

Significant differences were observed in laboratory values in rabbits with moderate to marked acanthocytosis or echinocytosis and with mild to moderate fragmentation (Table 3). Because few reticulocyte counts (n = 18) and band heterophils (n = 35) were reported, these analytes were not analyzed statistically.

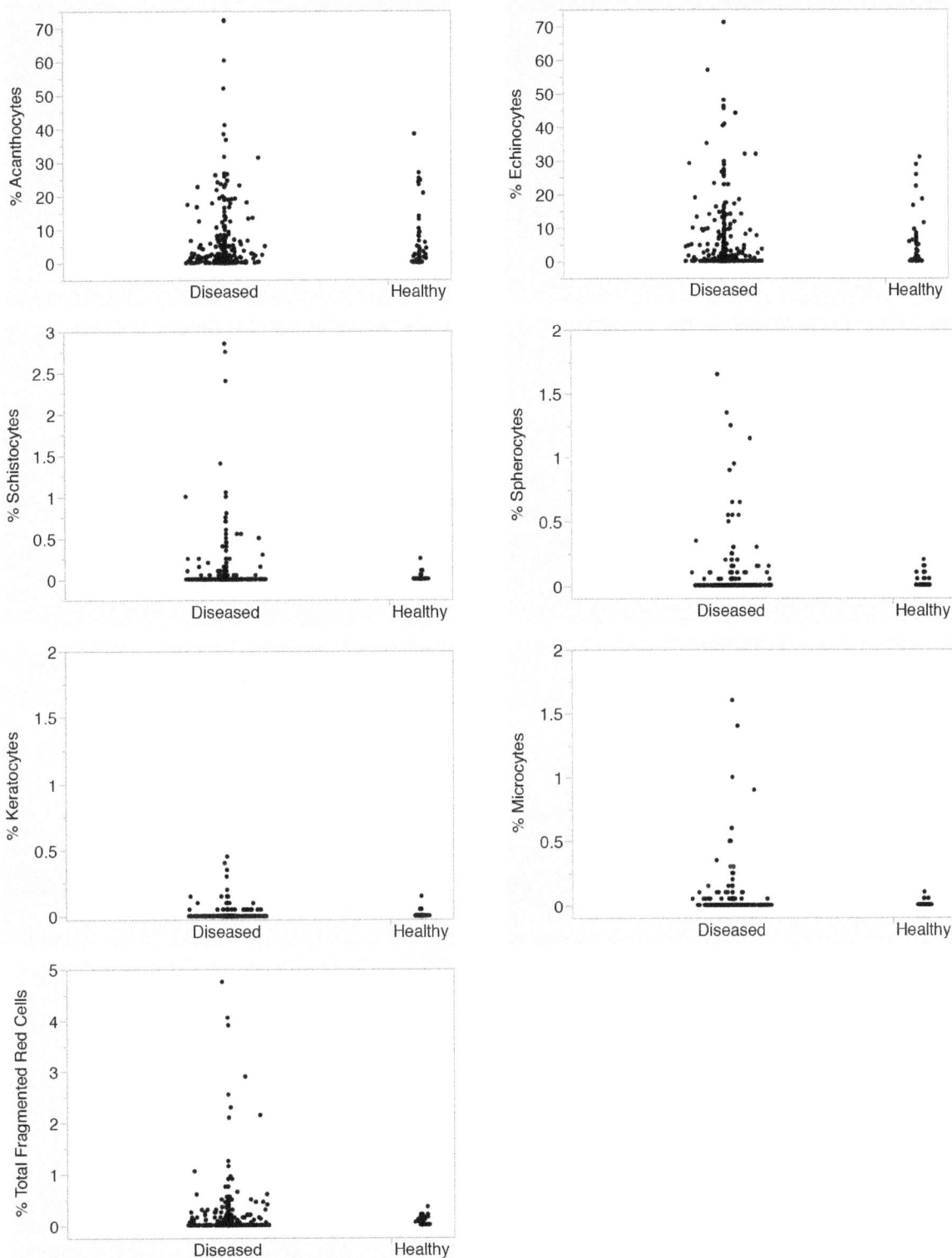

Figure 3. Dot plots of % poikilocytes in samples from healthy (n = 79) and diseased (n = 403) rabbits. Significant differences between healthy and diseased rabbits were observed for % schistocytes, % keratocytes, % microcytes, and % total fragmented cells (P<.05, Wilcoxon).

Based on Spearman rank correlation for all rabbits combined, % acanthocytes correlated positively with % polychromasia, red cell distribution width (RDW), and mean platelet volume (MPV) (P<0.02); % echinocytes correlated positively with RBC count, hematocrit (HCT), hemoglobin concentration (HGB), mean cell hemoglobin concentration (MCHC), MPV, anion gap, and sodium, potassium, chloride, and creatinine concentrations, and negatively with bicarbonate and glucose concentrations (P<0.01);

Table 1. Primary diagnosis by organ system for the 482 rabbits in the study (1990 to 2010).

Organ System	Disease	Clinical Diagnosis	Pathology Diagnosis	Total
Bone and joint	Fracture	14	0	14
	Degenerative joint disease	5	2	7
	Luxation	2	0	2
	Neoplasia (sarcoma, squamous cell carcinoma)	0	2	2
	Other (lameness, multifocal bony lesions)	2	0	2
Cardiovascular	Myxomatous valve degeneration	2	1	3
	Cardiomyopathy	1	1	2
	Arrythmia	1	0	1
Dental	Malocclusion/periodontitis	37	1	38
	Mandibular abscessation/osteomyelitis	29	9	38
Gastrointestinal	GI stasis	25	0	25
	Enteritis/gastritis/typhylitis/colitis	2	9	11
	Diarrhea	5	0	5
	Trichobezoar	0	3	3
	Abscess	1	1	2
	Neoplasia (papilloma, adenocarcinoma)	0	2	2
	Other (dysbiosis, cecal impaction)	4	0	4
Hemolymphatic	Mediastinal thymoma	2	2	4
	Lymphoma	0	3	3
	Regenerative anemia	1	0	1
Hepatic	Enzymopathy	4	0	4
	Hepatitis/cholangiohepatitis	0	3	3
	Torsion with necrosis	0	2	2
	Neoplasia (cystadenocarcinoma)	0	1	1
Neurologic	Encephalitozoonosis	0	6	6
	Ataxia/paresis/paralysis	6	0	6
	Myelopathy	5	0	5
	Vestibular disease	3	0	3
	CNS disease	3	0	3
	Neoplasia (pineocytoma)	0	1	1
	Bacterial meningoencephalitis	0	1	1
	Brain hemorrhage	0	1	1
	Other (lumbosacral disease, seizures, head trauma)	3	0	3
Ophthalmic	Keratitis/uveitis/ulcer	8	0	8
	Glaucoma/cataracts	5	0	5
	Chemosis/conjunctivitis	5	0	5
	Dacryocystitis	5	0	5
	Iris granuloma	3	0	3
	Other (corneal fibrosis, laceration, dystrichia, epicorneal membrane)	4	0	4
Reproductive	Uterine disease (endometritis, cysts, hydrometra, mass, varices)	4	1	5
	Neoplasia (testicular granular cell tumor)	0	1	1
Respiratory	Upper respiratory tract disease	20	3	23
	Bronchopneumonia	3	5	8
	Lung abscessation+pneumonia	0	4	4
	Neoplasia (carcinoma, granular cell tumor)	0	2	2
	Other (nasal mass, lung consolidation, stridor)	3	0	3
Skin/subcutis	Otitis	13	1	14
	Cellulitis (bite wounds, myiasis)	7	3	10
	Dermatitis, nonparasitic	9	5	14
	Dermatitis, parasitic	10	0	10

Table 1. Cont.

Organ System	Disease	Clinical Diagnosis	Pathology Diagnosis	Total
	Pododermatitis	6	0	6
	Abscess, soft tissue	3	3	6
	Laceration	6	0	6
	Neoplasia, malignant (sarcoma, squamous cell carcinoma)	0	7	7
	Neoplasia, benign (lipoma, polyp)	1	2	3
	Other (myositis/fibrosis, cutaneous mass)	3	0	3
Urinary	Renal failure	7	7	14
	Urolithiasis	8	0	8
	Urine sludge	7	0	7
	Cystitis	4	0	4
Other	Anorexia, weight loss	5	0	5
	Abdominal mass	1	0	1
	Hypercalcemia	1	0	1

% fragmented cells correlated positively with % polychromasia, MCHC, RDW, and heterophil, monocyte, and potassium concentrations, and negatively with bicarbonate and albumin concentrations (<0.02). Cholesterol correlated significantly with % acanthocytes ($P<0.0001$), % echinocytes ($P = 0.0069$), and % fragmented cells ($P = 0.0109$), but was not highly predictive (Spearman $\rho <0.2$).

We used principal component analysis to further visualize correlation patterns (Figure 4). In component 1, fragmented cells, and to a lesser extent acanthocytes, correlated positively with polychromasia, heterophils, monocytes, fibrinogen, globulins, and cholesterol; and negatively with albumin and HCT. In component 2, echinocytes correlated positively with azotemia, sodium, potassium, and anion gap; and negatively with bicarbonate.

Discussion

To our knowledge, this study is the first to quantify red cell morphology in a large population of rabbits. Acanthocytes and echinocytes comprised >3% of RBCs in about one-third of healthy and diseased rabbits and were slightly more frequent in healthy female than male rabbits. Fragmented red cells (schistocytes, microcytes, keratocytes, spherocytes) occurred in low numbers and were more frequently observed in diseased rabbits,

Table 2. The proportion of rabbits with specific diseases having moderate to marked acanthocytosis or echinocytosis and mild to moderate fragmentation as compared with healthy rabbits.

Disease[†]	Clinical Diagnosis	Pathologic Diagnosis	Acanthocytosis Mod-Mkd	Echinocytosis Mod-Mkd	Fragmentation Mild-Mod
Abscess	32	18	26/50 (52%)**	14/50 (28%)	7/50 (14%)***
Bronchopneumonia	3	9†	8/12 (67%)*	3/12 (25%)	1/12 (8%)**
Cellulitis§	7	3	7/10 (70%)**	4/10 (40%)	2/10 (20%)***
Dental (non-abscess)	37	1	11/38 (29%)	14/38 (36%)	2/38 (5%)*
Dermatitis	19	5	5/24 (21%)	6/24 (25%)	1/24 (4%)
Fracture	12	2	3/14 (21%)	2/14 (14%)	0/14 (0%)
GI inflammation§	2	9	4/11 (36%)	2/11 (18%)	1/11 (9%)**
GI stasis	25	0	5/25 (20%)	6/25 (24%)	0/25 (0%)
Neoplasia, malignant	0	22	5/22 (22%)	3/22 (14%)	2/22 (9%)**
Otitis	13	1	3/14 (21%)	3/14 (21%)	0/14 (0%)
Renal failure	7	7¶	4/14 (28%)	8/14 (57%)*	1/14 (7%)*
URTD	20	3	7/23 (30%)	7/23 (30%)	0/23 (0%)
Healthy	79	0	23/79 (29%)	19/79 (24%)	0/79 (0%)

*P<.05; **P<.01; ***P<.001.
†Four rabbits with bronchopneumonia also had lung abscessation; 4 had confirmed sepsis.
§Eight of 10 cases of cellulitis were septic (myiasis or bacterial); GI inflammation was septic in 7/11 cases (5 with intralesional bacteria, 1 with Coccidia, 1 with Coccidia and Giardia.
¶Two rabbits with renal failure also had pneumonia.
GI indicates gastrointestinal; URTD indicates upper respiratory tract disease.

Table 3. Hematologic and biochemical values (mean ± SEM) in 482 rabbits based on severity of poikilocytosis.

Analyte	Acanthocytosis			Echinocytosis			Fragmentation		
	Moderate-marked	None-mild	P value*	Moderate-marked	None-mild	P value*	Mild-moderate	None-rare	P value*
RBC (X10⁶/µl)	5.8±0.1	5.8±0.1	–	6.0±0.1	5.7±0.1	0.0055	5.3±0.2	5.8±0.1	0.0241
HCT (%)	36.7±0.5	37.2±0.3	–	38.5±0.5	36.6±0.3	0.0012	34.3±1.1	37.2±0.2	0.0124
HGB (g/dl)	12.3±0.1	12.5±0.1	0.0454	12.9±0.2	12.3±0.1	0.0055	11.1±0.4	12.5±0.1	0.0006
MCV (fl)	63.7±0.3	64.6±0.2	–	64.6±0.3	64.2±0.2	–	65.3±0.8	64.3±0.2	–
MCH (pg)	21.4±0.1	21.7±0.1	–	21.5±0.1	21.6±0.1	–	20.9±0.3	21.6±0.1	0.0243
MCHC (g/dl)	33.6±0.1	33.6±0.1	–	33.4±0.1	33.7±0.1	–	32.1±0.3	33.7±0.1	<0.0001
RDW (%)	13.8±0.1	13.2±0.1	0.0008	13.4±0.1	13.4±0.1	–	16.1±0.3	13.3±0.1	<0.0001
POLY (%)	1.3±0.1	1.2±0.04	–	1.3±0.1	1.2±0.04	–	1.8±0.1	1.2±0.03	0.0002
WBC (/µl)	7677±264	7509±178	–	8036±287	7393±171	–	8493±646	7510±151	–
HET (/µl)	3780±211	3663±142	–	4022±230	3585±137	–	4914±515	3632±120	0.0159
LYM (/µl)	2940±143	2970±96	–	3008±156	2944±93	–	2562±351	2983±82	–
MONO (/µl)	525±38	510±26	–	606±41	483±24	0.0116	679±94	506±22	–
EOS (/µl)	89±8	84±5	–	80±8	88±5	–	81±19	86±4	–
BASO (/µl)	314±19	261±13	0.0226	278±21	277±12	–	238±47	280±11	–
PLT (X10³/µl)	630±25	579±16	–	609±27	588±15	–	764±62	586±13	0.0057
MPV (fl)	7.4±0.2	7.2±0.1	–	7.7±0.2	7.1±0.1	0.0105	8.4±0.5	7.2±0.1	0.0228
TPP (g/dl)	7.2±0.1	7.1±0.04	–	7.3±0.1	7.1±0.1	–	7.1±0.1	7.2±0.04	–
FIB (mg/dl)	303±16	312±10	–	340±17	298±10	0.0377	408±38	304±9	0.0076
AG (mmol/L)	25.4±0.6	24.8±0.4	–	27.1±0.6	24.1±0.4	0.0001	26.3±1.7	25.0±0.3	–
Na (mmol/L)	144.0±0.4	143.6±0.2	–	144.6±0.4	143.4±0.2	0.0079	143.2±1.0	143.8±0.2	–
K (mmol/L)	4.6±0.1	4.4±0.1	0.0202	4.6±0.1	4.4±0.1	0.0271	5.0±0.2	4.4±0.04	0.0077
Cl (mmol/L)	102.9±0.4	102.5±0.3	–	103.6±0.5	102.3±0.3	0.0246	102.8±1.2	102.6±0.2	–
HCO3 (mmol/L)	20.3±0.5	20.9±0.3	–	18.5±0.4	21.6±0.3	<0.0001	19.1±1.2	20.8±0.2	–
CA (mg/dl)	14.7±0.1	14.4±0.1	–	14.5±0.1	14.5±0.1	–	14.2±0.3	14.5±0.1	–
PHOS (mg/dl)	3.6±0.2	3.7±0.1	–	4.0±0.2*	3.5±0.1	0.0331	3.5±0.5	3.7±0.1	–
BUN (mg/dl)	24.3±2.0	23.2±1.3	–	26.7±2.1	22.4±1.3	–	29.1±5.0	23.3±1.1	–
CREA (mg/dl)	1.3±0.1	1.4±0.1	–	1.7±0.1	1.3±0.1	0.0148	1.6±0.3	1.4±0.1	–
GLU (mg/dl)	164.7±4.0	166.4±2.7	–	158.3±4.3	168.6±2.6	0.0424	146.2±10.2	166.8±2.3	0.0482
T. PROT (g/dl)	7.3±0.2	6.9±0.1	–	7.0±0.2	7.1±0.1	–	6.9±0.5	7.1±0.1	–
ALB (g/dl)	5.3±0.1	5.2±0.1	–	5.1±0.1	5.2±0.1	–	4.4±0.2	5.3±0.04	<0.0001
GLOB (g/dl)	1.7±0.1	1.97±0.1	–	1.9±0.1	1.7±0.1	–	2.5±0.2	1.7±0.05	0.0010
CHOL (mg/dl)	58.1±3.9	43.5±2.6	0.0044	57.3±4.2	44.3±2.6	0.0094	93.5±9.9	45.6±2.2	<0.0001
T. BILI (mg/dl)	0.1±0.1	0.2±0.1	–	0.1±0.1	0.2±0.1	–	0.1±0.2	0.2±0.1	–
ALT (U/L)	50±17	81±11	–	57±18	77±11	–	66±44	71±10	–

Table 3. Cont.

Analyte	Acanthocytosis			Echinocytosis			Fragmentation		
	Moderate-marked	None-mild	P value*	Moderate-marked	None-mild	P value*	Mild-moderate	None-rare	P value*
AST (U/L)	44±62	129±42	–	64±67	116±41	–	63±159	104±36	–
ALP (U/L)	62±8	77±6	–	60±9	77±6	–	87±22	71±5	–
CK (U/L)	1244±430	2198±298	–	2429±465	1680±289	–	6567±1110	1658±246	<0.0001
GGT (U/L)	10±2	12±1	–	11±2	11±1	–	19±5	11±1	–
N	118–150	245–332	–	101–127	262–355	–	16–25	346–457	–

*Student's t test between rabbits having moderate-marked (>3% of RBCs) vs none-mild (≤3% of RBCs) acanthocytes or echinocytes, or mild-moderate (>0.5% of RBCs) vs none-rare (≤0.5% of RBCs) fragmented red cells. – indicates no significant difference.

especially those with abscesses, bronchopneumonia, cellulitits, gastrointestinal inflammation, and malignant neoplasia. In addition, moderate to marked echinocytosis was associated with renal failure and electrolyte abnormalities. These findings suggest common pathophysiologic mechanisms of poikilocyte formation in sepsis (fragmentation) and uremia (echinocytes). Our findings warrant further investigation into the pathogenesis of red cell shape change in rabbits and assessment of the diagnostic or prognostic value of poikilocytes.

Acanthocytes and echinocytes were the most frequent poikilocytes observed in rabbits in this study; they often occurred together and formed a morphologic spectrum that sometimes made differentiation difficult [12]. Acanthocytes have irregularly spaced, blunt-tipped projections, an irreversible shape change that usually results from altered membrane cholesterol or phospholipids [1,10–12]. Echinocytes have evenly spaced, narrow-tipped, reversible projections that form in the presence of fatty acids, lysophospholipids, and a variety of chemical agents [1,9,11]. Although acanthocytes (and sometimes echinocytes) are a pathologic finding, echinocytes (crenation) can be an artifact of excess EDTA, prolonged blood storage, or slow drying of smears [1]. Acanthocytes (or acantho-echinocytes) were first reported in healthy laboratory rabbits nearly 50 years ago [7] and have been observed anecdotally in companion rabbits. However, because of the frequent attribution of echinocytes to artifact [8,9] and because, based on our results, only a small proportion of rabbits had many acanthocytes and/or echinocytes, these poikilocytes may be overlooked or considered as insignificant in the routine examination of rabbit blood. Our findings emphasize the importance of documenting all poikilocytes, including echinocytes.

Rabbits fed high cholesterol (atherogenic) diets routinely develop acanthocytes ("spur cells") or echinocytes [16,17,21–23]. Serum cholesterol concentrations in the rabbits in this study also were associated with poikilocytes, especially acanthocytes, but low correlation coefficients suggested other factors were also involved. Cholesterol and phospholipid abnormalities in hepatic disease are another cause of acanthocyte or echinocyte formation [1,2,10,13,24]; we found no correlation with hepatic disease in this study, but the sample size was small. Whether the result of diet or disease, high plasma cholesterol causes cholesterol-enrichment of red cell membranes, expanding the outer leaflet of the phospholipid bilayer (forming membrane projections) and increasing membrane rigidity [18]. Decreased deformability and increased fragility shorten red cell lifespan and contribute to regenerative anemia [25].

An important finding in this study was the association of fragmentation with inflammation (often septic) and with malignant neoplasia in rabbits. This could be the result of bacterial toxins or microangiopathy, with endothelial fibrin deposition and microthrombi causing physical damage to erythrocytes [12,14]. Fragmented erythrocytes usually occurred together with acanthocytes, which can undergo mechanical or "budding" fragmentation and which have been associated with fragmentation in dogs with hemangiosarcoma and glomerulonephritis [1,12,15]. Addition of Staphylococcal alpha toxin to suspensions of rabbit erythrocytes resulted in multiple, discrete surface blebs and finger-like protrusions (i.e., acanthocytes) that suggested separation of the cell membrane from the cell surface; human red cells were more resistant to this shape change [26]. In a murine model of bacterial sepsis, schistocytes (<1% of red cells) were observed 14 days post-infection and attributed to mild microangiopathic hemolysis [27].

Sepsis and inflammation-mediated oxidative damage and cytokines also alter red cell membranes, reducing deformability and increasing phagocytosis by macrophages [22,27,28]. Corre-

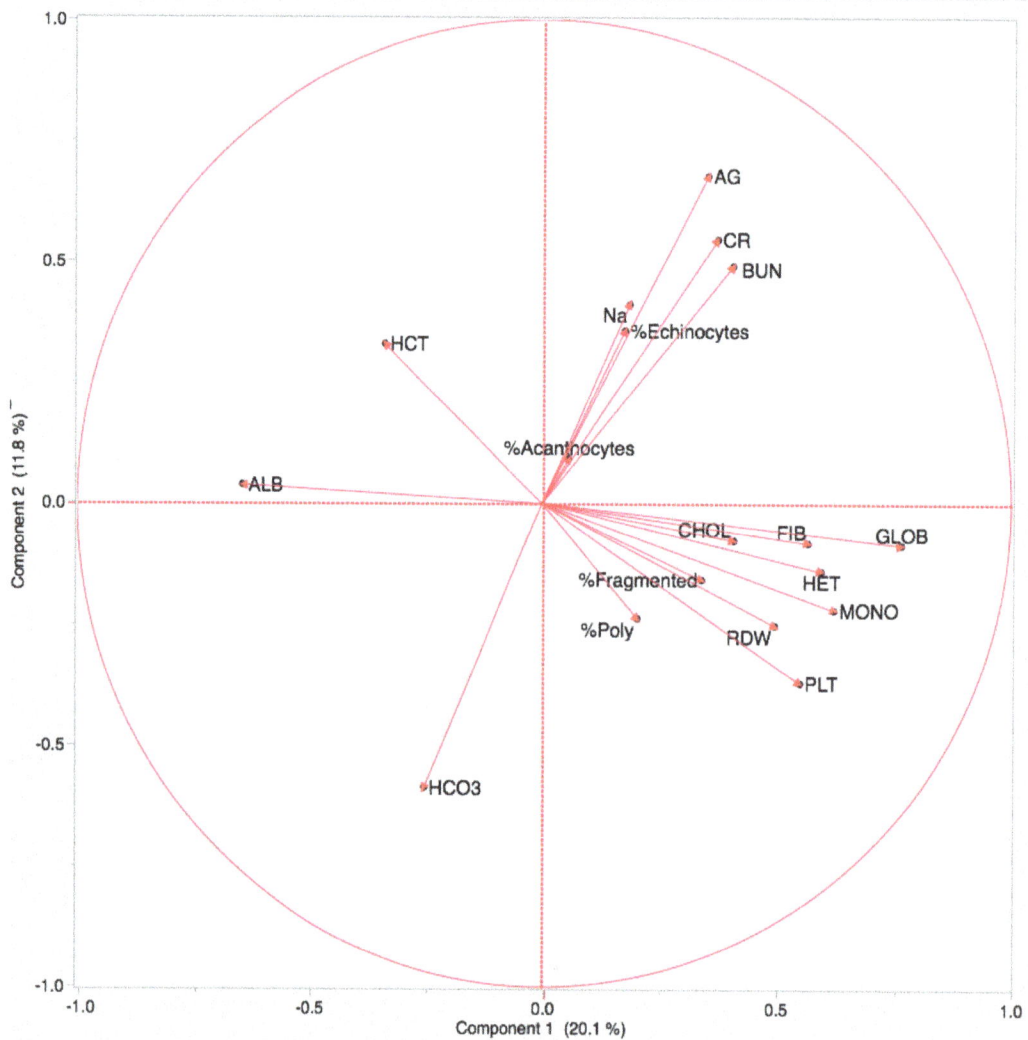

Figure 4. Principal component analysis of % poikilocytes and selected laboratory values. Two primary components were identified, in the right upper (component 2) and right lower (component 1) quadrants. The longer the arrow, the stronger the correlation. Analytes in left quadrants are negatively correlated with those in the diagonal quadrant.

lations between fragmentation and mild regenerative anemia and with heterophil, monocyte, fibrinogen, and globulins concentrations supported a relationship between bacterial infections, laboratory markers of inflammation, and red cell damage in the rabbits in our study. Lack of correlation of fragmented red cells with sample hemolysis was consistent with in vivo rather than in vitro fragment formation. Increased polychromatophils and fragments also contributed to high mean RDW and low MCH. High MPV and platelet counts supported reactive (inflammatory) thrombocytosis, in which IL-6-mediated thrombopoietin production stimulates platelet production [29]. False increases in MPV and platelet count from red cell fragments could have occurred in samples analyzed by the impedance analyzer in the first half of the study; however, the number of fragments was low.

Interestingly, high cholesterol diets can induce inflammation and oxidative stress together with acanthocyte formation in rabbits [30]. In one study [21] rabbits developed acanthocytes and fragments together with high concentrations of C-reactive protein, heterophils, and platelets, similar to our findings. The relationship between inflammation, hypercholesterolemia, and red cell mor-

phology in rabbits fed nonatherogenic diets is unclear, but warrants further study.

We combined spherocytes, keratocytes, microcytes, and schistocytes as fragmented red cells because they often appeared together and in low numbers [12]. No samples contained a predominance or high % of spherocytes, as in immune-mediated hemolytic anemia. Keratocytes form after rupture of "blister cells" (seen rarely in our rabbits) or due to mechanical trauma; they are considered schistocytes by the International Council for Standardization in Hematology [20] and are frequently observed in dogs with concurrent echinocytosis or acanthocytosis [1].

Strong associations between echinocytes, renal disease, and electrolyte abnormalities suggested uremia as one mechanism of moderate to marked echinocytosis in rabbits, as in other species [14,31–33]. Uremic toxins damage red cell membranes and lead to an influx of ionized calcium, externalization of phosphatidylserine in the lipid bilayer, and increased membrane rigidity concurrent with echinocyte formation [32–34]. In humans undergoing dialysis, % echinocytes correlated with intracellular calcium concentration and averaged 15–20% of RBCs [34]. The high anion gap in rabbits with echinocytosis and renal azotemia supported the presence of uremic acids. Increased echinocytes and red cell fragmentation in rabbits with renal disease also could have been associated with glomerulonephritis [1,9,12]. Increased plasma osmolality and hypernatremia (hypertonic dehydration) can also lead to echinocytosis, and may have been a factor in some rabbits in this study. Although smears in our laboratory are prepared soon after collection and dried rapidly, artifactual crenation likely contributed to echinocyte formation in some samples. Other disorders associated with echinocytosis in dogs (snakebite envenomation, lymphoma, cutaneous burns) [1,9], horses (total body cation depletion) [1,35], and rabbits (excess fluoride ingestion) [36] were not observed or associated with echinocytes in rabbits in this study.

A limitation of this retrospective study was the inability to verify underlying disease in all of the rabbits. In addition, we selected the primary disease process, but some rabbits had multiple problems. However, pathologic confirmation of disease was obtained in many of the rabbits, including diseases with potential relevance to poikilocyte formation. Further, many rabbits had diseases (such as fractures, dental malocclusion, and cystitis) that are readily diagnosed clinically or with imaging and laboratory tests. Despite this limitation, the large size of the database and consistent relationships between poikilocytes and clinicopathologic abnormalities helped support the primary findings of our study.

In conclusion, acanthocytes and echinocytes comprised >3% of erythrocytes in about one-third of healthy and diseased rabbits; a small proportion of rabbits had >30% poikilocytes. Echinocytosis also was associated with renal disease and electrolyte abnormalities, consistent with the effect of uremia on red cells. Rabbits with abscesses, other inflammatory disorders, and malignant neoplasia had more red cell fragmentation, which was associated with mild regenerative anemia and hematologic and biochemical evidence of inflammation. Serum cholesterol concentration also correlated poikilocytosis, but was not strongly predictive. Future research is warranted to prospectively evaluate the pathophysiologic mechanisms of poikilocyte formation, the role of diet, and the diagnostic and prognostic value of poikilocytes in rabbits.

Author Contributions

Conceived and designed the experiments: MMC MGH. Performed the experiments: MMC AGB. Analyzed the data: MMC. Contributed to the writing of the manuscript: MMC AGB MGH.

References

1. Harvey JW (2012) Veterinary hematology: A diagnostic guide and color atlas. St. Louis, MO: Elsevier Inc. 360 p.
2. Marks PW (2013) Hematologic manifestations of liver disease. Semin Hematol 50: 216–221.
3. Duranthon V, Beaujean N, Brunner M, Odening KE, Navarrete Santos A, et al. (2012) On the emerging role of rabbit as human disease model and the instrumental role of novel transgenic tools. Transgenic Res 21: 699–713.
4. Russell JC, Proctor SD (2006) Small animal models of cardiovascular disease: tools for the study of the roles of metabolic syndrome. Cardiovasc Path 15: 318–330.
5. Yanni AE (2004) The laboratory rabbit: an animal model of atherosclerosis research. Lab Anim 38: 246–256.
6. Moore DM (1986) Hematology of rabbits. In: Feldman BF, Zinkl JG, Jain NC, editors. Schalm's veterinary hematology, 5th ed. Baltimore, MD: Lippincott, Williams, and Wilkins. pp. 1100–1106.
7. Schermer S (1967) The blood morphology of laboratory animals, 3rd ed. Philadelphia: FA Davis Co. 200 p.
8. Sanderson JH, Phillips CE (1981) An atlas of laboratory animal hematology. Oxford, UK: Clarendon Press. 473 p.
9. Weiss DJ, Kristensen A, Papenfuss N, McClay CB (1990) Quantitative evaluation of echinocytes in the dog. Vet Clin Pathol 19: 114–118.
10. Palek J (1994) Acanthocytosis, stomatocytosis, and related disorders. IN: Williams, WJ, Beutler E, Erslev AJ, and Lichtman MA, editors. Williams hematology. New York: McGraw-Hill, Inc. pp. 557–558.
11. Lange Y, Steck TL (1984) Mechanism of red blood cell acanthocytosis and echinocytosis in vivo. J Membr Biol 77: 153–159.
12. Weiss DJ, Kristensen A, Papenfuss N (1993) Quantitative evaluation of irregularly spiculated red blood cells in the dog. Vet Clin Pathol 22: 117–121.
13. Christopher MM, Lee SE (1994) Red cell morphologic alterations in cats with hepatic disease. Vet Clin Pathol 23: 7–12.
14. Rebar AH, Lewis HB, Denicola DB, Halliwell WH, Boon GD (1981) Red cell fragmentation in the dog: an editorial review. Vet Pathol 18: 415–426.
15. Warry E, Bohn A, Emanuelli M, Thamm D, Lana S (2013) Disease distribution in canine patients with acanthocytosis: 123 cases. Vet Clin Pathol 42: 465–470.
16. Pinter GG, Bailey RE (1961) Anemia of rabbits fed a cholesterol-containing diet. Am J Physiol 200: 292–296.
17. Pessina GP, Paulesu L, Bocci V (1981) Red cell modifications in cholesterol-fed rabbits. Int J Biochem 13: 805–810.
18. Cooper RA, Leslie MH, Knight D, Detweiler DK (1980) Red cell cholesterol enrichment and spur cell anemia in dogs fed a cholesterol-enriched, atherogenic diet. J Lipid Res 21: 1082–1089.
19. Weiss DJ (1984) Uniform evaluation and semi quantitative reporting of hematologic data in veterinary laboratories. Vet Clin Pathol 13: 27–31.
20. Zini G, D'Onofrio G, Briggs C, Erber W, Jou JM, et al. (2012) ICSH recommendations for identification, diagnostic value, and quantification of schistocytes. Int J Lab Hematol 34: 107–116.
21. Karbiner MS, Sierra L, Minahk C, Fonio MC, de Bruno MP, et al. (2013) The role of oxidative stress in alterations of hematological parameters and inflammatory markers induced by early hypercholesterolemia. Life Sci 93: 503–508.
22. López-Revuelta A, Sánchez-Gallego JI, García-Montero AC, Hernández-Hernández A, Sánchez-Yagüe J, et al. (2007) Membrane cholesterol in the regulation of aminophospholipid asymmetry and phagocytosis in oxidized erythrocytes. J Free Radic Biol Med 42: 1106–1118.
23. Kanakaraj P, Singh M (1989) Influence of hypercholesterolemia on morphological and rhelogical characteristics of erythrocytes. Atherosclerosis 76: 209–218.
24. Owen JS, Brown DJC, Harry DS, McIntyre N (1985) Erythrocyte echinocytosis in liver disease. J Clin Invest 76: 2275–2285.
25. Morse EE (1990) Mechanisms of hemolysis in liver disease. Ann Clin Lab Sci 20: 169–174.
26. Klainer AS, Chang T-W, Weinstein L (1972) Effects of purified Staphylococcal alpha toxin on the ultrastructure of human and rabbit erythrocytes. Infect Immunol 5: 808–813.
27. Kim A, Fung E, Parikh SG, Valore EV, Gabayan V, et al. (2014) A mouse model of anemia of inflammation: complex pathogenesis with partial dependence on hepcidin. Blood 123: 1129–1136.
28. Straat M, van Bruggen R, de Korte D, Juffermans NP (2012) Red blood cell clearance in inflammation. Transfus Med Hemother 39: 353–360.
29. Kaser A, Brandacher G, Steurer W, Kaser S, Offner FA, et al. (2001) Interleukin-6 stimulates thrombopoiesis through thrombopoietin: role in inflammatory thrombocytosis. Blood 98: 2720–2725.
30. Kuwai T, Hayashi J (2006) Nitric oxide pathway activation and impaired red blood cell deformability with hypercholesterolemia. J Atheroscler Thromb 13: 286–294.
31. Christopher MM (2008) Of human loss and erythrocyte survival: uremia and anemia in chronic renal disease. Israel Journal of Veterinary Medicine 63: 4–11.
32. Sakthivel R, Farooq SM, Kalaiselevi P, Varalakshmi P (2007) Investigation on the early events of apoptosis in senescent erythrocytes with special emphasis on intracellular free calcium and loss of phospholipid asymmetry in chronic renal failure. Clin Chim Acta 382: 1–7.
33. Lichtman MA, Beutler E, Kipps TJ, Seligsohn E, Kaushansky K, Prchal J (2006) Williams hematology, 7th ed. New York: McGraw-Hill Inc. 2296 p.
34. Agroyannis B, Kopelias I, Fourtounas C, Paraskevopoulos A, Tzanatos H, et al. (2001) Relation between echinocytosis and erythrocyte calcium content in hemodialyzed uremic patients. Artif Organs 25: 486–502.
35. Weiss DJ, Geor R, Smith II CM, McClay CB (1992) Furosemide-induced electrolyte depletion associated with echinocytosis in horses. Am J Vet Res 53: 1769–1772.
36. Susheela AK, Jain SK (1985) Fluoride toxicity: erythrocyte membrane abnormality and "echinocyte" formation. Fluoride Research, Studies in Environmental Science 27: 231–239.

14

Cigarette Smoking Promotes Inflammation in Patients with COPD by Affecting the Polarization and Survival of Th/Tregs through Up-Regulation of Muscarinic Receptor 3 and 5 Expression

Ming-Qiang Zhang[1,⑨]**, Yong Wan**[2,⑨]**, Yang Jin**[1]**, Jian-Bao Xin**[1]**, Jian-Chu Zhang**[1]**, Xian-Zhi Xiong**[1]*****, Long Chen**[1]**, Gang Chen**[1]

1 Department of Respiratory and Critical Care Medicine, Key Laboratory of Pulmonary Diseases of Health Ministry, Union Hospital, Tongji Medical College, Huazhong University of Science and Technology, Wuhan, China, 2 Department of Respiratory and Critical Care Medicine WUHAN NO. 1 HOSPITAL, Wuhan, China

Abstract

Background: CD4[+] T cells in the lung are involved in the pathogenesis of chronic obstructive pulmonary disease (COPD), although CD4[+] T cell subsets and the direct effect of smoking on these cells, especially the expression of MRs, have not been comprehensively examined.

Methods: First, circulating CD4[+] T cell subsets in healthy nonsmokers, patients with SCOPD and patients with AECOPD were evaluated by flow cytometry. Then, differentiation experiments were carried out using RT-PCR, and Ki-67/Annexin V antibodies were used to measure proliferation and apoptosis. We also explored the impact of CSE on the differentiation and survival of CD4[+]Th/Tregs and examined the expression of MRs in healthy nonsmokers and patients with SCOPD.

Results: We found the percentages of circulating Th1 and Th17 cells were increased in patients with AECOPD, while the percentage of Th2 cells was decreased in patients with SCOPD. The percentages of Th10 cells were decreased in both patients with SCOPD and patients with AECOPD, while the percentages of Tregs were increased. In addition, the percentages of CD4[+]α-7[+] T cells were decreased in patients with SCOPD and patients with AECOPD. However, only the decrease observed in patients with AECOPD was significant. In vitro studies also revealed MR expression affected the polarization of T cells, with different CD4[+] T cell subtypes acquiring different MR expression profiles. The addition of CSE facilitated CD4[+] T cell polarization towards pro-inflammatory subsets (Th1 and Th17) and affected the survival of CD4[+] T cells and Treg cells by up-regulating the expression of MR3 and 5, resulting in an imbalance of CD4[+] T cell subsets.

Conclusions: Our findings suggest an imbalance of circulating CD4[+] T cell subsets is involved in COPD pathogenesis in smokers. Cigarette smoking may contribute to this imbalance by affecting the polarization and survival of Th/Tregs through the up-regulation of MR3 and MR5.

Editor: Yeonseok Chung, Seoul National University College of Pharmacy, Republic of Korea

Funding: This work was supported in part by a grant from the Science and Technology Program of Wuhan, China (No. 201052399660), and in part by a grant from the Natural Science Fund of Hubei Province, China (No. 2010CDB07805); and in part by a grant from the National Natural Science Foundation of China (No. 81370146). The funders had no role in study design, data collection and analysis, decision to publish, or preparation of the manuscript.

Competing Interests: The authors have declared that no competing interests exist.

* Email: xxz0508@hust.edu.cn

⑨ These authors contributed equally to this work.

Introduction

Chronic obstructive pulmonary disease (COPD) is characterized by persistent airflow limitation and progressive airway inflammation, and its prevalence is rapidly increasing worldwide. Inflammation in the airways is triggered by inhalation of hazardous gases and particles; tobacco smoking is the leading contributing factor for this type of inflammation [1]. Chronic smoking can lead to refractory inflammation in the lung, which eventually results in destruction of the alveolar space, loss of surface area for gas exchange and loss of elasticity (i.e., emphysema) [2]. However, the mechanisms underlying these changes following lung exposure to cigarette smoke have not been completely elucidated.

Increasing evidence indicates that adaptive immune responses are involved in the pathogenesis of COPD, and inflammation mediated by T cells has specifically been identified as a key component [3]. Although several studies have focused on CD4[+] T cells in the blood of patients with COPD [4,5], there are few comprehensive examinations of circulating CD4[+] T cell subsets in this disease. Recent research has shown that soluble components extracted from cigarette smoke (CSE) could significantly reduce T cell activation, proliferation and the expression of cytotoxic proteins, such as granzyme-B [6], thereby suppressing dendritic cell functions and favoring the development of T helper (Th)2 immunity [7]. However, other types of T cells, particularly the Th1 and Tc1 subsets, are present in the airways and parenchyma of smokers with COPD [8]. Thus, the precise influence of CSE on $CD4^+$ T cells, particularly whether cigarette smoke suppresses or facilitates the function and proliferation of these cells, remains unclear.

Recent emerging studies on the non-neuronal cholinergic system have shown that the cholinergic system is implicated in many diseases, such as arthritis, angiogenesis, cancer, non-healing wounds and inflammation [9]. Lymphocytes have been shown to both express cholinergic receptors, including muscarinic acetylcholine receptors (mAChRs), and serve as a source of Ach [10]. Indeed, accumulating evidence has further indicated that T cell-synthesized ACh acts as an autocrine and/or paracrine factor via ACh receptors on immune cells to modulate immune function [11]. COPD is a chronic inflammatory disease that is characterized by hyperfunction of the cholinergic system [12]. However, whether the cholinergic system is involved in the pathogenesis of COPD through the regulation of T cells remains unknown. In particular, whether smoking affects $CD4^+$ T cells through the cholinergic system, whether CSE enhances the expression of mAchR in $CD4^+$ T cells, and whether the effect of smoking could be decreased by blocking the mAchR are questions that have remained unanswered in the field.

To answer these questions, we examined and compared circulating $CD4^+$ T cell subsets (Th1, Th2, Th17, Tregs, Th10, and $CD4^+\alpha\text{-}7^+$ T cells) in healthy nonsmokers, patients with stable COPD, and patients with acute exacerbation in COPD. Then, in vitro experiments were carried out to investigate the effects of smoking and the muscarinic receptor (MR) signaling system on the differentiation and survival of $CD4^+$ Th/Tregs. Our results identified an imbalance of pro/anti-inflammatory $CD4^+$ T cell subsets in patients with COPD. Moreover, CSE affected the differentiation and survival of Th/Tregs through the up-regulation of MRs, resulting in an imbalance of Th/Tregs and the development of chronic inflammation in patients with COPD.

Materials and Methods

Subjects

The study was approved by Ethics Committee of the Tongji Medical School, Huazhong University of Science and Technology. All patients and volunteers were informed of the research process and signed informed consent forms. Based on the Global Initiative for Chronic Obstructive Lung Disease (GOLD) criteria [13], 24 patients with stable COPD (SCOPD), 14 patients with acute exacerbation COPD (AECOPD) (clinical characteristics listed in Table 1), and 14 healthy nonsmokers were enrolled (no smoking; age, sex, matched). Patients with AECOPD were diagnosed as the initiation of exacerbated COPD symptoms, which required hospitalization, in the previous 72 h without any new therapeutic intervention. The following examinations or tests were performed: medical history, physical examination, routine blood tests, liver and kidney functions tests, serum electrolytes and pulmonary function. Additionally, a chest X ray or helical computed tomography (CT) and electrocardiography (ECG) or heart ultrasound examination were performed to exclude other diseases. Peripheral blood samples were collected from all patients and volunteers.

Sample collection and isolation of peripheral blood T (PBT) cells

Peripheral blood samples were collected in heparin-treated tubes from each subject within 24 h of arrival to the hospital or during the medical examination for healthy nonsmokers. The blood samples were immediately immersed in ice and then centrifuged at 1,200×g for 5 min. After the peripheral blood mononuclear cells (PBMCs) were isolated from heparinized blood by Ficoll-Hypaque gradient centrifugation (Pharmacia, Uppsala, Sweden), PBT cells were recovered from the non-adherent cells after 24 h of PBMC culture, as previously described [14,15,16]. The recovered PBT cell fraction was greater than 85% $CD3^+$ cells, as assessed by flow cytometry. Isolated PBT cells were resuspended in complete medium RPMI 1640 (HyClone) plus 10% FBS (HyClone) and then placed in an incubator at 37°C in 5% CO_2 for subsequent experiments.

Flow cytometry

Surface marker expression and intracellular cytokine production by T cells were determined using flow cytometry. The staining was performed using anti-human-specific antibodies (Abs) conjugated with the following fluoresceins: isothiocyanate (FITC), phycoerythrin (PE), peridinin chlorophyll protein (PerCP)-cy5.5, allophycocyanin (APC), PE-CY7, or Alexa Fluor 647. These human Abs included anti-CD3, anti-CD4, anti-CD8, anti-CD25, anti-Foxp3, anti-IL-17A, anti-IL-10, anti–IFN-γ, anti-IL-4, and anti-Ki-67 mAbs, as well as isotype mAbs, which were purchased from BD Biosciences or eBioscience (San Diego, CA). The expression of nicotine receptor α7 on T cells was detected by its binding the alpha-bungarotoxin (Invitrogen, USA). Intracellular staining for IL-17-, IL-10-, IFN-γ-, and IL-4–producing T cells was performed on T cells stimulated with PMA (50 ng/ml; Sigma-Aldrich, St. Louis, MO) and ionomycin (1 μM; Sigma-Aldrich) in the presence of GolgiStop (BD Biosciences) for 5 h. Intracellular cytokines were then stained with the corresponding mAbs conjugated to fluoresceins after fixation and permeabilization (permeabilization kit, eBioscience) according to the manufacturer's instructions. Isotype controls were included to enable the correct compensation and confirm antibody specificity. Flow cytometry was performed using a fluorescence-activated cell sorter (FACS) Canto II (BD Biosciences) with BD FCSDiva software and FCS Express 4 (De Novo Software) software.

Preparation of CSE

Our preparation of CSE was performed according to the method of Blue and Janoff [17]. CSE was prepared by drawing cigarette smoke into a 50-ml plastic syringe and then slowly bubbling the smoke into a tube that contained 5 ml of sterile RPMI 1640 medium. Each 5 ml of CSE was produced using two cigarettes (Huang Helou, Wuhan China), and the concentration of the original CSE was considered to be 100%. All materials were sterile and used only once. Then, the solution of CSE was filtered through 0.22- μm filters. To ascertain the vitality of the substances in CSE, all CSE preparations were made within half an hour prior to each experiment. The concentrations of CSE used in the experiments were chosen according to the concentration gradient experiment.

Real-time quantitative PCR

Total RNA was prepared from T cells using TRIzol reagent (TaKaRa). In all, 2 μg of total RNA was reverse transcribed into 20 μl of complementary DNA using the cDNA reverse transcription kit (TaKaRa). Melting curves were generated to establish the

Table 1. Demographic and spirometric values of healthy nonsmokers, patients with SCOPD and patients with AECOPD.

	Healthy nonsmokers	SCOPD	AECOPD
Participants	14	24	14
Age (years)	65.6±7.8	66.5±7.2	69.1±9.6
Sex ratio (M/F)	12/2	19/5	11/3
Smoking history (pack, y)	0	41.9±17.6*	47.2±19.5*
FEV1 (% predicted)	104.6±10	47.7±24.2*	35.1±15.1*#
FEV1/FVC (%)	85.2±6.1	48.8±15.2*	47.9±10.1*

All data are presented as the mean±SD. FEV1: Forced expiratory volume in one second, measured post bronchodilatation and FVC: Forced vital capacity. *$P<0.05$ compared with healthy nonsmokers; #$P<0.05$ compared with SCOPD patients.

purity of the amplified band after 40 cycles of 30 s at 94°C, 30 s at 57°C, and 30 s at 72°C. Amplified fragments of the expected size were analyzed with a 2% agarose gel and were photographed under UV light. Q-PCR was performed on a StepOnePlus Real-Time PCR System (Applied Biosystems) in a 10- μl reaction that contained 1 μl of cDNA and SYBR Premix Ex Taq (TaKaRa). The following PCR parameters were used: 95°C for 3 min; 40 cycles of 95°C for 10 s and 60°C for 30 s; and a melting curve from 65°C to 95°C in increments of 0.5°C for 5 s. The expression level of GAPDH was used as an internal control. The relative expression was calculated with the comparative Ct method using StepOne Software v2.1 (Applied Biosystems) and was expressed as the fold change compared to the control. The specific primer pairs used to amplify genes are listed in Table 2.

Differentiation and polarization of T cell subsets

PBT cells (1×10^6) were cultured in 300 μl of complete medium in 96-well plates, and soluble anti-CD3 (1 μg/ml) and anti-CD28 Abs (1 μg/ml)(both from eBioscience) were added to achieve TCR stimulation via the TCR/CD3 complex. The cells were cultured in RPMI 1640 supplemented with 10% fetal calf serum in a 5% CO_2 humid atmosphere at 37°C for 5 days. To investigate the influence of cigarette smoke and the cholinergic system on the differentiation of T cells, CSE (0.33% = 1 μl of 100% CSE in 300 μl of medium) and an MR agonist or antagonist were added to the medium. The mAChRs were activated with muscarine (50 μM, the dose discussed in other papers was not suitable for our experimental conditions; this dose was selected based on a preliminary experiment, and toxicity and side effects were not observed at this dose). The mAChRs were inhibited with atropine (100 μM) from Sigma-Aldrich or Tocris. To derive Th1/Th2/

Table 2. Real-time RT-PCR primer sequences.

Target gene	Sequence (5'—3')
TBX21 (T-bet)	F:TGGTCCAAGTTTAATCAGCACCAG
	R:CCCGGCCACAGTAAATGACAG
GATA3	F:GAGATGGCACGGGACACTAC
	R:GGTCTGACAGTTCGCACAGG
RORC	F:CTGCAAGACTCATCGCCAAAG
	R:TTTCCACATGCTGGCTACACA
FOXP3	F:CTGGCAAATGGTGTCTGCAAGT
	R:CTGCCCTTCTCATCCAGAAGATG
GAPDH	F:GCACCGTCAAGGCTGAGAAC
	R:TGGTGAAGACGCCAGTGGA
MR1	F:AGGAAGTCAGGAGCCAGCAG
	R:GCACCATCTCACACCGCAATC
MR2	F:GTCAGAATGGAGATGAAAAGCAGA
	R:GAAAGCCAACAGAATAGCCAAGA
MR3	F:TCCGAGCAGATGGACCAAGA
	R:GAAGCTTGAGCACGATGGAGTAGA
MR4	F:AGATGGCAGGCCTCATGATTG
	R:CTGGGTTGGACAGGAACTGGA
MR5	F:ACAAGAGGAAGCACACTGGGTAA
	R:GCTGGTTCTCACTGGCACAAG

All of these primers were synthesized by TaKaRa in Dalian.

Th17/Treg cells, the following exogenous cytokines were added: 20 ng/ml IL-12 for Th1; 4 ng/ml IL-4 for Th2; 20 ng/ml IL-6 and 5 ng/ml TGF-β1 for Th17; and 2 ng/ml IL-2 and 5 ng/ml TGF-β1 for Treg. All of the aforementioned recombinant human cytokines were purchased from Peprotech.

Proliferation and apoptosis of T cells

PBT cells (1×10^6) were cultured in 300 μl of complete medium in 96-well plates. The cells were cultured in RPMI 1640 supplemented with 10% fetal calf serum in a 5% CO_2 humid atmosphere at 37°C. PBT cells were cultured in the presence of medium alone, CSE or mAChR agonist/antagonist. The mAChRs were activated with muscarine (50 μM) and inhibited with atropine (100 μM) (Sigma-Aldrich or Tocris). In the proliferation assays, 1 μg/ml PHA and 50 ng/ml PMA (both from Sigma-Aldrich, St. Louis, MO) were added to the medium to stimulate T cell proliferation. After 5 days, the cells were harvested and then stained with APC-conjugated Annexin V and propidium iodide (Annexin V Apoptosis Detection Kit APC; eBioscience) at room temperature in the dark for 10 min. Finally, the proportion of apoptotic T cells was determined by flow cytometry. For T cell proliferation assays, intracellular staining with Alexa Fluor 647 conjugated anti-human Ki-67 (eBioscience) was performed.

Statistics

The data are expressed as the mean ± SD (unless indicated in the figure legends). Comparisons of the data between different groups were performed using a Kruskal-Wallis one-way analysis of variance (ANOVA) with Tukey and Dunn post-hoc tests for between-group comparisons. Comparisons between healthy non-smokers and patients with SCOPD in the proliferation and apoptosis assays were performed using the Mann-Whitney U test. Data analysis was performed with GraphPad Prism V5.01 software (GraphPad Software, La Jolla, California), and two-tailed P-values of less than 0.05 were considered statistically significant.

Results

1 Changes in CD4$^+$ T cell subsets in the three patient populations

1.1 The percentages of Th1 and Th17 cells are increased in patients with AECOPD, while the percentage of Th2 cells is decreased in patients with SCOPD. To investigate the changes in pro-inflammatory CD4$^+$ T cells in COPD, we measured and analyzed the levels of Th1 cells (CD3$^+$CD8$^-$IFN-γ$^+$), Th2 cells (CD3$^+$CD8$^-$IL-4$^+$), and Th17 cells (CD3$^+$CD8$^-$IL-17A$^+$) in the blood among the three patient groups (Figure 1A). Due to the limited quantity in some samples, not all CD8$^+$ T cell subsets were detected.

As shown in Figure 1B, the percentages of Th1 and Th17 cells were remarkably elevated in patients with AECOPD (22.73±9.14%; 2.03±1.16%, respectively) compared to healthy nonsmokers (10.80±7.34%; 0.75±0.42%, respectively). There were no significant changes in the percentages of these cells in patients with SCOPD (17.15±12.28%; 0.86±0.44%, respectively). In addition, there were more Th17 cells in patients with AECOPD compared to patients with SCOPD (P<0.05). In addition, the percentage of Th2 cells was significantly reduced in patients with SCOPD (0.85±0.61%) compared to healthy nonsmokers (2.30±1.10%); however, no difference was observed was in patients with AECOPD (3.63±2.13%).

1.2 The percentages of Th10 and CD4$^+$α-7$^+$ T cells are lower and the percentages of Tregs are higher in patients with SCOPD and patients with AECOPD. To investigate the changes in the anti-inflammatory CD4$^+$ T cell population in patients with COPD, we detected and compared the percentages of the Tregs (CD3$^+$CD8$^-$CD25$^+$Foxp3$^+$), Th10 cells (CD3$^+$CD8$^-$IL-10$^+$), and CD4$^+$α-7$^+$T cells (CD3$^+$ CD8$^-$α-7$^+$) among the three groups (Figure 2). Due to the limited quantity in some samples, not all CD8$^+$ T cell subsets were detected.

Not surprisingly, the percentage of Th10 cells in patients with SCOPD or AECOPD (0.20±0.11%; 0.30±0.10%, respectively) was significantly reduced to approximately one-quarter of that in healthy nonsmokers (1.23±0.54%). Interestingly, the percentage of Tregs was only increased in patients with AECOPD (5.13±1.73%) compared to healthy nonsmokers and patients with SCOPD (2.62±0.86%; 3.08±3.01%, respectively). In contrast, the percentage of CD4$^+$α-7$^+$ T cells was significantly reduced in patients with AECOPD (0.23±0.11%) compared to healthy nonsmokers (1.48±0.95%). The percentage of CD4$^+$α-7$^+$ T cells was modestly decreased in patients with SCOPD (0.36±1.16%) compared to healthy nonsmokers, but the difference was not significant.

1.3 Comprehensive analysis of the relative percentages of CD4$^+$ T cell subsets. To clarify the precise changes in CD4$^+$ T cell subsets in patients with COPD, we performed a comprehensive analysis of the relative proportion of each subset. As shown in Figure 3, Th1 cells accounted for most of the pro-inflammatory CD4$^+$ T cells in both the SCOPD and AECOPD groups (77% and 67%, respectively), and both of these percentages were higher than that observed in healthy nonsmokers (60%). The percentage of Th2 cells was clearly reduced in patients with SCOPD (4%) but were detected at nearly normal levels in patients with AECOPD (11%) compared to healthy nonsmokers (13%). Interestingly, the percentage of Th17 cells was only increased in the AECOPD group (6%) compared to the healthy nonsmoker (5%) and SCOPD (4%) groups. Although the percentage of Tregs was not lower in the SCOPD (14%) and AECOPD (15%) groups compared to healthy nonsmokers (15%), the percentage of Th10 cells was remarkably decreased in both the SCOPD (1%) and AECOPD (1%) groups compared to healthy nonsmokers (7%). As a result, the overall percentage of anti-inflammatory CD4$^+$ T cells (Tregs plus Th10 cells) was reduced in patients with AECOPD (16%) and progressively decreased in patients with SCOPD (15%) compared to healthy nonsmokers (22%).

In addition, as indicated in Figure 3B, the Th1/Th2 ratio was notably, although not significantly, elevated in patients with SCOPD (mean value 19.9:1), but not in patients with AECOPD (mean value 7.9:1), compared to healthy nonsmokers (mean value 7.8:1). Interestingly, the Th1/Th17 ratio was modestly increased in patients with SCOPD (mean value 22.9:1), whereas it was decreased in patients with AECOPD (mean value: 14.2:1) compared to healthy nonsmokers (mean value: 20.2:1). In addition, the pro-inflammatory index (<Th1+Th2+Th17> / < Tregs+Th10>) was modestly increased in patients with SCOPD and AECOPD (mean value: 7.8:1 and 6.3:1, respectively) compared to healthy nonsmokers (mean value: 5.1:1).

In total, this comprehensive analysis showed that, compared with healthy nonsmokers, there were relatively more Th1 cells and fewer Th2 and Th10 cells in patients with SCOPD and patients with AECOPD. Additionally, the percentage of Th17 cells was increased in patients with AECOPD, but not in patients with SCOPD. Although the relative percentage of Tregs was normal, the overall levels of anti-inflammatory CD4$^+$ T cells were insufficient in these two groups, which lacked Th10 cells. In addition, there was an imbalance in the Th1/Th2 ratio in patients with SCOPD, Th1/Th17 ratio in patients with AECOPD, and the pro/anti-inflammatory ratio in both groups.

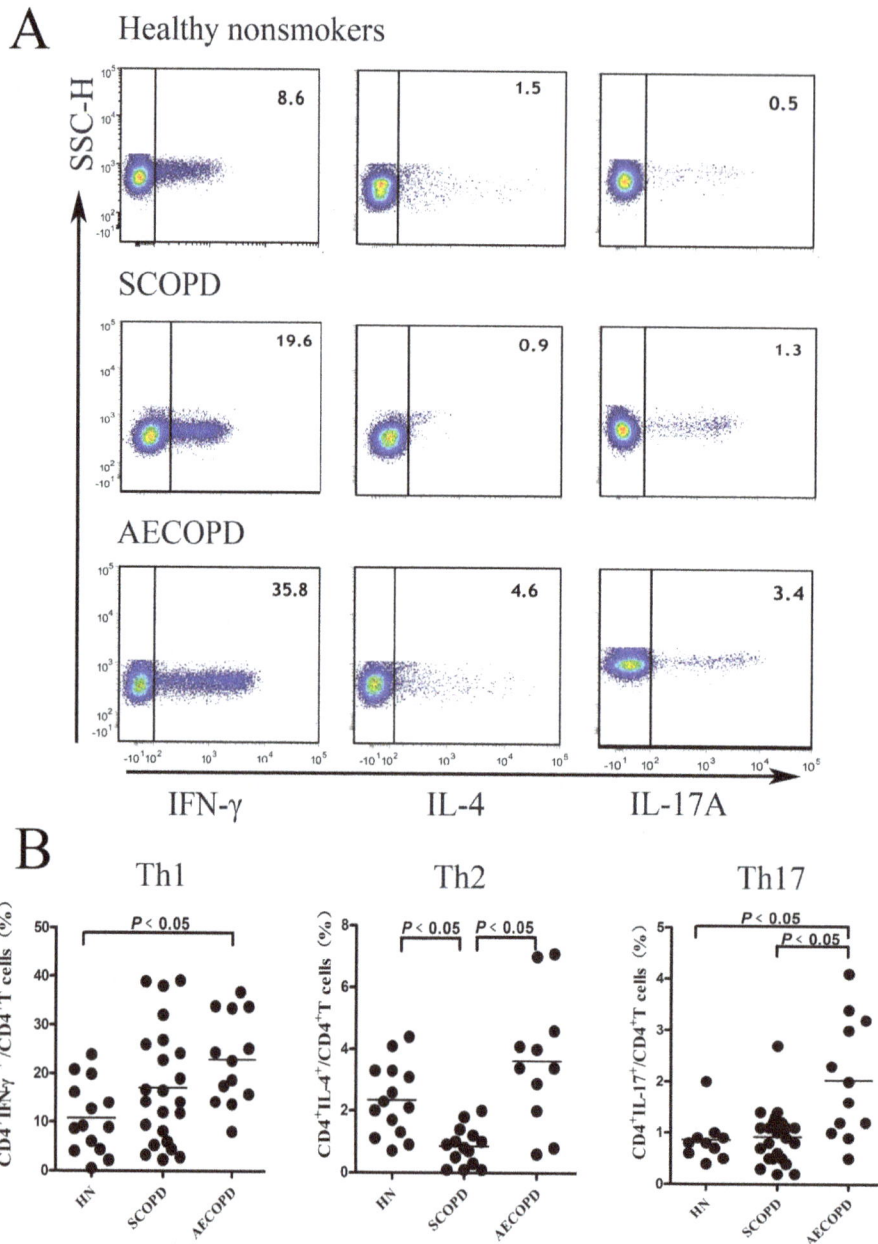

Figure 1. The percentages of Th1 and Th17 cells are increased in patients with AECOPD, while the percentage of Th2 cells is decreased in patients with SCOPD. (**A**) Representative flow cytometric dot-plots of Th1, Th2 and Th17 cells (*Th1: CD3+CD8⁻ IFN-γ+ T cells, Th2: CD3+CD8⁻ IL-4+T cells, Th17: CD3+CD8⁻ IL-17A+T cells*) in healthy nonsmokers (HN), patients with SCOPD and patients with AECOPD are shown. (**B**) Comparisons of the percentages of Th1, Th2 and Th17 cells in healthy nonsmokers, patients with SCOPD and patients with AECOPD (*n = 14, 24, 14, respectively*) are shown. Horizontal bars indicate the mean value. The comparisons were made using a Kruskal-Wallis one-way ANOVA on ranks.

2 CD4+ T cell subsets express different mAChR subtypes

Cigarette smoking is the leading factor contributing to the pathogenesis of COPD. Therefore, we asked whether cigarette smoking caused the imbalance in pro- and anti-inflammatory activity by directly affecting the differentiation of CD4+ T cells and Tregs through the up-regulation of the mAchRs. In particular, we examined the mRNA expression of mAchRs and performed differentiation assays with PBT cells obtained from patients with SCOPD and healthy nonsmokers.

2.1 CD4+ T cell subsets express different mAChR subtypes. As indicated in Figure 4A, PBT cells expressed

MR1-MR5 mRNA, but the RT-PCR results showed that only the expression of MR3, MR4, and MR5 mRNA was relatively stable (data not shown). Compared to unstimulated T cells, the mRNA expression levels of RORC and FOXP3 were significantly increased, whereas those of T-bet and GATA3 were reduced following stimulation with anti-CD3/anti-CD28 Abs, indicating that activation of the TCR facilitates the polarization of naïve T cells to Treg and Th17 cells.

To investigate whether different CD4+ T cell subsets express different mAChR subtypes, various exogenous cytokines were used to derive Th1/Th2/Th17/Treg cells. We confirmed the successful

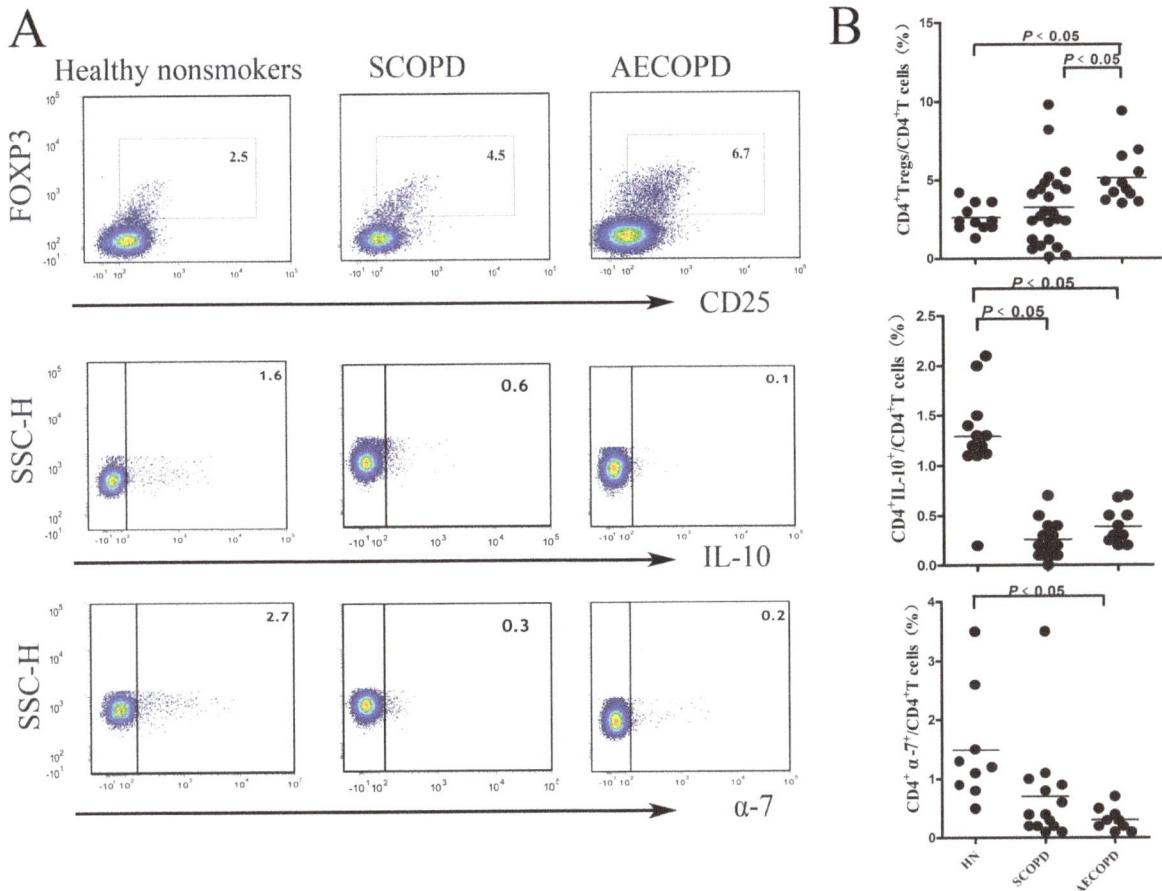

Figure 2. The percentage of Tregs is increased in patients with AECOPD, and the percentages of Th10 and CD4$^+$α7$^+$ T cells are decreased in both patients with SCOPD and patients with AECOPD. (**A**) Representative flow cytometric dot-plots of Tregs, Th10 and CD4$^+$α7$^+$ T cells (*Tregs: CD3$^+$CD8$^-$CD25$^+$FOXP3$^+$ T cells, Th10: CD3$^+$CD8$^-$ IL-10$^+$T cells, and CD4$^+$α7$^+$ T: CD3$^+$CD8$^-$ α7$^+$ T cells*) in healthy nonsmokers, patients with SCOPD and patients with AECOPD are shown. (**B**) Comparisons of the percentages of Th1, Th2 and Th17 cells in healthy nonsmokers, patients with SCOPD and patients with AECOPD (*n = 14, 24, and 14, respectively*) are shown. Horizontal bars indicate the mean value. The comparisons were made using a Kruskal-Wallis one-way ANOVA on ranks.

polarization of these subsets by their expression of specific nuclear transcription factors, including T-bet, GATA3, RORC, and FOXP3, respectively (Figure 5A). Our data revealed that, in both healthy nonsmokers and patients with SCOPD, the expression of MR3 and MR5 mRNA was significantly up-regulated in Th1 cells (P<0.05) and modestly increased in Th17 cells; MR4 mRNA was modestly increased in Tregs; and there was no significant change in mAchR expression in Th2 cells, although MR5 expression was increased.

2.2 MRs affect the differentiation of CD4$^+$T cells. To assess whether MRs influence the differentiation of CD4$^+$ T cells, we performed a differentiation experiment. We found that activation of mAChRs by muscarine significantly enhanced GATA3 mRNA expression (P<0.05) in healthy nonsmokers while up-regulating T-bet, RORC and FOXP3 mRNA expression (P< 0.05) in patients with SCOPD, and both effects could be blocked by addition of the mAChR antagonist atropine. Thus, activation of mAChRs promoted the polarization of Th2 cells in healthy nonsmokers and that of Th1, Th17 and Treg cells in patients with SCOPD (Fig. 6A, B).

2.3 CSE affects the mAChR expression and differentiation of CD4$^+$ T cells. Our data are the first to show that CSE enhances MR3 and MR5 mRNA expression in T cells in both

healthy nonsmokers and patients with SCOPD (P<0.05). Importantly, the increased MR3 and MR5 expression could be blocked by atropine in patients with SCOPD compared to the unchallenged group (Fig. 5B, C). Additionally, CSE significantly increased the T-bet and RORC mRNA expression (P<0.05) in healthy nonsmokers while up-regulating T-bet, RORC and FOXP3 mRNA expression (P<0.05) in patients with SCOPD, and both effects could be blocked by the addition of the mAChR antagonist atropine (Fig. 6A, B). Thus, CSE facilitated the polarization of Th1 and Th17 cells in healthy nonsmokers as well as that of Th1, Th17 and Treg cells in patients with SCOPD via the increased expression of MR3 and MR5 mRNA.

3 CSE affects the proliferation and apoptosis of CD4$^+$ T cells through MRs

To investigate the effects of cigarette smoking on the proliferation and apoptosis of CD4$^+$ T cells and Tregs, we carried out proliferation and apoptosis assays with PBT cells obtained from patients with SCOPD and healthy nonsmokers.

First, various concentrations of CSE were added to lymphocyte cultures (Fig. 7). CSE promoted the proliferation of CD4$^+$ T cells at a low concentration (0.033% = 0.1 μl of 100% CSE in 300 μl of medium in one well of a 96-well plate), while a high concentration

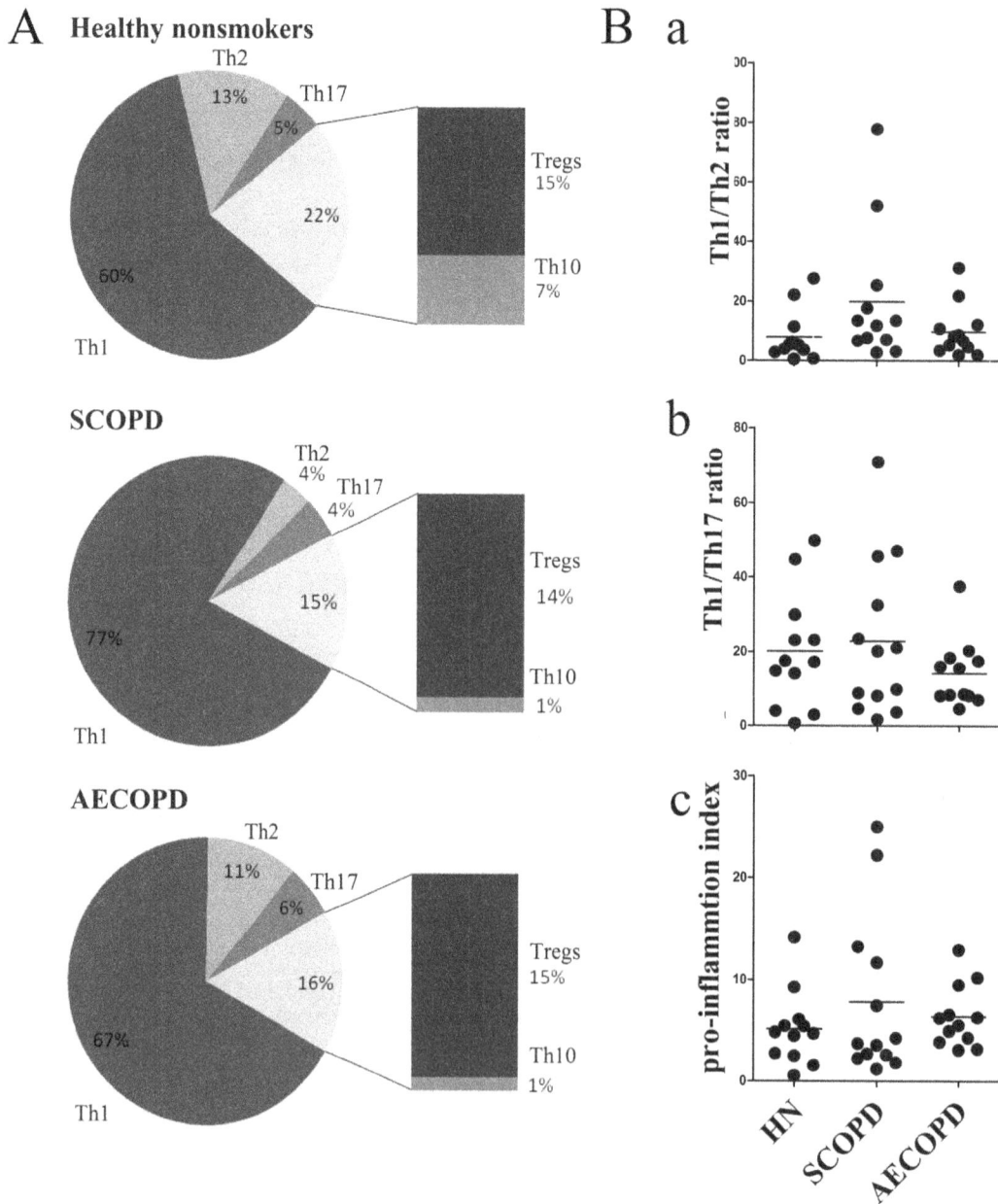

Figure 3. Comprehensive analyses of the relative percentages of CD4$^+$ T cell subsets. (A) The relative percentages of Th1, Th2, Th17, Treg and Th10 cells in healthy nonsmokers, patients with SCOPD and patients with AECOPD were calculated from their mean values. Anti-inflammatory CD4$^+$ T cells consisted of Tregs and Th10 cells. The data are presented in a pie graph. **(B)** The Th1/Th2 ratio (a), Th1/Th17 ratio (b), and pro-inflammatory index (c) in healthy nonsmokers (HN), patients with SCOPD and patients with AECOPD are presented, and the pro-inflammatory index was calculated by dividing the percentage of (Th1+Th2+Th17) by that of (Tregs and Th10).

of CSE had the opposite effect (Fig. 7Ba). Therefore, this low concentration of CSE was used in the proliferation assays, and the Ki-67 expression level was used to measure cellular proliferation (Fig. 7A). For the proliferation assays, we also found that various concentrations of CSE affected the apoptosis of CD4$^+$ T cells (Fig. 7Bb). CSE facilitated the apoptosis of CD4$^+$ T cells even at the concentration of 0.17%, and this pro-apoptotic effect increased at higher concentrations. Therefore, we selected this concentration of CSE to use in the apoptosis assays. PI-negative, Annexin V-positive cells were identified as apoptotic cells (Fig. 7A). In addition, we observed that Treg proliferation and apoptosis were increased compared with those of CD4$^+$ T cells. In addition, the

effects of CSE on Treg proliferation and apoptosis were similar to those observed in CD4$^+$ T cells. However, Tregs appear to be less sensitive to low concentrations of CSE.

3.1 CSE promotes the proliferation of CD4$^+$ T cells in healthy nonsmokers and facilitates the apoptosis of CD4$^+$ T cells in patients with SCOPD. As shown in Figure 8, CSE and mAChR agonists strikingly promoted the proliferation of CD4$^+$ T cells (excluding CD3$^+$CD8$^-$Foxp3$^+$ T cells) from healthy nonsmokers and patients with SCOPD. Additionally, this pro-proliferative effect could be neutralized with the mAChR antagonist atropine. We also noted that atropine inhibited the

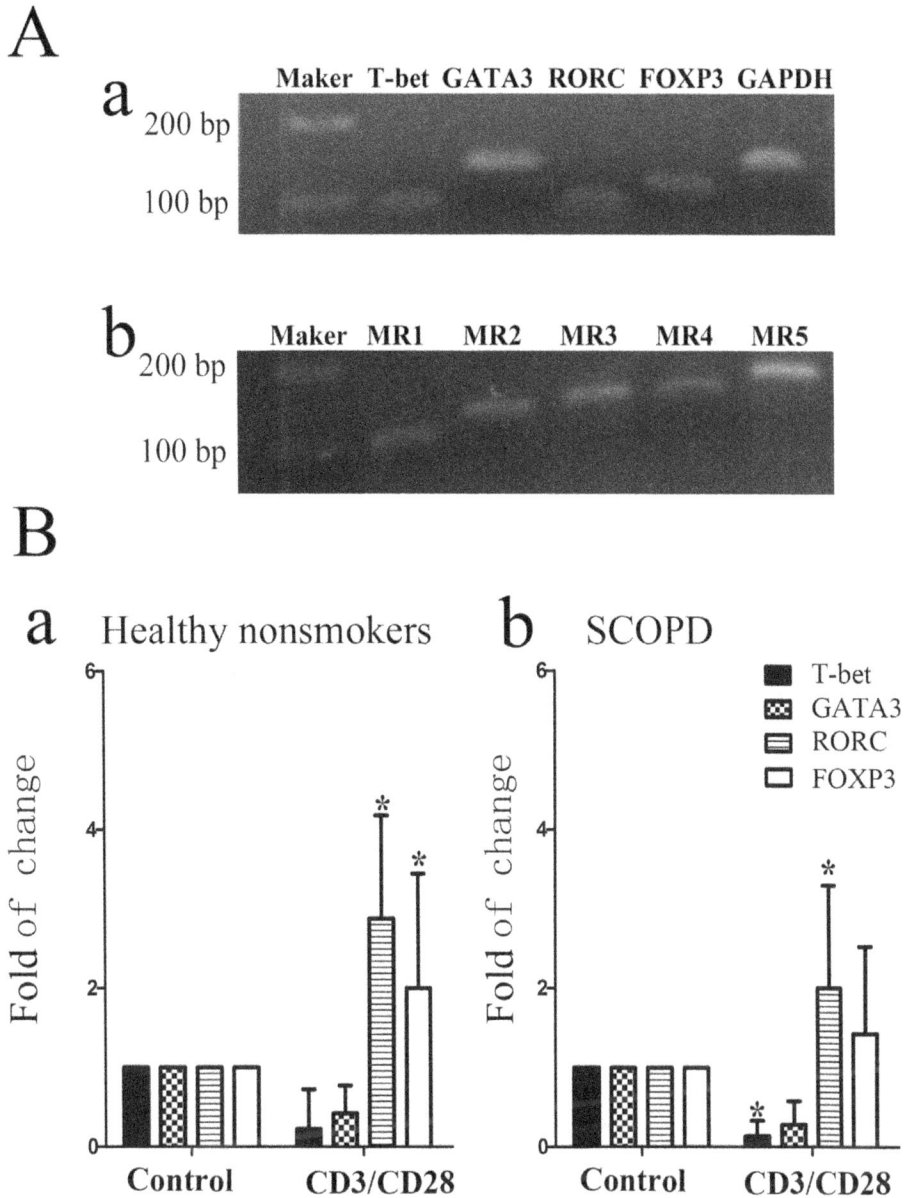

Figure 4. T-bet, GATA3, RORC, FOXP3, and mAChR (MR1–5) mRNA expression in human T cells. (A) Nuclear transcription factors (T-bet, GATA3, RORC, and FOXP3) and mAChR (MR1–5) mRNA expression in T cells was confirmed by PCR. **(B)** PBT cells from the healthy nonsmokers (**a**) or patients with SCOPD (**b**) were analyzed either immediately upon isolation or after stimulation with anti-CD3 and anti-CD28 Abs for 5 days, as detailed in the Materials and Methods. The data from 7 independent experiments are expressed as the mean ± SD of the mRNA in question relative to that in unstimulated T cells (control), which is taken as 1. The comparisons were determined by the Kruskal-Wallis one-way analysis of variance on ranks. *P< 0.05 compared with the relevant control.

proliferation of $CD4^+$ T cells, and this effect was less significant in patients with SCOPD.

In regards to apoptosis, CSE facilitated the apoptosis of $CD4^+$ T cells (excluding $CD3^+$ $CD8^-CD25^{++}$ T cells) from patients with SCOPD but not healthy nonsmokers. Moreover, the activation of mAChRs by muscarine reduced the apoptosis of $CD4^+$ T cells in healthy nonsmokers, and this effect could be completely abolished by treatment with the antagonist atropine (Fig. 9).

In addition, further analysis indicated that CSE promoted the proliferation and inhibited the apoptosis of $CD4^+$ T cells in healthy nonsmokers, while modestly facilitating apoptosis in cells from patients with SCOPD (Table 3).

3.2 CSE significantly promotes the apoptosis of Tregs from patients with SCOPD. We further analyzed the proliferation of $CD3^+CD8^-Foxp3^+$ Tregs (Fig. 7A). As indicated in Figure 10, CSE and the mAChR agonist did not significantly affect the proliferation of Tregs in either the healthy nonsmokers or patients with SCOPD. However, stimulation of mAChRs with the agonist muscarine led to the enhanced proliferation of Tregs in healthy nonsmokers but not in patients with SCOPD; furthermore, treatment with the antagonist could counteract this effect.

Considering that the cell membrane must be intact when measuring apoptosis with PI and Annexin V, we used $CD3^+CD8^-CD25^{++}$ as an expression signature for Tregs

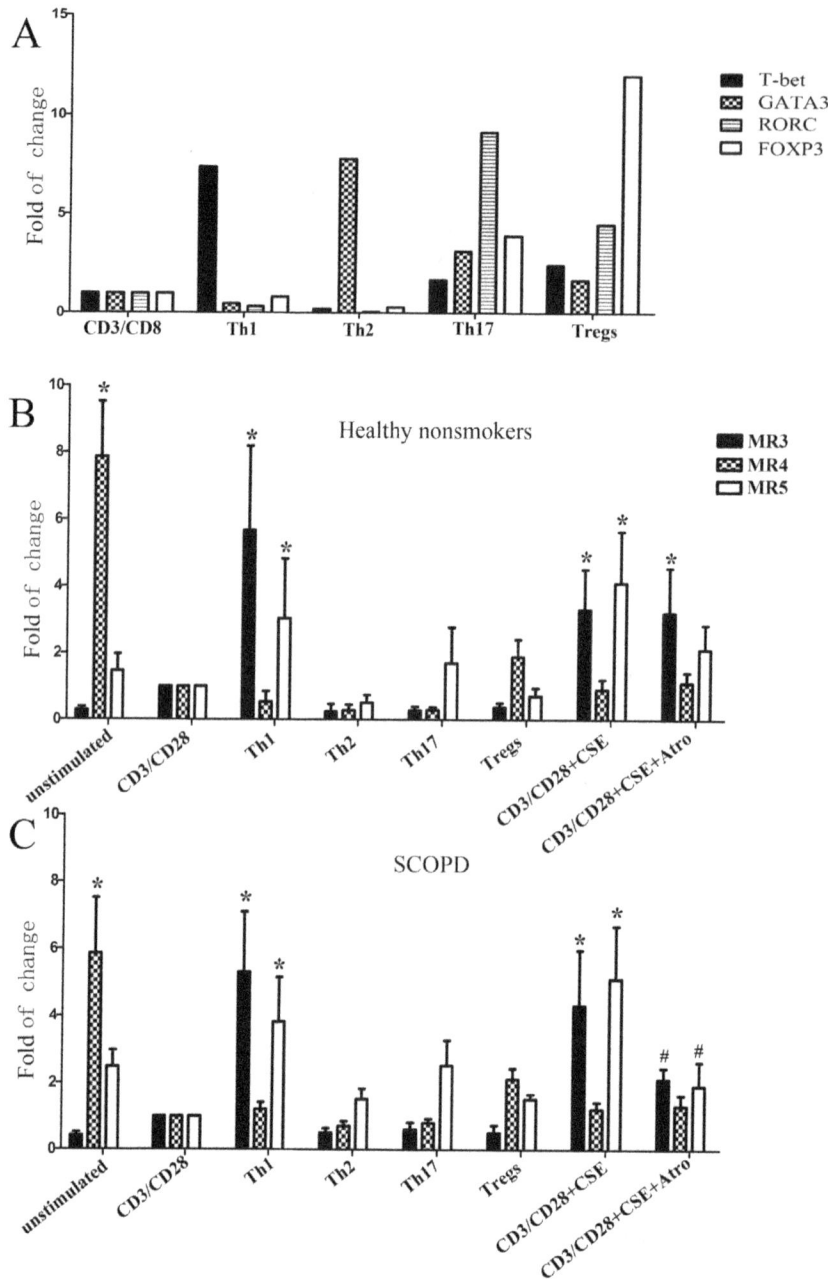

Figure 5. The mAChR subtype changes with polarization into different T cell subsets. PBT cells from healthy nonsmokers (**B**) or patients with SCOPD (**C**) were cultured in conditioned media for polarization towards the Th1, Th2, Th17 and Treg lineages or in the presence of CSE with or without a mAChRs antagonist, and the polarized cells were analyzed by qPCR for the relative levels of mAChR (MR3, MR4, and MR5) mRNA. (**A**) The polarization of T cells was confirmed by the expression of specific nuclear transcription factor mRNA. The data from 7 independent experiments are expressed as the mean ± SD of the mRNA in question relative to that in stimulated T cells (CD3/CD28), which was set as 1. The comparisons were determined by the Kruskal-Wallis one-way analysis of variance on ranks. *P<0.05 compared with the relevant control. #P<0.05 compared with CD3/CD28 plus CSE.

(Fig. 7A). As shown in Figure 11, CSE promoted the apoptosis of Tregs in patients with SCOPD, and the mAChR antagonist could not completely neutralize this effect. Moreover, stimulating mAChRs did not significantly affect the apoptosis of Tregs in these two groups.

Our analysis showed that CSE modestly facilitates the proliferation and inhibits the apoptosis of Treg cells in healthy nonsmokers when used at a low concentration, whereas it

significantly promotes apoptosis in cells obtained from patients with SCOPD (Table 3).

Discussion

Alterations of T subsets in the three patient groups

Early and recent studies have demonstrated that abnormalities in the immune system play a major role in the development of COPD [18,19]. In particular, decreased numbers of CD4⁺ T cells

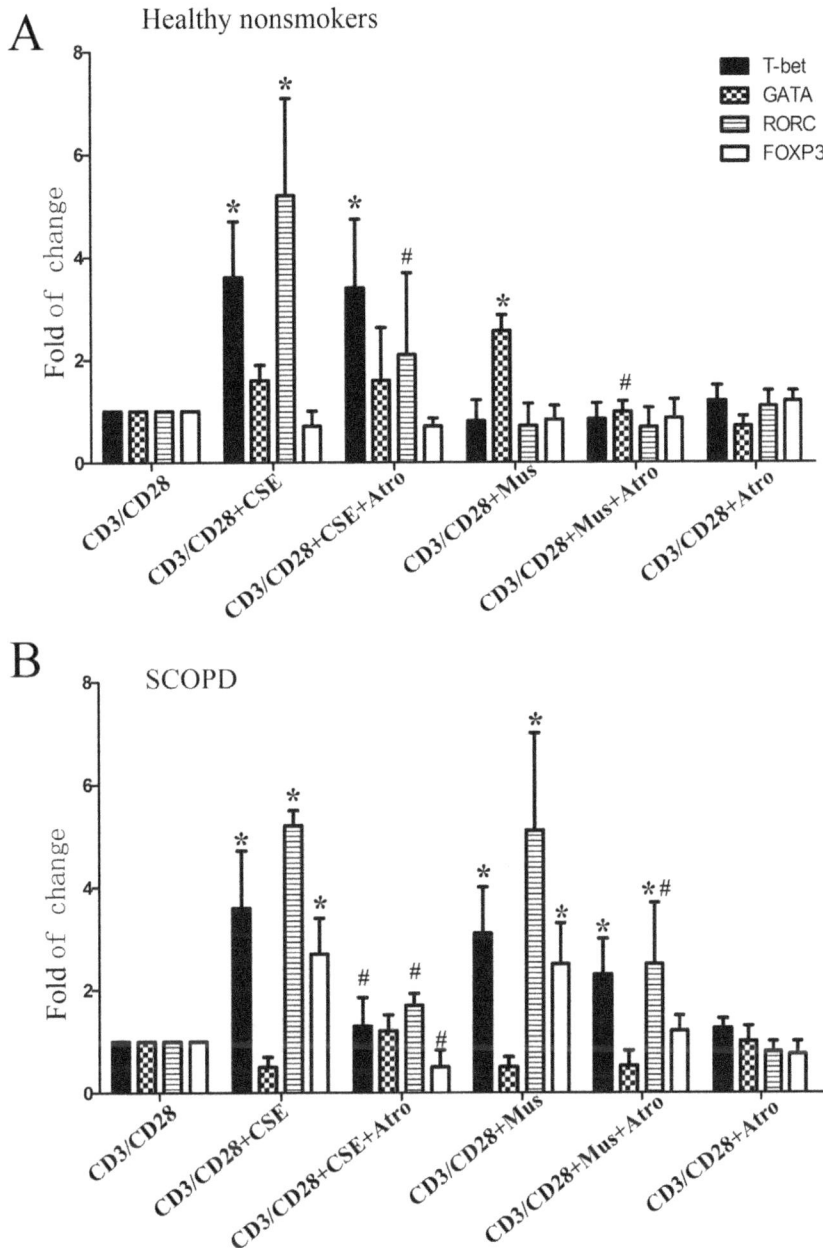

Figure 6. MRs and CSE affect the expression of T cell subset nuclear transcription factors. PBT cells from healthy nonsmokers (**A**) or patients with SCOPD (**B**) were cultured and stimulated with anti-CD3 and anti-CD28 Abs in the presence of CSE, mAChR agonist/antagonist, or combinations of these factors (*as shown in bottom panels*). The agonist and antagonist of mAChRs were muscarine (Mus) and atropine (Atro), respectively. After 5 days in culture, the cells were harvested, and the total RNA was extracted. The expression levels of nuclear transcription factor mRNA, namely that of T-bet, GATA3, RORC, and FOXP3, were detected by qPCR, with GAPDH serving as an internal control. The data from 7 independent experiments are expressed as the mean ± SD of the mRNA in question relative to that in unstimulated T cells (controls), which was set as 1. The comparisons were determined by the Kruskal-Wallis one-way analysis of variance on ranks.*P<0.05 compared with the relevant control. # P<0.05 compared with CD3/CD28 plus CSE or CD3/CD28 plus Muscarine (Mus).

and CD8[+] T cells and a decreased ratio of CD4[+]/CD8[+] T cells with an abnormal ratio of T helper cells/Tregs and Th17/Tregs have been observed in the peripheral blood in patients with COPD [20]. This reported diversity likely originates from the heterogeneity of peripheral blood T cells in patients with COPD.

Our data indicate that different stages of COPD present disparate alterations in the subsets of T cells and Tregs in the peripheral blood. A remarkable increase in the percentage of Th1 cells with a prominent decrease in the percentage of Th2 cells was observed in patients with SCOPD. In addition, a small increase in the percentage of Th17 cells and an imbalance of Th1/Th2 cells were observed in these patients. Therefore, our data are consistent with previous reports that indicate that COPD is a disease that is predominantly characterized by Th1 responses [21], which is consistent with increased levels of IFN-γ in the airways. Therefore, these features of systemic inflammation in both the local airway and peripheral blood distinguish COPD from asthma, which predominantly involves Th2 responses.

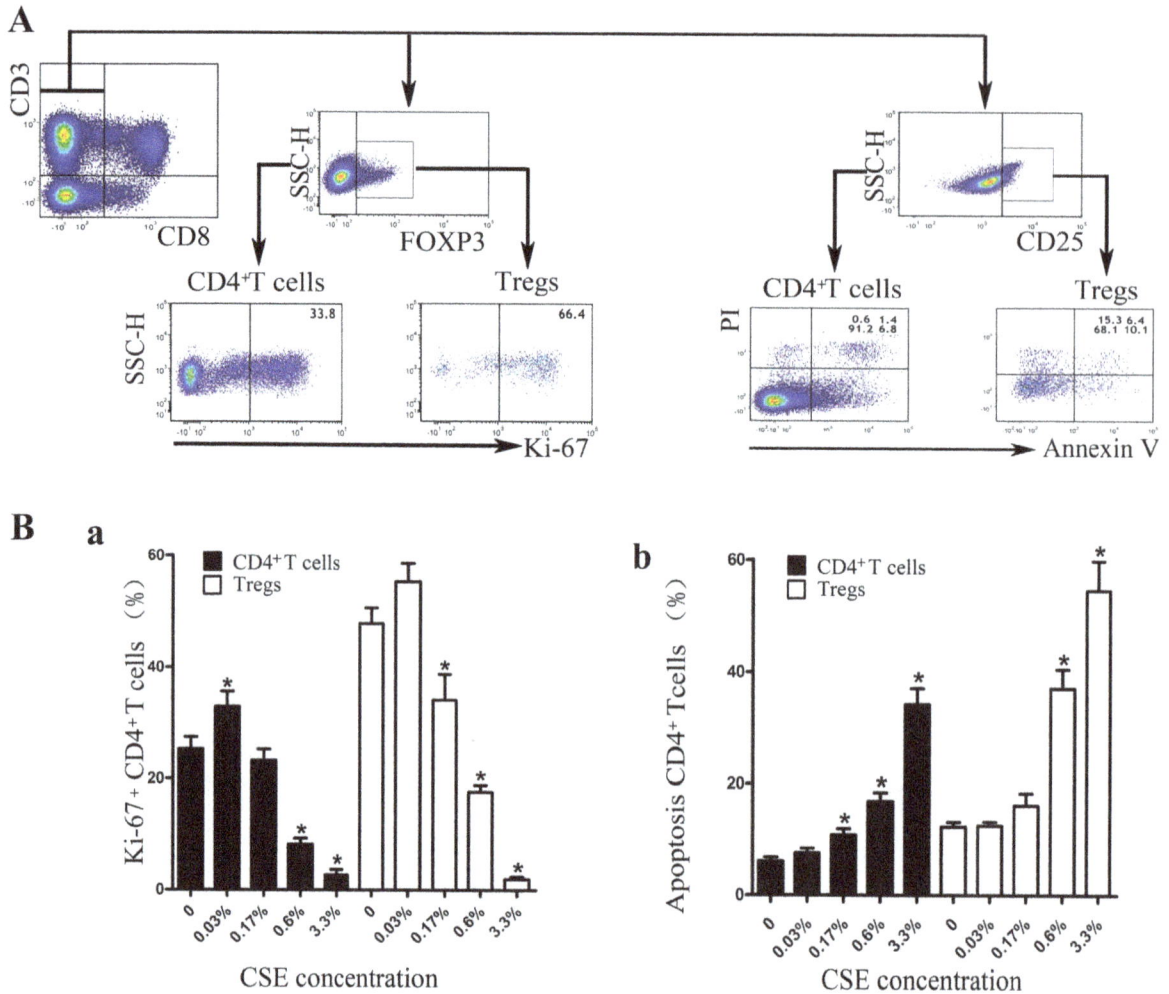

Figure 7. CSE affects the proliferative response and apoptosis of CD4$^+$ T cells/Tregs. (A) Representative dot-plots showing the analysis strategy. In the proliferation assays, Tregs were gated from CD4$^+$T cells (*CD3$^+$CD8$^-$*) by their positive expression of Foxp3. Then, the expression levels of Ki-67 by CD4$^+$T cells and Treg cells were further analyzed. However, in the apoptosis assays, Tregs were gated from CD4$^+$T cells (*CD3$^+$CD8$^-$*) by the high expression of CD25. Then, the apoptosis of CD4$^+$T cells and Tregs was further analyzed. **(B)** Various concentrations (0.03%, 0.17%, 0.6% and 3.3%) of CSE were cultured with T cells (PHA and PMA were added in the proliferation assays) for 5 days; then, the expression of Ki-67 was determined by flow cytometry in the proliferation assays (a), while the expression of Annexin V and PI was determined in the apoptosis assays (b). The results are reported as the mean ± SEM from 5 independent experiments. The comparisons were determined by the Kruskal-Wallis one-way analysis of variance on ranks. *P<0.05 compared with control.

For patients with AECOPD, the inflammatory outburst is mainly due to infection, which leads to a substantial increase in Th1, Th2 and Th17 cells compared to that observed in healthy nonsmokers. Th17 cells play a significant role in pro-inflammatory immune responses against pathogens, and increases in Th1 and Th2 cells facilitate normal immune functions that are similar to those in healthy individuals.

By contrast, we found that the ratio of Th1/Th17 cells was even lower in patients with COPD than healthy controls, which implies that there is an insufficient immune-inflammatory reaction that likely develops into chronic inflammation.

The anti-inflammatory role of the pathogenesis of COPD has attracted increasing attention since the discovery of Tregs. Indeed, different lesion locations in COPD show a variety of changes in the quantity and function of Tregs [22]. Our observations revealed a small increase in the percentage of Tregs, a reduction in the percentage of Th10 cells and a conspicuous decrease in percentage of Th10 cells in the peripheral blood of patients with

SCOPD. In summary, the anti-inflammatory response is decreased in patients with SCOPD compared to healthy nonsmokers. Furthermore, there were more Tregs in patients with AECOPD than in healthy nonsmokers and patients with SCOPD; nevertheless, the percentage of Th10 cells was significantly reduced (accompanied by a decrease in the percentage of α-7+ T cells.) compared to healthy nonsmokers but higher than that in patients with SCOPD.

Our data illustrate the role of Treg cell expansion in AECOPD, which we posit is a compensatory reaction in response to inflammation, as Treg differentiation can be induced by LPS [23] and there is plasticity between Th17 cells and Tregs [24]. Moreover, we demonstrated that the MR4 and MR5 are the major MRs expressed by Tregs and Th17 cells, respectively. This result indicates that ACh could serve as a differentiation regulator in the local inflammatory environment.

Th10 cells can produce IL-10, which decreases the number of Tregs and induces the proliferation of Tr1 cells [25]. Due to

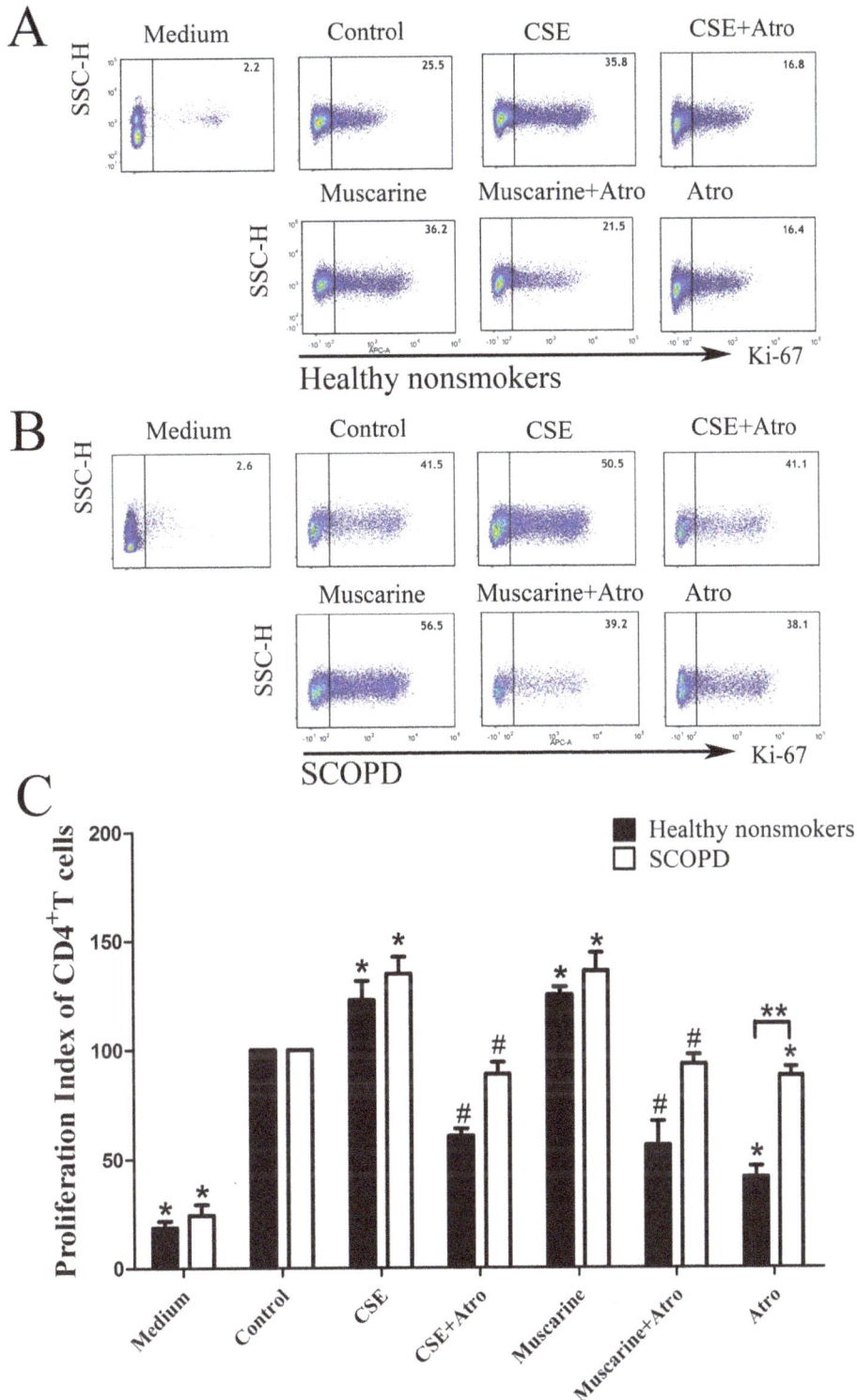

Figure 8. Effects of CSE and MRs on the proliferative response of CD4⁺ T cells. (**A, B**) T cells from healthy nonsmokers and patients with SCOPD were cultured in the presence of CSE, mAChR agonist/antagonist, or combinations of these factors (*top panels*) under stimulation with PMA and PHA for 5 days. Ki-67⁺CD4⁺T cells (*excluding Tregs*) were determined by flow cytometry, and the representative flow cytometric dot-plots are shown. (**C**) The proliferation index was calculated by dividing the percentage of Ki-67⁺CD4⁺ T cells of various groups by the percentage of Ki-67⁺CD4⁺T cells stimulated with PMA and PHA alone, and the proliferation index of control was considered to be 100. Comparisons of the proliferation of CD4⁺T cells from the healthy nonsmokers (*solid bars*) or patients with SCOPD (*open bars*) in various trial groups were made; the results are reported as the mean ± SEM from 5 independent experiments. The comparisons were determined by the Kruskal-Wallis one-way analysis of variance on ranks or Mann-Whitney U test. *P<0.05 compared with control, **P<0.05 in the comparison between healthy nonsmokers and patients with SCOPD. # P< 0.05 indicates CSE plus Atro compared with CSE alone and Muscarine plus Atro compared with Muscarine alone.

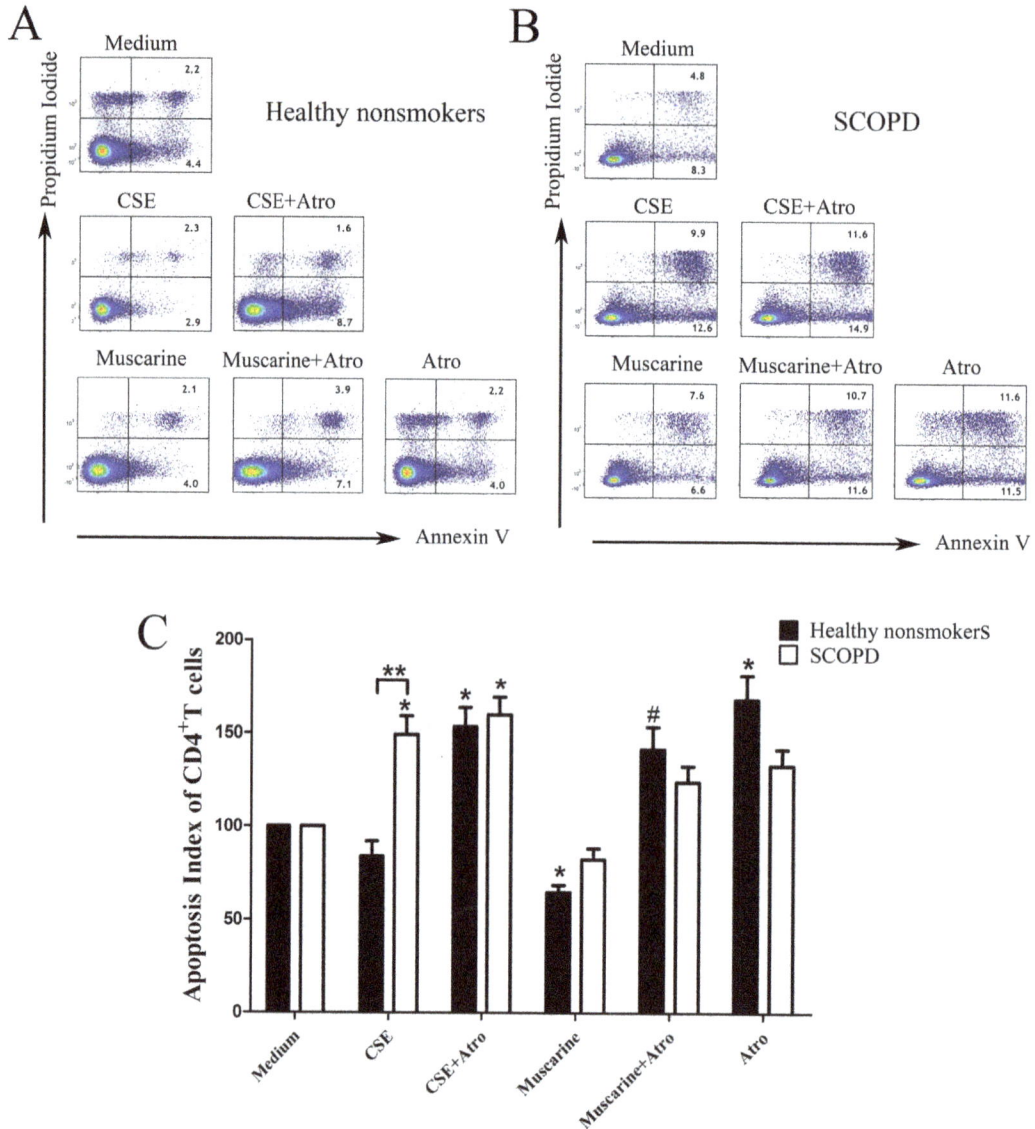

Figure 9. Effects of CSE and MRs on the apoptosis of CD4⁺ T cells. T cells from healthy nonsmokers and patients with SCOPD were cultured in the presence of medium alone, CSE, mAChR agonist/antagonist or combinations of these factors (*top panels*) for 5 days. (**A, B**) The representative flow cytometric dot-plots show Annexin V/PI co-staining for the identification of apoptotic CD4⁺ T cells. (**C**) The apoptosis index was calculated by dividing the percentage of apoptotic CD4⁺ T cells in various groups by the percentage of apoptotic CD4⁺ T cells in the medium alone, and the proliferation index of the controls was 100. Comparing the apoptotic CD4⁺T (*excluding Tregs*) cells from healthy nonsmokers (*solid bars*) or patients with SCOPD (*open bars*) in each group, the results were reported as the mean ± SEM from 5 independent experiments. The comparisons were determined by the Kruskal-Wallis one-way analysis of variance on ranks or Mann-Whitney U test. *P<0.05 compared with control, **P<0.05 comparison between healthy nonsmokers and patients with SCOPD. # P<0.05 indicates CSE plus Atro compared with CSE alone and Muscarine plus Atro compared with Muscarine alone.

Table 3. The net effect of CSE on the survival of CD4⁺ T cells and Tregs.

		Proliferation index	Apoptosis index	Total effect
Healthy nonsmokers	**CD4⁺ T cells**	122.9	83.8	Significantly promote proliferation and inhibit apoptosis
	Tregs	115.9	90.9	Modestly promote proliferation and inhibit apoptosis
SCOPD	**CD4⁺ T cells**	134.9	149.2	Modestly facilitate apoptosis
	Tregs	109.3	154.8	Significantly facilitate apoptosis

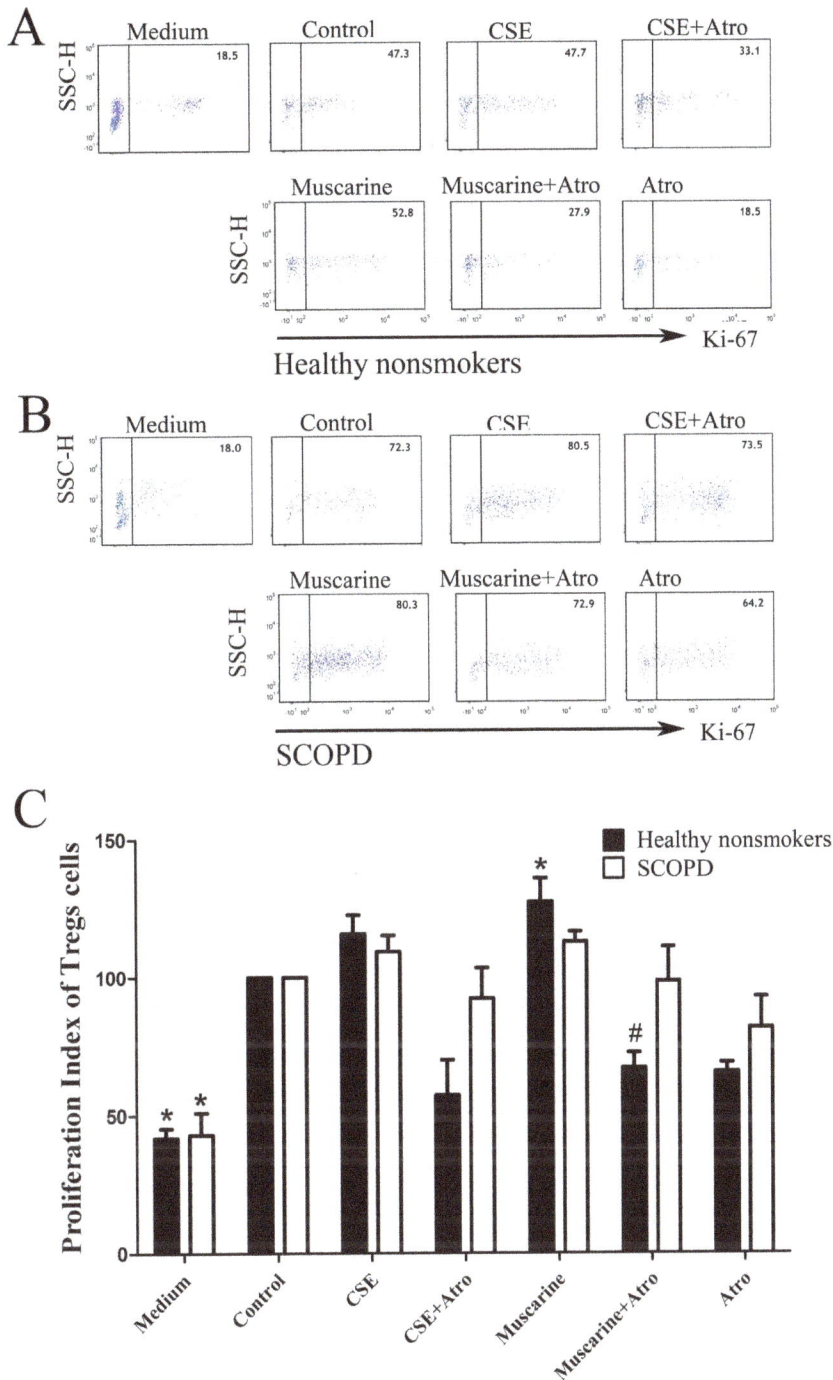

Figure 10. Effects of CSE and MRs on the proliferative response of Tregs. (A, B) The proliferation of Tregs was further analyzed by flow cytometry, and the representative flow cytometric dot-plots are shown. **(C)** The proliferation index was calculated by dividing the percentage of Ki-67+Tregs cells of various groups by the percentage of Ki-67+Tregs cells under the stimulation of PMA and PHA alone, and the proliferation index of controls was considered 100. Comparisons of the proliferation of Tregs from the healthy nonsmokers (*solid bars*) or patients with SCOPD (*open bars*) in various trial groups were made; the results were reported as the mean ± SEM from 5 independent experiments. The comparisons were determined by the Kruskal-Wallis one-way analysis of variance on ranks or the Mann-Whitney U test. *P<0.05 compared with control, **P<0.05 for the comparison between healthy nonsmokers and patients with SCOPD. # P<0.05 indicates CSE plus Atro compared with CSE; Muscarine plus Atro compared with Muscarine.

technical issues, CD4+CD25+Foxp3+IL-10+ T cells could hardly be detected in our experiments; however, the increased percentage of Tregs and the decreased percentage of Th10 cells reveal the possibility of the down-regulation of Treg or Tr1 cell activities in the context of COPD. This result was in accordance with an *in vitro* experiment indicating impaired Treg function in COPD patients [26]. In addition, an imbalance between the anti-

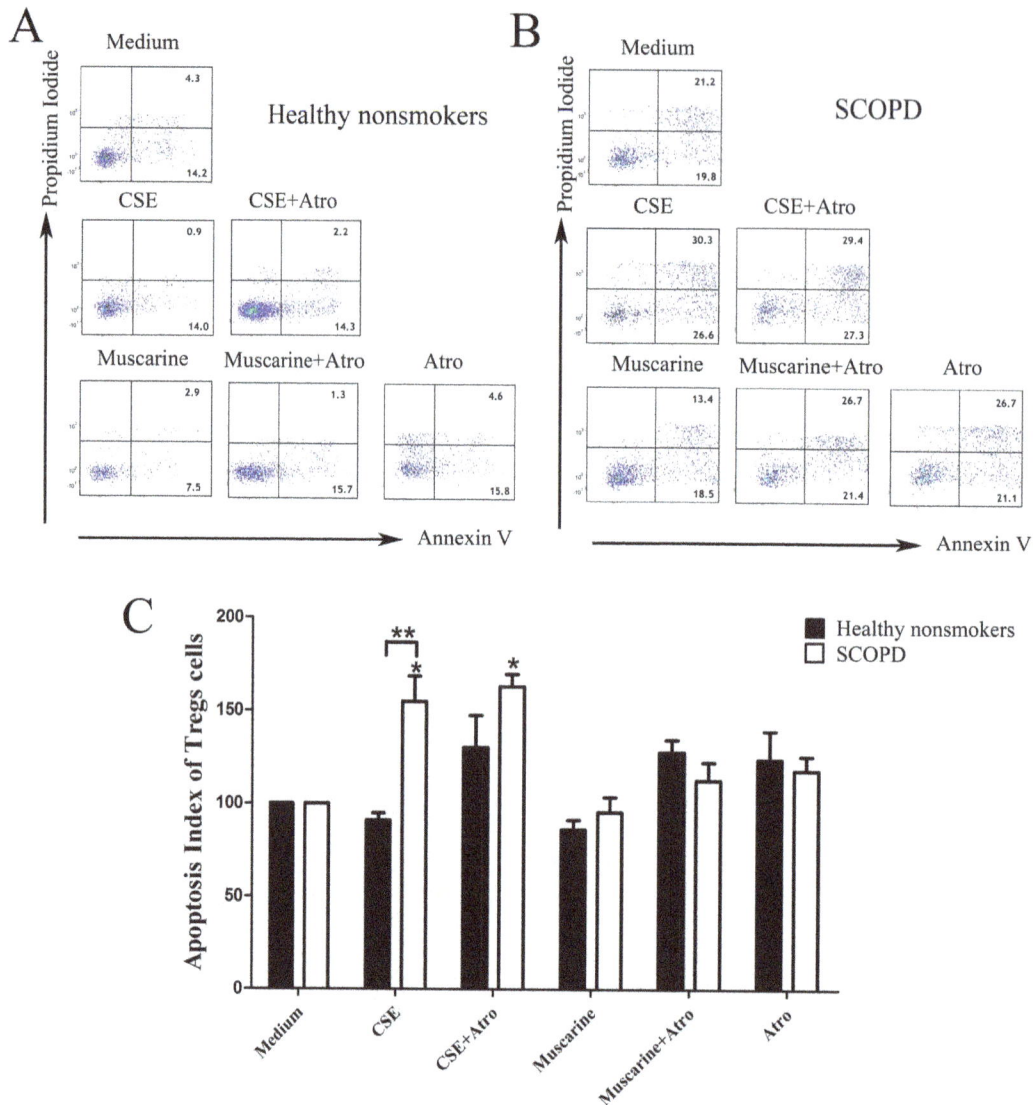

Figure 11. Effects of CSE and MRs on the apoptosis of Tregs. (A, B) The apoptosis of Tregs was further analyzed by flow cytometry, and the representative flow cytometric dot-plots were shown. (C) The apoptosis index was calculated by dividing the percentage of apoptotic Tregs from various groups by the percentage of apoptotic Treg cells in the medium alone, and the apoptosis index of controls was considered to be 100. Comparisons of the apoptosis of Tregs from the healthy nonsmokers (*solid bars*) or patients with SCOPD (*open bars*) in the various trial groups were made. The results are reported as the mean ± SEM from 5 independent experiments. The comparisons were determined by the Kruskal-Wallis one-way analysis of variance on ranks or Mann-Whitney U test. *P<0.05 compared with control, **P<0.05 comparison between healthy nonsmokers and patients with SCOPD. # P<0.05 indicates CSE plus Atro compared with CSE alone and Muscarine plus Atro compared with Muscarine alone.

inflammatory and pro-inflammatory subsets of Tregs was noted in COPD patients [27].

There are various subtypes of nicotinic acetylcholine receptors expressed on the surface of T cells, and these receptors have a series of complex functions [28]. The high expression of the α-7 subtype can inhibit Th1 and Th17 responses, leading to the induction of Treg in inflammatory bowel disease. In contrast, smoking downregulates the α-7 nicotinic receptor and decreases the levels of IL-10 and Tregs [29,30]. Both observations show the anti-inflammatory function of the α-7 nicotinic receptor; however, the expression of the α-7 nicotinic receptor in PBT cells of patients with COPD remains unclear. To the best of our knowledge, this is the first report of the expression of the α-7 nicotinic receptor in T cells from patients with COPD. Our results match the features of the T cell subsets of COPD, particularly SCOPD, wherein the

Th1 response dominates the microenvironment, which is followed by increasing levels of IFN-γ and IL-12. The subdued Th2 response leads to a reduction in IL-4, which results in lower expression of the α-7 nicotinic receptor. A stronger Th1 response has been correlated with a further reduction in the expression of the α-7 nicotinic receptor, which is more pronounced in patients with AECOPD. In addition, the variation of α-7 T cells is different from that of Tregs and may be related to the diversity in the expression of MRs between Th and Treg cells, although further studies are needed to clarify these findings.

The extent of inflammation depends on the battle between pro-inflammatory and anti-inflammatory forces, and the balance of Th1/Th2, CD4/CD8, and Th17/Treg cells has been proposed as the foundation of the immune response. The emergence of novel technology makes it possible to analyze new subtypes of T cells, such as the nicotinic α-7[+] T cells. In general, the balance of pro-inflammatory factors and anti-inflammatory factors has been shown to play a major role in inflammation. The balances of the Th1/Th2, CD4/CD8 and Th17/Treg ratios are mainly controlled by Th1, CD8[+] and Th17 [20,21], respectively. As shown in Fig. 3, our results suggest that there are minor Th1/Th2 and Th1/Th17 alterations in patients with COPD compared to healthy controls; however, the small number of cases examined may have biased the results.

The pro-inflammatory index is simply defined by the ratio of the percentage of Th1, Th2, and Th17 cells to that of Treg and Th10 cells. We observed an increase in the pro-inflammatory index in patients with AECOPD and in patients with SCOPD, with a higher increase found in patients with SCOPD, which indicates that the characteristics of inflammation in patients with SCOPD are pro-inflammatory and that the Th1 response occupies the dominant role without influencing inflammatory compensation. Nevertheless, an intense Th1 response causes damage to the lung and airway tissue instead of resisting infection. Therefore, inhaled corticosteroids may reduce the local differentiation of CD4[+] and CD8[+] T cells and the production of IFN-γ, thereby mitigating local inflammation and suppressing the immune response in patients with SCOPD [5].

The MR system and the effect of CSE on COPD

Early studies on lymphocytes in the extra neuronal cholinergic system primarily focused on the expression of mAChRs and nAChRs [31,32,33]. MR3 has also been reported in patients with COPD [14,29], but the expression of MRs in subsets of T cells in patients with COPD remains unknown. As shown in Fig. 4, our study is the first to show that MR3 and MR5 are mainly expressed in Th1 and Th17 cells, respectively. In Treg cells, MR4 was dominantly expressed, with a minor expression level of M5. Additionally, we detected the expression of MR5 in Th2 cells. More importantly, CSE not only enhanced the expression of MR3 and MR5 in human lymphocytes but was also inhibited by the M receptor blocker atropine. This blocking effect reached a statistically significant level in patients with SCOPD without exerting an obvious effect on MR4, which differs from murine splenic T cells that mainly expresses MR1 and MR5 [34]. However, MR1, MR3 and MR5 all facilitated cellular proliferation.

In the process T cell subset differentiation, muscarine chiefly induces a Th2 response in healthy individuals that can be blocked by atropine; however, it also induces the proliferation of Th1, Th17 and Treg cells in patients with COPD. Although atropine can restrain this proliferation, an obvious inhibitory effect could only be observed on Th17 cells. This result indicates that the M receptor could also promote the differentiation Th1 and Th17 cells, which forms a positive feedback loop between the M receptor and the induced differentiation of Th cells. Our study is the first to report this finding.

In our study, CSE induced the differentiation and proliferation of Th1, Th17 and Treg cells in both healthy controls and patients with COPD. Furthermore, these processes could be partially inhibited by atropine; the SCOPD group showed a significant inhibition of these processes by atropine. These results verify that the expression of MR1 and MR5 can be induced by CSE, thus promoting the differentiation of Th1 and Th17 cells. Hence, for the first time, we report positive feedback between Th1/Th17 cells and the expression of MR1/MR5 in patients with COPD. In both trials, there were no significant alterations in Th2 cells or MR4 expression, which is consistent with our previous report of the use of an MR3 receptor blocker, tiotropium bromide, to treat patients

with COPD [35]. The proportion of CD4[+] and CD25[+] decreases remarkably after the blockage of MR3, i.e., the differentiation of Th1 and Th17 was inhibited, which is in line with recent reports [36].

Our results disagree with those in murine splenic T cells [34], which is mainly due to differences between species. Murine spleens mostly express MR1 and MR5 with scarce expression of MR3. Our data verify that Th1 cells in humans express MR3 and MR5, whereas the expression of MR3, MR4 and MR5 was rare in Th2 cells. Following stimulation by muscarine, the Th2 response becomes dominant, although this effect could be inhibited by atropine. These observations are in agreement with earlier reports showing dominant expression of Th2 cells in the fetus of women who smoked during pregnancy [37]. However, the increases in the proportion of Th1, Th17 and Treg cells caused by stimulation with muscarine seemed to be more prominent in patients with COPD, which was different from that observed in healthy groups. Based on our results, this difference may be due to lack of the α7 nicotinic receptor in patients with COPD.

Influence of CSE on the proliferation and apoptosis of CD4[+] Th/Tregs

The data presented in Fig. 8 show that muscarine significantly promoted the proliferation of CD4[+]T cells in both healthy nonsmokers and patients with SCOPD by activating the mAChRs, and the pro-proliferation effect could be neutralized by atropine. Thus, activation or hyperfunction of mAChRs leads to the enhanced proliferation of CD4[+] T cells. CSE could similarly facilitate the proliferation of CD4[+]T cells in both groups, and the pro-proliferation effect could also be counteracted by atropine, indicating that CSE may affect the proliferation of CD4[+]T cells through the muscarine system. Previous research demonstrated a cholinergic system in lymphocytes, and muscarine was shown to promote the proliferation of the CD4[+] T cells by enhancing the production of IL-2 [38]. Subsequently, a study reported that both muscarinic and nicotinic receptors regulate the proliferation and apoptosis of CD4[+] T cells in animals and humans [39,40]. With respect to the current knowledge, our study is the first to show that CSE could facilitate the proliferation of CD4[+] T cells through up-regulating the muscarine system, thereby aggravating the inflammation present in the airways of patients with COPD.

Our data also show that muscarine could inhibit the apoptosis of CD4[+]T cells in healthy nonsmokers (Fig. 9), while atropine had an opposing pro-apoptotic effect, demonstrating that activation of mAChRs could reduce the apoptosis of CD4+ T cells. Interestingly, CSE promoted the apoptosis of CD4+T cells from patients with SCOPD but not in healthy nonsmokers, and this effect could not be neutralized by atropine. CSE-induced apoptosis is potentially mediated by a variety of mechanisms, including increased oxidative stress, Bax protein accumulation, mitochondrial dysfunction, mitochondrial cytochrome c release and NF-κB inhibition [41,42,43,44,45,46]. It is unknown why CD4[+] T cells from healthy nonsmokers and patients with SCOPD react differently to CSE with respect to apoptosis. However, we speculate that CD4[+] T cells may present alterations during the development of the disease, such as enhanced reactivity to oxidative stress, up-regulation of receptors that are sensitive to apoptosis or down-regulation of receptors with inhibitory functions, resulting in a distinct apoptotic response.

We found that the MR system had a pro-proliferative effect on Tregs in healthy nonsmokers, which could be blocked by atropine (Fig. 10), suggesting a reliance of Tregs on mAChRs. However, this phenomenon was not obvious in patients with COPD, who showed no responses to muscarine and atropine; the reason for these differences is not yet known but is potentially related to the reduction of nicotinic receptor α-7 expression. Additionally, CSE only modestly, but not significantly, enhanced the proliferation of Tregs in healthy nonsmokers and patients with SCOPD, and this effect could not be offset by atropine. As a result, the MR system may not have pro-proliferative effects on Tregs in patients with SCOPD.

Our results imply that neither muscarine nor atropine significantly affect the apoptosis of Tregs (Fig. 11). Therefore, the muscarine system may not be involved in the apoptosis of Tregs. However, CSE robustly promoted the apoptosis of Tregs in patients with SCOPD, and atropine could not completely reverse this effect, indicating that CSE induces the apoptosis of these cells without affecting the muscarine system. The following potential mechanisms may explain these findings: 1) oxidative stress, 2) poisonous substances contained in CSE, and 3) abnormal alterations in the Tregs of patients with SCOPD. Considering that apoptosis of Tregs from healthy nonsmokers was not affected by CSE, there may be substantial changes in these cells during the development of COPD. Taken together, our data indicate that CSE modestly facilitates the proliferation and inhibits the apoptosis of Tregs in healthy nonsmokers, but it also significantly promotes apoptosis in cells from patients with SCOPD. Further studies are needed to clarify the mechanisms underlying the different reactions to CSE in different populations.

In summary, our current research identifies an imbalance of pro/anti-inflammatory CD4$^+$ T subsets in patients with COPD, with increased percentages of Th17 cells (only in AECOPD) and Th1 cells and reduced percentages of Th2 cells (only in SCOPD) and Th10 cells, as well as a reduced quantity and impaired capacity of Tregs. Our study is the first to report the expression of MRs in T cell subsets from the peripheral blood in these three patient groups, and our results reveal a positive feedback loop between the MR and the induced differentiation of Th cells. We also speculate there is a lack of α-7 nicotinic receptor expression in patients with COPD. The different reactions to smoke observed in our study indicate that there are differences in the genetic sensitivity between healthy individuals and patients with COPD, although further studies need to be conducted to acquire a full explanation of these interesting phenomena.

Acknowledgments

We thank Liang Shi for excellent flow cytometric assistance; Zhi-jian Ye, Ming-Li Yuan and Wen Yin for helpful suggestions and discussion; Xia Yang and Dan Yang for assistance in patient recruitment; and Xiao-Nan Tao for administrative support.

Author Contributions

Conceived and designed the experiments: XZX. Performed the experiments: MQZ YW. Analyzed the data: YJ LC GC. Contributed reagents/materials/analysis tools: JBX JCZ. Wrote the paper: JBX JCZ.

References

1. Hogg JC, Chu F, Utokaparch S, Woods R, Elliott WM, et al. (2004) The nature of small-airway obstruction in chronic obstructive pulmonary disease. N Engl J Med 350: 2645–2653.

2. Barnes PJ, Shapiro SD, Pauwels RA (2003) Chronic obstructive pulmonary disease: molecular and cellular mechanisms. Eur Respir J 22: 672–688.

3. Saetta M, Di Stefano A, Maestrelli P, Ferraresso A, Drigo R, et al. (1993) Activated T-lymphocytes and macrophages in bronchial mucosa of subjects with chronic bronchitis. Am Rev Respir Dis 147: 301–306.

4. Glader P, von Wachenfeldt K, Lofdahl CG (2006) Systemic CD4+ T-cell activation is correlated with FEV1 in smokers. Respir Med 100: 1088–1093.

5. Zhu X, Gadgil AS, Givelber R, George MP, Stoner MW, et al. (2009) Peripheral T cell functions correlate with the severity of chronic obstructive pulmonary disease. J Immunol 182: 3270–3277.

6. Glader P, Moller S, Lilja J, Wieslander E, Lofdahl CG, et al. (2006) Cigarette smoke extract modulates respiratory defence mechanisms through effects on T-cells and airway epithelial cells. Respir Med 100: 818–827.

7. Vassallo R, Tamada K, Lau JS, Kroening PR, Chen L (2005) Cigarette smoke extract suppresses human dendritic cell function leading to preferential induction of Th-2 priming. J Immunol 175: 2684–2691.

8. Saetta M, Baraldo S, Corbino L, Turato G, Braccioni F, et al. (1999) CD8+ve cells in the lungs of smokers with chronic obstructive pulmonary disease. Am J Respir Crit Care Med 160: 711–717.

9. Grando SA, Kawashima K, Kirkpatrick CJ, Meurs H, Wessler I (2012) The non-neuronal cholinergic system: basic science, therapeutic implications and new perspectives. Life Sci 91: 969–972.

10. Fujii T, Takada-Takatori Y, Kawashima K (2008) Basic and clinical aspects of non-neuronal acetylcholine: expression of an independent, non-neuronal cholinergic system in lymphocytes and its clinical significance in immunotherapy. J Pharmacol Sci 106: 186–192.

11. Kawashima K, Fujii T, Moriwaki Y, Misawa H, Horiguchi K (2012) Reconciling neuronally and nonneuronally derived acetylcholine in the regulation of immune function. Ann N Y Acad Sci 1261: 7–17.

12. Gross NJ, Skorodin MS (1984) Role of the parasympathetic system in airway obstruction due to emphysema. N Engl J Med 311: 421–425.

13. Rabe KF, Hurd S, Anzueto A, Barnes PJ, Buist SA, et al. (2007) Global strategy for the diagnosis, management, and prevention of chronic obstructive pulmonary disease: GOLD executive summary. Am J Respir Crit Care Med 176: 532–555.

14. Profita M, Riccobono L, Montalbano AM, Bonanno A, Ferraro M, et al. (2012) In vitro anticholinergic drugs affect CD8+ peripheral blood T-cells apoptosis in COPD. Immunobiology 217: 345–353.

15. Inatsu A, Kogiso M, Jeschke MG, Asai A, Kobayashi M, et al. (2011) Lack of Th17 cell generation in patients with severe burn injuries. J Immunol 187: 2155–2161.

16. Pace E, Gagliardo R, Melis M, La Grutta S, Ferraro M, et al. (2004) Synergistic effects of fluticasone propionate and salmeterol on in vitro T-cell activation and apoptosis in asthma. J Allergy Clin Immunol 114: 1216–1223.

17. Blue ML, Janoff A (1978) Possible mechanisms of emphysema in cigarette smokers. Release of elastase from human polymorphonuclear leukocytes by cigarette smoke condensate in vitro. Am Rev Respir Dis 117: 317–325.

18. Wouters EF (2005) Local and systemic inflammation in chronic obstructive pulmonary disease. Proc Am Thorac Soc 2: 26–33.

19. Cosio MG, Saetta M, Agusti A (2009) Immunologic aspects of chronic obstructive pulmonary disease. N Engl J Med 360: 2445–2454.

20. Wang H, Ying H, Wang S, Gu X, Weng Y, et al. (2014) Imbalance of peripheral blood Th17 and Treg responses in patients with chronic obstructive pulmonary disease. Clin Respir J.

21. Hodge G, Nairn J, Holmes M, Reynolds PN, Hodge S (2007) Increased intracellular T helper 1 proinflammatory cytokine production in peripheral blood, bronchoalveolar lavage and intraepithelial T cells of COPD subjects. Clin Exp Immunol 150: 22–29.

22. Isajevs S, Taivans I, Strazda G, Kopeika U, Bukovskis M, et al. (2009) Decreased FOXP3 expression in small airways of smokers with COPD. Eur Respir J 33: 61–67.

23. D'Alessio FR, Tsushima K, Aggarwal NR, West EE, Willett MH, et al. (2009) CD4+CD25+Foxp3+ Tregs resolve experimental lung injury in mice and are present in humans with acute lung injury. J Clin Invest 119: 2898–2913.

24. Noack M, Miossec P (2014) Th17 and regulatory T cell balance in autoimmune and inflammatory diseases. Autoimmun Rev 13: 668–677.

25. Lane N, Robins RA, Corne J, Fairclough L (2010) Regulation in chronic obstructive pulmonary disease: the role of regulatory T-cells and Th17 cells. Clin Sci (Lond) 119: 75–86.

26. Tan DB, Fernandez S, Price P, French MA, Thompson PJ, et al. (2014) Impaired function of regulatory T-cells in patients with chronic obstructive pulmonary disease (COPD). Immunobiology.

27. Hou J, Sun Y, Hao Y, Zhuo J, Liu X, et al. (2013) Imbalance between subpopulations of regulatory T cells in COPD. Thorax.

28. De Rosa MJ, Esandi MC, Garelli A, Rayes D, Bouzat C (2005) Relationship between alpha 7 nAChR and apoptosis in human lymphocytes. J Neuroimmunol 160: 154–161.

29. Kolahian S, Gosens R (2012) Cholinergic regulation of airway inflammation and remodelling. J Allergy (Cairo) 2012: 681258.

30. Lee J, Taneja V, Vassallo R (2012) Cigarette smoking and inflammation: cellular and molecular mechanisms. J Dent Res 91: 142–149.

31. Hellstrom-Lindahl E, Nordberg A (1996) Muscarinic receptor subtypes in subpopulations of human blood mononuclear cells as analyzed by RT-PCR technique. J Neuroimmunol 68: 139–144.

32. Sato KZ, Fujii T, Watanabe Y, Yamada S, Ando T, et al. (1999) Diversity of mRNA expression for muscarinic acetylcholine receptor subtypes and neuronal

nicotinic acetylcholine receptor subunits in human mononuclear leukocytes and leukemic cell lines. Neurosci Lett 266: 17–20.

33. Kawashima K, Fujii T (2000) Extraneuronal cholinergic system in lymphocytes. Pharmacol Ther 86: 29–48.

34. Qian J, Galitovskiy V, Chernyavsky AI, Marchenko S, Grando SA (2011) Plasticity of the murine spleen T-cell cholinergic receptors and their role in in vitro differentiation of naive CD4 T cells toward the Th1, Th2 and Th17 lineages. Genes Immun 12: 222–230.

35. Zhang J, Deng L, Xiong X, Wang P, Xin J, et al. (2011) Effect of tiotropium bromide on expression of CD(8) (+)CD (25) (+)FoxP (3) (+) regulatory T cells in patients with stable chronic obstructive pulmonary disease. J Huazhong Univ Sci Technolog Med Sci 31: 463–468.

36. Profita M, Albano GD, Riccobono L, Di Sano C, Montalbano AM, et al. (2014) Increased levels of Th17 cells are associated with non-neuronal acetylcholine in COPD patients. Immunobiology 219: 392–401.

37. Noakes PS, Holt PG, Prescott SL (2003) Maternal smoking in pregnancy alters neonatal cytokine responses. Allergy 58: 1053–1058.

38. Kawashima K, Fujii T (2003) The lymphocytic cholinergic system and its contribution to the regulation of immune activity. Life Sci 74: 675–696.

39. Kawashima K, Fujii T, Moriwaki Y, Misawa H (2012) Critical roles of acetylcholine and the muscarinic and nicotinic acetylcholine receptors in the regulation of immune function. Life Sci 91: 1027–1032.

40. Wessler I, Kilbinger H, Bittinger F, Kirkpatrick CJ (2001) The biological role of non-neuronal acetylcholine in plants and humans. Jpn J Pharmacol 85: 2–10.

41. Fujihara M, Nagai N, Sussan TE, Biswal S, Handa JT (2008) Chronic cigarette smoke causes oxidative damage and apoptosis to retinal pigmented epithelial cells in mice. PLoS One 3: e3119.

42. Carnevali S, Petruzzelli S, Longoni B, Vanacore R, Barale R, et al. (2003) Cigarette smoke extract induces oxidative stress and apoptosis in human lung fibroblasts. Am J Physiol Lung Cell Mol Physiol 284: L955–L963.

43. Menon R, Fortunato SJ, Yu J, Milne GL, Sanchez S, et al. (2011) Cigarette smoke induces oxidative stress and apoptosis in normal term fetal membranes. Placenta 32: 317–322.

44. Baglole CJ, Bushinsky SM, Garcia TM, Kode A, Rahman I, et al. (2006) Differential induction of apoptosis by cigarette smoke extract in primary human lung fibroblast strains: implications for emphysema. Am J Physiol Lung Cell Mol Physiol 291: L19–L29.

45. Tagawa Y, Hiramatsu N, Kasai A, Hayakawa K, Okamura M, et al. (2008) Induction of apoptosis by cigarette smoke via ROS-dependent endoplasmic reticulum stress and CCAAT/enhancer-binding protein-homologous protein (CHOP). Free Radic Biol Med 45: 50–59.

46. Zhong CY, Zhou YM, Pinkerton KE (2008) NF-kappaB inhibition is involved in tobacco smoke-induced apoptosis in the lungs of rats. Toxicol Appl Pharmacol 230: 150–158.

15

Impact of Protein Domains on PE_PGRS30 Polar Localization in Mycobacteria

Flavio De Maio[1,9], Giuseppe Maulucci[2,9], Mariachiara Minerva[1], Saber Anoosheh[4], Ivana Palucci[1], Raffaella Iantomasi[1], Valentina Palmieri[2], Serena Camassa[1], Michela Sali[1], Maurizio Sanguinetti[1], Wilbert Bitter[3], Riccardo Manganelli[4], Marco De Spirito[2], Giovanni Delogu[1]*

1 Institute of Microbiology, Universita' Cattolica del Sacro Cuore, Rome, Italy, 2 Institute of Physics, Universita' Cattolica del Sacro Cuore, Rome, Italy, 3 Department of Medical Microbiology and Infection Control, VU University Medical Center, Amsterdam, Netherlands, 4 Department of Molecular Medicine, University of Padua, Padua, Italy

Abstract

PE_PGRS proteins are unique to the *Mycobacterium tuberculosis* complex and a number of other pathogenic mycobacteria. PE_PGRS30, which is required for the full virulence of *M. tuberculosis* (*Mtb*), has three main domains, *i.e.* an N-terminal PE domain, repetitive PGRS domain and the unique C-terminal domain. To investigate the role of these domains, we expressed a GFP-tagged PE_PGRS30 protein and a series of its functional deletion mutants in different mycobacterial species (*Mtb*, *Mycobacterium bovis* BCG and *Mycobacterium smegmatis*) and analysed protein localization by confocal microscopy. We show that PE_PGRS30 localizes at the mycobacterial cell poles in *Mtb* and *M. bovis* BCG but not in *M. smegmatis* and that the PGRS domain of the protein strongly contributes to protein cellular localization in *Mtb*. Immunofluorescence studies further showed that the unique C-terminal domain of PE_PGRS30 is not available on the surface, except when the PGRS domain is missing. Immunoblot demonstrated that the PGRS domain is required to maintain the protein strongly associated with the non-soluble cellular fraction. These results suggest that the repetitive GGA-GGN repeats of the PGRS domain contain specific sequences that contribute to protein cellular localization and that polar localization might be a key step in the PE_PGRS30-dependent virulence mechanism.

Editor: Ann Rawkins, Public Health England, United Kingdom

Funding: This work was funded by the EU (FP7/2007–2013) under grant agreement n°201762 awarded to GD and RM and by MIUR (Ministero dell'istruzione, Università e Ricerca of the Italian Governement) (project number PRIN 2008 Y8RZTF) awarded to GD and RM. The funders had no role in study design, data collection and analysis, decision to publish, or preparation of the manuscript.

Competing Interests: The authors have declared that no competing interests exist.

* Email: gdelogu@rm.unicatt.it

9 These authors contributed equally to this work.

Introduction

Despite many research and sanitary efforts, tuberculosis (TB) remains one of the deadliest human infectious diseases far from being defeated [1]. The poor knowledge of the biology of its causative agent, *Mycobacterium tuberculosis* (*Mtb*), is a main obstacle toward the development of improved control strategies [2,3]. In this context, a better understanding of surface exposed, secreted and cell wall associated proteins is classically a key step to dissect the mechanisms of pathogenesis of bacteria and to identify antigens that may serve as candidate vaccines [4,5]. The complexity of the mycobacterial cell wall is such that only recently it has been possible to solve its structure [6,7], including a peculiar outer membrane referred to as mycomembrane. Consequently, we still have limited knowledge regarding the proteins and protein apparatuses localizing in the mycomembrane and the molecular determinants mediating host-pathogen interactions [8]. The recent discovery of the ESX secretion systems is shedding light on the mechanism whereby *Mtb* translocate effector proteins that are secreted or exposed on its surface and that can interfere with host components [9–12]. The results of these studies are leading to the

development of new vaccines and drug targets [13,14], emphasizing the impact that this line of research may have in the control of TB.

Among the cell wall associated proteins are the PE_PGRSs, a family of around 60 proteins found only in members of the *Mtb* complex, in *Mycobacterium ulcerans* and *Mycobacterium marinum* [15–18]. PE_PGRSs are characterized by a highly conserved PE domain, a central polymorphic PGRS domain and a unique C-terminal domain that may vary in size from few to up to 300 amino acids [17]. Studies carried out with PE_PGRS33 showed that the PE domain is required for the correct protein localization in the mycobacterial cell wall [19–21], although only the PGRS domain appears to be properly exposed for interaction with host components [22]. Indeed, PE_PGRS33 shows immunomodulatory properties thanks to its ability to interact with TLR2, which may trigger macrophage cell death [16,23–26].

Among the few PE_PGRSs for which experimental evidences are available, PE_PGRS30 is required for the full virulence of *Mtb* [27]. PE_PGRS30, encoded by the gene Rv1651c in *Mtb* H37Rv, is a protein of 1011 amino acids composed by a PE domain (90 aa), followed by a domain of 39 amino acids containing the highly conserved GRPLI motif (TM, trans-membrane domain) that is probably involved in the anchorage of the protein to the mycobacterial cell wall [17,27,28]. The central region of the protein is formed by the PGRS domain (566 aa), which is followed by a large unique C-terminal domain (316 aa). While we await a functional characterization of the different protein domains, it was with surprise that the large unique C-terminal domain was found dispensable for the PE_PGRS30-dependent virulence phenotype [27].

The role and precise localization of PE_PGRS proteins is still elusive as well as the role of their different domains in this process. Objective of this study is the characterization of the domains involved in the cellular localization of PE_PGRS30.

Materials and Methods

Construction of plasmids expressing PE_PGRS30 and its chimeras fused with green fluorescent protein (GFP)

The PE_PGRS30 full length gene and selected fragments of its open reading frame were amplified from the *Mtb* H37Rv genomic DNA [15] using primers indicated in table S1 and cloned using standard procedures. Briefly, the forward primer was designed to anneal to the upstream region of the Rv1651c so to amplify its putative promoter sequence and contained the *Hind*III restriction site adaptor sequence. Reverse primers were designed to anneal to different positions of the Rv1651c coding sequence and contained the *Xba*I adaptor sequence. PCR products were amplified using Vent polymerase (New England Biolab, Beverly, MA) and cloned in pCR blunt vector (Life technologies). The GFP gene was amplified from the pJWtPAGFP vector [29] using primers containing the *Nhe*I and *Bam*HI restriction sites at 5' and 3', respectively. The PE_PGRS30-derived fragments were inserted in the pMV206 medium copy episomal plasmid [30] in frame and upstream of the GFP coding sequence. The gene cassettes, containing the Rv1651c putative promoter sequence and the PE_PGRS30-derived fragments, were also inserted in the integrative plasmid pMV361 downstream of the *hsp*60 promoter sequence and upstream and in frame with the sequence coding the haemagglutinin (HA) epitope.

Bacterial strains

The constructed recombinant plasmids were used to transform *Mtb* H37Rv, *Mycobacterium bovis* BCG Pasteur and *Mycobacterium smegmatis* mc^{2}155 using standard procedures [19]. Transformants were selected on 7H11 agar media supplemented with 10% OADC (Microbiol, Cagliari, Italy) containing 50 µg/ml hygromycin B (Sigma–Aldrich, Saint Louis, MO). Single individual antibiotic-resistant colonies were isolated and subcultured in a 7H9 media supplemented with 10% ADC (Microbiol, Cagliari, Italy) and 0,05% Tween 80 containing hygromycin B (50 µg/ml) and incubated at 37°C. Mycobacteria cultures were stocked at −80°C in 20% glycerol.

Construction of the DNA plasmid vector encoding the PE_PGRS30 C-terminal unique domain (ptPA-30^{Cter})

A plasmid DNA coding the C-terminal domain of PE_PGRS30 was constructed following standard procedures. Briefly, a 918 bp fragment corresponding to the coding sequence of the C-terminus 306 amino acids domain of PE_PGRS30 was amplified using the primers indicated in table S1. The DNA fragment was amplified from the *Mtb* H37Rv genomic DNA using Vent polymerase and cloned in pCRblunt (Life Technologies). The DNA fragment was then cleaved with *Nhe*I and *Bam*HI and cloned in pJW4303 to obtain ptPA^{30Cter} [29]. Endotoxin-free plasmid DNA was prepared and purified with the Qiagen EndoFree Plasmid Maxi Kit (Qiagen, Chatsworth, US) for the ptPA^{30Cter} and ptPA-GFP constructs [29].

Immunization of mice

Specified pathogen-free female BALB/c mice were obtained from Enclosure Labs of the Università Cattolica del Sacro Cuore, Rome and immunized at the age of eight weeks. The animals were housed in a temperature-controlled environment with 12 h light/dark cycles, and received food and water ad libitum. All animal experiments were authorized by the Ethical Committee of the Università Cattolica del Sacro Cuore and performed in compliance with the legislative decree of the Italian Government 27 January 1992, n. 116 and the Health Minister memorandum 14 May 2001, n. 6. All manipulations were performed under isoflurane anesthesia, and all efforts were made to minimize suffering. Three Balb/c mice per group (pTPA-GFP and ptPA^{30Cter}, total six mice) were immunized by three intramuscular injection of 100 µg of plasmid DNA and bled 4–10 weeks following the third immunization by the tail vein to collect sera, as previously indicated [31].

Immunoblotting

The *Mtb* recombinant strains were cultured in 7H9 media containing Tween80 (without ADC) until mid-log phase and cells harvested by centrifugation [32]. To obtain whole cell lysates, cell pellets were washed with PBS and directly re-suspended in Laemmli buffer and boiled for 10 minutes. To obtain the cytosolic fraction, cell pellets were resuspended in lysis buffer (10 mM Tris-HCl, 5 mM EDTA, protease inhibitors cocktail, pH 9.5) containing 0,1 mm Silica/Zirconia beads (Biospec products) and subjected to three cycles of homogenization with the Mini-Beadbeater (Biospec products). After centrifugation to remove the insoluble fraction supernatants were filtered through 0.22 µm filters (Cellulose acetate membrane sterile syringe filter, VWR International). Proteins samples were separated by SDS-PAGE and transferred to nitrocellulose membranes by western blot. Membranes were probed with polyclonal sera (1:200) obtained from mice immunized with ptPA^{30Cter} or ptPA-GFP and then anti-mouse IgG-Peroxidase (Sigma–Aldrich, Saint Louis, MO) was used as a secondary antibody. Immunoblot developed using Supersignal West Dura Extended Duration Substrate (Thermo scientific). Membranes were probed with polyclonal sera (1:200) obtained from mice immunized with ptPA^{30Cter} or monoclonal anti-HA epitope antibody (Covance).

Immunofluorescence

Recombinant *Mtb* strains, expressing PE_PGRS30 and its chimera $_{30}$PE_Ct tagged with HA epitope, were plated in chamber slides as indicated above and then fixed with 4% paraformaldehyde and washed with PBS. After blocking with BSA 0.3%, plates were incubated with anti-HA epitope (1:200) (Covance). After washing with PBS, slides were probed with the secondary antibody Alexa Fluor 546 donkey anti-mouse (Life technologies) and then Prolong gold anti-fade reagent (Life technologies) was added before closing the slides. Chamber slides were observed with a confocal microscope.

Cells cultures and mycobacteria infection

J774 cells (ATCC) were grown in RPMI-1640 medium (Euroclone Milan, Italy) supplemented with 10% fetal calf serum (FCS), glutamine (2 mM), and sodium pyruvate (1 mM) (Euroclone Milan, Italy) and kept in a humidified atmosphere

A

B

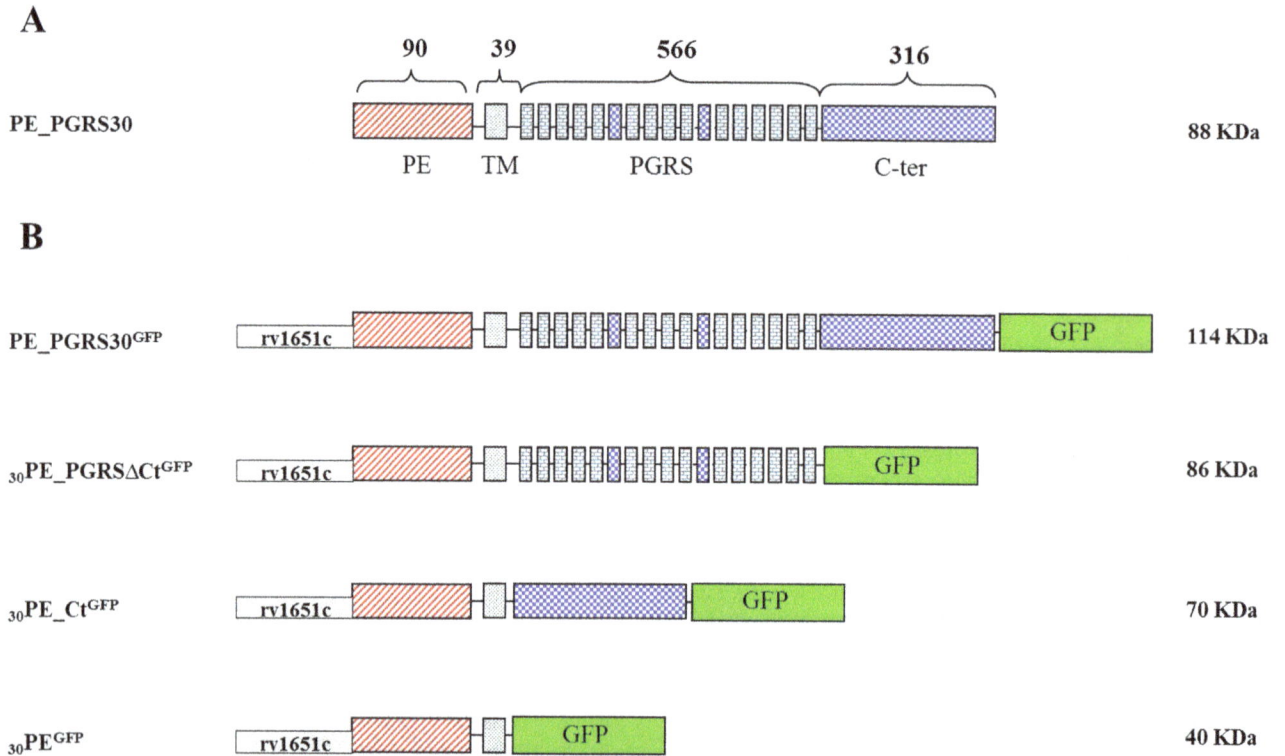

Figure 1. Scheme showing the constructs expressing PE_PGRS30 used in this study. Schematic representation of native full length PE_PGRS30 gene with the indication of the different protein domains (A). List of constructs generated in pMV206 and expressing the PE_PGRS30 functional chimeras, tagged with green fluorescent protein (B). The constructs were transformed in *Mtb* H37Rv, *M. smegmatis* and *M. bovis* BCG.

containing 5% CO_2 at 37°C [27]. Cells were plated in chamber slides ($1,2 \times 10^6$ cell/ml) in media without antibiotics and then infected with the recombinant *Mtb* strains expressing the GFP-tagged proteins at a multiplicity of infection (MOI) of 5:1. After 1 hour of incubation, cells were washed with warm PBS and after adding fresh media (RPMI 2% FCS without antibiotics) plates were incubated at 37°C (5% CO2). At different time points, cells were washed with PBS, fixed with 4% paraformaldehyde and chamber slides closed and observed at the confocal microscope as indicated above.

Confocal microscopy and image analysis

The recombinant mycobacterial strains (*M. tuberculosis* H37Rv, *M. bovis* BCG and *M. smegmatis* mc[155]) expressing PE_PGRS30 and its chimeras fused with GFP, were grown in 7H9/ADC/Tween80 and at mid-log phase these strains were plated on chamber slides pre-treated with polylisine (Sigma–Aldrich, Saint Louis, MO). Subsequently chamber slides were incubated for 24 hours at 37°C, then fixed with 4% parafolmaldehyde and washed with phosphate buffered saline (PBS). Chamber slides were closed and observed with a confocal microscope.

Images were collected by using an inverted confocal microscope (DMIRE2, Leica Microsystems, Wetzlar, Germany) equipped with a 40× oil immersion objective (NA 1.25). For GFP excitation a He/Ne laser at 476 nm was used. Internal photon multiplier tubes collected 8-bit unsigned images at 400 Hz scan speed in an emission range comprised between 500 nm and 550 nm. Imaging was performed at room temperature. Image processing was performed with ImageJ software; image background values

(defined as intensities below 7% of the maximum intensity) were set to zero and colored in black [33]. Intensity profiles were measured on bacteria entire length with 'line profile' tool [34]. To obtain a representative index of protein polar localization, a ratio R was calculated as follows: $R = I_{pole}/I_{cyto}$ where I_pole is the GFP emission intensity at bacterium pole, considered as the value in correspondence of the border of the bacterium and I_{cyto} is the GFP emission intensity in the middle part of the bacterium (measured at the 50% of the bacterium length). At least 20 line profiles were analyzed for each construct. R values are reported for each line profile and their mean ± standard deviation (SD) were determined and utilized for two-tailed Student's *t*-test analysis (GraphPad).

Localization of the anti-mouse AlexaFluor-546-tagged antibodies (Life technologies) outside the mycobacterial cell was assessed by acquiring images with a 63× oil immersion objective (NA 1.4) using an excitation wavelength of 543 nm (Ar/ArKr laser) and with photomultiplier emission range comprised between 560 and 700 nm. Image background was corrected as defined above and fluorophore localization was evaluated with ImageJ software using overlap between red channel and transmission images.

Results

Expression of PE_PGRS30-derived GFP chimeras in mycobacterial strains

To determine PE_PGRS30 localization in the mycobacterial cell and the impact of the different protein domains on this process, the PE_PGRS30 native gene, and its functional deletion mutants [27], were fused to the GFP coding sequence in the medium copy number plasmid pMV206 (figure 1) [30]. These plasmids were electroporated in *Mtb* H37Rv, *M. bovis* BCG and

M. smegmatis mc^{2}155 to obtain strains expressing PE_PGRS30-derived GFP-tagged proteins. Expression of these chimeras was under the control of the PE_PGRS30 (Rv1651c) putative promoter [27]. Correct protein expression was demonstrated by immunoblot using an anti-GFP antibody on whole cell lysates of recombinant *Mtb*, *M. smegmatis* and BCG strains (Figure S1).

PE_PGRS30 localize at cellular poles in *Mtb* and in *M. bovis* BCG but not in *M. smegmatis*

The recombinant *Mtb* strains expressing PE_PGRS30 and its chimeras fused with GFP were grown until mid-log phase and plated in chamber slides and then observed at fluorescence confocal microscope. As shown in figure 2A, polarization of the GFP signal was observed for the strain expressing PE_PGRS30^{GFP} and a similar pattern was observed for *Mtb*-$_{30}$PE_PGRSΔCT^{GFP} and, to a lesser extent, for *Mtb*-$_{30}$PE_CT^{GFP}. Conversely, a fluorescence diffused throughout the mycobacterial cell was observed for the *Mtb*-$_{30}$PE^{GFP}. Analysis of the fluorescence pattern was performed using line profile software (ImageJ software), in order to evaluate the polar localization of the protein spatial distribution. As shown in the line profile (figure 2B), comparison of the fluorescence pattern indicated a less pronounced polarization in the *Mtb*-$_{30}$PE^{GFP} strain compared with the full length PE_PGRS30 chimera and the other two chimeras. R values (mean ± SD) are reported in figure 2C for each sample and in table S2, with higher R values indicating more pronounced polar localization of the GFP-tagged protein. A significant difference is observed only for *Mtb*-$_{30}$PE^{GFP} and *Mtb*-$_{30}$PE_CT^{GFP}.

As shown in figure S2, the BCG recombinant strains expressing PE_PGRS30 and its chimeras fused with GFP were analyzed as for *Mtb* and the results obtained indicate a similar pattern of protein localization to that observed in *Mtb*, though a less pronounced polar localization was observed for the $_{30}$PE_CT^{GFP} chimera.

Figure 3A shows the results obtained with the *M. smegmatis* recombinant strains expressing the chimeras under study. Interestingly, expression and localization profiles in this species were radically different; expression of the full length protein (PE_PGRS30^{GFP}), of $_{30}$PE_CT^{GFP} and $_{30}$PE^{GFP} resulted in a diffused fluorescence with little or no polarization (figure 3B).

Taken together these results indicate that expression of the PE_PGRS30 chimeras in *Mtb* and BCG follows a similar pattern, which is different to what observed in *M. smegmatis*, and that the PE domain does not contain the information sufficient to warrant polar localization of the full PE_PGRS30 protein.

The PGRS domain contributes to PE_PGRS30 cellular localization in *Mtb*

Compared with most PE_PGRS proteins, PE_PGRS30 contains, downstream of the PGRS domain, a large unique C-terminal domain (306 aa) of unknown function, and whose role in mediating protein localization has not been investigated. A plasmid DNA expressing only the PE_PGRS30 C-terminal domain (figure S3A) was used to immunize mice following standard procedures [29] and the antiserum raised was used to probe in immunoblots whole cell lysates of *Mtb* containing the different PE_PGRS30 constructs (figure 4A). A band of ≈90 kDa was detected in the whole lysate of *Mtb* expressing PE_PGRS30, that was not detected in any other of the *Mtb* strains tested (figure 4A), indicating that PE_PGRS30 cannot be detected in immunoblots with this polyclonal sera unless the protein is overexpressed as in *Mtb*-PE_PGRS30, where overexpression is warranted by the presence, upstream of the gene cassette inserted

in pMV361, of the *hsp60* promoter. Interestingly, in all the *Mtb* strains a much stronger signal at 52 kDa was detected, probably corresponding to the gene product of Rv3812, which is a PE-unique protein containing a C-terminal domain highly homologous to that of PE_PGRS30 [35,36]. The whole cell lysate of *Mtb*-$_{30}$PE_CT, expressing the functional deletion mutant under similar conditions as the full length protein (pMV361), showed a band of ≈50 kDa, theoretically corresponding to the expected size of the $_{30}$PE_CT chimera, and with a signal intensity similar to that observed for the Rv3812 gene product (figure S3B). Immunoblot analysis carried out on the soluble fraction of the *Mtb* lysates (figure 4B), showed the presence of the PE_CT chimera with the anti-HA and anti-Ct sera, though the full length protein and the other chimeras could not be detected. Again, the anti-Ct sera identified a band at ≈50 kDa as in figure 4A. These results suggest that the full length protein remains mostly associated with cellular debris compared with the $_{30}$PE_CT chimera.

The C-terminal domain of PE_PGRS30 is not exposed on the mycobacterial surface

To assess whether the large unique C-terminal domain was available on the mycobacterial surface, the recombinant *Mtb* expressing PE_PGRS30 and *Mtb* expressing PE_CT fused with the HA epitope were assayed in immunofluorescence studies using the anti-HA antibody. As shown in figure 5A, analysis at the fluorescence confocal microscope indicated that no significant signal was detected on the surface of *Mtb* expressing full length PE_PGRS30 using an anti-HA primary antibody. Conversely, *Mtb* expressing $_{30}$PE_CT^{HA} chimeras showed a fluorescence along the outside mycobacterial cell wall (figure 5B). These results suggest that the C-terminal domain of PE_PGRS30 is not available on the mycobacterial surface, unless the PGRS domain is lacking as in *Mtb* $_{30}$PE_CT^{HA}, further establishing the key role of the PGRS domain for the correct localization of PE_PGRS30.

PE_PGRS30 and PE_PGRS33 have different localization in *Mtb*

Previous studies demonstrated that the PE domain of PE_PGRS33 contains the information sufficient to drive localization of the protein to the mycobacterial cell wall [19–21] and that it is possible to use this domain to deliver protein or protein domains to the mycobacterial surface [37]. To investigate whether the pattern of protein polarization observed for PE_PGRS30 was similar to that observed for another well studied PE_PGRS protein (PE_PGRS33), we generated a plasmid expressing the PE_PGRS33^{GFP} chimera under the control of its physiological promoter (p$_{rv1818c}$) (figure 6A, B). This construct is different from that used in previous studies where PE_PGRS33^{GFP} was overexpressed under the control of the *hsp60* promoter [19]. The *Mtb* strain transformed with this plasmid was analyzed by confocal microscopy and protein polarization measured with the line profile software (figure 6C). Surprisingly, differently from what observed with *Mtb*-PE_PGRS30^{GFP}, no polarization was observed for the *Mtb*-PE_PGRS33^{GFP}, where fluorescence was found diffused throughout the cell. To assess whether the differential polarization was due to the PE domain, an *Mtb* strain expressing the first 140 amino acids of PE_PGRS33 fused to GFP, under the control of the Rv1818c promoter, was generated and analyzed at confocal fluorescence microscopy (figure 6D). The $_{33}$PE^{GFP} showed a strong polarization (figure 6B), that was not observed for $_{30}$PE^{GFP} (figure 1A), clearly indicating that under physiological conditions the PGRS domain of PE_PGRS33 contributes to protein localization on the mycobacterial cell wall.

A

B

C

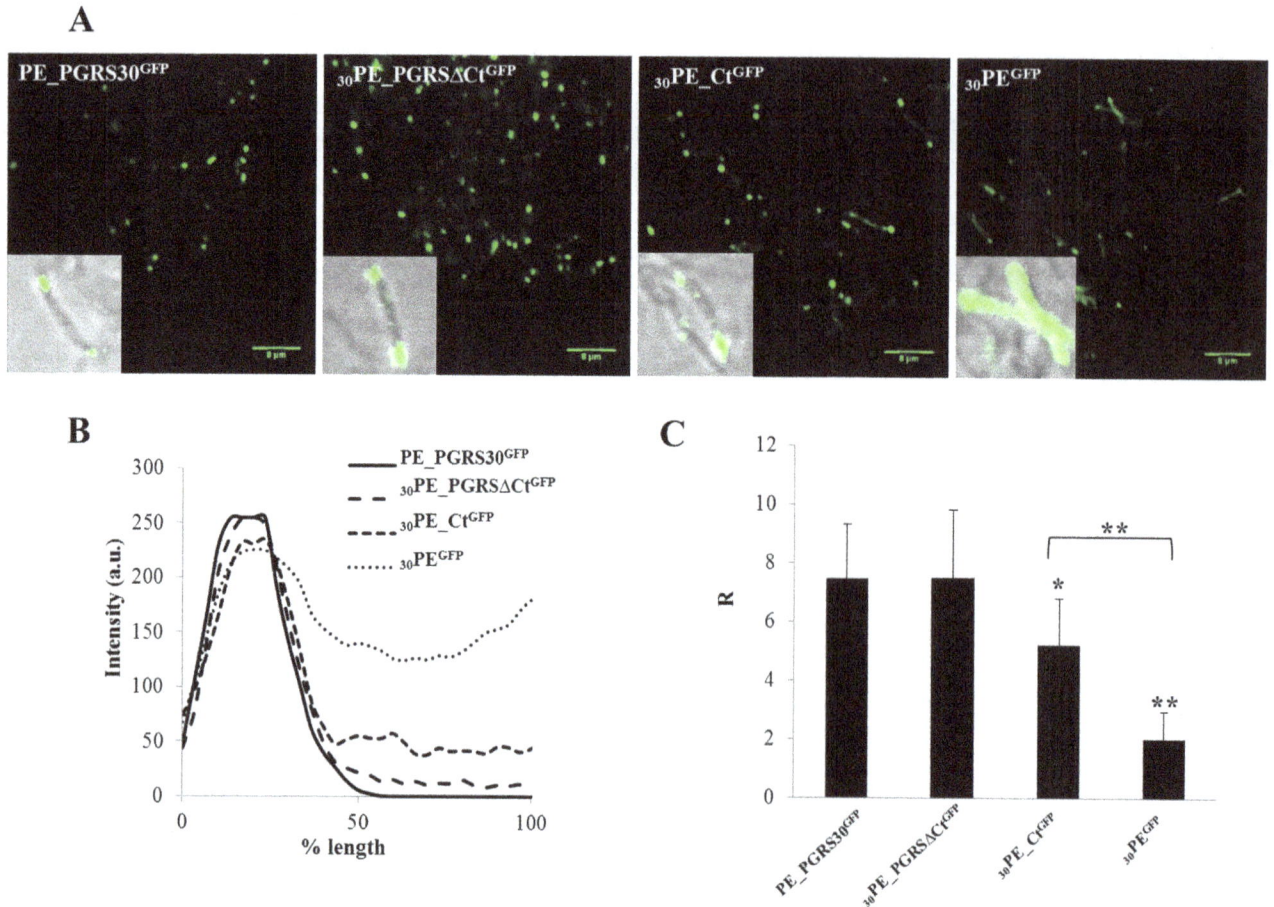

Figure 2. Polar localization of PE_PGRS30^{GFP} spatial distribution in *Mtb*. A) Confocal images of *Mtb* H37Rv expressing PE_PGRS30^{GFP} and its functional GFP-tagged chimeras obtained with a 63× objective. In the inbox, a 100× image obtained overlapping green channel and transmission image is shown. B) Sample line profile obtained quantifying the fluorescence along mycobacterial cell. C) Ratio between the GFP emission intensity at bacterium pole (considered as the value 200 nm far from the bacterium border) and GFP emission intensity in the cytoplasm (measured at the 50% of the bacterium length). Twenty R values were analyzed for each *Mtb* strain under study. Two-tailed Student's *t*-test was used to analyze R ratio (* $p < 0.05$, ** $p < 0.01$).

The different degree of polarization observed for $_{30}$PE^{GFP} and $_{33}$PE^{GFP} suggests that amino acids differences in the PE domain may also impact protein localization (figure S4).

PE_PGRS30 and PE_PGRS33 have a different polar localization during infection

Protein localization in mycobacteria may be affected by expression level or by interaction with other protein partners or cellular components, which in turn depend on the environment [38]. To assess protein localization in conditions mimicking the intracellular environment typically encountered by bacteria, *Mtb* expressing PE_PGRS30^{GFP} and PE_PGRS33^{GFP} were used to infect the murine macrophages cell line J774. An *Mtb* strain expressing GFP only was used as a control. Infected cells were fixed at different time points (1 hour and 6 days post-infection, and day 1 post-reinfection) and then observed at the confocal microscope as previously described. The first two time points mimic the early (1 hour) and the late (6 days) phase of infection, respectively. As expected, infection with the *Mtb*^{GFP} control strain resulted in bacteria showing diffused and homogeneous fluorescence throughout the bacilli, and no changes in fluorescence diffusion were observed between 1 hour and 6 days post-infection

(figure 7). A clear polarization was observed in *Mtb*-PE_PGRS30^{GFP} infecting macrophages at the early time point, and the polar localization was found more pronounced at 6 days post-infection. Conversely, diffused fluorescence was observed at 1 hour and 6 days post-infection for the *Mtb*-PE_PGRS33^{GFP} strain (figure 7). Since bacteria used to infect cells were obtained from glycerol stocks prepared from cultures grown in axenic media, it cannot be excluded that protein localization observed at 1 hour post-infection may represent the *Mtb* status in axenic media rather than a physiological situations. Hence, we collected the supernatants of the macrophage-infected culture at 6 days post-infection, that contain many bacteria released by dying macrophages, and used it to infect fresh macrophages. One day after infection, macrophages were fixed and analyzed at the confocal microscope. Polarization of PE_PGRS30^{GFP} was found even more pronounced under this condition, while *Mtb*-PE_PGRS33^{GFP} showed a diffused and homogenous fluorescence throughout the cell.

Discussion

Since their identification in the *Mtb* genome, PE_PGRS proteins have been implicated in the mechanism of pathogenesis

A

B

C

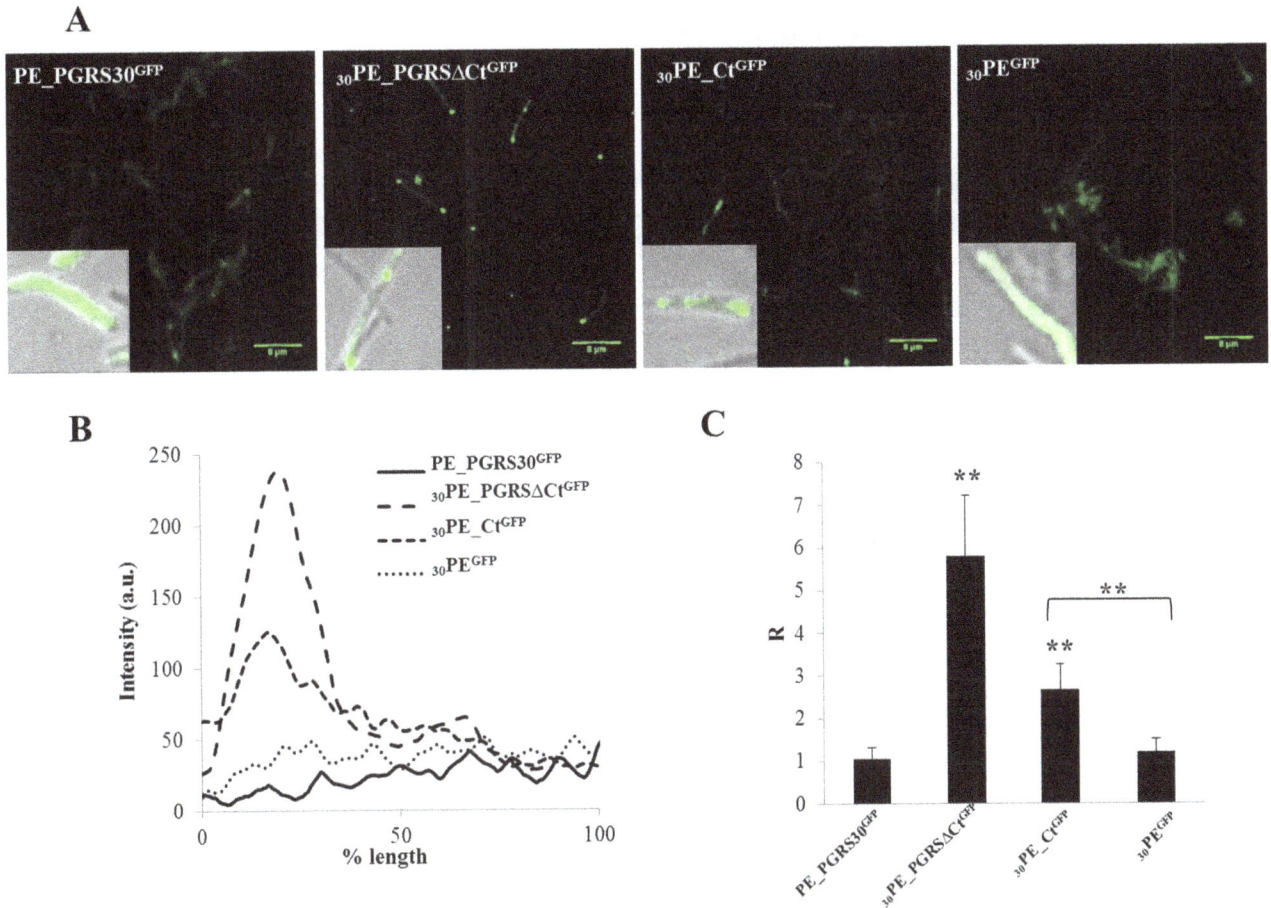

Figure 3. Polar localization of PE_PGRS30^{GFP} spatial distribution in *M. smegmatis.* A) Confocal images of *M. smegmatis* expressing PE_PGRS30^{GFP} and its functional GFP-tagged chimeras obtained with a 63× objective. In the inbox, a 100× image obtained overlapping green channel and transmission image is shown. B) Sample line profile obtained quantifying the fluorescence along mycobacterial cell. C) Ratio between the GFP emission intensity at bacterium pole (considered as the value 200 nm far from the bacterium border) and GFP emission intensity in the cytoplasm (measured at the 50% of the bacterium length). Twenty R values were analyzed for each *M. smegmatis* strain under study. Two-tailed Student's *t*-test was used to analyze R ratio (* $p<0.05$, ** $p<0.01$).

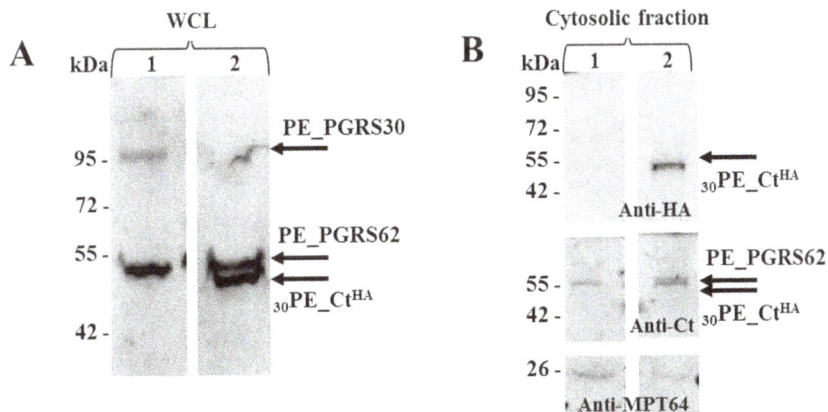

A

B

Figure 4. Immunoblot showing expression of PE_PGRS30 by *Mtb.* A) Immunoblot analysis on whole cell lysates of *Mtb* expressing PE_PGRS30 and its HA-tagged chimeras with anti-C-terminal domain primary antibody. B) Immunoblot analysis on cytoplasmatic fraction of *Mtb* expressing PE_PGRS30 and its HA_tagged chimeras probed with anti-HA antibody, anti-C-terminal domain and anti-MPT64 sera; 1: *Mtb*-PE_PGRS30^{HA}; 2: *Mtb*-$_{30}$PE_CT^{HA}; Arrows indicate the band corresponding to PE_PGRS30^{HA} and PE_CT^{HA} and PE_PGRS62.

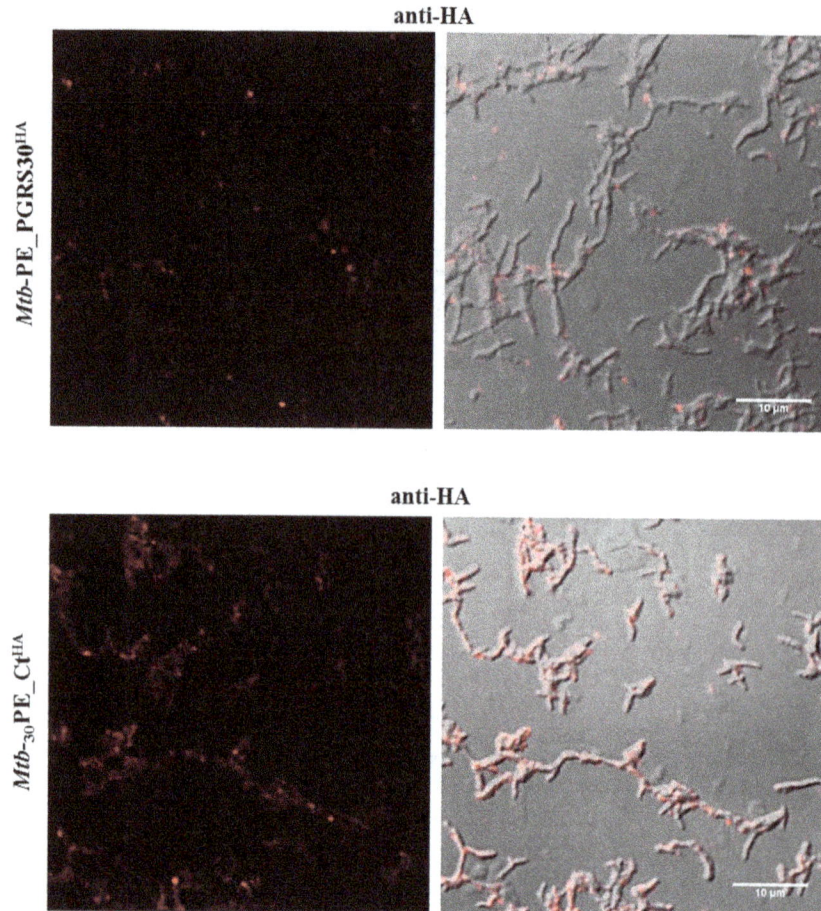

Figure 5. Immunofluorescence using anti-HA antibodies. *Mtb*-PE_PGRS30[HA] (A) and *Mtb*-30PE_CT[HA] (B) were subjected to immunofluorescence using anti-HA antibodies. Confocal images were acquired with a 63× oil immersion objective and localization was evaluated with ImageJ software using overlap between red channel (left panel) and transmission images.

of TB and included in an hypothetical panel of surface mycobacterial antigens involved in immune evasion strategies [15–17]. In this study, using a panel of GFP-tagged proteins, we investigate the localization of PE_PGRS30 in three mycobacterial species (*Mtb*, *M. bovis* BCG and *M. smegmatis*) and analyzed the impact of the different protein domains on protein polarization on the bacterial cells. We show that both the PGRS and C-terminal unique domain of PE_PGRS30 contribute to protein localization and that the C-terminal domain is not available on the mycobacterial surface. Moreover, using GFP-protein chimeras we demonstrate that PE_PGRS30 localize at the bacterial poles during infection in macrophages, while PE_PGRS33 remains homogeneously distributed on the mycobacterial surface. These results provide further insights on PE_PGRS protein localization and suggest the functional diversity between PE_PGRS proteins.

Recent data obtained using an *Mtb* mutant strain demonstrated that PE_PGRS30 is required for the full virulence of *Mtb* and for intracellular survival of the bacilli in macrophages [27]. While the exact mechanism whereby PE_PGRS30 exerts its activity remains to be elucidated, some results obtained in *M. marinum* suggest that PE_PGRS proteins may be secreted as effector molecules through the ESX5 apparatus, a type seven secretion system (T7SS) [9,39]. These results are in line with the discovery that in MTB complex, *M. marinum* and *M. ulcerans*, PE_PGRS (and PPE_MPTR) proteins emerged and coevolved in parallel with the ESX5

secretion system [40,41], suggesting a functional link between the most recent T7SS (ESX5) and these two protein subfamilies [10]. Indeed, ESX-5 was elegantly shown to be required for the export of several immunogenic PE and PPE proteins and for the full virulence of *Mtb* [42,43]. In this context, PE_PGRSs would be a substrate for ESX5 which mediates protein secretion or translocation to the surface, as it has been shown in *M. marinum* [9,44]. However, ESX5-dependent PE_PGRS secretion in *Mtb* is still debated, with some experimental data supporting the ESX5-dependent secretion of PE_PGRSs [45] and other suggesting that inactivation of ESX5 in *Mtb* has no obvious effect on exposure of PE_PGRSs in the mycobacterial surface [13]. The finding that surface localization of PE_PGRS proteins could be achieved in *M. smegmatis* which lacks ESX5 [20,46], further questions the need of ESX5 for proper PE_PGRS cellular localization.

In order to investigate PE_PGRS30 localization in different mycobacterial species, we expressed in *M. smegmatis*, *M. bovis* BCG and *Mtb* the PE_PGRS30[GFP] protein under the control of its own putative promoter [27]. Surprisingly, PE_PGRS30[GFP] polarized at the bacterial poles when expressed in *Mtb* and *M. bovis* BCG but not in *M. smegmatis*, contrary to what previously observed when PE_PGRS30 was overexpressed under the control of the *hsp60* promoter in *M. smegmatis* [46,47]. These results highlight the impact that protein expression has on polarization and most importantly, that segregation of PE_PGRS30 at the

A

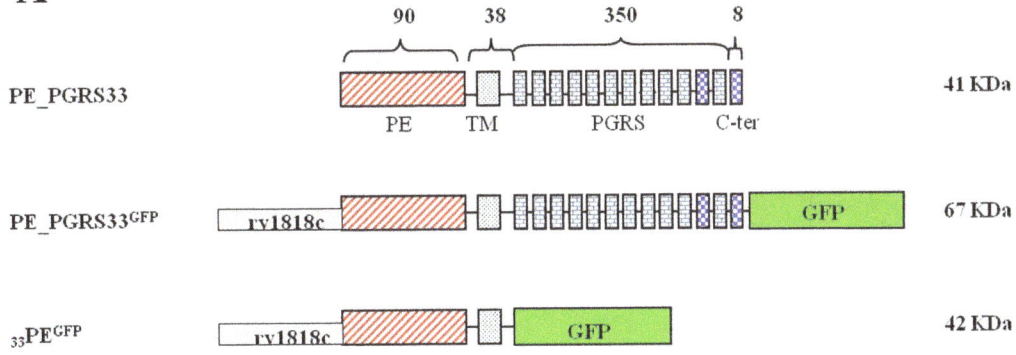

B

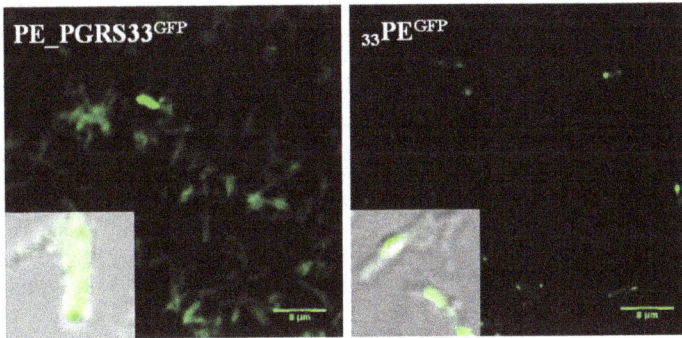

C

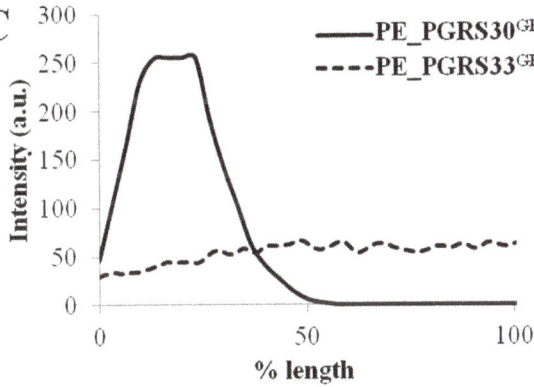
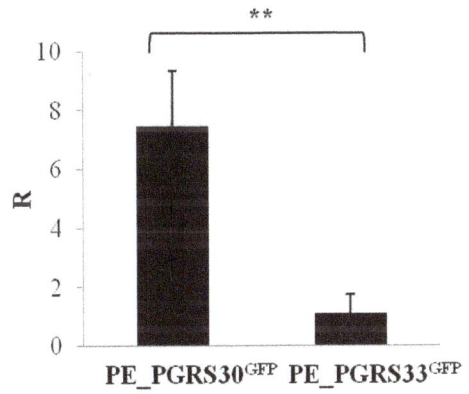

D

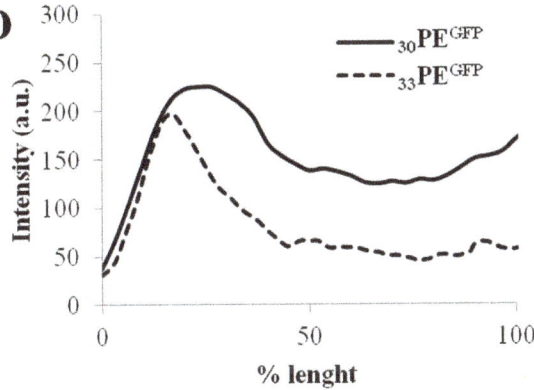
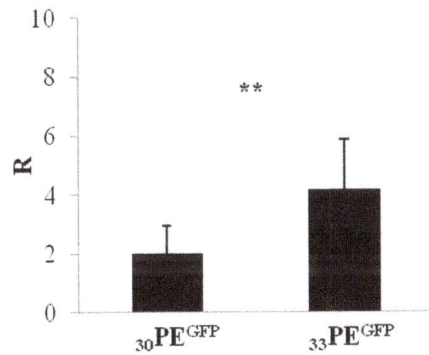

Figure 6. Differential polar localization between PE_PGRS30 and PE_PGRS33 spatial distribution in *Mtb*. A) Schematic representation of the PE_PGRS33-derived chimeras expressed in *Mtb* H37Rv. B) Confocal images of *Mtb* H37Rv expressing PE_PGRS33^{GFP} and $_{33}$PE^{GFP} using a 63× objective. In the inbox, a 100× image obtained overlapping green channel and transmission image is shown. Sample line profile and ratio between the GFP emission intensity at the bacterium pole and the GFP emission intensity in the cytoplasm between PE_PGRS30^{GFP} and PE_PGRS33^{GFP} (C) and between $_{30}$PE^{GFP} and $_{33}$PE^{GFP} (D). Twenty R values were analyzed for each *Mtb* strain under study. Two-tailed Student's *t*-test was used to analyze R ratio (* $p<0.05$, ** $p<0.01$).

bacterial poles occurs in members of MTB complex, which naturally express PE_PGRS, but not in *M. smegmatis*, which does not express any PE_PGRS, and as such may miss some of the protein partners [28,48] or cellular components involved in MTB complex in PE_PGRS cellular localization [9]. It remains to be seen whether polarization of PE_PGRS30 is dependent upon interaction with ESX-5 components and expression of the chimeras used in this study in *Mtb* ΔESX5 mutants [13,49] will shed light on the molecular mechanism of this process. The fact that a similar pattern of protein localization for PE_PGRS30 and its functional deletion chimeras was observed in *Mtb* and BCG suggests that lack of ESX-1 or other region of deletions in BCG [45,50] does not impact PE_PGRS30 localization.

PE_PGRS30 polarization was observed also for the $_{30}$PE_PGRSΔCT^{GFP}, indicating that the unique 306 amino acids C-terminal domain is not necessary for proper localization of the protein on the mycobacterial cell wall. These results are in line with our previous finding that the C-terminal unique domain is dispensable for the PE_PGRS30-dependent virulence [27] and imply that the PGRS domain is properly exposed or available to deploy its function in *Mtb* regardless of the C-terminal domain. Conversely, deletion of the PGRS central domain, as in the $_{30}$PE^{GFP} and $_{30}$PE_Ct^{GFP} chimeras, results in a partial loss of the

polar phenotype, suggesting that both the PE and PGRS domains are important for proper PE_PGRS30 localization. Since the first 140 amino acids of the protein (PE domain) are likely responsible for protein translocation [19–21], but not sufficient to mediate polar localization, it implies that the PGRS region downstream of the GRPLI domain plays a key role in protein polarization.

The importance of the PGRS region and of the GRPLI domain is further highlighted by the analysis of the *Mtb* cell lysates expressing the PE_PGRS30^{HA} and its functional HA-tagged chimeras in immunoblot using antiserum directed against the C-terminal domain. A clear band of 52 kDa was detected in all *Mtb* lysates, corresponding probably to the gene product of Rv3812, which was annotated as PE_PGRS62 [15] although it lacks both the typical PGRS domain and the GRPLI anchoring domain, highly conserved in all PE_PGRS proteins [18,35,51]. While the signal of the 52 kDa band was very similar in intensity to that corresponding to $_{30}$PE_CT^{HA}, a much lower signal was detected at ≈88 kDa, which corresponds to the full length PE_PGRS30. Since the level of fluorescence in *Mtb* was found similar between PE_PGRS30^{GFP} and $_{30}$PE_CT^{GFP} (figure 2), indicating similar level of protein expression, it is possible that PE_PGRS30 remains associated with the non-soluble cellular debris, suggesting a tight anchoring to the mycobacterial cell wall. Conversely, the

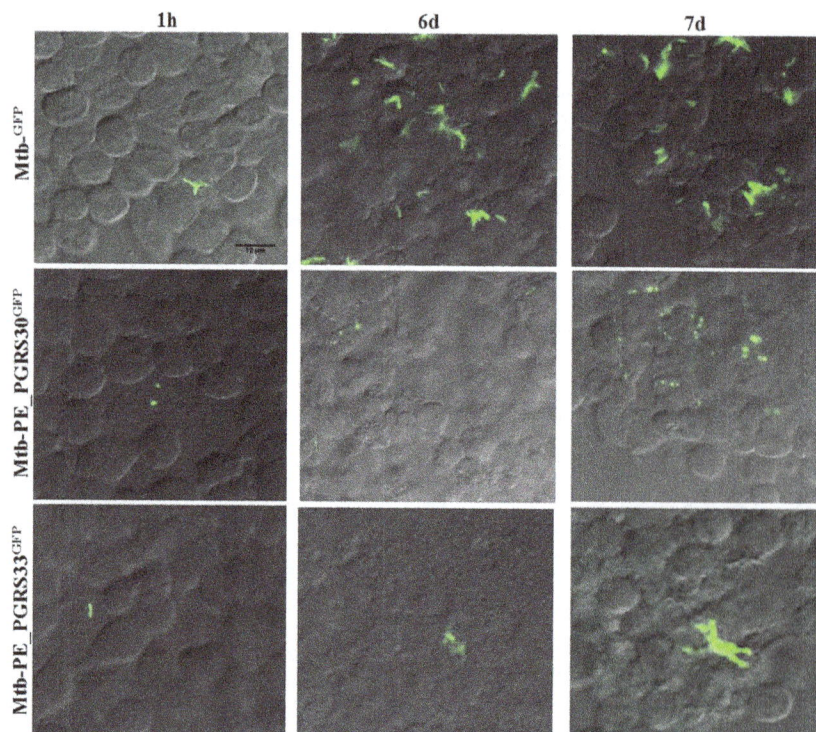

Figure 7. Polar localization of PE_PGRS30 during *Mtb* macrophage infection. Macrophages (J774) were infected with the *Mtb*^{GFP}, *Mtb*-PEGRS30^{GFP} and *Mtb*-PE_PGRS33^{GFP} and cells washed and fixed at 1 h and 6 days post-infection. Supernatants from infected macrophages at 6 days post-infection were harvested and used to infect fresh J774 macrophages, that 1 day later were washed and harvested. Slides containing infected macrophages harvested at the different time-points were analyzed at the confocal microscopy and images were obtained using a 63× objective.

$_{30}$PE_CT^{HA}, similarly to the Rv3812 gene product, appears to be more soluble, further highlighting the importance of PGRS for proper cellular localization.

Indeed, immunofluorescence studies showed that in *Mtb* the $_{30}$PE_CT^{HA} chimera is exposed on the mycobacterial surface while the full length protein (PE_PGRS30^{HA}) is not. Hence, while the results obtained with the $_{30}$PE_CT^{HA} support previous findings showing that the PE domain of PE_PGRS33 contains the information sufficient to drive an heterologous antigen to the mycobacterial surface [20,37], the results obtained with the full length protein suggest that the unique C-terminal domain of PE_PGRS30 localizes in the periplasm or is tightly embedded in the mycomembrane. The lack of any information on the potential function of the 306 amino acids long C-terminal domain prevents further hypothesis and the 40% identity (ClustalW2 software) with the C-terminal domain of Rv3812 is not high enough to exclude a different function.

Under physiological conditions of expression, PE_PGRS30^{GFP} and PE_PGRS33^{GFP} showed a different localization pattern in *Mtb*, with the former strongly polarizing and the latter homogeneously dispersed throughout the bacterial cell. Surprisingly, $_{33}$PE^{GFP} polarized at the cell poles but not $_{30}$PE^{GFP}. These results indicate that concentration of PE_PGRS30 at the bacterial poles depends upon the PGRS domain and not on the PE domain. Differences in amino acids sequences (figure S4) between the $_{30}$PE and $_{33}$PE may help explain the differential pattern of polarization observed between $_{30}$PE^{GFP} and $_{33}$PE^{GFP}, though we should remind that no such proteins, that is PE domain containing the GRPLI motif but lacking the PGRS domain (corresponding to the first $\approx$140 amino acids of PE_PGRSs), are naturally expressed by *Mtb* and as such these functional deletion chimeras may be missing key protein domains required to reach the natural cellular localization. Genomic analysis of MTB complex and *M. marinum* indicate that PE_PGRS30 is much more conserved than PE_PGRS33, with orthologous proteins found in *M. canettii* and *M. marinum*. Conversely, the gene encoding PE_PGRS33 was found only in the MTB complex genome but not in the smooth tubercle bacilli genome [52] nor in *M. marinum* genome, despite the large number of PE_PGRS genes present in the latter [18]. This evolutionary context may help explain the different cellular localization observed in this study between the two PE_PGRS proteins.

Concentration at one bacterial pole of proteins and enzymes involved in peptidoglycan synthesis [53] and virulence, such as the ESX1 secretory apparatus [54,55] is known to be important in mycobacteria. Concentration at a pole of virulence associated proteins or protein scaffolds may be a key step to evade from phagosome or eject from host cells [56]. Indeed, the ESX1 T7SS apparatus was shown to accumulate at the bacterial pole [54,55] and this process may be instrumental to produce holes in the phagosome that warrant cytoplasm access to *Mtb* [57]. Our finding indicating that PE_PGRS30 strongly accumulate at the bacterial poles in *Mtb* infecting macrophages and replicating intracellularly suggests that polarization may be a key step in the PE_PGRS30-dependent virulence mechanism. Since PE_PGRS30 is required for the survival and replication of *Mtb* in macrophages [27], it may be hypothesized that PE_PGRS30, alone or in combination with other yet undefined effectors, concentrates at one bacterial pole to maximize its activity. Conversely, PE_PGRS33^{GFP} was homogeneously distributed throughout the bacterial cells during *Mtb* infection in macrophages, indicating that different PE_PGRS proteins show a different

localization pattern. These findings further support the view that the PE_PGRS family includes a heterogeneous, differentially regulated group of proteins which, despite their similarities, exert different roles and functions in *Mtb* biology [58]. The repetitive GGA-GGN repeats of the PGRS domain are intercalated by protein-specific sequences which provide each PE_PGRS with a specific role and function. The results of this study highlight the role of the PGRS domain in the cellular localization of an *Mtb* virulence factor as PE_PGRS30.

Supporting Information

Figure S1 Immunoblots showing expression of PE_PGRS30 chimeras tagged with green fluorescent protein (GFP) in *Mycobacterium smegmatis* (A) and in *Mycobacterium tuberculosis* (B). Immunoblot analysis of whole cell lysates were probed with anti-GFP primary antibody.

Figure S2 Polar localization of PE_PGRS30^{GFP} spatial distribution in *M. bovis* BCG. A) Confocal images of *M. bovis* BCG expressing PE_PGRS30^{GFP} and its functional GFP-tagged chimeras obtained with a 63× objective. In the inbox, a 100× image obtained overlapping green channel and transmission image is shown. B) Sample line profile obtained quantifying the fluorescence along mycobacterial cell. C) Ratio between the GFP emission intensity at bacterium pole (considered as the value 200 nm far from the bacterium border) and GFP emission intensity in the cytoplasm (measured at the 50% of the bacterium length). Twenty R values were analyzed for each *M. bovis* strain under study. Two-tailed Student's *t*-test was used to analyze R ratio (* $p<0.05$, ** $p<0.01$).

Figure S3 A) Schematic representation showing the DNA construct ptPA^{30Cter} used to immunize mice and obtain specific polyclonal serum against the unique C-terminal domain of PE_PGRS30. B) Schematic showing the protein domains of PE_PGRS30 and PE_PGRS62.

Figure S4 Alignment of amino acid sequence of $_{30}$PE and $_{33}$PE using *ClustalW2 software* and *ESPripte software*.

Table S1 Primers used in this work.

Table S2 R indicates the index of the polarization of the protein distribution calculated with the ratio I_{pole}/I_{cyto} where I_pole is the GFP emission intensity at bacterium pole, considered as the value in correspondence of the border of the bacterium, and I_{cyto} is the GFP emission intensity in the middle part of the bacterium (measured at the 50% of the bacterium length).

Author Contributions

Conceived and designed the experiments: FDM GM RM MDS GD. Performed the experiments: FDM GM MM SA IP RI VP SC M. Sali. Analyzed the data: FDM GM WB RM M. Sanguinetti MDS GD. Contributed reagents/materials/analysis tools: WB RM MDS GD. Wrote the paper: FDM GM WB RM MDS GD.

References

1. World Health Organization (2012) Global Tuberculosis report 2012.

2. Dorhoi A, Reece ST, Kaufmann SH (2011) For better or for worse: the immune response against Mycobacterium tuberculosis balances pathology and protection. Immunol Rev 240: 235–251.

3. Ottenhoff TH, Kaufmann SH (2012) Vaccines against tuberculosis: where are we and where do we need to go? PLoS Pathog 8: e1002607.

4. Delogu G, Manganelli R, Brennan MJ (2014) Critical research concepts in tuberculosis vaccine development. Clin Microbiol Infect 20 Suppl 5: 59–65.

5. Morandi M, Sali M, Manganelli R, Delogu G (2013) Exploiting the mycobacterial cell wall to design improved vaccines against tuberculosis. J Infect Dev Ctries 7: 169–181.

6. Zuber B, Chami M, Houssin C, Dubochet J, Griffiths G, et al. (2008) Direct visualization of the outer membrane of mycobacteria and corynebacteria in their native state. J Bacteriol 190: 5672–5680.

7. Hoffmann C, Leis A, Niederweis M, Plitzko JM, Engelhardt H (2008) Disclosure of the mycobacterial outer membrane: cryo-electron tomography and vitreous sections reveal the lipid bilayer structure. Proc Natl Acad Sci U S A 105: 3963–3967.

8. Moreno-Altamirano MM, Paredes-Gonzalez IS, Espitia C, Santiago-Maldonado M, Hernandez-Pando R, et al. (2012) Bioinformatic identification of Mycobacterium tuberculosis proteins likely to target host cell mitochondria: virulence factors? Microb Inform Exp 2: 9. 2042-5783-2-9 [pii];

9. Abdallah AM, Verboom T, Weerdenburg EM, Gey van Pittius NC, Mahasha PW, et al. (2009) PPE and PE_PGRS proteins of Mycobacterium marinum are transported via the type VII secretion system ESX-5. Mol Microbiol 73: 329–340.

10. Bitter W, Houben EN, Bottai D, Brodin P, Brown EJ, et al. (2009) Systematic genetic nomenclature for type VII secretion systems. PLoS Pathog 5: e1000507.

11. Stoop EJ, Bitter W, van der Sar AM (2012) Tubercle bacilli rely on a type VII army for pathogenicity. Trends Microbiol 20: 477–484. S0966-842X(12)00117-5.

12. Daleke MH, Ummels R, Bawono P, Heringa J, Vandenbroucke-Grauls CM, et al. (2012) General secretion signal for the mycobacterial type VII secretion pathway. Proc Natl Acad Sci U S A 109: 11342–11347. 1119453109

13. Bottai D, Di LM, Majlessi L, Frigui W, Simeone R, et al. (2012) Disruption of the ESX-5 system of Mycobacterium tuberculosis causes loss of PPE protein secretion, reduction of cell wall integrity and strong attenuation. Mol Microbiol.

14. Campuzano J, Aguilar D, Arriaga K, Leon JC, Salas-Rangel LP, et al. (2007) The PGRS domain of Mycobacterium tuberculosis PE_PGRS Rv1759c antigen is an efficient subunit vaccine to prevent reactivation in a murine model of chronic tuberculosis. Vaccine 25: 3722–3729.

15. Cole ST, Brosch R, Parkhill J, Garnier T, Churcher C, et al. (1998) Deciphering the biology of Mycobacterium tuberculosis from the complete genome sequence. Nature 393: 537–544.

16. Banu S, Honore N, Saint-Joanis B, Philpott D, Prevost MC, et al. (2002) Are the PE-PGRS proteins of Mycobacterium tuberculosis variable surface antigens? Mol Microbiol 44: 9–19.

17. Brennan MJ, Delogu G (2002) The PE multigene family: a 'molecular mantra' for mycobacteria. Trends Microbiol 10: 246–249.

18. Delogu G, Cole ST, Brosch R (2008) The PE and PPE Protein Families of Mycobacterium tuberculosis. In: Kaufmann SH, Rubin E, editors. Handbook of Tuberculosis. Weinheim: Wiley-VCH Verlag GmbH%Co. KGaA. pp.131–150.

19. Delogu G, Pusceddu C, Bua A, Fadda G, Brennan MJ, et al. (2004) Rv1818c-encoded PE_PGRS protein of Mycobacterium tuberculosis is surface exposed and influences bacterial cell structure. Mol Microbiol 52: 725–733.

20. Cascioferro A, Delogu G, Colone M, Sali M, Stringaro A, et al. (2007) PE is a functional domain responsible for protein translocation and localization on mycobacterial cell wall. Mol Microbiol 66: 1536–1547.

21. Cascioferro A, Daleke MH, Ventura M, Dona V, Delogu G, et al. (2011) Functional dissection of the PE domain responsible for translocation of PE_PGRS33 across the mycobacterial cell wall. PLoS ONE 6: e27713.

22. Brennan MJ, Delogu G, Chen Y, Bardarov S, Kriakov J, et al. (2001) Evidence that mycobacterial PE_PGRS proteins are cell surface constituents that influence interactions with other cells. Infect Immun 69: 7326–7333.

23. Singh PP, Parra M, Cadieux N, Brennan MJ (2008) A comparative study of host response to three Mycobacterium tuberculosis PE_PGRS proteins. Microbiology 154: 3469–3479.

24. Cadieux N, Parra M, Cohen H, Maric D, Morris SL, et al. (2011) Induction of cell death after localization to the host cell mitochondria by the Mycobacterium tuberculosis PE_PGRS33 protein. Microbiology 157: 793–804.

25. Zumbo A, Palucci I, Cascioferro A, Sali M, Ventura M, et al. (2013) Functional dissection of protein domains involved in the immunomodulatory properties of PE_PGRS33 of Mycobacterium tuberculosis. Pathog Dis 69: 232–239.

26. Balaji KN, Goyal G, Narayana Y, Srinivas M, Chaturvedi R, et al. (2007) Apoptosis triggered by Rv1818c, a PE family gene from Mycobacterium tuberculosis is regulated by mitochondrial intermediates in T cells. Microbes Infect 9: 271–281.

27. Iantomasi R, Sali M, Cascioferro A, Palucci I, Zumbo A, et al. (2012) PE_PGRS30 is required for the full virulence of Mycobacterium tuberculosis. Cell Microbiol 14: 356–367.

28. Strong M, Sawaya MR, Wang S, Phillips M, Cascio D, et al. (2006) Toward the structural genomics of complexes: crystal structure of a PE/PPE protein complex from Mycobacterium tuberculosis. Proc Natl Acad Sci U S A 103: 8060–8065.

29. Sali M, Clarizio S, Pusceddu C, Zumbo A, Pecorini G, et al. (2008) Evaluation of the anti-tuberculosis activity generated by different multigene DNA vaccine constructs. Microbes Infect. 10(6): 605–12.

30. Stover CK, de lC, V, Fuerst TR, Burlein JE, Benson LA, et al. (1991) New use of BCG for recombinant vaccines. Nature 351: 456–460.

31. Delogu G, Howard A, Collins FM, Morris SL (2000) DNA Vaccination against Tuberculosis: Expression of a Ubiquitin- Conjugated Tuberculosis Protein Enhances Antimycobacterial Immunity. Infect Immun 68: 3097–3102.

32. Daleke MH, Cascioferro A, de PK, Ummels R, Abdallah AM, et al. (2011) Conserved PE and PPE protein domains target LipY lipases of pathogenic mycobacteria to the cell surface via ESX-5. J Biol Chem.

33. Maulucci G, Pani G, Labate V, Mele M, Panieri E, et al. (2009) Investigation of the spatial distribution of glutathione redox-balance in live cells by using Fluorescence Ratio Imaging Microscopy. Biosens Bioelectron 25: 682–687.

34. Balogh G, Maulucci G, Gombos I, Horvath I, Torok Z, et al. (2011) Heat stress causes spatially-distinct membrane re-modelling in K562 leukemia cells. PLoS ONE 6: e21182.

35. Huang Y, Wang Y, Bai Y, Wang ZG, Yang L, et al. (2010) Expression of PE_PGRS 62 protein in Mycobacterium smegmatis decrease mRNA expression of proinflammatory cytokines IL-1beta, IL-6 in macrophages. Mol Cell Biochem 340: 223–229.

36. Thi EP, Hong CJ, Sanghera G, Reiner NE (2013) Identification of the Mycobacterium tuberculosis protein PE-PGRS62 as a novel effector that functions to block phagosome maturation and inhibit iNOS expression. Cell Microbiol 15: 795–808.

37. Sali M, Di SG, Cascioferro A, Zumbo A, Nicolo C, et al. (2010) Surface expression of MPT64 as a fusion with the PE domain of PE_PGRS33 enhances Mycobacterium bovis BCG protective activity against Mycobacterium tuberculosis in mice. Infect Immun 78: 5202–5213.

38. Delogu G, Sanguinetti M, Pusceddu C, Bua A, Brennan MJ, et al. (2006) PE_PGRS proteins are differentially expressed by Mycobacterium tuberculosis in host tissues. Microbes Infect 8: 2061–2067.

39. Abdallah AM, Gey van Pittius NC, Champion PA, Cox J, Luirink J, et al. (2007) Type VII secretion—mycobacteria show the way. Nat Rev Microbiol 5: 883–891.

40. Gey van Pittius NC, Sampson SL, Lee H, Kim Y, van Helden PD, et al. (2006) Evolution and expansion of the Mycobacterium tuberculosis PE and PPE multigene families and their association with the duplication of the ESAT-6 (esx) gene cluster regions. BMC Evol Biol 6: 95.

41. Soldini S, Palucci I, Zumbo A, Sali M, Ria F, et al. (2011) PPE_MPTR genes are differentially expressed by Mycobacterium tuberculosis in vivo. Tuberculosis(Edinb).

42. Bottai D, Di LM, Majlessi L, Frigui W, Simeone R, et al. (2012) Disruption of the ESX-5 system of Mycobacterium tuberculosis causes loss of PPE protein secretion, reduction of cell wall integrity and strong attenuation. Mol Microbiol 83: 1195–1209.

43. Sayes F, Sun L, Di LM, Simeone R, Degaiffier N, et al. (2012) Strong immunogenicity and cross-reactivity of Mycobacterium tuberculosis ESX-5 type VII secretion: encoded PE-PPE proteins predicts vaccine potential. Cell Host Microbe 11: 352–363.

44. Sani M, Houben EN, Geurtsen J, Pierson J, de PK, et al. (2010) Direct visualization by cryo-EM of the mycobacterial capsular layer: a labile structure containing ESX-1-secreted proteins. PLoS Pathog 6: e1000794.

45. Houben EN, Bestebroer J, Ummels R, Wilson L, Piersma SR, et al. (2012) Composition of the type VII secretion system membrane complex. Mol Microbiol 86: 472–484.

46. Chatrath S, Gupta VK, Dixit A, Garg LC (2011) The Rv1651c-encoded PE-PGRS30 protein expressed in Mycobacterium smegmatis exhibits polar localization and modulates its growth profile. FEMS Microbiol Lett 322: 194–199.

47. Chatrath S, Gupta VK, Garg LC (2014) The PGRS domain is responsible for translocation of PE_PGRS30 to cell poles while the PE and the C-terminal domains localize it to the cell wall. FEBS Lett 588: 990–994.

48. Riley R, Pellegrini M, Eisenberg D (2008) Identifying cognate binding pairs among a large set of paralogs: the case of PE/PPE proteins of Mycobacterium tuberculosis. PLoS Comput Biol 4: e1000174.

49. Daleke MH, van der Woude AD, Parret AH, Ummels R, de Groot AM, et al. (2012) Specific Chaperones for the Type VII Protein Secretion Pathway. J Biol Chem 287: 31939–31947.

50. Brosch R, Gordon SV, Marmiesse M, Brodin P, Buchrieser C, et al. (2002) A new evolutionary scenario for the Mycobacterium tuberculosis complex. Proc Natl Acad Sci U S A 99: 3684–3689.

51. McEvoy CR, Cloete R, Muller B, Schurch AC, van Helden PD, et al. (2012) Comparative analysis of Mycobacterium tuberculosis pe and ppe genes reveals high sequence variation and an apparent absence of selective constraints. PLoS ONE 7: e30593.

52. Supply P, Marceau M, Mangenot S, Roche D, Rouanet C, et al. (2013) Genomic analysis of smooth tubercle bacilli provides insights into ancestry and pathoadaptation of Mycobacterium tuberculosis. Nat Genet 45: 172–179.

53. Hett EC, Chao MC, Rubin EJ (2010) Interaction and modulation of two antagonistic cell wall enzymes of mycobacteria. PLoS Pathog 6: e1001020.

54. Carlsson F, Joshi SA, Rangell L, Brown EJ (2009) Polar localization of virulence-related Esx-1 secretion in mycobacteria. PLoS Pathog 5: e1000285.

55. Wirth SE, Krywy JA, Aldridge BB, Fortune SM, Fernandez-Suarez M, et al. (2012) Polar assembly and scaffolding proteins of the virulence-associated ESX-1 secretory apparatus in mycobacteria. Mol Microbiol 83: 654–664.

56. Hagedorn M, Rohde KH, Russell DG, Soldati T (2009) Infection by tubercular mycobacteria is spread by nonlytic ejection from their amoeba hosts. Science 323: 1729–1733.

57. Simeone R, Bobard A, Lippmann J, Bitter W, Majlessi L, et al. (2012) Phagosomal rupture by Mycobacterium tuberculosis results in toxicity and host cell death. PLoS Pathog 8: e1002507.

58. Copin R, Coscolla M, Seiffert SN, Bothamley G, Sutherland J, et al. (2014) Sequence diversity in the pe_pgrs genes of Mycobacterium tuberculosis is independent of human T cell recognition. MBio 5: e00960–13.

16

Involvement of TNF-α Converting Enzyme in the Development of Psoriasis-Like Lesions in a Mouse Model

Kenji Sato[1,2], Mikiro Takaishi[1], Shota Tokuoka[2], Shigetoshi Sano[1]*

1 Department of Dermatology, Kochi Medical School, Kochi University, Nankoku, Japan, **2** Pharmacology Department, Drug Research Center, Kaken Pharmaceutical Co., Ltd., Kyoto, Japan

Abstract

TNF-α plays a crucial role in psoriasis; therefore, TNF inhibition has become a gold standard for the treatment of psoriasis. TNF-α is processed from a membrane-bound form by TNF-α converting enzyme (TACE) to soluble form, which exerts a number of biological activities. EGF receptor (EGFR) ligands, including heparin-binding EGF-like growth factor (HB-EGF), amphiregulin and transforming growth factor (TGF)-α are also TACE substrates and are psoriasis-associated growth factors. Vascular endothelial growth factor (VEGF), one of the downstream molecules of EGFR and TNF signaling, plays a key role in angiogenesis for developing psoriasis. In the present study, to assess the possible role of TACE in the pathogenesis of psoriasis, we investigated the involvement of TACE in TPA-induced psoriasis-like lesions in K5.Stat3C mice, which represent a mouse model of psoriasis. In this mouse model, TNF-α, amphiregulin, HB-EGF and TGF-α were significantly up-regulated in the skin lesions, similar to human psoriasis. Treatment of K5.Stat3C mice with TNF-α or EGFR inhibitors attenuated the skin lesions, suggesting the roles of TACE substrates in psoriasis. Furthermore, the skin lesions of K5.Stat3C mice showed down-regulation of tissue inhibitor of metalloproteinase-3, an endogenous inhibitor of TACE, and an increase in soluble TNF-α. A TACE inhibitor abrogated EGFR ligand-dependent keratinocyte proliferation and VEGF production in vitro, suggesting that TACE was involved in both epidermal hyperplasia and angiogenesis during psoriasis development. These results strongly suggest that TACE contributes to the development of psoriatic lesions through releasing two kinds of psoriasis mediators, TNF-α and EGFR ligands. Therefore, TACE could be a potential therapeutic target for the treatment of psoriasis.

Editor: Akihiko Yoshimura, Keio University School of Medicine, Japan

Funding: This study was funded in part by Kaken Pharmaceuticals Co. Ltd. KS, ST, SS received the funding. This study was additionally funded by grants-in-aid from the Ministry of Education, Culture, Sports, Science and Technology of Japan; and by a grant for Research on Intractable Diseases from the Ministry of Health, Labour, and Welfare of Japan. The funders had no role in study design, data collection and analysis, decision to publish, or preparation of the manuscript.

Competing Interests: The authors have read the journal's policy and have the following competing interests: KS and ST are employees of Kaken Pharmaceuticals Co. Ltd.

* Email: sano.derma@kochi-u.ac.jp

Introduction

Psoriasis is one of the most common inflammatory disorders and affects >2% of the population in Western countries. It has been demonstrated that TNF-α is involved in the development of psoriasis, as evidenced by the therapeutic efficacy of TNF-α inhibitors on psoriasis [1,2]. TNF-α has multiple functions and is one of the most important proinflammatory cytokines in psoriasis, linking innate immunity to adaptive immunity [3]. Indeed, previous studies suggested that TNF-α production from dendritic cells (DCs) is essential for activation of the pathogenic IL-23/Th17 axis in psoriasis [4].

TNF-α is produced as a membrane-bound form and is processed by TNF-α converting enzyme (TACE) to become a soluble form that exerts biological activity [5–7]. In addition to TNF-α, membrane-bound EGFR ligands, including amphiregulin, heparin-binding EGF (HB-EGF) and transforming growth factor (TGF)-α, are TACE substrates. More importantly, these EGFR ligands are known to contribute to the pathogenesis of psoriasis [8–10]. Furthermore, TACE is expressed by epidermal keratinocytes and inflammatory cells in the dermis in psoriatic lesions [11].

However, it remains unclear whether TACE is involved in the pathogenesis of psoriasis.

We previously reported that Stat3 is activated in keratinocytes in the majority of human psoriatic lesions [12]. K5.Stat3C transgenic mice, in which Stat3 is constitutively active in keratinocytes, develop psoriasis-like lesions following wounding stimuli or topical treatment with the tumor promoter 12-O-tetradecanoylphorbol-13-acetate (TPA), which strongly suggests that Stat3 activation is required for the development of psoriasis. The skin lesions of K5.Stat3C mice closely resemble psoriasis and provide a relevant animal model of psoriasis based on clinical, histological, immunophenotypic and biological criteria [12,13]. For example, the skin lesions in K5.Stat3C mice show epidermal hyperplasia, infiltration of immune cells into the dermis and abscess formation in the epidermis, which represent shared pathologic features with human psoriasis [12,14]. Furthermore, the skin lesions in K5.Stat3C mice are attenuated by administration of an anti-IL-17A antibody or anti-IL-12/23p40 antibody, similar to human psoriasis [14]. Therefore, K5.Stat3C mice provide a platform for screening potential therapeutic targets for the treatment of psoriasis.

Angiogenesis is a hallmark of psoriasis and the psoriasis-like skin lesions in K5.Stat3C mice [12]. VEGF plays a key role in angiogenesis and wound healing [15], and is a potential target for the treatment of psoriasis [16]. Upon wounding, keratinocytes produce VEGF, which is also strongly up-regulated in the epidermis of psoriatic lesions [17]. Previous studies have demonstrated that VEGF production by keratinocytes is regulated by TNF-α or HB-EGF [18,19]. Therefore, it is likely that TACE plays a role in VEGF production from keratinocytes not only during wound healing but also in psoriasis. In this regard, TACE is a post-translational regulator for the release of multiple soluble mediators required for psoriasis.

In the present study, we investigated the expression of TACE and its related molecules in psoriasis-like skin lesions in K5.Stat3C mice, and addressed the question as to how TACE inhibition impacts the release of cytokines/growth factors and keratinocyte proliferation. The sum of our results suggests TACE inhibition as a potential strategy for the treatment of psoriasis.

Materials and Methods

Patients and normal controls

The study protocol was conducted in accordance with the guidelines of the World Medical Association's Declaration of Helsinki and was approved by the Institute Ethical Review Board of the Kochi Medical School, Kochi University. Written informed consent was obtained from subjects after explaining the purpose of the study.

Mice

All experimental procedures performed on mice were approved by the Institutional Animal Care and Use Committee of Kochi Medical School. K5.Stat3C mice were generated as previously reported [20]. Briefly, Stat3C cDNA (a gift from Dr. J. Bromberg, Memorial Sloan Kettering Cancer Center) was ligated into the pBK5 construct, followed by digestion with EcoRI. The construct was then used to generate transgenic founder mice on an FVB/N background.

TPA-induced psoriasis-like lesions in the ears of K5.Stat3C mice

The generation of psoriasis-like lesions in the ears of K5.Stat3C mice was conducted as previously described [14,21]. In brief, the skin lesions were generated by topical application of 0.68 nmol TPA (Wako) in 20 μl acetone to all surfaces of the left and right ears at day 0 and 2. Etanercept (Pfizer) (1 mg/mouse) was intravenously injected on day 0 and 2. The dosage of etanercept was decided as previously described [22]. AG1478 (LC laboratories) was dissolved in acetone to prepare a 0.016% solution. Following this, 20 μl AG1478 solution was topically applied to all surfaces of the left and right ears twice a day. The concentration of AG1478 was decided as previously described [23]. Ear thickness was measured every day from day 0 to 3. The mice were sacrificed and ear skins were collected for gene and protein expression analysis and histological analysis. All mouse experiments were performed with strict adherence to institutional guidelines for minimizing distress.

Histology

Ear tissues were fixed in 20% formalin and then embedded in paraffin. Sections were obtained from the paraffin blocks and stained by hematoxylin and eosin (H&E) using standard methods. Epidermal thickness was measured at 12 spots in the interfollicular epidermis in each slide.

Immunohistochemical staining

Formalin-fixed slides were deparaffinized with xylene and rehydrated in an alcohol gradient. Slides were autoclaved in 10 mmol/l citrate (pH 6.0) at 115°C for 5 min to retrieve antigen, then incubated for 40 min at room temperature. Endogenous peroxidase was quenched using 3% hydrogen peroxide, then non-specific antibody reaction was blocked using protein block serum free (DAKO) at room temperature for 30 min. Slides were incubated with specific primary antibodies, rabbit anti-human TACE antibody (QED Bioscience) or rabbit anti-human TNF-α (IHC-world), at 4°C overnight. Slides were washed with PBS and subjected to horseradish peroxidase-conjugated secondary antibody (DAKO) for 30 min at 37°C. The slides were washed with PBS, then detected by diaminobenzidine substrate kit (Life Technologies). All slides were counterstained with hematoxylin.

Quantitative real-time PCR

Ear tissues were minced with scissors into small pieces on ice, and were then disrupted by sonication in RNA lysis buffer contained in an RNA isolation kit (Promega). For some experiments, primary keratinocytes were stimulated with 20 ng/ml IL-17A (R&D Systems) and 10 ng/ml TNF-α (R&D Systems) for 24 h and peritoneal macrophages were stimulated with 100 ng/ml LPS (Sigma) for 0.5, 6 and 24 h pretreated with or without 10 μmol/l TAPI-1 (Enzo Life Sciences), for 30 min prior to stimulation. Total RNAs were extracted using an RNeasy Mini kit (Qiagen) according to the manufacturer's protocol. RNAs were reverse transcribed using M-MLV reverse transcriptase with random oligonucleotide hexamers (Life Technologies). Quantitative PCR reactions were performed using Taqman Master Mix or Power SYBR Green PCR Master Mix (Life Technologies). Amplification conditions were as follows: 50°C for 2 min, 90°C for 10 min for 1 cycle, followed by 40 cycles of 95°C for 15 sec and 60°C for 1 min. Primers used were described elsewhere [14] and those for HPRT (Mm01545399_m1), TNF-α (Mm00443258_m1), amphiregulin (Mm00437583_m1), HB-EGF (Mm00439306_m1), TGF-α (Mm00446232_m1) and TIMP-3 (Mm00441826_m1), all from Life Technologies. The quantity of each transcript was analyzed using the 7300 Fast System Software (Life Technologies) and was normalized to hypoxanthine phosphoribosyltransferase (HPRT), according to the ΔΔ Ct method.

Determination of TNF-α in skin samples

For measurement of TNF-α in skin, ear biopsy samples were taken using a punch (a diameter of 8 mm, Kai Industries Co. Ltd.). Ear tissues were minced with scissors into small pieces on ice in cold PBS containing protease inhibitor cocktail, phosphatase inhibitor cocktail 2 and 3 (Sigma), and were disrupted by sonication. The homogenized tissues were centrifuged at 20,000 g for 20 min at 4°C, and supernatants were harvested. TNF-α in the supernatants was measured using ELISA for TNF-α (R&D Systems).

Measurement of in vivo TACE activity

TACE activity was determined by the SensoLyte 520 TACE Activity Assay Fluorimetric Kit (AnaSpec), according to the manufacturer's instructions. In brief, Ear skins were minced with scissors into small pieces in cold assay buffer containing 0.1% TritonX-100 and were homogenized. The lysates were centrifuged at 2,000 g for 15 min at 4°C, and supernatants were harvested. TACE activity from 25 μg of total protein was measured using the kit for TACE activity.

Western blot

The protein extraction from ear skins was performed as described above. The protein concentration of each supernatant was measured with the Bio-Rad protein assay system (Bio-Rad). The supernatants were separated on 4–20% SDS/PAGE according to the method as previously described [24], under reducing conditions. Recombinant TNF-α (eBioscience) was loaded as a positive control in some experiments. Separated proteins were electrophoretically transferred to polyvinylidene difluoride membranes and blocked with 5% skim milk in TBS with 0.1% Tween 20 (TBST) for 1 h at room temperature. Membranes were incubated with specific primary antibodies, goat anti-mouse TNF-α antibody (Antigenix America) or rabbit anti-mouse TIMP-3 antibody (Millipore), at 4°C overnight. Membranes were washed with TBST and subjected to horseradish peroxidase-conjugated secondary antibodies against goat (SantaCruz) and rabbit (GE Healthcare) for 45 min at room temperature. The membranes were washed with TBST, then detection for TNF-α and TIMP-3 were performed using SuperSignal West Femto (Thermo Fisher Scientific) and ECL plus Western Blotting Detection System (GE Healthcare), respectively. The membranes were stripped by Restore Western blot stripping buffer (Thermo Fisher Scientific) and reprobed with mouse anti-mouse fiactin (Sigma) for 1 h at room temperature. The membranes were washed with TBST, then subjected to corresponding horseradish peroxidase-conjugated secondary antibodies (GE Healthcare). The membranes were washed with TBST, then detected with ECL plus Western Blotting Detection System.

Preparation of bone marrow derived dendritic cells (BMDCs), peritoneal macrophages and keratinocytes

BMDCs were generated as previously described [25]. Briefly, bone marrow cells taken from wild-type FVB/N mice were suspended in RPMI 1640 (Life Technologies) containing 10 ng/ml GM-CSF (Peprotech), antibiotic-antimycotic (Life Technologies) and 10% FBS (Nichirei Bioscience). BMDCs were harvested 9 d later and plated at $5×10^4$ cells/well in 96-well plates. Peritoneal macrophages were isolated as previously described [26] with modifications. Briefly, wild-type FVB/N mice were injected i.p. with 500 μL 4% sterile thioglycolate (Becton Dickinson) solution in PBS, and cells were harvested by peritoneal lavage 4 d later. Cells were plated at $5×10^4$ cells/well in 96-well plates. For gene expression analysis, cells were plated at $2.5×10^5$ cells/well in 24-well plates. Primary keratinocytes were isolated from the skin of K5.Stat3C newborn mice as described [12]. In brief, epidermis was isolated by overnight digestion of dorsal skin from K5.Stat3C newborn mice with dispase (Becton Dickinson) at 4°C. The epidermis was incubated with 0.25% trypsin (Life Technologies) for 5 min at 37°C. After stopping the trypsin reaction with FBS, the keratinocyte suspension was passed through a 70 μm cell strainer. Freshly isolated primary keratinocytes were plated at $2.5×10^5$ cells/well in 24-well plates for the detection TNF-ted wiamphiregulin or $1.5×10^5$ cells/well in 48-well plates for the detection VEGF in DMEM-Glutamax (Life Technologies) containing antibiotic-antimycotic and 10% FBS. Three hours later, the medium and floating cells were removed, and attached cells were refed with Epilife (Life Technologies) supplemented with Hu-Media KG (Kurabo). Cells were cultured until they were subconfluent, then used for the detection of TNF-α, amphiregulin and VEGF. For the proliferation assay, freshly isolated primary keratinocytes were plated at $6×10^4$ cells/well in 48-well plates. A medium change was performed as described above, then cells were cultured for 2 days.

Production of TNF-α, amphiregulin and VEGF in vitro

BMDCs and peritoneal macrophages from wild-type FVB/N mice were stimulated with 100 ng/ml LPS. Primary keratinocytes isolated from K5.Stat3C newborn mice were stimulated with 100 nmol/l TPA for 24 h. Cells were pretreated with or without TAPI-1 for 30 min prior to stimulation. The concentrations of cytokines and growth factors in the culture medium were examined by ELISA for TNF-α (eBioscience), amphiregulin (R&D Systems) and VEGF (R&D Systems).

Keratinocyte proliferation assay and Cytotoxic assay

Primary keratinocytes were treated with or without 100 μmol/l TAPI-1 or 100 nmol/l AG1478. HB-EGF (BioVision) or amphiregulin (R&D Systems) (all at 100 ng/ml) were added at 30 min after TAPI-1 or AG1478 treatment, then cultured for 3 days. Keratinocyte proliferation was assessed using 3-(4,5-dimethylthiazol-2-yl)-5-(3-carboxymethoxyphenyl)-2-(4-sulfophenyl)-2H-tetrazolium, inner salt (MTS) assay (Promega) on day 0 to 3, or bromodeoxyuridine (BrdU) ELISA (Roche) on day 2. Toxicity effects and adverse reactions to chemical compounds were assessed by measuring lactate dehydrogenase (LDH) release in the culture medium (Promega), and Triton X-100 (Wako) was used as a positive control.

Statistical analysis

Statistical differences were evaluated by Student's t-test, Tukey-Kramer's test or Duunett's test. p values less than 0.05 were considered significant.

Results

Expression of TACE and TNF-α in human psoriatic skin and in psoriasis-like skin lesions of K5.Stat3C mice

As previously described, TACE was expressed in all layers of the epidermis, blood vessels and appendages in human psoriatic lesions as well as in uninvolved human skin (Fig. 1A, middle panels) [11,27]. However, dermal inflammatory cells in psoriatic lesions strongly expressed TACE (Fig. 1A, right middle panel) [11,27]. TNF-α was expressed in the epidermis and inflammatory cell infiltrates of psoriatic lesions (Fig. 1A, right bottom panel), whereas uninvolved skin did not express TNF-α (Fig. 1A, left bottom panel) as previously reported [28]. Topical treatment with TPA resulted in the emergence of psoriasis-like lesions in K5.Stat3C mice, but not in wild-type mice (Fig. 1B–D) [14]. The histopathology of skin lesions in K5.Stat3C included epidermal hyperplasia, a number of inflammatory cell infiltrates in the dermis, and abscess formation in the epidermis, all of which resemble psoriasis (Fig. 1A–B, top panels). Similar to human psoriasis, TPA-induced psoriasis-like lesions in K5.Stat3C mice were positive for TACE in the epidermis, inflammatory cells, blood vessels and appendages (Fig. 1A–B, middle panels). It is noteworthy that the neutrophilic abscess in the epidermis showed strong TACE expression (Fig. 1B, arrow). Furthermore, as found in human psoriasis [28] (Fig. 1A, bottom panels), TNF-α was overexpressed in psoriasis-like skin lesions of K5.Stat3C mice, although virtually no TNF-α was found in untreated control skin (Fig. 1B, bottom panels). However, TPA treatment induced TNF-α expression in the epidermis of wild-type mice as well (Fig. 1C, bottom). This was supported by the results of RT-PCR (Fig. 1E) and ELISA (Fig. 1F) showing that TPA-treated skins of wild-type mice showed increased TNF-α expression as well as K5.Stat3C mice on day 3. Taken together, elevated levels and distribution of TACE and TNF-α in skin lesions of K5.Stat3C mice are similar to those in human psoriasis.

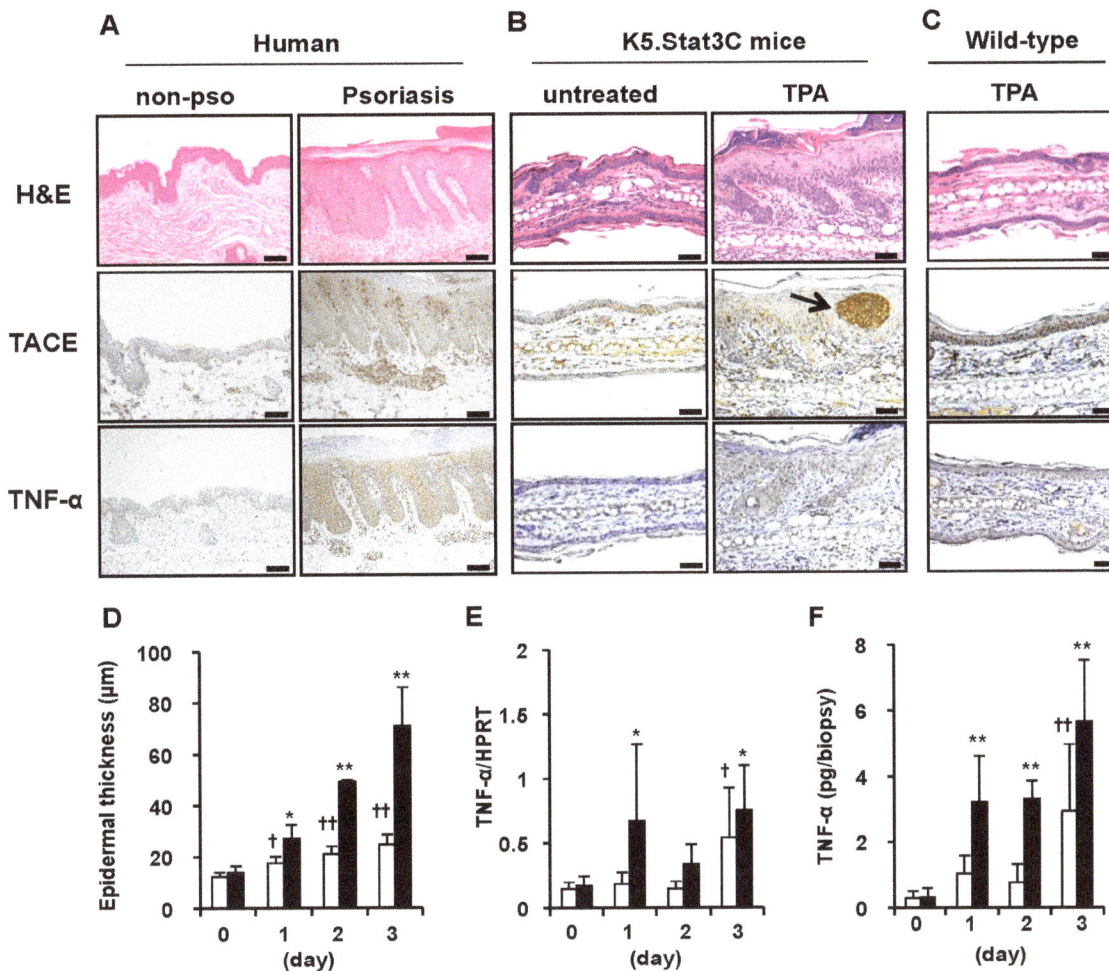

Figure 1. Expression of TACE and TNF-α in the development of psoriasis-like skin lesions in K5.Stat3C mice. (A–C), Representative histology and immunohistochemistry of human skins (A), ear skins in K5.Stat3C mice (B), and wild-type mice (C). non-pso, non-psoriasis control; TPA, TPA-treated ear skins sampled at day 3; Hematoxylin and eosin staining (H&E, top panels), Immunohistochemical staining for TACE (middle panels) and TNF-α (bottom panels). Arrow, intraepidermal pustule of neutrophils. Bars = 100 μm (human), 50 μm (mouse). (D–F), epidermal thickness (D), TNF-α mRNA expression (E) and TNF-α protein levels (F) in the TPA-treated ear skins of K5.Stat3C mice (black bars) and wild-type mice (white bars). Data represent means ± SD of 3 to 8 mice. *$p<0.05$, **$p<0.01$, versus K5.Stat3C mice at day 0, †$p<0.05$, ††$p<0.01$, versus wild-type mice at day 0, by Dunnett's test.

TNF-α is involved in the development of psoriasis-like skin lesions in K5.Stat3C mice

To examine whether TNF-α is involved in the development of skin lesions, we intravenously injected a TNF-α inhibitor, etanercept, to K5.Stat3C mice before topical TPA application. Etanercept attenuated the TPA-induced thickening of ear skins (Fig. 2A) as well as epidermal hyperplasia (Fig. 2B–C). In addition, etanercept lowered the TPA-induced gene expression of IL-17A and IL-12/23p40 in the skin lesions (Fig. 2D–E). These results suggest that the inhibition of TNF-α signaling attenuates the psoriasis-like phenotype in K5.Stat3C mice through down-regulation of the IL-23/Th17 axis as found in patients with psoriasis treated with TNF-α inhibitors [4]. These results suggest that the inhibition of TNF-α attenuates the psoriasis-like phenotype in K5.Stat3C mice as occurs in patients with psoriasis treated with TNF-α inhibitors.

EGFR signaling is involved in the development of skin lesions in K5.Stat3C mice

EGFR ligands, including amphiregulin, HB-EGF and TGF-α, all of which are TACE substrates, have been shown to be up-regulated in psoriatic lesions [29]. We analyzed the gene expression of EGFR ligands during the development of psoriasis-like skin lesions in K5.Stat3C mice. Transcriptional levels of amphiregulin, HB-EGF and TGF-α were increased at day 1, and remained elevated until day 3, whereas the increase in levels of those genes in wild-type mouse skin was much less pronounced during 3 days of topical TPA application (Fig. 3A). This result indicated that up-regulation of EGFR ligands was associated with Stat3 activation in keratinocytes [13]. To assess whether EGFR signaling is involved in TPA-induced psoriasis-like skin lesions, we topically treated K5.Stat3C mice with AG1478, an EGFR inhibitor. AG1478 attenuated the epidermal thickness (Fig. 3B–C), which suggests that the EGFR signaling by the aforementioned EGFR ligands contributed, at least in part, to the generation of lesions in K5.Stat3C mice.

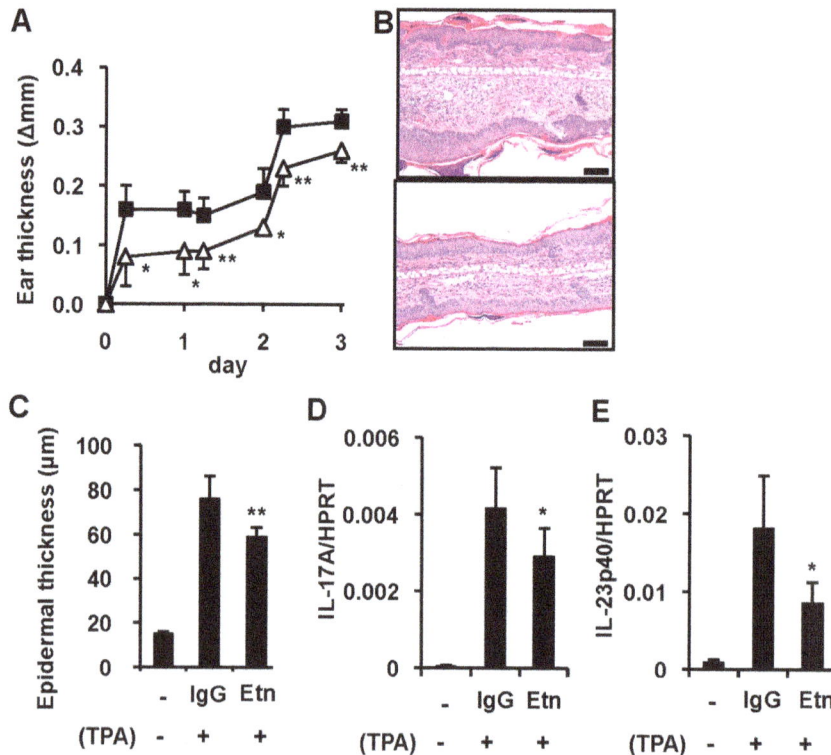

Figure 2. Involvement of TNF-α in the development of psoriasis-like skin lesions in K5.Stat3C mice. (A), Ear thickness (Δmm) ± SD following topical TPA in mice treated with control IgG (n=6, squares) and etanercept (n=6, triangles). *p<0.05, **p<0.01, versus control IgG, by Student's t-test. (B), Representative histology of ear skins from K5.Stat3C mice treated with control IgG (top) and etanercept (bottom). H&E staining. Bar=100 μm. (C–E), Inhibitory effect of etanercept (Etn) on TPA-induced epidermal hyperplasia (C), gene expression of IL-17A (D), and IL-12/23p40 (E) in ear skins. Data represent means ± SD of 3 to 6 mice. *p<0.05, **p<0.01, versus control IgG, by Student's t-test.

Down-regulation of TIMP-3, an endogenous TACE inhibitor, and increased TACE enzymatic activity in psoriasis-like skin lesions of K5.Stat3C mice

Tissue inhibitor of metalloproteinase-3 (TIMP-3) has been reported as the negative regulator of the enzymatic activity of TACE [30–32]. Gene expression of TIMP-3 in the ear skin of K5.Stat3C mice was decreased in a time-dependent manner during the generation of TPA-induced lesions (Fig. 4A, black bars), while this decline was much less pronounced in wild-type mice (Fig. 4A, white bars). Strikingly, Western blot analysis revealed that TIMP-3 protein levels in the ear skin of K5.Stat3C mice were almost completely abrogated as early as 6 h of TPA application (Fig. 4B), and in turn, soluble TNF-α emerged around 17 kDa of molecular weight (Fig. 4C), through TACE-mediated processing of its membrane-bound form. In contrast, soluble TNF-α was hardly detected from the lysates of wild-type mice at this early time point (Fig. 4C). However, the gene expression of TACE was not different between wild-type mice and K5.Stat3C mice, or not increased by TPA treament (data not shown), suggesting that the post-transcriptional function of TACE might be enhanced likely by down-regulation of TIMP-3. Indeed, the skin of K5.Stat3C mice at baseline showed higher enzymatic activity of TACE than wild-type mice, and it was further increased following TPA treatment (Fig. 4D). Taken collectively, these results implicated that TACE was favorably activated in the skin of K5.Stat3C mice, at least in part, due to down-modulation of TIMP-3, leading to lesion development.

TACE releases TNF-α from various cells

TNF-α is produced by various cells in psoriasis, including keratinocytes, dendritic cells, macrophages and lymphocytes [33,34]. To assess whether TACE plays a role in releasing TNF-α from these cells, we added a relatively selective inhibitor of TACE, TAPI-1 [35], to an in vitro culture of bone marrow-derived dendritic cells (BMDCs), peritoneal macrophages and primary keratinocytes. TAPI-1 significantly and dose-dependently suppressed the LPS- or TPA-induced release of TNF-α from BMDCs and macrophages from wild-type FVB/N mice and keratinocytes of K5.Stat3C newborn mice, respectively (Fig. 5A–C). The release of TNF-α from T lymphocytes was also abrogated by TAPI-1 (data not shown). It should be noted that TNF-α mRNA levels in macrophages were increased by LPS stimulation but not affected by TAPI-1 treatment (Fig. S1), verifying that TAPI-1 inhibited the release of TNF-α post-transcriptionally. Collectively, these results clearly indicate that the release of soluble TNF-α from a variety of cells is dependent on TACE activity.

TACE induces the release of EGFR ligands from keratinocytes

EGFR ligands are produced by keratinocytes, and thereby an auto-stimulation loop is formed to generate psoriatic changes in an autocrine and paracrine fashion [10,36]. To assess whether TACE activity is required for the release of EGFR ligands as well as TNF-α, we evaluated the effects of TAPI-1 using primary cultured keratinocytes isolated from K5.Stat3C mice. Like TNF-α, amphiregulin was released by TACE from keratinocytes in response to TPA, since it was significantly suppressed by TAPI-1

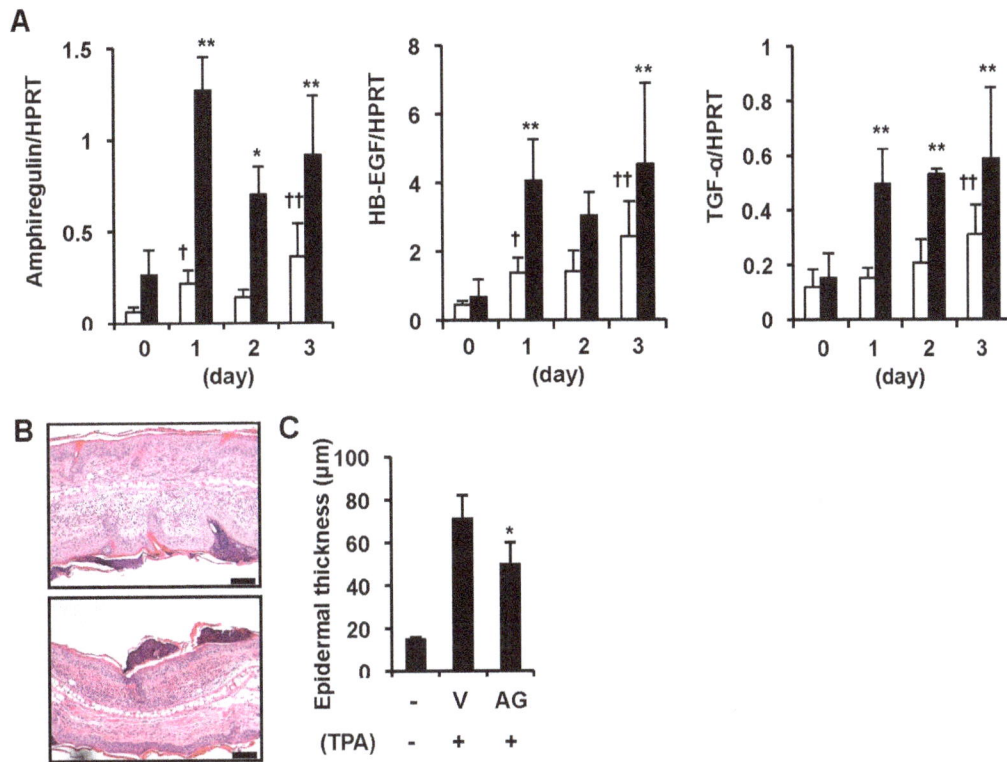

Figure 3. Involvement of EGFR signaling in the development of psoriasis-like skin lesions in K5.Stat3C mice. (A), Gene expression of amphiregulin, HB-EGF and TGF-α in the TPA-treated ear skins of K5.Stat3C mice (black bars) and wild-type mice (white bars). Data represent means ± SD of 3 to 8 mice. *$p<0.05$, **$p<0.01$, versus K5.Stat3C mice at day 0, †$p<0.05$, ††$p<0.01$, versus wild-type mice at day 0, by Dunnett's test. (B), Representative histology of ear skins from K5.Stat3C mice treated with vehicle alone (top) and AG1478 (bottom). Bars = 100 μm. (C), Suppression of TPA-induced epidermal hyperplasia by treatment with AG1478 (AG) at day 3. Data represent means ± SD of 3 to 5 mice, *$p<0.05$ versus vehicle alone (V) by Student's t-test.

in a dose-dependent manner (Fig. 5D). EGFR stimulation leads to keratinocyte proliferation, and contributes to epidermal hyperplasia in psoriasis [29,37] and the skin phenotypes of K5.Stat3C mice as well (Fig. 3). We next examined whether TACE is directly required for keratinocyte proliferation in response to the endogenous EGFR ligands. In vitro keratinocyte proliferation was suppressed by TAPI-1 and AG1478 (Fig. 5E). The inhibitory effects of both reagents on cell proliferation were confirmed using a BrdU incorporation assay (Fig. S2A). TAPI-1 or AG1478 did not raise lactate dehydrogenase levels in the culture supernatants compared with the vehicle control, thus ruling out cytotoxicity as a possible cause of impaired keratinocyte proliferation (Fig. S2B). The suppression of keratinocyte proliferation by TAPI-1 was reversed by the addition of amphiregulin, suggesting that TACE is involved in keratinocyte proliferation via EGFR stimulation with soluble amphiregulin (Fig. 5E). Although the underlying mechanism is not known, HB-EGF seemed to augment the TAPI-1-induced suppression of keratinocyte proliferation. VEGF is an angiogenetic factor, and is involved in the pathogenesis of psoriasis [17,38,39]. Psoriatic lesions in K5.Stat3C mice showed increased levels of VEGF [12] (Fig. S3). Furthermore, TAPI-1 and AG1478 inhibited the TPA-induced VEGF production from K5.Stat3C keratinocytes to a similar extent (Fig. 5F). Suppression of VEGF production by TAPI-1 was reversed by the addition of HB-EGF, but not by amphiregulin (Fig. 5F). These results demonstrate that TACE-dependent HB-EGF stimulation leads to VEGF produc-

tion by K5.Stat3C keratinocytes. Taken together, TACE is required for the release of soluble EGFR ligands from keratinocytes, thereby promoting keratinocyte proliferation and VEGF production, which are required for the development of psoriasis.

Discussion

The auto-stimulation loop of cytokine/growth factors within the epidermis and its bidirectional interaction with immunocytes play critical roles in the development of psoriasis. One of the proinflammatory cytokines, TNF-α, and growth factors of the EGFR ligand family represent essential mediators for the pathogenesis of psoriasis. TNF-α and EGFR ligands are overexpressed in plaque psoriasis compared with uninvolved skin or healthy control skin [28,29]. Our current study highlights the role of TACE, by which both TNF-α and growth factors for EGFR are shed to form soluble ligands. Here we took advantage of K5.Stat3C mice, which develop skin lesions that closely resemble human psoriasis with respect to clinical features, histopathology, immunological abnormalities and sensitivities to biologics [12,14,40].

The role for TNF-α in psoriasis has been well documented, and is supported by a number of studies showing successful therapeutic effects of its inhibitors [1,2]. It was suggested that TNF-α stimulation of DCs results in IL-23 production, which is required for Th17 cell activation [4,41]. Indeed, a comparison of gene expression in psoriasis patients between responders to etanercept,

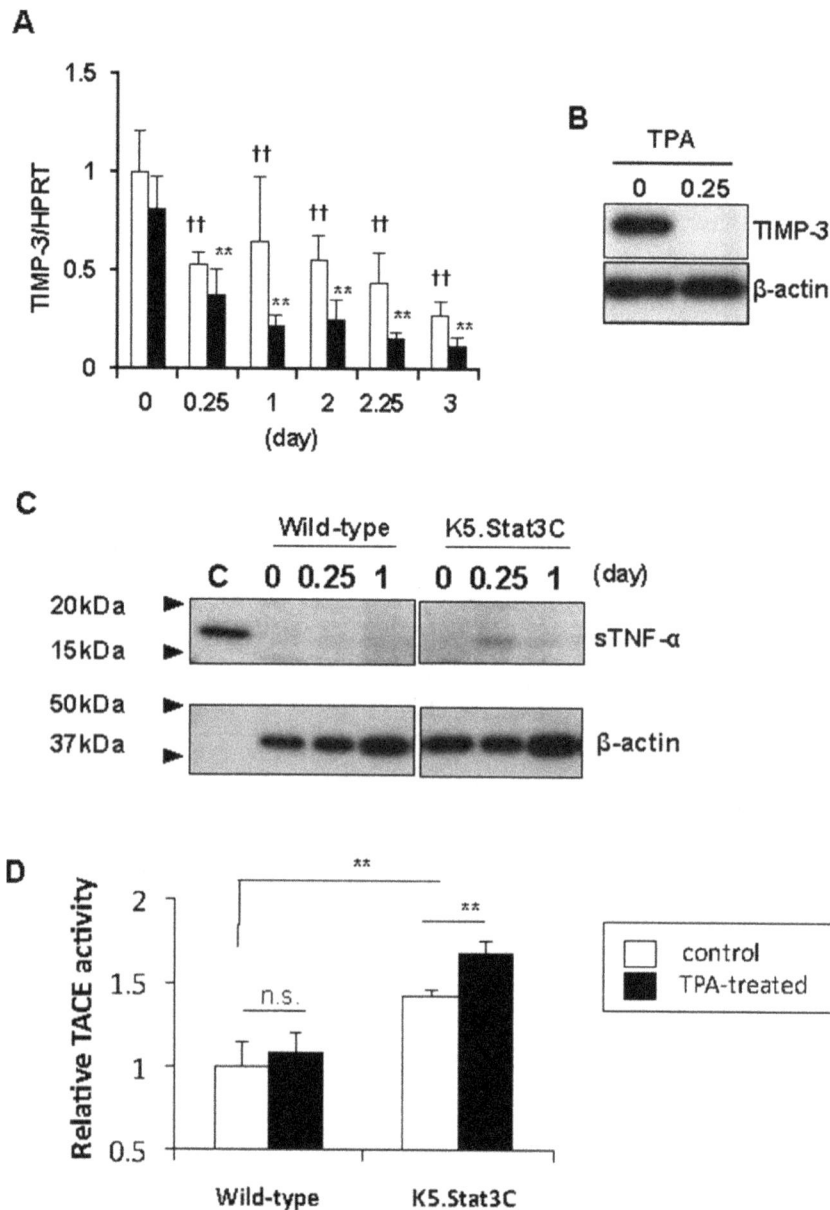

Figure 4. Down-regulation of TIMP-3, an endogenous TACE inhibitor, and TACE enzymatic activity in the development of psoriasis-like skin lesions. (A), Gene expression of TIMP-3 in the TPA-treated ear skins of K5.Stat3C mice (black bars) and wild-type mice (white bars). Data represent means ± SD of 3 to 8 mice. **$p<0.01$, versus K5.Stat3C mice at day 0, ††$p<0.01$, versus wild-type mice at day 0, by Dunnett's test. (B), Western blot analysis of TIMP-3 in ear skins of K5.Stat3C mice collected before TPA application (0) or 6 h (0.25) after TPA application. (C), Western blot analysis of soluble TNF-α (sTNF-α), which is around 17 kDa of molecular size, in the lysates from ear skins of K5.Stat3C mice compared with wild-type mice. The ear skins were collected before TPA application (0) or at 6 h (0.25) and 1 day (1) after TPA application. C, Control of soluble TNF-α. (D), Enzymatic activity of TACE in ear skins of K5.Stat3C mice versus wild-type mice; untreated control (white bars) and TPA-treated at 6h of the second TPA application (black bars). Enzymatic activity in skins was indicated as ratio to that in untreated wild-type skins. Data represent means ± SD of 4 to 5 mice, **$p<0.01$; n.s., not significant by Tukey-Kramer's test.

a TNF-α inhibitor, and non-responders revealed that the responsiveness is dependent on inactivation of the Th17 immune response [42]. We showed that TNF-α stimulation enhances the production of IL-12/IL-23p40, one of the IL-23 subunits, from murine bone marrow-derived DCs (BMDCs) (data not shown). TNF-α inhibition also abrogates Th17 differentiation in vitro [43]. Furthermore, TNF-α synergistically augments IL-17A stimulation of gene expression by keratinocytes, including IL-24 (a member of IL-20 subfamily cytokines), IL-17C, TNF-α, HB-EGF, TGF-α, S100A7, S100A8, S100A9, β-defensin-3 and β-defensin-14 (Fig.

S4). Thus, TNF-α stimulation impacts a variety of cells that release mediators required for the pathogenesis of psoriasis. In the experimental setting of the present study, however, treatment with etenercept (Etn) resulted in significant but insufficient attenuation of psoriatic phenotype of K5.Stat3C mice. The incomplete in vivo effect of Etn might be due to insufficient local concentrations of Etn in the skin lesions or lymphoid organs, where TNF-α was required for immune cell activation to drive psoriatic change.

EGFR signaling participates in psoriasis through its promotion of keratinocyte proliferation [44,45], and production of growth

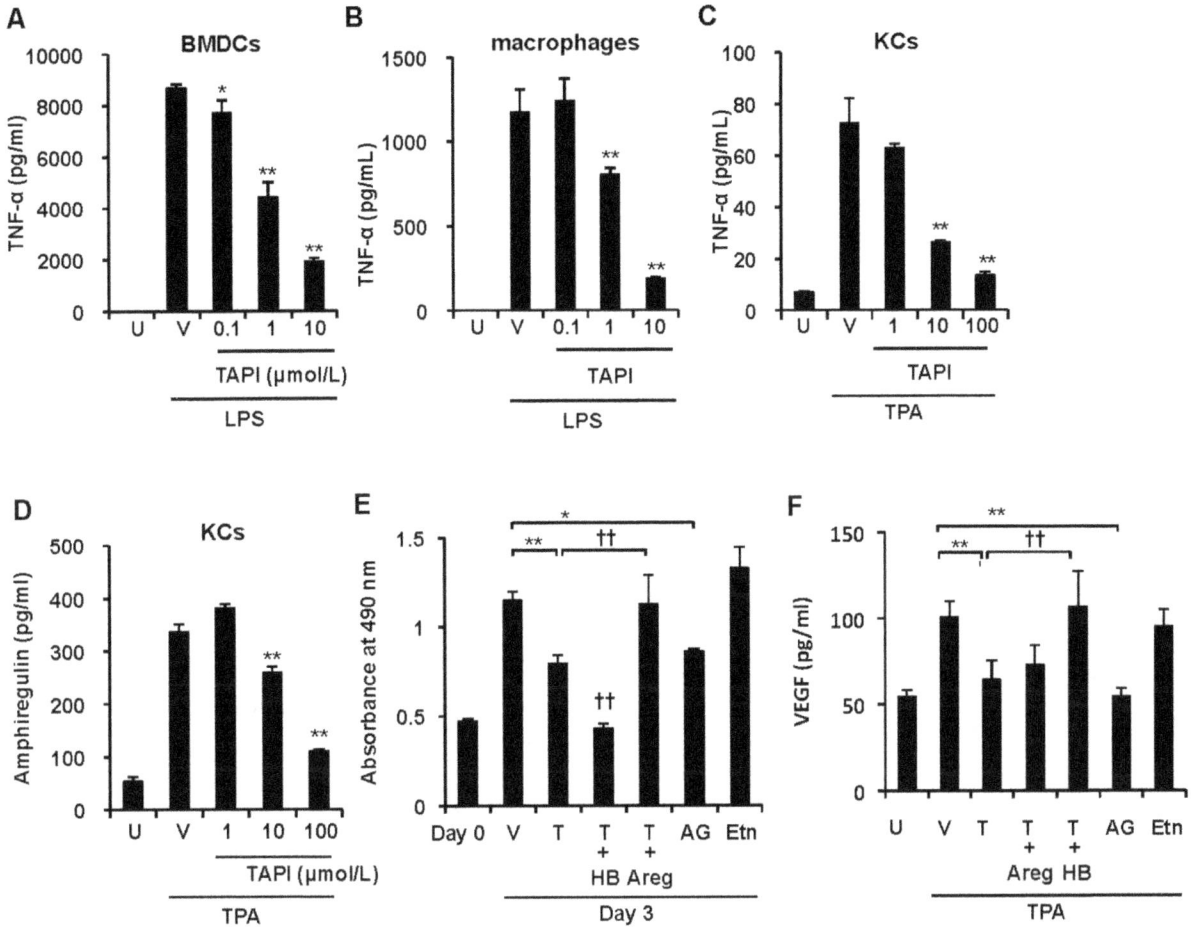

Figure 5. Contribution of TACE to the production of soluble TNF-α and EGFR ligands from murine cells. (A–C), TNF-α proteins in the 24 h culture supernatants of cells pretreated with or without TAPI-1 (TAPI) at the indicated concentrations. LPS-stimulated bone marrow derived dendritic cells (BMDCs) from wild-type FVB/N mice (A), LPS-stimulated thioglycolate-elicited peritoneal macrophages from wild-type FVB/N mice (B), and TPA-stimulated primary keratinocytes from K5.Stat3C newborn mice (C). Cells were pretreated with or without TAPI-1 (TAPI) for 30 min prior to stimulation. (D), Production of amphiregulin from TPA-treated primary keratinocytes of K5.Stat3C newborn mice for 24 h. Cells were pretreated with or without TAPI-1 (TAPI) at the indicated concentrations for 30 min prior to stimulation. U, unstimulated control. V, vehicle alone. Data represent means ± SD of triplicate wells. *$p<0.05$, **$p<0.01$, versus vehicle alone by Dunnett's test. (E), Keratinocyte proliferation evaluated by MTS assay with absorbance at 490 nm. Cells were untreated or treated with TAPI-1 (100 μmol/l) (T) and cultured in the absence or presence of HB-EGF (HB), amphiregulin (Areg), AG1478 (AG) or etanercept (Etn) for 3 days. (F), VEGF production from primary keratinocytes. Cells were stimulated with TPA for 24 h treated with or without reagents as described. Data represent means ± SD from triplicate wells. *$p<0.05$, **$p<0.01$ versus vehicle alone, ††$p<0.01$ versus TAPI-1 alone by Tukey-Kramer's test.

factors such as VEGF [18,19]. Indeed, EGFR inhibitors improve lesions in patients with psoriasis [46,47], as also shown in skin lesions of K5.Stat3C mice in the present study. Previous studies demonstrated that topical TPA application led to EGFR activation followed by Stat3 activation in keratinocytes [48]. Therefore, it was suggested that EGFR signaling was involved in the amplification of Stat3 signaling and contributed to the development of the skin lesions in this murine model. Similar to previous studies showing that amphiregulin promotes human keratinocyte proliferation [36,37], we showed here that the TACE inhibitor-induced attenuation of murine keratinocyte proliferation was reversed by the inclusion of amphiregulin but not by HB-EGF. Specifically, HB-EGF-mediated EGFR triggering led to VEGF production by HaCat cells [19]. VEGF plays a critical role in angiogenesis of psoriatic lesions [15], which are attenuated by treatment with an anti-VEGF antibody [39]. Likewise, we confirmed the role of HB-EGF-mediating EGFR signaling in inducing VEGF production by keratinocytes from K5.Stat3C

mice, since TACE inhibition reduced the production of VEGF, which was reversed by the addition of recombinant HB-EGF, but not by amphiregulin. Thus, EGFR-mediated biological outcomes were determined by distinct ligands, all of which were sensitive to TACE inhibition. Therefore, results in the present study is, at least in part, reproduced previous studies demonstrating that TACE mediated context-dependent function of amphiregulin and HB-EGF; cell proliferation and migration possibly through VEGF signaling, respectively [37,49].

Psoriatic lesions both in humans and in K5.Stat3C mice demonstrated a similar distribution pattern of TACE and its substrate TNF-α. Interestingly, an endogenous TACE inhibitor, TIMP-3 was found to be decreased in psoriatic lesions compared with uninvolved skin and healthy control skin [50]. It was demonstrated that mice lacking Jun-B/c-Jun in the epidermis showed a down-regulation of TIMP-3, resulting in the generation of a psoriasis-like phenotype through massive TNF-α shedding by TACE activation [32]. Likewise, TIMP-3 expression in the skin of

K5.Stat3C mice was attenuated as the psoriasis-like lesions developed by TPA application. TACE enzymatic activity was elevated in the skin of K5.Stat3C mice at baseline, compared with wild-type mice, and it was further increased by TPA treatment. Since TACE mRNA levels were not elevated in K5.Stat3C mice, this finding suggested that Stat3 signaling contributed to enhanced TACE activity via post-transcriptional regulation. Most recently, it has been reported that microRNA-21 (miR-21) targeted *TIMP-3* and was functionally involved in the pathogenesis of psoriasis [51]. Most interestingly, miR-21 expression was up-regulated by the Stat3 signaling [52], supporting our data using K5.Stat3C keratinocytes, which showed acute decline of *TIMP-3* upon TPA treatment, thereby TACE activity might be elevated, followed by release of the TACE substrates. In other words, Stat3 is not only a transcriptional but post-transcriptional regulator for TACE ligands.

The results of the present study strongly suggest that TACE is involved in the pathogenesis of psoriasis through the release of TNF-α and EGFR ligands. Therefore, TACE inhibitors in clinical use may be relevant to both TNF-α and EGFR inhibitors. Our preliminary data showed that topical treatment with TAPI-1 mildly but significantly attenuated skin lesion development in K5.Stat3C mice. We are now under seeking for more potent and specific TACE inhibitors than TAPI-1, so that they should be relevant to clinical use for treatment of psoriasis.

Supporting Information

Figure S1   Effect of TAPI-1 treatment on TNF-α gene expression in LPS-stimulated peritoneal macrophages. Cells were pretreated with or without 10 μM TAPI-1 (TAPI) for 30 min prior to 100 ng/ml LPS stimulation and harvested at 0.5, 6 and 24 h. Data represent means ± SD of triplicate wells.

Figure S2   Inhibition of keratinocyte proliferation by TAPI-1. (A) BrdU incorporation of primary keratinocytes from K5.Stat3C mice. (B) LDH assay using keratinocyte culture supernatants. Cells were treated with or without 100 μmol/l TAPI-1 (TAPI), 100 nmol/l AG1478 (AG) or 1% TritonX-100 (Triton) and cultured for 2 days. BrdU incorporation was quantified by ELISA. Data represent means ± SD of triplicate wells. **p<0.01, versus vehicle alone (V), by Dunnett's test. n.s., not significant.

Figure S3   VEGF production in the skin lesions of K5.Stat3C mice. VEGF production was determined by ELISA using untreated or TPA treated ear skins. TPA treated skins were sampled at day 3. Data represent means ± SD of 4 to 5 mice. **p<0.01, versus the untreated group, by Student's *t*-test.

Figure S4   Expression of psoriasis-related genes in primary murine keratinocytes by synergistic stimulation with TNF-α and IL-17A. Primary keratinocytes were stimulated with 20 ng/ml IL-17A and 10 ng/ml TNF-α for 24 h. Data represent means ± SD of triplicate wells. **p<0.01, by Tukey-Kramer's test.

Acknowledgments

We thank Kimiko Nakajima for helpful discussion; Reiko Kamijima, Chisa Fujimoto and Tomoko Nagayama for technical assistance; Keiko Udaka and Toshihiro Komatsu for technical advice for BMDC preparation.

Author Contributions

Conceived and designed the experiments: KS ST SS. Performed the experiments: KS MT. Analyzed the data: KS MT SS. Contributed reagents/materials/analysis tools: ST SS. Contributed to the writing of the manuscript: KS SS.

References

1. Menter A, Feldman SR, Weinstein GD, Papp K, Evans R, et al. (2007) A randomized comparison of continuous vs. intermittent infliximab maintenance regimens over 1 year in the treatment of moderate-to-severe plaque psoriasis. J Am Acad Dermatol 56: 31 e31–15.
2. Gordon K, Papp K, Poulin Y, Gu Y, Rozzo S, et al. (2012) Long-term efficacy and safety of adalimumab in patients with moderate to severe psoriasis treated continuously over 3 years: results from an open-label extension study for patients from REVEAL. J Am Acad Dermatol 66: 241–251.
3. Gaspari AA (2006) Innate and adaptive immunity and the pathophysiology of psoriasis. J Am Acad Dermatol 54: S67–80.
4. Zaba LC, Cardinale I, Gilleaudeau P, Sullivan-Whalen M, Suarez-Farinas M, et al. (2007) Amelioration of epidermal hyperplasia by TNF inhibition is associated with reduced Th17 responses. J Exp Med 204: 3183–3194.
5. Black RA, Rauch CT, Kozlosky CJ, Peschon JJ, Slack JL, et al. (1997) A metalloproteinase disintegrin that releases tumour-necrosis factor-alpha from cells. Nature 385: 729–733.
6. Moss ML, Jin SL, Milla ME, Bickett DM, Burkhart W, et al. (1997) Cloning of a disintegrin metalloproteinase that processes precursor tumour-necrosis factor-alpha. Nature 385: 733–736.
7. Blaydon DC, Biancheri P, Di WL, Plagnol V, Cabral RM, et al. (2011) Inflammatory skin and bowel disease linked to ADAM17 deletion. N Engl J Med 365: 1502–1508.
8. Vassar R, Fuchs E (1991) Transgenic mice provide new insights into the role of TGF-alpha during epidermal development and differentiation. Genes Dev 5: 714–727.
9. Cook PW, Piepkorn M, Clegg CH, Plowman GD, DeMay JM, et al. (1997) Transgenic expression of the human amphiregulin gene induces a psoriasis-like phenotype. J Clin Invest 100: 2286–2294.
10. Piepkorn M, Pittelkow MR, Cook PW (1998) Autocrine regulation of keratinocytes: the emerging role of heparin-binding, epidermal growth factor-related growth factors. J Invest Dermatol 111: 715–721.
11. Kawaguchi M, Mitsuhashi Y, Kondo S (2005) Overexpression of tumour necrosis factor-alpha-converting enzyme in psoriasis. Br J Dermatol 152: 915–919.
12. Sano S, Chan KS, Carbajal S, Clifford J, Peavey M, et al. (2005) Stat3 links activated keratinocytes and immunocytes required for development of psoriasis in a novel transgenic mouse model. Nat Med 11: 43–49.
13. Sano S, Chan KS, DiGiovanni J (2008) Impact of Stat3 activation upon skin biology: a dichotomy of its role between homeostasis and diseases. J Dermatol Sci 50: 1–14.
14. Nakajima K, Kanda T, Takaishi M, Shiga T, Miyoshi K, et al. (2011) Distinct roles of IL-23 and IL-17 in the development of psoriasis-like lesions in a mouse model. J Immunol 186: 4481–4489.
15. Ferrara N (2004) Vascular endothelial growth factor: basic science and clinical progress. Endocr Rev 25: 581–611.
16. Weidemann AK, Crawshaw AA, Byrne E, Young HS (2013) Vascular endothelial growth factor inhibitors: investigational therapies for the treatment of psoriasis. Clin Cosmet Investig Dermatol 6: 233–244.
17. Detmar M, Brown LF, Claffey KP, Yeo KT, Kocher O, et al. (1994) Overexpression of vascular permeability factor/vascular endothelial growth factor and its receptors in psoriasis. J Exp Med 180: 1141–1146.
18. Frank S, Hubner G, Breier G, Longaker MT, Greenhalgh DG, et al. (1995) Regulation of vascular endothelial growth factor expression in cultured keratinocytes. Implications for normal and impaired wound healing. J Biol Chem 270: 12607–12613.
19. Nakai K, Yoneda K, Moriue T, Igarashi J, Kosaka H, et al. (2009) HB-EGF-induced VEGF production and eNOS activation depend on both PI3 kinase and MAP kinase in HaCaT cells. J Dermatol Sci 55: 170–178.
20. Sano S, Chan KS, Kira M, Kataoka K, Takagi S, et al. (2005) Signal transducer and activator of transcription 3 is a key regulator of keratinocyte survival and proliferation following UV irradiation. Cancer Res 65: 5720–5729.
21. Hirai T, Kanda T, Sato K, Takaishi M, Nakajima K, et al. (2013) Cathepsin K is involved in development of psoriasis-like skin lesions through TLR-dependent Th17 activation. J Immunol 190: 4805–4811.

22. Murakawa M, Yamaoka K, Tanaka Y, Fukuda Y (2006) Involvement of tumor necrosis factor (TNF)-alpha in phorbol ester 12-O-tetradecanoylphorbol-13-acetate (TPA)-induced skin edema in mice. Biochem Pharmacol 71: 1331–1336.

23. Chun KS, Lao HC, Trempus CS, Okada M, Langenbach R (2009) The prostaglandin receptor EP2 activates multiple signaling pathways and beta-arrestin1 complex formation during mouse skin papilloma development. Carcinogenesis 30: 1620–1627.

24. Laemmli UK (1970) Cleavage of structural proteins during the assembly of the head of bacteriophage T4. Nature 227: 680–685.

25. Feng T, Qin H, Wang L, Benveniste EN, Elson CO, et al. (2011) Th17 cells induce colitis and promote Th1 cell responses through IL-17 induction of innate IL-12 and IL-23 production. J Immunol 186: 6313–6318.

26. Gais P, Tiedje C, Altmayr F, Gaestel M, Weighardt H, et al. (2010) TRIF signaling stimulates translation of TNF-alpha mRNA via prolonged activation of MK2. J Immunol 184: 5842–5848.

27. Kawaguchi M, Mitsuhashi Y, Kondo S (2004) Localization of tumour necrosis factor-alpha converting enzyme in normal human skin. Clin Exp Dermatol 29: 185–187.

28. Terajima S, Higaki M, Igarashi Y, Nogita T, Kawashima M (1998) An important role of tumor necrosis factor-alpha in the induction of adhesion molecules in psoriasis. Arch Dermatol Res 290: 246–252.

29. Johnston A, Gudjonsson JE, Aphale A, Guzman AM, Stoll SW, et al. (2011) EGFR and IL-1 signaling synergistically promote keratinocyte antimicrobial defenses in a differentiation-dependent manner. J Invest Dermatol 131: 329–337.

30. Lee MH, Verma V, Maskos K, Becherer JD, Knauper V, et al. (2002) The C-terminal domains of TACE weaken the inhibitory action of N-TIMP-3. FEBS Lett 520: 102–106.

31. Mohammed FF, Smookler DS, Taylor SE, Fingleton B, Kassiri Z, et al. (2004) Abnormal TNF activity in Timp3−/− mice leads to chronic hepatic inflammation and failure of liver regeneration. Nat Genet 36: 969–977.

32. Guinea-Viniegra J, Zenz R, Scheuch H, Hnisz D, Holcmann M, et al. (2009) TNFalpha shedding and epidermal inflammation are controlled by Jun proteins. Genes Dev 23: 2663–2674.

33. Lowes MA, Russell CB, Martin DA, Towne JE, Krueger JG (2013) The IL-23/T17 pathogenic axis in psoriasis is amplified by keratinocyte responses. Trends Immunol 34: 174–181.

34. Johansen C, Funding AT, Otkjaer K, Kragballe K, Jensen UB, et al. (2006) Protein expression of TNF-alpha in psoriatic skin is regulated at a posttranscriptional level by MAPK-activated protein kinase 2. J Immunol 176: 1431–1438.

35. Kim S, Beyer BA, Lewis C, Nadel JA (2013) Normal CFTR inhibits epidermal growth factor receptor-dependent pro-inflammatory chemokine production in human airway epithelial cells. PLoS One 8: e72981.

36. Stoll SW, Johnson JL, Li Y, Rittie L, Elder JT (2010) Amphiregulin carboxy-terminal domain is required for autocrine keratinocyte growth. J Invest Dermatol 130: 2031–2040.

37. Stoll SW, Johnson JL, Bhasin A, Johnston A, Gudjonsson JE, et al. (2010) Metalloproteinase-mediated, context-dependent function of amphiregulin and HB-EGF in human keratinocytes and skin. J Invest Dermatol 130: 295–304.

38. Xia YP, Li B, Hylton D, Detmar M, Yancopoulos GD, et al. (2003) Transgenic delivery of VEGF to mouse skin leads to an inflammatory condition resembling human psoriasis. Blood 102: 161–168.

39. Akman A, Yilmaz E, Mutlu H, Ozdogan M (2009) Complete remission of psoriasis following bevacizumab therapy for colon cancer. Clin Exp Dermatol 34: e202–204.

40. Miyoshi K, Takaishi M, Nakajima K, Ikeda M, Kanda T, et al. (2011) Stat3 as a therapeutic target for the treatment of psoriasis: a clinical feasibility study with STA-21, a Stat3 inhibitor. J Invest Dermatol 131: 108–117.

41. Gottlieb AB, Chamian F, Masud S, Cardinale I, Abello MV, et al. (2005) TNF inhibition rapidly down-regulates multiple proinflammatory pathways in psoriasis plaques. J Immunol 175: 2721–2729.

42. Zaba LC, Suarez-Farinas M, Fuentes-Duculan J, Nograles KE, Guttman-Yassky E, et al. (2009) Effective treatment of psoriasis with etanercept is linked to suppression of IL-17 signaling, not immediate response TNF genes. J Allergy Clin Immunol 124: 1022–1010 e1021–1395.

43. Sugita S, Kawazoe Y, Imai A, Yamada Y, Horie S, et al. (2012) Inhibition of Th17 differentiation by anti-TNF-alpha therapy in uveitis patients with Behcet's disease. Arthritis Res Ther 14: R99.

44. Peus D, Hamacher L, Pittelkow MR (1997) EGF-receptor tyrosine kinase inhibition induces keratinocyte growth arrest and terminal differentiation. J Invest Dermatol 109: 751–756.

45. Tokumaru S, Higashiyama S, Endo T, Nakagawa T, Miyagawa JI, et al. (2000) Ectodomain shedding of epidermal growth factor receptor ligands is required for keratinocyte migration in cutaneous wound healing. J Cell Biol 151: 209–220.

46. Neyns B, Meert V, Vandenbroucke F (2008) Cetuximab treatment in a patient with metastatic colorectal cancer and psoriasis. Curr Oncol 15: 196–197.

47. Oyama N, Kaneko F, Togashi A, Yamamoto T (2012) A case of rapid improvement of severe psoriasis during molecular-targeted therapy using an epidermal growth factor receptor tyrosine kinase inhibitor for metastatic lung adenocarcinoma. J Am Acad Dermatol 66: e251–253.

48. Chan KS (2004) Epidermal Growth Factor Receptor-Mediated Activation of Stat3 during Multistage Skin Carcinogenesis. Cancer Research 64: 2382–2389.

49. Maretzky T, Evers A, Zhou W, Swendeman SL, Wong PM, et al. (2011) Migration of growth factor-stimulated epithelial and endothelial cells depends on EGFR transactivation by ADAM17. Nat Commun 2: 229.

50. Zibert JR, Lovendorf MB, Litman T, Olsen J, Kaczkowski B, et al. (2010) MicroRNAs and potential target interactions in psoriasis. J Dermatol Sci 58: 177–185.

51. Guinea-Viniegra J, Jimenez M, Schonthaler HB, Navarro R, Delgado Y, et al. (2014) Targeting miR-21 to Treat Psoriasis. Sci Transl Med 6: 225re221.

52. Iliopoulos D, Jaeger SA, Hirsch HA, Bulyk ML, Struhl K (2010) STAT3 activation of miR-21 and miR-181b-1 via PTEN and CYLD are part of the epigenetic switch linking inflammation to cancer. Mol Cell 39: 493–506.

17

Enhanced Tissue Factor Expression by Blood Eosinophils from Patients with Hypereosinophilia: A Possible Link with Thrombosis

Massimo Cugno[1,2]*, **Angelo V. Marzano**[3], **Maurizio Lorini**[1], **Vincenzo Carbonelli**[1], **Alberto Tedeschi**[4]

1 Dipartimento di Fisiopatologia Medico-Chirurgica e dei Trapianti, Università degli Studi di Milano, Milano, Italy, 2 Medicina Interna, Fondazione IRCCS Ca' Granda, Ospedale Maggiore Policlinico, Milano, Italy, 3 Unità Operativa di Dermatologia, Fondazione IRCCS Ca' Granda, Ospedale Maggiore Policlinico, Milano, Italy, 4 Unità Operativa di Allergologia e Immunologia Clinica, Fondazione IRCCS Ca' Granda, Ospedale Maggiore Policlinico, Milano, Italy

Abstract

Thrombotic risk is increased in eosinophil-mediated disorders, and several hypotheses have been proposed to link eosinophilia and thrombosis. In particular, eosinophils have been described as source of tissue factor (TF), the main initiator of blood coagulation; however, this aspect is still controversial. This study was aimed to evaluate whether TF expression varies in eosinophils isolated from normal subjects and patients with different hypereosinophilic conditions. Eosinophils were immunologically purified from peripheral blood samples of 9 patients with different hypereosinophilic conditions and 9 normal subjects. Western blot analysis and real-time polymerase chain reaction (RT-PCR) were performed to test eosinophil TF expression. For comparison, TF expression was evaluated in monocytes from blood donors and in human endothelial (ECV304) and fibroblast (IMR90) cell lines. Western blot analysis revealed a major band of 47,000 corresponding to native TF in homogenates of purified eosinophils with a higher intensity in the 9 patients than in the 9 controls (p< 0.0001). According to RT-PCR cycle threshold (Ct), TF gene expression was higher in eosinophils from patients than in those from controls, median (range) 35.10 (19.45–36.50) vs 37.17 (35.33–37.87) (p = 0.002), and was particularly abundant in one patient with idiopathic hypereosinophilic syndrome and ischemic heart attacks (Ct: 19.45). TF gene expression was moderate in monocytes, Ct: 31.32 (29.82–33.49) and abundant in endothelial cells, Ct: 28.70 (27.79–29.57) and fibroblasts, Ct: 22.77 (19.22–25.05). Our results indicate that human blood eosinophils contain variable amounts of TF. The higher TF expression in patients with hypereosinophilic disorders may contribute to increase the thrombotic risk.

Editor: Simon Patrick Hogan, Cincinnati Children's Hospital Medical Center, University of Cincinnati College of Medicine, United States of America

Funding: This work was supported by "Ricerca corrente", Fondazione IRCCS Ca' Granda, Ospedale Maggiore Policlinico, Milano, Italy. The funder had no role in study design, data collection and analysis, decision to publish, or preparation of the manuscript.

Competing Interests: The authors have declared that no competing interests exist.

* Email: massimo.cugno@unimi.it

Introduction

Eosinophils are leukocytes involved in host protection against parasite infection and in allergic reactions [1]. During T-helper 2-type immune response, they are recruited at sites of inflammation where they produce an array of cytokines and lipid mediators, and release toxic granule proteins [2,3]. Thus, they induce and amplify inflammatory changes and contribute to tissue damage. Besides these well known functions, several lines of evidence now indicate eosinophils as multifunctional leukocytes involved in tissue homeostasis, adaptive immune responses, innate immunity [2–4] and coagulation [5]. An increase in blood eosinophil number can occur in several disorders [6] presenting with a wide spectrum of manifestations, ranging from asymptomatic conditions to multi-organ involvement [7,8]. In particular, it has been observed that in eosinophil-mediated disorders there is an increased risk of thrombosis [9–13], and several hypotheses have been proposed to link eosinophilia and thrombosis, involving endothelium damage, platelet activation and coagulation. Endothelial cells may be damaged by eosinophil peroxidase products. Moreover,

peroxidase and several additional proteins contained in eosinophil granules, such as eosinophil cationic protein and major basic protein, can stimulate platelet activation and aggregation [14–18]. Eosinophils express CD40 ligand, which is involved in initiation and progression of thrombosis through amplification of the inflammatory network [16]. Finally, it has been shown that eosinophils store tissue factor (TF), which is mainly embodied within their specific granules and is exposed upon activation [5]. However, some of these aspects remain controversial because Sovershaev et al. did not confirm tissue factor expression in highly purified preparations of human eosinophils [19].

With this background, we evaluated TF expression by eosinophils isolated from blood samples of normal subjects and patients with different hypereosinophilic conditions. For this purpose, western blot analysis and real-time polymerase chain reaction (RT PCR) for TF were performed. For comparison, TF expression was also evaluated in cells commonly recognized as source of TF, i.e. monocytes from blood donors and human endothelial and fibroblast cell lines.

Subjects and Methods

Subjects

Nine normal subjects (6 men and 3 women, age range 40–72 years) and 9 patients with different hypereosinophilic conditions (2 with idiopathic hypereosinophilic syndrome, 2 with bullous pemphigoid, 1 with Churg Strauss syndrome, 2 with eosinophilic asthma, and 2 with nematodes infestation; 7 men and 2 women, age range 40–78 years) were studied (Table 1). All the patients were evaluated in an active phase of their disease, before starting any systemic treatment aimed at reducing eosinophil number. Their blood pressure and cholesterol levels were within the normal range. The two patients with idiopathic hypereosinophilic syndrome (patients n. 5 and 6 in Table 1) also suffered from ischemic heart attacks that disappeared after the normalization of eosinophil count obtained with corticosteroid treatment. Eosinophils were isolated from peripheral blood of both patients and controls. Proteins and RNA from eosinophils were used for western blot and real-time PCR, respectively.

The study was approved by the local Review Board of Internal Medicine, Dermatology, Allergy and Clinical Immunology of the University of Milan, Italy, and all of the subjects gave their written informed consent.

Eosinophil isolation

Leukocyte suspensions were obtained by dextran sedimentation of peripheral blood anticoagulated with 3.75% Na_2EDTA (Sigma-Aldrich St Louis, Mo, USA) diluted 1:2 in 0.9% sodium chloride. Dextran sedimentation (3 g D-Glucose, Sigma-Aldrich St Louis, Mo, USA; 3 g Dextran T500, Carl Roth Gmbh, Karlsruhe, Germany) lasted 90 minutes at room temperature. Twenty ml of leukocyte-enriched plasma were layered over 12 ml of a density gradient medium (sodium diatrizoate 9.1%; polysaccharide 5.7%; $\rho = 1.077$ g/ml, Fresenius Kabi, Oslo, Norway) in 50 ml conical tube and centrifuged at $600 \times g$ for 20 minutes at 20°C. The cell pellet containing eosinophils and neutrophils was collected and the contaminating red cells were eliminated by hypotonic ammonium chloride lysis solution (155 mM NH_4Cl_4, 10 mM $KHCO_3$ and 0,1 mM Na_2EDTA, Sigma-Aldrich St Louis, Mo, USA) for 10 minutes at 4°C. Contaminating neutrophils were removed using a magnetic-activated cell sorting system (Miltenyi Biotec Gmbh, Bergish Gladbach, Germany), containing a cocktail of biotin-conjugated monoclonal antibodies against CD2, CD14, CD16, CD19, CD56, CD123 and CD235a (Glycophorin A). Percentage purification of eosinophils recovered ranged from 95 to 99%, as assessed by differential count of 500 cells on May Grunwald

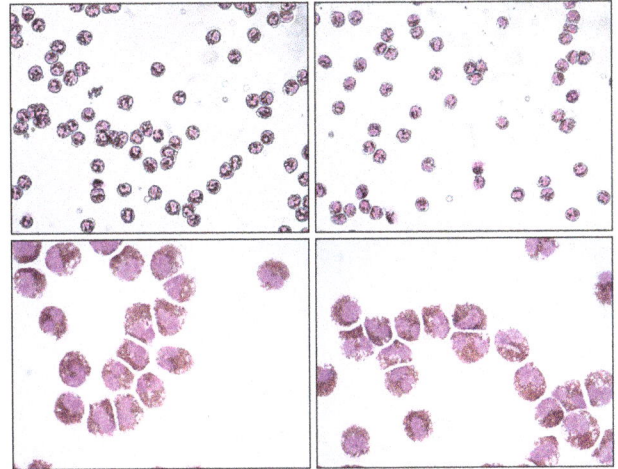

Figure 1. Representative cytocentrifuge smears of two high purity eosinophil preparations obtained from peripheral blood samples. May-Grünwald-Giemsa staining, original magnification: X 400 in the upper panels and X 1000 (immersion) in the lower panels.

Giemsa-stained cytocentrifuge smears (Figure 1). For protein extraction and western-blot analysis, 10^7 cells were used in each experiment. For RNA extraction, 3×10^6 cells were used in each experiment.

Monocyte isolation

Monocytes were isolated from peripheral blood mononuclear cells using a monocyte isolation kit from Miltenyi Biotec Gmbh (Bergish Gladbach, Germany), an indirect magnetic labeling system. Non-monocytes, such as T cells, NK cells, B cells, dendritic cells, and basophils, are indirectly magnetically labeled using a cocktail of biotin-conjugated antibodies and anti-biotin microbeads. Highly pure unlabeled monocytes are obtained by depletion of the magnetically labeled cells. For protein extraction and western-blot analysis, 10^7 cells were used in each experiment. For RNA extraction, 10^6 cells were used for each experiment.

Endothelial cell culture

Human ECV304 endothelial cells, European Collection of Cell Cultures (ECACC) No. 92091712, were grown in M199 supplemented with 10% fetal bovine serum, penicillin 50 U/mL and

Table 1. Demographic and clinical characteristics of patients with hypereosinophilia.

N	Age (years)	Sex	Diagnosis	Blood eosinophils (n/μl)
1	71	F	Bullous pemphigoid	1680
2	40	M	Asthma with eosinophilia	3080
3	78	M	Bullous pemphigoid	1620
4	77	F	Churg-Strauss syndrome	2140
5	44	M	Asthma with eosinophilia	1600
6	55	M	Strongyloidiasis	3100
7	48	M	Ascariasis	3260
8	69	M	Idiopathic hypereosinophilic syndrome	6210
9	63	M	Idiopathic hypereosinophilic syndrome	2870

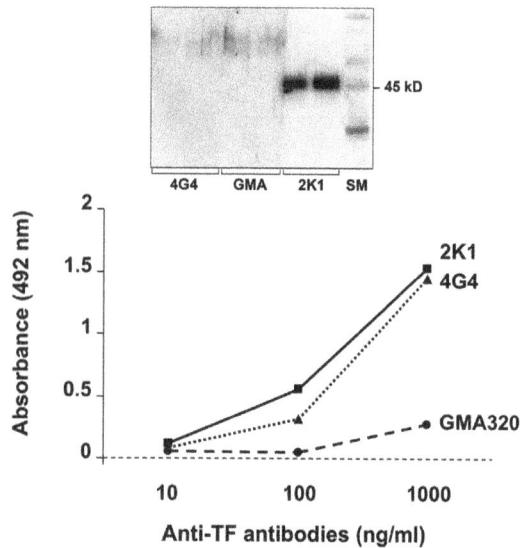

Figure 2. Binding of human recombinant tissue factor (TF) by three commercial anti-TF antibodies (2K1, 4G4 and GMA) evaluated by western blot (upper panel) and enzyme immunoassay (lower panel) methods. Only 2K1 efficiently recognizes TF with both methods. The last lane of western blotting refers to the size markers (SM). In enzyme immunoassay experiments, data represent the mean of three different measurements.

streptomycin 100 µg/ml at 37°C in humidified air with 5% CO2. When endothelial cells reached over 90% of the flask, 2 ml of trypsin 0.02% with EDTA 0.02% (Sigma-Aldrich, St Louis, Mo, USA) was instilled and left in humidified incubator for 10 minutes. Five ml of culture medium, supplemented with 10% fetal bovine serum, were added to cells to neutralize the enzymatic action of trypsin. For protein extraction and western-blot analysis, 10^7 cells were used in each experiment. For RNA extraction, 10^6 cells were used for each experiment.

Fibroblast culture

Human IMR-90 fibroblast cells, American Type Culture Collection (ATCC) No. CCL-186, were grown in 10 ml of Dulbecco's Modified Eagle's medium (DMEM) with 10% fetal bovine serum (Sigma-Aldrich, St Louis, Mo, USA), penicillin (100 UI/ml) and streptomycin (100 µg/ml) (Sigma-Aldrich, St Louis, Mo, USA) at 37°C. Cell cultures were maintained in humidified incubator at 37°C with 5% CO_2, until fibroblasts reached over 95% of confluence. Then, 2 ml of 0.25% trypsin with 0.02% EDTA (Sigma-Aldrich, St Louis, Mo, USA) was instilled in the Petri dish and left in humidified incubator for 10 minutes. Five ml of culture medium, supplemented with 10% fetal bovine serum, were added to cells to neutralize the enzymatic action of trypsin. For protein extraction and western-blot analysis, 10^7 cells were used in each experiment. For RNA extraction, 10^6 cells were used for each experiment.

Western blot analysis of Tissue Factor

Western blot analysis for TF was performed on cell lysates. Cells (10^7) were lysed with 0.5 ml ice cold RIPA (radio-immunoprecipitation assay) buffer (Thermo Scientific, Rockford, IL, USA) with freshly added protease and phosphatase inhibitors. After lysis, total protein levels were measured using the bicinchoninic acid assay (Pierce Biotechnology, Thermo Scientific, Rockford, IL, USA). Equal protein amounts (20 µg) were warmed at 95–98°C with 2-

βmercaptoethanol bromophenol blue buffer (Bio-Rad Laboratories, Hercules, CA, USA), subjected to 11% sodium dodecyl sulfate-polyacrylamide gel electrophoresis (SDS-PAGE), transferred by electroblotting onto nitrocellulose membranes (Whatmann, Dassel, Germany) and incubated with blocking buffer (free protein blocking buffer T20, Pierce Biotechnology, Thermo Scientific, Rockford, IL, USA). As control, recombinant human TF purified from SF9 cells (Haematologic Technologies Inc, Essex, VT, USA) was also loaded. Western blotting was performed with 1:1000 mouse monoclonal anti-TF antibody (2K1 Abcam, Cambridge, UK) corresponding to the concentration of 1000 ng/ml. Protein loading was controlled by probing the membranes with 1:10000 monoclonal antibodies against β-actin (AC-74 Sigma-Aldrich, St Louis, MO, USA). Bands were visualized by incubation of membranes with horseradish peroxidase–conjugated rabbit anti-mouse secondary antibody (Sigma-Aldrich, St Louis, MO, USA) and a chemiluminescence-based detection system (ECL WB GE Healthcare, Amersham, Little Chalfont, UK). Density of the bands was evaluated by computerized image analysis (Image Master; Pharmacia, Uppsala, Sweden) and expressed as the ratio to the density of the band corresponding to standard recombinant TF. The choice of 2K1 as anti-TF primary antibody derived from a comparative evaluation with two other monoclonal antibodies (GMA-320, Upstate, Lake Placid, NY, USA and 4G4 Abnova, Taipei, Taiwan), as shown below.

Western blot analysis to test the binding of anti-TF antibodies to TF

Ten microliters of recombinant human TF purified from SF9 cells (Haematologic Technologies Inc, Essex, VT, USA), at the concentration of 140 ng/ml, were sujected to 11% SDS-PAGE in three different lanes and transferred by electroblotting onto nitrocellulose membranes. TF was identified in each lane with one of the three monoclonal anti-TF antibodies (2K1, 4G4 and GMA320) and revealed with horseradish peroxidase–conjugated rabbit anti-mouse secondary antibody.

Immunoassay to test the binding of anti-TF antibodies to TF

Recombinant human TF purified from SF9 cells (Haematologic Technologies Inc, Essex, VT, USA) was adsorbed to microtitration plates by overnight incubation of protein diluted 10 µg/ml in PBS (phosphate buffered saline) pH 7.4 at 4°C. After block with BSA (bovine serum albumin) and washing, scalar dilutions of the tested antibody (from 1000 ng/ml to 10 ng/ml) were incubated 1 hour at room temperature, and then detected by a peroxidase-conjugated goat anti-mouse antibody (Sigma-Aldrich, St Louis, MO, USA).

Real-Time PCR System

For total RNA extraction, isolated cells (10^6) were treated using a high pure RNA isolation kit (Roche Diagnostics GmbH, Mannheim, Germany) according to the manufacturer's instructions.

For cDNA construction, 300 ng of total RNA were processed using a high capacity RNA-to-cDNA kit (Life Technologies, Carlsbad, CA, USA) for 60 minutes at 37°C and stopping the reaction at 95°C for 5 minutes.

Real-time amplification was performed as follows: cDNA (1 to 9 µl) was amplified using TaqMan Gene Expression Master Mix with primers and probes of beta-actin and TF genes (Life Technologies, Carlsbad, CA, USA), respectively housekeeping and target. The sequence detection systems consisted in an

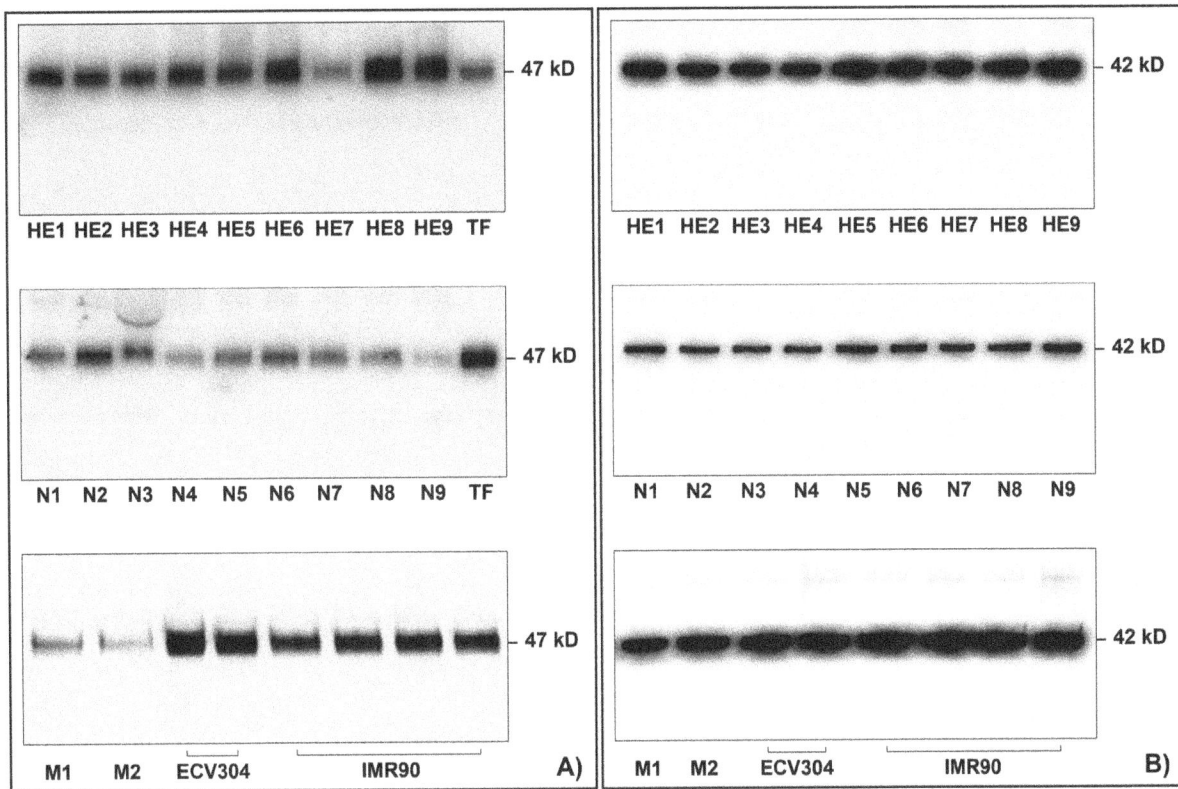

Figure 3. Panel A shows the western blot analysis of tissue factor (TF) in homogenate samples of purified eosinophils from 9 patients with hyperosinophilic conditions (HE) (top), purified eosinophils from 9 normal controls (N) (middle), and purified monocytes from 2 normal controls (M), purified endothelial cells from 2 samples of cell line ECV304 and purified fibroblasts from 4 samples of cell line IMR90 (bottom). A major band with Mr of 47,000 corresponding to the native TF was found in the eosinophil homogenates from the 9 patients and the 9 controls, with a higher intensity in the former than in the latter. The intensity of the TF band was weaker in monocytes (M1, M2) than in endothelial cells (ECV304) and in fibroblasts (IMR90). Panel B shows the western blot analysis of the ubiquitary protein beta-actin, which was well represented in all patients, normal subjects and positive controls.

activation of 2 minutes at 50°C, UNG (Uracil N-Glycosylase) - UDG (uracil-DNA glycosylase) incubation, 10 minutes at 95°C, 40 cycles at 95°C for 10 seconds each, 1 minute at 60°C (anneal/extend). The accumulation of fluorescent signal was detected. The number of cycles required for the fluorescent signal to exceed the threshold over the background level is defined cycle threshold [20]. Levels of cycle threshold are inversely proportional to the amount of target nucleic acid in the sample (i.e. the lower the cycle threshold level the greater the amount of target nucleic acid in the sample). A strong positive reaction, indicative of abundant target nucleic acid in the sample, corresponds to cycle thresholds lower than 29. Cycle thresholds of 30–37 are positive reactions indicative of moderate amounts of target nucleic acid. Cycle thresholds of 38–40 are weak reactions indicative of minimal amounts of target nucleic acid which could represent an environmental contamination. Moreover, we analysed PCR data of TF considering for each individual value its beta actin control, and the results were calculated with the equation: $2^{\Delta Ct} = 2^{(Ct\ TF-\ Ct\ Actin)}$ according to Zhu et al. [21].

Statistical analysis

Results were expressed as median and [range]. Mann-Whitney U test for unpaired values was used to assess the statistical significance of the differences between groups. A P value of <0.05 was considered statistically significant. Differences in frequencies of TF expression were evaluated by Chi-square test. All analyses were performed by the SPSS PC statistical package, version 20.00 (IBM SPSS, Armonk, NY, USA).

Results

Detection of tissue factor in isolated eosinophils

We tested the ability to detect native TF of 3 commercial anti TF antibodies by both western blot (Figure 2, upper panel) and enzyme immunoassay (Figure 2, lower panel) methods. On the basis of the results of these experiments, we chose the antibody 2K1 which efficiently recognizes TF with both methods.

As demonstrated by western blot analysis, TF was present in homogenates of purified eosinophils from patients with hyper-osinophilic disorders (Figure 3, panel A). A major band with Mr of 47,000 corresponding to the native TF was found in the eosinophil homogenates from the 9 patients and the 9 controls. The intensity of the bands, expressed as the ratio to the band of standard recombinant TF, was significantly higher in patients with hypereosinophilic disorders than in normal subjects, median (range) 1.77 (0.82–2.63) vs 0.49 (0.25–0.75) (p<0.0001) (Figure 3, panel A and B). As positive control we evaluated TF by western blot in 2 homogenate samples of purified monocytes, in 2 homogenate samples of purified endothelial cells from line ECV304 and in 4 homogenate samples of purified fibroblasts from cell line IMR90 (Figure 3, panel A, bottom).

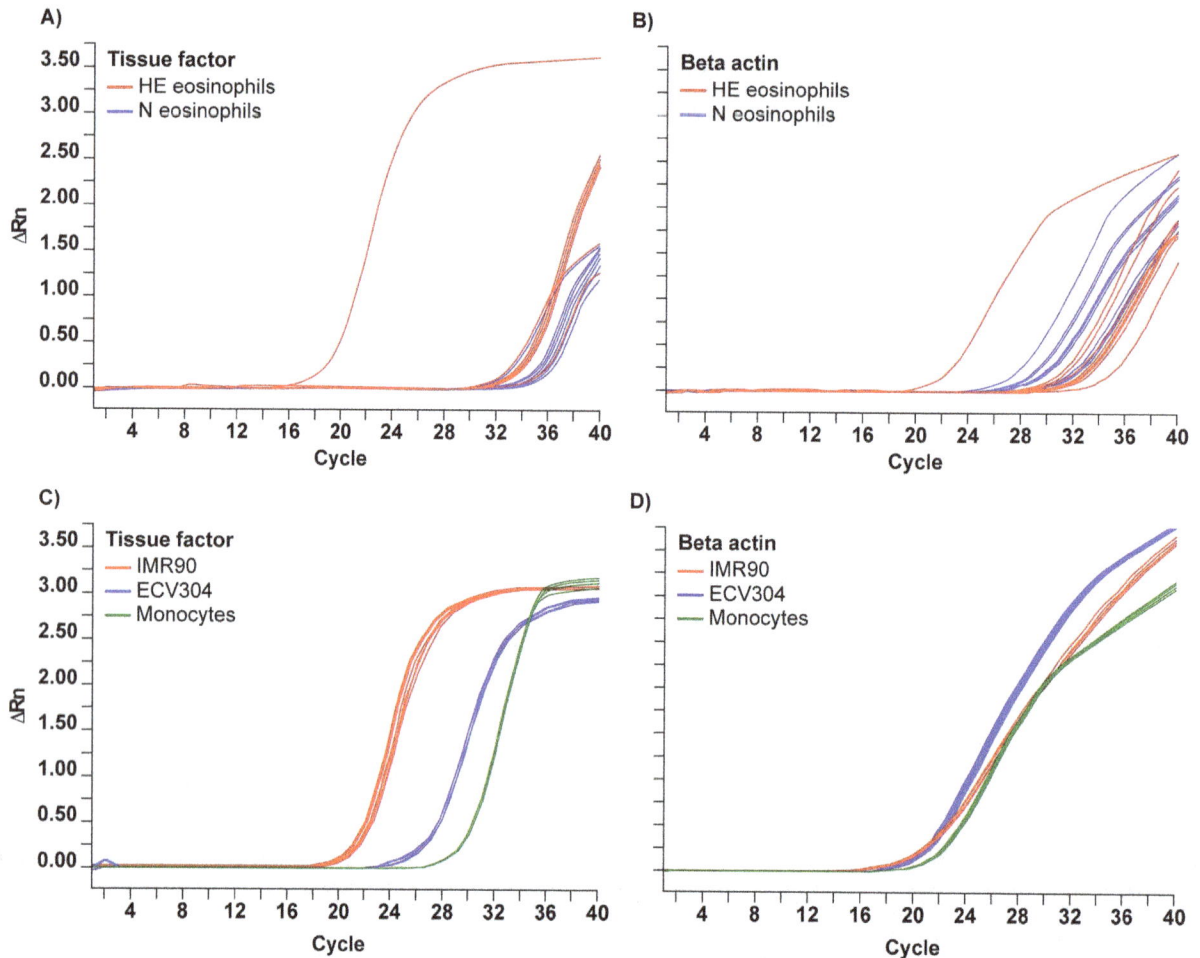

Figure 4. Panel A shows real-time polymerase chain reaction (RT-PCR) analysis of tissue factor (TF) in purified eosinophils from 9 patients with hyperesinophilia (HE, red lines) and 9 normal controls (N, blue lines). Panel B shows RT-PCR analysis of beta-actin in purified eosinophils from 9 patients with hyperesinophilia (HE, red lines) and 9 normal controls (N, blue lines). Panel C shows RT-PCR analysis of TF in purified monocytes from 4 normal controls (green lines), in 4 samples of endothelial cell line ECV304 (blue lines) and in 8 samples of fibroblast cell line IMR90 (red lines). Panel D shows RT-PCR analysis of beta-actin in purified monocytes from 4 normal controls (green lines), in 4 samples of endothelial cell line ECV304 (blue lines) and in 8 samples of fibroblast cell line IMR90 (red lines).

To rule out the possibility that low levels of TF found in some samples were due to the reduction of total proteins; in the same samples, we evaluated by western blot the ubiquitary protein actin, which was well represented in all patients, normal subjects and positive controls (Figure 3, panel B).

Evaluation of tissue factor mRNA in isolated eosinophils

Real-time polymerase chain reaction (RT-PCR) analysis revealed different amplifications in 9 patients with hypereosinophilia using TF specific sets of primers and probes (Figure 4). As shown in table 2 and in figure 4, TF cycle threshold was significantly lower in patients with hypereosinophilia than in healthy subjects, median (range) 35.10 (19.45–36.50) vs 37.17 (35.33–37.87) (p = 0.002), indicating that TF gene expression was higher in hypereosinophilic disorders. Interestingly, the two patients with idiopathic hypereosinophilic syndrome and ischemic heart attacks, showed the lowest TF cycle threshold (19.45 and 33.68) indicating an enhanced TF gene expression. The cycle thresholds of the housekeeping gene beta actin in patients and controls ranged between 27.79 and 36.31, without any significant differences between the two groups (Table 2). Considering the

beta-actin controls, the relative quantification of PCR data confirmed a significantly higher expression of TF mRNA in patients with hypereosinophilia than in normal subjects (Table 2).

We also analyzed TF expression in 4 samples of monocytes, cycle threshold: median (range) 31.32 (29.82–33.49), corresponding to moderate amount, in 4 samples of endothelial cell line ECV304, cycle threshold: 28.70 (27.79–29.57), corresponding to abundant amount, and in 8 samples of fibroblast cell line IMR90, cycle threshold: 22.77 (19.22–25.05), corresponding to abundant amount.

Discussion

The results of the present study show that TF is detectable in high-purity preparations of immunologically isolated eosinophils from healthy subjects and patients with different hypereosinophilic conditions. TF gene expression was higher in eosinophils from patients with hypereosinophilic disorders than in those from normal subjects (on the basis of RT-PCR cycle threshold). Western blot analysis revealed that a strong expression of TF by eosinophils was significantly more frequent in patients with hyperosinophilia.

Table 2. Expression of target (tissue factor) and housekeeping (beta-actin) genes in purified eosinophils obtained from 9 patients with hypereosinophilia and 9 normal controls.

N	Condition	Tissue factor Ct	Beta-actin Ct	$2^{\Delta Ct}$
	Patients with hypereosinophilia			
1	Bullous pemphigoid	36.50	31.27	0.43
2	Asthma with eosinophilia	35.20	36.31	2.16
3	Bullous pemphigoid	33.72	31.56	0.45
4	Churg-Strauss syndrome	35.10	31.04	0.51
5	Asthma with eosinophilia	34.91	28.98	0.52
6	Strongyloidiasis	35.67	33.12	0.37
7	Ascariasis	35.54	30.10	0.49
8	Idiopathic hypereosinophilic syndrome	19.45	27.79	20.25
9	Idiopathic hypereosinophilic syndrome	33.68	32.25	0.56
	Median	35.10 *	31.27	0.51**
	Range	19.45–36.50	27.79–36.31	
	Normal controls			
1	Healthy	37.18	31.66	0.02
2	Healthy	36.04	33.65	0.19
3	Healthy	35.33	33.23	0.23
4	Healthy	37.87	30.47	0.01
5	Healthy	37.25	33.89	0.10
6	Healthy	36.62	31.76	0.03
7	Healthy	37.17	29.57	0.01
8	Healthy	37.23	31.95	0.03
9	Healthy	36.12	30.28	0.02
	Median	37.17	31.76	0.03
	Range	35.33–37.87	29.57–33.89	0.01–0.23

Gene expression was analysed by real-time polymerase chain reaction and reported as cycle threshold (Ct) and as corrected Ct ($2^{\Delta Ct} = 2^{Ct \ tissue \ factor \ - \ Ct \ beta \ actin}$).
* Median value of tissue factor cycle threshold (Ct) was significantly lower in patients with hypereosinophilia than in healthy subjects (p = 0.002). **Median value of tissue factor Ct corrected for beta actin Ct (using the equation $2^{\Delta Ct} = 2^{Ct \ tissue \ factor \ - \ Ct \ beta \ actin}$) was significantly higher in patients with hypereosinophilia than in healthy subjects (p = 0.0001). Both analyses indicate an increased mRNA espression of tissue factor in patients with hypereosinophilia.

Although eosinophil immunoreactivity with antibodies to TF could be due, at least in part, to internalization and storage of TF produced by other cells, namely monocytes [22], our data indicate that eosinophils themselves are able to produce TF in variable amounts, and TF content seems to be increased in hypereosinophilic conditions. These observations are in keeping with studies showing that eosinophils produce, store and rapidly transfer TF to the cell membrane during activation [5]. However, Sovershaev et al. [19] have failed to find TF expression by purified blood eosinophils. Different reasons have been advocated to explain these discrepancies. Firstly, antibodies used in the immunoassays may have different sensitivity and specificity in TF detection, as demonstrated by our results (Figure 2) and by those of Basavaraj et al. [23]. Secondly, immunochemical detection of TF in eosinophils may be due to attachment and uptake of monocyte-derived TF, as demonstrated in granulocytes by Egorina et al. [22]. Finally, the detection of TF mRNA in purified eosinophils could be due to non-specific amplification during the late cycles of PCR or contamination of the eosinophil fraction with monocytes, as hypothesized by Sovershaev et al. [19]. However, in the present study this last possibility is unlikely given the high purity of our eosinophil preparations (Figure 1). In our experiments, we have compared three different antibodies to TF and we have chosen the most efficient in TF binding to test blood eosinophils. The observation that immunoreactivity for TF in purified eosinophils was variable in different subjects being almost absent in 2 out of 9 normal controls renders unlikely a non-specific binding of the antibody and supports interindividual differences in TF expression. In contrast, a strong reactivity was observed in 8 out of 9 patients with hypereosinophilic conditions. We cannot exclude that part of the TF detected in purified eosinophils is the result of uptake of monocyte-derived TF; however, the detection of TF mRNA in purified eosinophils suggests that it is, at least in part, produced by eosinophils themselves. The very high level of TF mRNA detected in eosinophils from one patient with idiopathic hypereosinophilic syndrome indicates that TF production by eosinophils is variable and can be markedly increased in pathological conditions. The reasons of the enhanced TF expression by blood eosinophils from patients with hypereosinophilia are as yet unknown; however, a candidate effector molecule may be interleukin-5 (IL-5) due to its pivotal role in promoting survival and activation of eosinophils [24]. Future studies are needed to investigate whether stimulation of eosinophils with IL-5 upregulates TF expression.

Previously, we demonstrated by immunohistochemical methods that TF is expressed by inflammatory cells present in the infiltrate of chronic urticaria skin lesions [25]. The nature of the TF-expressing cell was revealed by performing double-staining studies that showed co-localization of TF and eosinophil cationic protein, a classic cell marker of the eosinophil [26]. The strong expression of TF in chronic urticaria lesional skin may be due to eosinophil activation, even if patients with chronic urticaria virtually never show peripheral eosinophilia, probably because TF specifically facilitates the early transendothelial migration of the eosinophils [5]. Further immunohistochemical studies, carried out in patients with bullous pemphigoid, an autoimmune blistering disease characterized by skin and peripheral blood eosinophilia, showed a strong TF expression in lesional skin [27]. Immunofluorescence studies using laser scanning confocal microscopy showed that, in patients with bullous pemphigoid, most of the cells making up the inflammatory infiltrate co-expressed TF and the eosinophil marker CD125, thus indicating that they were eosinophils [27,28].

Considering that TF is the main activator of blood coagulation, the demonstration that eosinophils produce and store TF raises the possibility that they are involved in coagulation activation. Thus, they may contribute to induce thrombosis, even if other eosinophil-related pathophysiologic mechanisms may be operating, including endothelium damage and platelet activation. Eosinophils may damage endothelial cells by releasing peroxidase, and stimulate platelet activation and aggregation through several additional proteins contained in their granules, such as eosinophil cationic protein and major basic protein [14,15]. Furthermore, eosinophils express CD40 ligand, which is involved in initiation and progression of thrombosis through amplification of the inflammatory network [16,17]. Finally, platelet activating factor (PAF), a lipid mediator generated after eosinophil stimulation [18], induces the activation of platelets, leukocytes and endothelial cells. It would be interesting to determine if the increase of TF observed in eosinophils of patients with hypereosinophilia occurs primarily inside the cell or at transmembrane level. The latter possibility

could be relevant to the increase of thrombotic risk due to the interaction of transmembrane TF with the other blood components. Our results do not allow to distinguish between intracellular and transmembrane TF since the antibody used recognizes the extracellular domain of TF which is shared by the two forms. Thus, to define the subcellular localization of TF in hypereosinophilic conditions further methods are needed using the approach of Moosbauer et al. with electronic microscopy [5] or that of Mandal et al. and Peña et al. with confocal microscopy [29,30].

Some hypereosinophilic conditions such as idiopathic hypereosinophilic syndrome, Churg-Strauss syndrome and bullous pemphigoid are characterized by an increased incidence of thrombotic events [9,10,31,32]. It is conceivable that TF expression by eosinophils has an important role in increasing the thrombotic risk of patients with hypereosinophilic conditions. Although the amount of TF generated by and stored in peripheral blood eosinophils is variable and may be small or moderate compared to other cell types (i.e. monocytes and endothelial cells), the presence of large numbers of eosinophils in hypereosinophilic conditions may markedly amplify the TF effect on coagulation. The observation that two of our patients with idiopathic hypereosinophilic syndrome experienced ischemic heart attacks, healed after steroid-induced normalization of the eosinophil count, further supports a link between eosinophils and cardiovascular events.

Author Contributions

Conceived and designed the experiments: MC AT. Performed the experiments: ML VC. Analyzed the data: MC AT ML VC AVM. Contributed reagents/materials/analysis tools: MC AT ML VC AVM. Wrote the paper: MC AT AVM. Collection of clinical and laboratory data: MC AT AVM.

References

1. Hogan SP, Rosenberg HF, Moqbel R, Phipps S, Foster PS, et al. (2008) Eosinophils: biological properties and role in health and disease. Clin Exp Allergy 38: 709–750.

2. Rosenberg HF, Dyer KD, Foster PS (2013) Eosinophils: changing perspectives in health and disease. Nat Rev Immunol 13: 9–22.

3. Kita H (2013) Eosinophils: multifunctional and distinctive properties. Int Arch Allergy Immunol, 161 Suppl 2: 3–9.

4. Blanchard C, Rothenberg ME (2009) Biology of the eosinophil. Adv Immunol 101: 81–121.

5. Moosbauer C, Morgenstern E, Cuvelier SL, Manukyan D, Bidzhekov K, et al. (2007) Eosinophils are a major intravascular location for tissue factor storage and exposure. Blood 109: 995–1002.

6. Roufosse F, Weller PF (2010) Practical approach to the patient with hypereosinophilia. J Allergy Clin Immunol 126: 39–44.

7. Valent P, Klion AD, Horny HP, Roufosse F, Gotlib J, et al. (2012) Contemporary consensus proposal on criteria and classification of eosinophilic disorders and related syndromes. J Allergy Clin Immunol 130: 607–612.

8. Chen YY, Khoury P, Ware JM, Holland-Thomas NC, Stoddard JL, et al. (2014) Marked and persistent eosinophilia in the absence of clinical manifestations. J Allergy Clin Immunol 133: 1195–202.

9. Ames PR, Margaglione M, Mackie S, Alves JD (2010) Eosinophilia and thrombophilia in Churg Strauss syndrome: a clinical and pathogenetic overview. Clin Appl Thromb Hemost 16: 628–636.

10. Ogbogu PU, Rosing DR, Horne MK 3rd (2007) Cardiovascular manifestations of hypereosinophilic syndromes. Immunol Allergy Clin North Am 27: 457–475.

11. Maino A, Rossio R, Cugno M, Marzano AV, Tedeschi A (2012) Hypereosinophilic syndrome, Churg-Strauss syndrome and parasitic diseases: possible links between eosinophilia and thrombosis. Curr Vasc Pharmacol 10: 670–675.

12. Slungaard A, Vercellotti GM, Tran T, Gleich GJ, Key NS (1993) Eosinophil cationic granule proteins impair thrombomodulin function: a potential mechanism for thromboembolism in hypereosinophilic heart disease. J Clin Invest 91: 1721–1730.

13. Marzano AV, Tedeschi A, Rossio R, Fanoni D, Cugno M (2010) Prothrombotic state in Churg-Strauss syndrome: a case report. J Investig Allergol Clin Immunol 20: 616–619.

14. Wang JG, Mahmud SA, Thompson JA, Geng JG, Key NS, et al. (2006) The principal eosinophil peroxidase product, HOSCN, is a uniquely potent phagocyte oxidant inducer of endothelial cell tissue factor activity: a potential mechanism for thrombosis in eosinophilic inflammatory states. Blood 107: 558–565.

15. Rohrbach MS, Wheatley CL, Slifman NR, Slifman NR, Gleich GJ (1990) Activation of platelets by eosinophil granule proteins. J Exp Med 172: 1271–1274.

16. Gauchat JF, Henchoz S, Fattah D, Mazzei G, Aubry JP, et al. (1995) CD40 ligand is functionally expressed on human eosinophils. Eur J Immunol 25: 863–865.

17. Santilli F, Basili S, Ferroni P, Davi G (2007) CD40/CD40L system and vascular disease. Intern Emerg Med 2: 256–268.

18. Ojima-Uchiyama A, Masuzawa Y, Sugiura T, Waku K, Fukuda T (1991) Production of platelet-activating factor by human normodense and hypodense eosinophils. Lipids 26: 1200–1203.

19. Sovershaev MA, Lind KF, Devold H, Jørgensen TØ, Hansen JB, et al. (2008) No evidence for the presence of tissue factor in high-purity preparations of immunologically isolated eosinophils. J Thromb Haemost 6: 1742–1749.

20. Caraguel CG, Stryhn H, Gagné N, Dohoo IR, Hammell KL (2011) Selection of a cutoff value for real-time polymerase chain reaction results to fit a diagnostic purpose: analytical and epidemiologic approaches. J Vet Diagn Invest 23: 2–15.

21. Zhu L, Gao D, Yang J, Li M (2012) Characterization of the phenotype of high collagen-producing fibroblast clones in systemic sclerosis, using a new modified limiting-dilution method. Clin Exp Dermatol 37: 395–403.

22. Egorina EM, Sovershaev MA, Olsen JO, Østerud B (2008) Granulocytes do not express but acquire monocyte-derived tissue factor in whole blood: evidence for a direct transfer. Blood 111: 1208–1216.

23. Basavaraj MG, Olsen JO, Østerud B, Hansen JB (2012) Differential ability of tissue factor antibody clones on detection of tissue factor in blood cells and microparticles. Thromb Res 130: 538–546.

24. Ackerman SJ, Bochner BS (2007) Mechanisms of eosinophilia in the pathogenesis of hypereosinophilic disorders. Immunol Allergy Clin North Am 27: 357–375.

25. Asero R, Tedeschi A, Coppola R, Griffini S, Paparella P, et al. (2007) Activation of the tissue factor pathway of blood coagulation in patients with chronic urticaria. J Allergy Clin Immunol 119: 705–710.

26. Cugno M, Marzano AV, Tedeschi A, Fanoni D, et al. (2009) Expression of tissue factor by eosinophils in patients with chronic urticaria. Int Arch Allergy Immunol 148: 170–174.

27. Marzano AV, Tedeschi A, Fanoni D, Bonanni E, Venegoni L, et al. (2009) Activation of blood coagulation in bullous pemphigoid: role of eosinophils and local and systemic implications. Br J Dermatol 160: 266–272.

28. Marzano AV, Tedeschi A, Berti E, Fanoni D, Crosti C, et al. (2011) Activation of coagulation in bullous pemphigoid and other eosinophil-related inflammatory skin diseases. Clin Exp Immunol 165: 44–50.

29. Mandal SK, Pendurthi UR, Rao LV (2006) Cellular localization and trafficking of tissue factor. Blood 107: 4746–4753.

30. Peña E, Arderiu G, Badimon L (2012) Subcellular localization of tissue factor and human coronary artery smooth muscle cell migration. J Thromb Haemost 10: 2373–2382.

31. Langan SM, Hubbard R, Fleming K, West J (2009) A population-based study of acute medical conditions associated with bullous pemphigoid. Br J Dermatol 161: 1149–1152.

32. Yang YW, Chen YH, Xirasagar S, Lin HC (2011) Increased risk of stroke in patients with bullous pemphigoid: a population-based follow-up study. Stroke 42: 319–323.

18

Adoptive Immunotherapy of Cytokine-Induced Killer Cell Therapy in the Treatment of Non-Small Cell Lung Cancer

Min Wang[1][⑨][¶], **Jun-Xia Cao**[1][⑨][¶], **Jian-Hong Pan**[2], **Yi-Shan Liu**[1], **Bei-Lei Xu**[1], **Duo Li**[1], **Xiao-Yan Zhang**[1], **Jun-Li Li**[1], **Jin-Long Liu**[1], **Hai-Bo Wang**[1], **Zheng-Xu Wang**[1]*

1 Biotherapy Center, General Hospital of Beijing Military Command, Beijing, China, 2 Department of Biostatistics, Peking University Clinical Research Institute, Peking University Health Science Center, Beijing, China

Abstract

Aim: The aim of this study was to systemically evaluate the therapeutic efficacy of cytokine-induced killer (CIK) cells for the treatment of non-small cell lung cancer.

Materials and Methods: A computerized search of randomized controlled trials for CIK cell-based therapy was performed. The overall survival, clinical response rate, immunological assessment and side effects were evaluated.

Results: Overall, 17 randomized controlled trials of non-small cell lung cancer (NSCLC) with a total of 1172 patients were included in the present analysis. Our study showed that the CIK cell therapy significantly improved the objective response rate and overall survival compared to the non-CIK cell-treated group. After CIK combined therapy, we observed substantially increased percentages of CD3$^+$, CD4$^+$, CD4$^+$CD8$^+$, CD3$^+$CD56$^+$ and NK cells, whereas significant decreases were noted in the percentage of CD8$^+$ and regulatory T cell (Treg) subgroups. A significant increase in Ag-NORs was observed in the CIK-treated patient group ($p = 0.00001$), whereas carcinoembryonic antigen (CEA) was more likely to be reduced to a normal level after CIK treatment ($p = 0.0008$). Of the possible major side effects, only the incidence of fever in the CIK group was significantly higher compared to the group that received chemotherapy alone.

Conclusion: The CIK cell combined therapy demonstrated significant superiority in the overall survival, clinical response rate, and T lymphocytes responses and did not present any evidence of major adverse events in patients with NSCLC.

Editor: Nupur Gangopadhyay, University of Pittsburgh, United States of America

Funding: This research work was supported by the National Natural Science Foundation of China (No. 31171427 and 30971651 to Zheng-Xu Wang), Beijing Municipal Science & Technology Project; Clinical characteristics and Application Research of Capital (No. Z121107001012136 to Zheng-Xu Wang) and the Postdoctoral Foundation of China (No. 20060400775 to Jun-Xia Cao). Zheng-Xu Wang designed the research; Jun-Xia Cao is one of the people who performed the research and wrote the paper. The funders had no role in study design, data collection and analysis, decision to publish, or preparation of the manuscript.

Competing Interests: The authors have declared that no competing interests exist.

* Email: zhxwang18@hotmail.com

⑨ These authors contributed equally to this work.

¶ These authors are co-first authors on this work.

Introduction

Lung cancer is the leading cause of cancer-related mortality worldwide [1]. According to the 2012 Chinese cancer registration annual report, more than 3 million new cases of lung cancer will be diagnosed every year, and the approximately 2.7 million deaths from lung cancer will account for 13% of allmortalities. There is no doubt that the incidence and mortality of lung cancer are far too prevalent [2]. In patients with advanced lung disease, 1-year survival rates are typically 35%, and 2-year survival rates were shown to approach 15%-20% in recent studies [3]. At best, the 5-year overall survival rate of localized cancer is 15.9%, and only half of extended-stage patients have a 3.7% chance of surviving 5 years [4]. Most NSCLC patients have locally advanced or metastatic cancer at stage IIIB-IV at the time of diagnosis, leaving only palliative therapeutic options. Based on the existing clinical data, chemotherapy appears to have limited benefits and disappointed prognoses [5].

The novel approach of adoptive cell immunotherapy relies on an ex vivo expansion of the autologous tumor-specific effector cells before their reinfusion into the host [6]. Since the development of this immunotherapy, a number of immunological effector cells have been employed to treat cancer and eliminate residual tumor cells after surgery, such as CIK cells, lymphokine-activated killer cells (LAKs), tumor-infiltrating lymphocytes (TILs), natural killer cells (NKs), and cytotoxic T lymphocyte cells (CTLs) [7,8]. Among them, LAKs, which are a mixture of lymphokine-activated CD3$^+$ T lymphocytes and CD3$^-$CD56$^+$CD16$^+$ NK cells, were cultured with recombinant interleukin-2 (rIL-2) for 3 days, and CTLs were isolated from a patient's own tissues, including peripheral blood mononuclear cells (PBMCs), TILs, draining lymph nodes, or PBMCs after vaccination with irradiated autologous tumor cells (ATCs) [7,8]. After adoptive cell immunotherapy made great strides due to the efforts of several generations of researchers, CIK cells were found to possess greater proliferative and cytolytic capacities than NK or LAK cells. CIK cells are MHC-unrestricted cytotoxic lymphocytes that can be generated in vitro from PBMCs and cultured with the addition of IFN-γ, IL-2 and CD3 monoclonal antibody (CD3mAb). Anti-tumor cytotoxic activity is represented by surface markers for both T cells (TCR-α/β, CD3) and NKT cells (CD3$^+$CD56$^+$) [9].

The first clinical trial using CIK cell therapy for cancer patients was reported in 1999 [10]. Soon afterward, a growing number of clinical trials have suggested that CIK therapy yields highly compelling objective clinical responses in several solid carcinomas compared to other immunological effectors. A pooled analysis of 792 patients with solid carcinomas indicated that treatment with CIK cells is associated with a significant prolonging of the mean survival time and disease control rate [11]. Recently, both chinese clinical trials with 563 patients and international registered clinical trials with 426 cases of CIK cell therapy provided evidence for a broad clinical application based on a positive evaluation of the immunological and clinical responses [12,13]. Some systematic reviews have analyzed CIK cell therapy and shown it to be safe and efficient to treat renal cell carcinoma, hepatocellular carcinoma, and colon cancer [14–16]. Furthermore, CIK cell therapy has been perceived to have significant survival benefits in a few NSCLC clinical trials [17–22]. These studies showed that the immunotherapy of cancers with CIK cells may improve immunological and clinical responses, promote the quality of life (QoL) of cancer patients, and extend their life spans under certain conditions. However, there is no systematic review to assess the therapeutic efficacy of CIK cell therapies combined with chemotherapy in NSCLC; therefore, we performed a systematic meta-analysis of CIK cell therapy with randomized controlled trials on NSCLC. Our large-scale CIK cell immunotherapy clinical trials systematically analyzed the clinical efficiency and safety considering the overall survival, clinical response, immunological assessments and side effects.

Methods

Study design, search strategy and eligibility criteria

The relevant studies were identified by searching PubMed, the Cochrane Center Register of Controlled Trials, Science Direct, Embase, and China National Knowledge Infrastructure for randomized controlled trials (RCT) in the most recent decades. The search strategy included the keywords 'non-small-cell lung cancer,' 'adoptive immunotherapy,' and 'cytokine induced killer cells' adoptive immunotherapy arms with no adjuvant treatment in NSCLC patients except those who had undergone the same chemotherapy compared with control arms. In addition, we manually searched a website of clinical trials for ongoing trials. We searched keywords 'non-small-cell lung cancer' and 'cytokine induced killer cells' on the website http://www.clinicaltrials.gov/. The registered clinical trials with publication citations are displayed at the bottom of the Full Text View tab of a study record, under the More Information heading. Reference lists of previously published trials and relevant review articles were examined for other eligible trials. No language restriction was applied. Review papers and postgraduate theses were also examined for published results. Furthermore, we performed manual searches in reference lists and conference proceedings of the American Society of Clinical Oncology (ASCO) annual

meetings and the European Cancer Conference (ECCO). We excluded abstracts that were never subsequently published as full papers and studies on animals and cell lines.

Data selection criteria

Data extraction was independently conducted by two reviewers (Min Wang and Jun-Xia Cao) using a standardized approach. Disagreement was adjudicated by a third reviewer (Zheng-Xu Wang) after referring back to the original publications. The selection criteria were as follows: (1) English language studies on human clinical trials with patients at all stages of NSCLC were included; (2) RCT with CIK cell-based immunotherapy combined with chemotherapy versus chemotherapy alone for the treatment of NSCLC were included; (3) all trials approved by the local ethical committee and in which all patients signed a study-specific consent form prior to study entry were included; (4) case studies, review articles, and studies involving fewer than 10 patients were excluded; (5) uncontrolled metabolic disease, inadequate hepatic function, renal dysfunction, neurological disorders and other infectious diseases were excluded from the study; and (6) blood samples receiving any chemotherapy or radiotherapy within one month before treatment were excluded.

The overall quality of each included paper was evaluated by the Jadad scale [23]. A few of the major criteria were employed as a grading scheme: (1) randomization; (2) allocation concealment; (3) blinding; (4) lost to follow up; (5) ITT (intention to treat); and (6) baseline. We also used a funnel plot to evaluate the publication bias.

Definition of outcome measures

The primary clinical endpoints in RCT for cancer therapies employed the measures of median survival time (MST) and progression-free survival (PFS). The time to progression (TTP) may not consider those patients who die from other causes but is often used as equivalent to PFS. The secondary endpoints were the clinical response rate, including the objective response rate (ORR) and disease control rate (DCR). The ORR was defined as the sum of the partial rates (PRs) and complete response rates (CRs), and the DCR was defined as the sum of the stable disease (SD), PR and CR, according to the World Health Organization criteria. The side effects and toxicity were graded according to the National Cancer Institute Common Toxicity Criteria. The data were either obtained directly from the articles or calculated using the graphed data in articles using Photoshop and a software graph digitizer scout.

Statistical analysis

The analysis was performed using Review Manager Version 5.0 (Nordic Cochran Centre, Copenhagen, Denmark). Heterogeneity was assessed to determine which model should be used. To assess the statistical heterogeneity between the studies, the Cochran Q-test was performed using a predefined significance threshold of 0.1. The treatment effects are reflected by odds ratios (ORs), which were obtained using a method reported by Mantel and Haenszel. To evaluate whether the results of the studies were homogeneous, Cochran's Q test was performed. We also calculated the quantity I^2, which describes the percentage of variation across studies that is due to heterogeneity rather than chance. The OR was obtained using a fixed-effect model with no statistically significant heterogeneity; otherwise, a random-effects model was employed. P-values <0.05 were considered statistically significant. All reported P-values were two-sided.

Results

Selection of the trials

The data searches yielded 167 references, 91 of which were considered ineligible for different reasons (44 non-CIK immunotherapy, 19 multiple cancer analyses, 18 reviews, and 10 animal models). The remaining 76 articles were further evaluated, and 59 trials were excluded due to language, lack of an RCT, and insufficient data. The final 17 articles were included in the meta-analysis with RCTs of CIK cell-based therapy for the treatment of NSCLC (Figure 1, also see the checklist S1).

The quality assessment of the 17 studies is summarized in Table 1. We also used a funnel plot to evaluate the publication bias. In our analysis, overall survival, clinical response rate, and side effects suffered low published bias. However, immunological assessment and T cell subgroups observed a high published bias (Figure 2), which demonstrated that the node of the vertical line does not meet the horizontal one at the midpoint by analysis with Review Manager Version 5.0.

Characteristics of CIK cell-based therapy

The characteristics of the 17 trials are listed in Table 2. Our selected 17 trials with a total of 1172 NSCLC patients in stage I-IV were included in the present analysis, and 90% of them included metastatic or locally advanced NSCLC. The enrolled ages were between 28 and 82 years of age, with a median age greater than 50.

In all 17 trials, the control arm was chemotherapy or cyberknife alone, whereas the treatment arm was chemotherapy or cyberknife combined with CIK cell therapy. In each trial, all of the patients in the CIK group were treated identically to those in the chemotherapy group in terms of chemotherapy doses and cycles. In all 17 trials of the treatment arm, most of the patients were treated with CIK cells plus DC immunotherapy combined with chemotherapy, although patients in four of the trials were injected with CIK cells combined with chemotherapy [6,30,38,39]. Most of the CIK groups used DCs without pulse, i.e., the DCs were only induced to become mature before co-culture with CIK cells. In 4 out of 17 studies, the DCs were injected while being pulsed with lung cancer antigens or tumor lysate [17,22,33,37]. Some of the necessary cytokines were supplied in a culture of CIK, IL-2, IFN-γ, and CD3mAb in a variety of culture media. The patients received cell infusions of 1×10^9 to 2×10^{12} cells per course, mostly at a 10^9 order of magnitude. Most of the treatments with repeated CIK cell infusions were administered for at least 2 weeks, and some of them lasted over 1 month. The injected route for immunotherapy was mainly intravenous for CIK cells and via subcutaneous injection for DCs (File S1 and File S2).

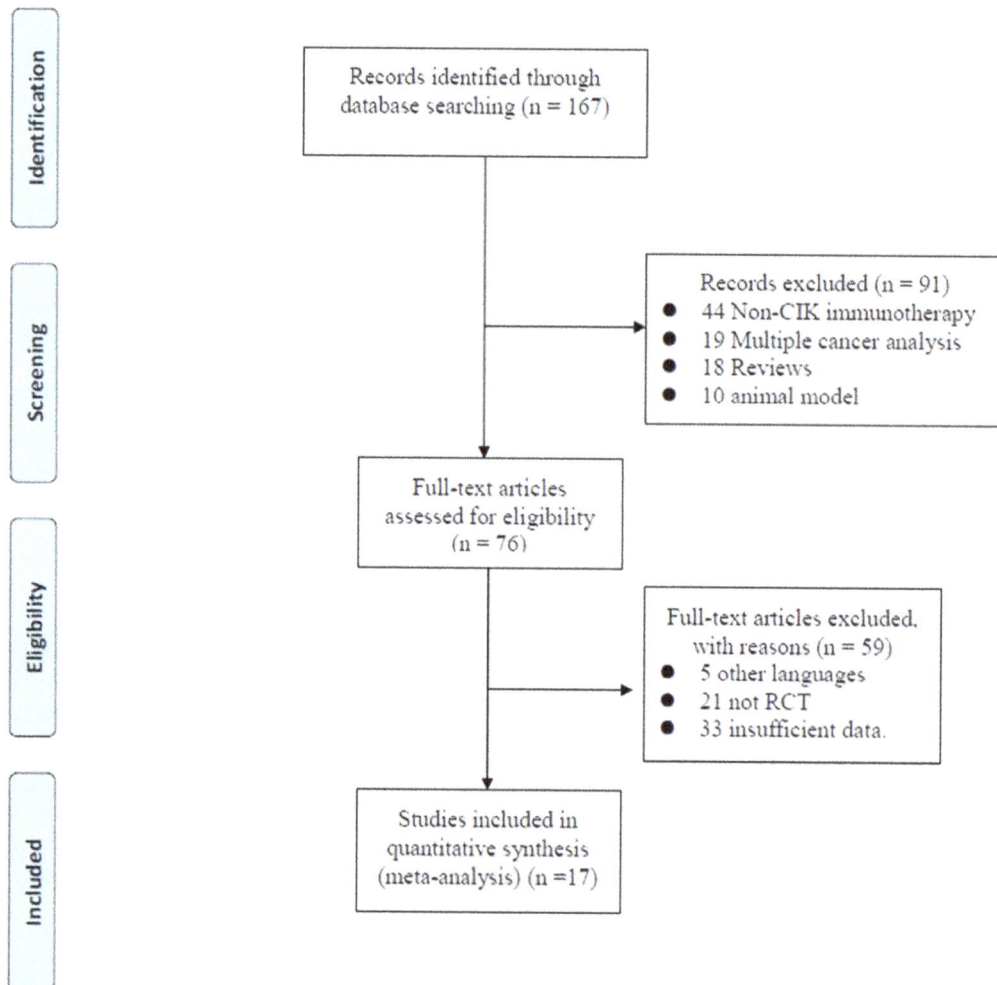

Figure 1. Flow diagram of the study selection process.

Table 1. Jadad Scale for the 17 randomized controlled studies.

Included studies	Randomization	Allocation concealment	Blinding	Lost to follow up	ITT analysis	Baseline	Quality grading
Li 2009 [17]	Yes	Unclear	Unclear	No	Yes	Similar	B
Li 2012 [30]	Yes	Unclear	Unclear	No	Yes	Similar	B
Mo 2010 [18]	Yes	Unclear	Unclear	Yes	Unclear	Unclear	C
Peng 2012 [19]	Yes	Unclear	Unclear	No	Yes	Similar	B
Sheng 2011 [20]	Yes	Unclear	Unclear	No	Yes	Similar	B
Shi 2012 [21]	Yes	Unclear	Unclear	No	Yes	Similar	B
Wang 2013 [39]	Yes	Unclear	Unclear	Yes	Yes	Similar	B
Wu 2008 [6]	Yes	Unclear	Unclear	No	Yes	Similar	B
Xu 2010 [31]	Yes	Unclear	Unclear	No	Yes	Similar	B
Xu 2011 [32]	Yes	Unclear	Unclear	No	Yes	Similar	B
Yang 2013 [33]	Yes	Unclear	Unclear	No	Yes	Similar	B
You 2012 [34]	Yes	Unclear	Unclear	Yes	Yes	Unclear	B
Yuan 2011 [35]	Yes	Unclear	Unclear	Yes	Yes	Unclear	C
Zhang 2012 [36]	Yes	Unclear	Unclear	No	Yes	Similar	B
Zheng 2012 [38]	Yes	Unclear	Unclear	No	Yes	Similar	B
Zhong 2008 [37]	Yes	Unclear	Unclear	No	Yes	Similar	B
Zhong 2011 [22]	Yes	Unclear	No	No	Yes	Similar	B

ITT: intention-to-treat. A: adequate, with correct procedure; B: unclear, without a description of the methods; C: inadequate procedures, methods, or information. Each criterion was graded as follows: Yes, adequate, with correct procedure; Unclear, without a description of the methods; No, inadequate procedures, methods, or information. Each involved study was graded as follows: A, studies with a low risk of bias and which were scored as grade of A for all items; B, studies with a moderate risk of bias, with one or more grades of B; and C, studies with a high risk of bias, with one or more grades of C.

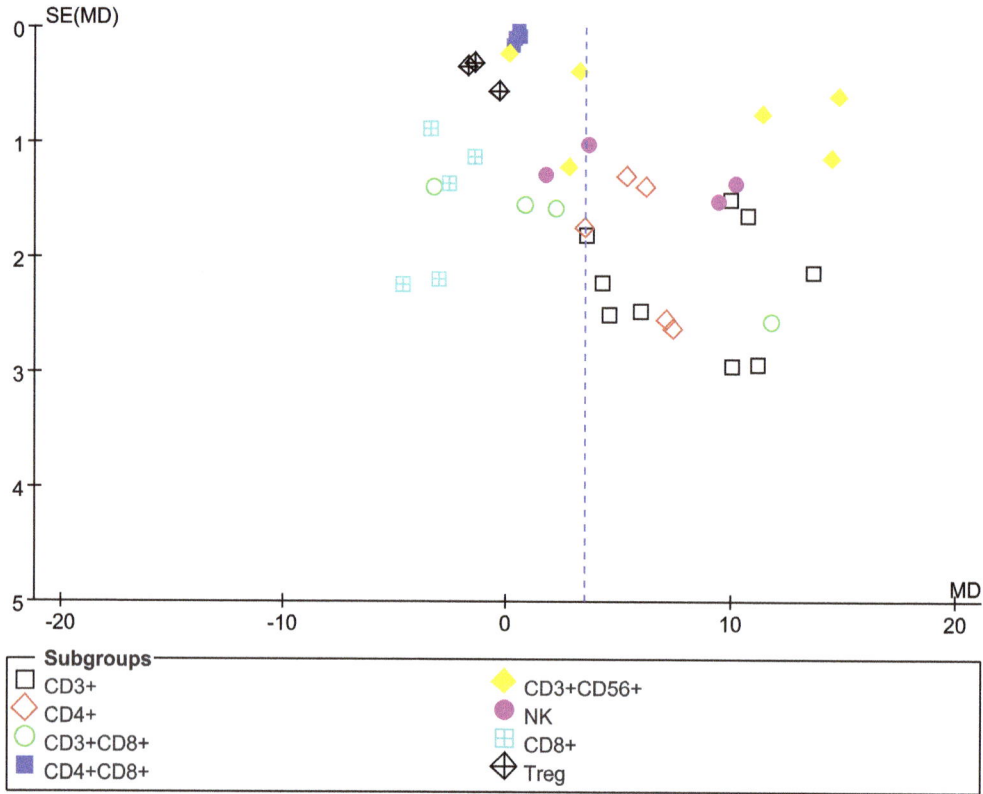

Figure 2. Funnel plot to evaluate the publication bias of T-cell subgroups. The analysis was performed using Review Manager Version 5.0.

Survival

The patients in the CIK group had significantly prolonged MST compared with those in the non-CIK group (95%CI −7.45 to −0.66, $p = 0.02$) (Table 3). The results of the pooled analysis showed that the CIK arm significantly extended overall survival at the end of follow-up, compared with the non-CIK group (Table 4). Three subgroups of patients of the CIK cell-based therapy group at 1-year survival, 2-year survival, and 3-year survival presented significant survival benefits compared to the patients in the non-CIK group (OR 0.64, 95%CI 0.46–0.91, $p = 0.01$; OR 0.36, 95%CI 0.22–0.59, $p < 0.0001$; OR 0.37, 95%CI 0.20–0.70, $p = 0.002$, respectively), which was consistent with the overall survival (OR 0.50, 95%CI 0.39–0.64, $p < 0.0001$). Based on the results of our analysis, the short-term survival subgroup showed a significant difference at the 1-year and 2-year survivals. The 1-year survival for the 282 patients in the CIK group was 56%, whereas a slightly lower 1-year survival rate was found for the non-CIK group (45% of 278 patients). A significant difference was also demonstrated in the 2-year survival group, which was 43.22% for 236 patients in the CIK group and 27.47% of 233 patients without the CIK cell treatment. The long-term survival rates in the CIK group showed a slight decrease compared with the short-term survival rate; however, a significant difference in the long-term survival rates was found compared to the non-CIK group ($p = 0.002$).

Concerning the median PFS, the CIK group did not produce any significant improvement compared with the corresponding control groups (95%CI −13.27 to 3.89, $p = 0.28$), whereas the median TTP clearly prolonged the median time to disease progression in the CIK group (95%CI −2.70 to −0.47, $p = 0.005$) (Table 3).

Response rate

The CIK cell-based therapy group showed favorable results when subjected to both analysis of the ORR (OR 0.58, 95%CI 0.44–0.78, $p = 0.00003$) and the DCR (OR 0.41, 95%CI 0.29–0.58, $p < 0.0001$), compared with the corresponding control arms. With no significant heterogeneity, a fixed-effect model was used in the ORR and DCR analyses (Table 4). Cochran's Q test resulted in a statistically significant P-value, and the corresponding quantity for I^2 was 0% for both groups, indicating that there was no evidence of heterogeneity among the individual studies.

Immunological assessment of T-cell subgroups

When heterogeneity was observed in the T-cell subgroups, a random-effects model was applied for the overall and subgroup analysis of T-cell immunological assessments (Table 5). The results demonstrated a substantially increased ratio of $CD3^+$ (MD 8.21, 95%CI 5.79–10.64, $p < 0.00001$), $CD4^+$ (MD 5.59, 95%CI 4.10–7.07, $p < 0.00001$), $CD4^+CD8^+$ (MD 0.49, 95%CI 0.37–0.61, $p < 0.00001$), $CD3^+CD56^+$ (MD 7.80, 95%CI 2.61–12.98, $p = 0.003$) and NK cells ($CD3^-CD16^+CD56^+$) (MD 6.21, 95%CI 2.25–10.17, $p = 0.002$), whereas the ratio of $CD3^+CD8^+$ (MD 2.55, 95%CI −2.46 to 7.56, $p = 0.32$) generated no statistical improvement after CIK treatment. In addition, the pooled analysis showed a significant decrease in the percentage of $CD8^+$ (MD −2.75, 95%CI −3.88 to −1.63, $p < 0.00001$) and Treg ($CD4^+CD25^+CD127^-$) (MD −1.26, 95%CI −1.94 to −0.58,

Table 2. Clinical information from the eligible trials in the meta-analysis.

Trials	Age	No. of pts	Operative method	Tumor Stage	CIK regimens	CIK culture	DC modification
Li 2009 [17]	40–80; (M61)	42;42	Chemo; Chemo+DC-CIK	I-IIIA	1.3×10^9/course, 4 treatments at intervals of a month	X-Vivo 20, IL-1α, IL-2, IFN-γ, CD3	ATL (100 µg/ml)
Li 2012 [30]	UK	37; 37	Chemo; Chemo+ CIK	III-IV	13×10^9/course, twice in a cycle, at least 3 cycles	X-Vivo 20,IL-1α, IL-2, IFN-γ, CD3	NO DC
Mo 2010 [18]	39–77; (M60)	20;21	Chemo; Chemo+ DC-CIK	IV	$2-6\times10^6$/course, 6 times every second day	RPMI1640, IL-1α, IL-2, IFN-γ, CD3mAb	NI-DC
Peng 2012 [19]	65–79; (M71)	23; 24	Chemo; Chemo+ DC-CIK	III-IV	$1\times10^{10}-2\times10^{12}$/course, 2–3 times a week, 7 days intervals for 4 cycles	CM, IL-1α, IL-2, IFN-γ, CD3	NI-DC
Sheng 2011 [20]	35–65; (M54)	33; 32	Chemo; Chemo+ DC-CIK	III-IV	5×10^9/course, 4 treatments in a week for 2 weeks	RPMI1640, IL-1α, IL-2, IFN-γ, CD3	NI-DC
Shi 2012 [21]	UK	30; 30	Chemo; Chemo+ DC-CIK	III-IV	5 times every second day	RPMI1640, IL-1, IL-2, CD3	NI-DC
Wang 2013 [39]	UK	11; 11	CK; CK+ CIK	AS	2×10^{10}/course, 2 courses in 2 months	UK	No DC
Wu 2008 [6]	38–78; (M60)	30; 29	Chemo; Chemo+ CIK	III-IV	1×10^9/course, 5 times every second day	RPMI1640, IL-1α, IL-2, IFN-γ, CD3	No DC
Xu 2010 [31]	47–75; (M59.6)	40; 38	Chemo; Chemo+ DC-CIK	III-IV	1.6×10^9/course, 2 times a week in next following 4–5 weeks	RPMI1640, IL-2, IFN-γ, CD3	NI-DC
Xu 2011 [32]	45–73; (M59)	40; 45	Chemo; Chemo+ DC-CIK	III	1.3×10^9/course, 2 times a week in 5–6 weeks	RPMI1640, IL-2, IFN-γ, CD3	NI-DC
Yang 2012 [33]	28–82; (M63.5)	61; 61	Chemo; Chemo + DC-CIK	III-IV	1.2×10^9/course, 30day intervals for 4 cycles	X-vivo 20, IFN-γ,IL-1α,IL-2,CD3McAb	ATL (100 µg/ml)
You 2012 [34]	M 52	50; 55	Chemo; Chemo+ DC-CIK	III-IV	5×10^9/course, 4 times a cycle, 2–6 cycles	RPMI1640, IL-1α, IL-2, IFN-γ, CD3mAb	NI-DC
Yuan 2011 [35]	M 66	32; 32	Chemo; Chemo+ DC-CIK	AS	4 times a cycle	Unknown	NI-DC
Zhang 2012 [36]	35–72; (M57)	50; 50	Chemo; Chemo+ DC-CIK	III-IV	28day intervals for 2 cycles	GT-T551,IL-2, IFN-γ, CD3	NI-DC
Zheng 2012 [38]	M 59	36; 36	γK; γK +CIK	III	1×10^{10}/course, 1 month intervals for 2 cycles	RPMI1640, IL-1α, IL-2,IFN-γ, CD3mAb	No DC
Zhong 2008 [37]	M 53.6	44; 22	Chemo; Chemo+ DC-CIK	IB	2 times in 4 days	UK	CEA PI-DC
Zhong 2011 [22]	40–65	14; 14	Chemo; Chemo+ DC-CIK	IIIB- IV	$1-1.7\times10^9$/course,30day intervals for 4 cycles	CM, IFN-γ, IL-2,CD3McAb	CEA, PI-DC (10 µg/ml)

M: median; UK: unknown; AS: advanced stage; Chemo: chemotherapy; CK: cyberknife; γK: γ-knife; NI-DC: non-impulsed DC; ATL: Autologous tumor lysate; PI-DC: peptide impulse DC; Pts: Patients. The selective data include the authors' names, year of publication, trial period, sample size per arm, regimen used, median or mean age of patients, cell preparation, CIK-based therapy treatment and information pertaining to the study design.

Table 3. Comparison of MTTP, MST, and MPFS between the non-CIK and CIK groups.

Event	No. of Trials [Ref]	No. of pts Non-CIK CIK		Mean Difference	95% CI	P value	Heterogeneity (I²)
MTTP	4 [6,21,31,36]	97	100	−1.59	−2.70 to −0.47	0.005	0%
MST	4 [6,31,32,37]	154	134	−4.06	−7.45to −0.66	0.02	0%
MPFS	3 [21,30,37]	161	139	−4.69	−13.27to 3.89	0.28	56%

MTTP: median time to progression; MST: median survival time; MPFS: median progression-free survival; Pts: patients; 95%CI: 95% confidence interval; significant difference: P value <0.05.

Table 4. Comparison of OS, ORR and DCR between the non-CIK and CIK groups.

Event	No. of Trials [Ref]	No. pts of Non-CIK CIK		Odds Ratio (OR)	95% CI	P value	Heterogeneity (I²)
1 yr OS	8 [6,18,19,22,31,32,33,36]	278	282	0.64	0.46 to 0.91	0.01	0%
2 yr OS	6 [6,17,18,31–33]	233	236	0.36	0.22 to 0.59	<0.0001	0%
3 yrOS	4 [17,20,31,37]	154	136	0.37	0.20 to 0.70	0.002	13%
ORR	11 [6,18–20,31–36,38]	401	410	0.58	0.44 to 0.78	0.0003	0%
DCR	10 [6,18–20,31–34,36,38]	369	378	0.41	0.29 to 0.58	<0.00001	0%

Forest plot comparing the 1-, 2- and 3-year OS between the non-CIK and CIK groups.OR, odds ratio; OS, overall survival. Due to the low heterogeneity detected, the fixed-effect model was used in this OS meta-analysis. Comparison of the ORR and the DCR between the non-CIK group and CIK group. OR, odds ratio; ORR, objective response rate; DCR, disease control rate. Due to the lack of heterogeneity, the fixed-effect model was used. OS: overall survival; ORR: objective response rate; DCR: disease control rate.

Table 5. Comparison of CD3+, CD4+, CD3+CD8+, CD4+CD8+, CD3+CD56+, NK, CD8+ and Treg before CIK treatment and after CIK therapy.

Event	No. of Trials [Ref]	No. of pts Before-CIK	CIK	Mean Difference	95% CI	P value	Heterogeneity (I^2)
CD3+	9 [6,17,20,21,31–33,35,36]	359	359	8.21	5.79 to 10.64	<0.00001	67%
CD4+	5 [6,21,31,32,35]	174	174	5.59	4.10 to 7.07	<0.0001	0%
CD3+CD8+	4 [17,18,33,36]	174	174	2.55	−2.46 to 7.56	0.32	89%
CD4+CD8+	4 [6,31,32,35]	144	144	0.49	0.37 to 0.61	<0.00001	53%
CD3+CD56+	6 [6,18,19,30,36,38]	222	222	7.80	2.61 to 12.98	0.003	99%
NK	4 [6,21,32,36]	154	154	6.21	2.25 to 10.17	0.002	90%
CD8+	5 [6,21,31,32,35]	174	174	−2.75	−3.88 to −1.63	<0.00001	0%
Treg	3 [17,33,36]	153	153	−1.26	−1.94 to −0.58	0.0003	58%

Forest plot for the comparison of T-cell subgroups, before and after treatment with the CIK cell-based therapy. The random-effects meta-analysis model was used in this analysis.

$p = 0.0003$) subgroups after treatment with CIK cell-based therapy.

Immunological assessment of Ag-NORs and CEA expression

Due to the limited data presented in the published papers, only some of the immunological assessments, e.g., Ag-NORs (argyrophilic nucleolar organizer regions), and NSCLC tumor markers, e.g., CEA, were subjected to analysis. Heterogeneity was observed, and a random-effects model was therefore applied for the analysis of the subgroups and the overall analysis. The analysis showed that the CIK group significantly improved the patients' T lymphocyte immune activity, showing better Ag-NORs (MD −0.71, 95%CI − 0.94 to −0.47, $p = 0.00001$) compared with the non-CIK therapy group (Table 6). The CEA expression level in the analysis was based on two trials [38,39]. The plasma CEA was markedly decreased in the CIK group compared to the non-CIK group (MD 3.96, 95%CI 1.64–6.28, $p = 0.0008$) (Table 6).

Toxicity and adverse reactions

The patients in the CIK group observed fewer severe side effects from chemotherapy, such as fewer cases of grade III and IV leucopenia, gastrointestinal adverse reactions, anemia and liver dysfunction (Figure 3). Without significant heterogeneity, a fixed-effect model (Mantel-Haenszel method) was used for the side effect analysis.

After CIK cell transfusion, most of the patients developed a slight fever, between 37.5 and 39 degrees, but the patients recovered within a few days without severe side effects. Four types of serious chemotherapy side effects could lead to toxic reactions in both groups of patients. The pooled analysis showed that the adverse effects of gastrointestinal adverse reactions (OR 1.77, 95%CI 1.20–2.59, $p = 0.004$) and anemia (OR 2.80, 95%CI 1.37–5.73, $p = 0.005$) generated a significant difference, with fewer episodes in the CIK group. Leucopenia and liver dysfunction were observed less frequently in the patients receiving the CIK treatment, but neither set of data displayed a significant difference compared with the non-CIK group (OR 1.59, 95% CI 0.93–2.72, $p = 0.09$; OR 1.11, 95%CI 0.60–2.06, $p = 0.73$).

Discussion

Immunotherapy has benefited from an increased understanding of tumor immunology and genetics. A number of studies have confirmed that immunotherapy is a safe and feasible treatment option for cancer patients [12–16]. Therefore, conventional therapy combined with adoptive cell immunotherapy is associated with a favorable prognosis compared to chemotherapy alone [18]. Our analysis was designed to elucidate the effects of CIK cell therapy on improving the therapeutic efficacy and safe treatment of NSCLC patients based on a variety of evaluation indexes, including clinical survival outcomes, clinical response rates, immunophenotypes and adverse effects.

In our study, 17 trials were selected for the analysis of the culture of CIK cells and treatment regimens. Most of the trials collected 50–100 ml of autologous peripheral blood and separated the mononuclear cells for further induction. Some of the necessary cytokines were supplied to the cultures of CIK cells, such as IL-2, IFN-γ, and CD3mAb, in 1640 or serum-free medium. Based on our study, most of the treatments with repetitive infusions of 1×10^9 to 2×10^{12} CIK cells were administered for at least 2 weeks on every second day for a minimum of two treatment cycles. However, the different doses and cycles of CIK cell transfusions may lead to different outcomes and immune responses.

Table 6. Comparison of the immunological assessment of Ag-NORs and CEA expression between the CIK and non-CIK group.

Event	No. of Trials [Ref]	No. of pts Non-CIK	CIK	Mean Difference	95% CI	P value	Heterogeneity (I^2)
Ag-NORs	2 [20,38]	69	68	−0.71	−0.94 to −0.47	0.00001	33%
CEA	2 [38,39]	47	47	3.96	1.64–6.28	0.0008	0%

Summary of the significant points in the Ag-NORs and CEA expression level between the CIK group and the non-CIK group with meta-analysis. The random-effects model was used for the calculations. Ag-NORs: argyrophilic nucleolar organizer regions; CEA: carcinoembryonic antigen; Pts: patients; 95%CI: 95% confidence interval; significant difference: P value <0.05.

In the present study, the CIK cell-based therapy group was associated with favorable results based on an evaluation of both the overall survival and clinical responses (Table 4). The 1-year survival (OR 0.64, 95%CI 0.46–0.91, $p = 0.01$), 2-year survival (OR 0.36, 95%CI 0.22–0.59, $p<0.0001$), and 3-year survival (OR 0.37, 95%CI 0.20–0.70, $p = 0.002$) showed significantly prolonged durations in the CIK cell therapy group. A favorable DCR and ORR were also observed in patients receiving CIK cell therapy ($p<0.0001$). The MTTP and MST also showed significant improvements in the CIK group ($p = 0.005$, $p = 0.02$). CIK cells, which are also known as NKT cells, exhibit both the cytotoxicity activities of T-lymphocytes and the restrictive tumor-killing activity by non-MHC of NK cells, among which the main effectors are CD3$^+$CD56$^+$ cells [7]. In total, 4 of 17 trials used DCs pulsed with lung cancer antigens or tumor lysate, whereas 9 trials used mature DCs co-cultured with CIK cells (Table 2). DCs possess antigen-presenting activities on the extracellular surface and are able to activate the proliferation of T cells and CIK cells. Therefore, considering the poor immunogenicity of NSCLC, CIK infusion with an immunoadjuvant or tumor-specific antigen pulsed DCs boosted the immune responses [24]. Therefore, CIK cell-based therapy even acting through completely different mechanisms for fighting cancer cells, can lead to an improvement in the clinical objective responses based on the assessment of traditional RECIST criteria [40].

The human immune response against cancer cells is mainly dependent on cellular immunity. Previous studies have found that the numerical ratios of T-lymphocyte subsets in the peripheral blood are disordered in tumor patients [17]. In the present study, we observed a substantially increased percentage of CD3$^+$ and CD4$^+$ ($p<0.001$), the ratio of CD4$^+$CD8$^+$ and CD3$^+$CD56$^+$ ($p< 0.001$) and NK cells ($p = 0.002$), but a significant decrease in the percentage of the CD8$^+$ ($p<0.001$) and Treg ($p = 0.0003$) subgroups after DC-CIK treatment by meta-analysis. Many studies have demonstrated that CIK cells possess strong cytotoxicity against a variety of T-lymphocyte populations, among which CD3$^+$CD56$^+$ is mainly responsible for the MHC unrestricted antitumor activity [8]. In addition, the number of CD4$^+$ and CD8$^+$ T-cells plays an important role in affecting clinical outcomes in NSCLC. The activation of CD4$^+$ T cells contributes to the secretion of immune regulatory cytokines, including IL-2, IL-12, and IFN-γ, which in turn facilitate an elevation in the cytolytic CD8$^+$ T cell responses, thereby inducing tumor cell death [25]. The activation of CD4$^+$ T cells also enhances the killing activity of NK cells and the phagocytic activity of macrophages, triggering a humoral immune response that leads to antibody production, thus CD4$^+$ and CD8$^+$ have a synergistic relationship in immune responses. Our meta-analysis demonstrated that CD3$^+$, CD4$^+$, CD4$^+$CD8$^+$, CD3$^+$CD56$^+$ and NK cells were increased after DC-CIK treatment, therefore suggesting the improvement of immune function after immunotherapy in the NSCLC patients.

In addition, we should note that CD8$^+$ T cells were not significantly increased after the immunotherapy, which also showed the varied immunophenotypes compared with the results of other T-cell assessments by the CIK treatment in different solid carcinomas [11–13]. Naïve CD4$^+$ T lymphocytes undergo cell differentiation in the presence of antigen, co-stimulatory molecules and cytokines, and these cells can be divided into several major groups: Th1, Th2 and Treg cells [26]. Th1 helper cells are the host immunity effectors against intracellular bacteria and protozoa. These are triggered by IL-12, IL-2 and the effector cytokine IFN-γ. The main effector cells of Th1 immunity are macrophages, CD8 T cells, IgG B cells, and CD4 T cells. Th2 helper cells are the host immunity effectors against multicellular helminthes [26]. The

Study or Subgroup	Non-CIK Events	Total	CIK Events	Total	Weight	Odds Ratio M-H, Fixed, 95% CI	Odds Ratio M-H, Fixed, 95% CI
4.1.1 Leucopenia							
Xu 2010	32	40	31	38	5.5%	0.90 [0.29, 2.79]	
Xu 2011	33	40	36	45	5.2%	1.18 [0.39, 3.52]	
Zheng 2012	28	36	20	36	3.9%	2.80 [1.01, 7.80]	
Zhong 2008	10	44	4	22	3.6%	1.32 [0.36, 4.82]	
Zhong 2011	13	14	10	14	0.6%	5.20 [0.50, 54.05]	
Subtotal (95% CI)		174		155	18.8%	1.59 [0.93, 2.72]	
Total events	116		101				
Heterogeneity: Chi² = 3.49, df = 4 (P = 0.48); I² = 0%							
Test for overall effect: Z = 1.70 (P = 0.09)							
4.1.2 Gastrointestinal adverse reaction							
Peng 2012	5	23	2	24	1.3%	3.06 [0.53, 17.66]	
Xu 2010	30	40	29	38	6.5%	0.93 [0.33, 2.62]	
Xu 2011	32	40	37	45	6.1%	0.86 [0.29, 2.57]	
You 2012	15	50	13	55	7.5%	1.38 [0.58, 3.30]	
Zhang 2012	27	50	16	50	6.4%	2.49 [1.11, 5.63]	
Zheng 2012	19	36	10	36	4.1%	2.91 [1.09, 7.74]	
Zhong 2008	6	44	2	22	2.0%	1.58 [0.29, 8.55]	
Zhong 2011	13	14	9	14	0.6%	7.22 [0.72, 72.70]	
Subtotal (95% CI)		297		284	34.5%	1.77 [1.20, 2.59]	
Total events	147		118				
Heterogeneity: Chi² = 6.93, df = 7 (P = 0.44); I² = 0%							
Test for overall effect: Z = 2.90 (P = 0.004)							
4.1.3 Anemia							
Zhang 2012	36	50	22	50	5.4%	3.27 [1.42, 7.52]	
Zhong 2008	1	44	0	22	0.6%	1.55 [0.06, 39.65]	
Zhong 2011	6	14	4	14	2.0%	1.88 [0.39, 9.01]	
Subtotal (95% CI)		108		86	7.9%	2.80 [1.37, 5.73]	
Total events	43		26				
Heterogeneity: Chi² = 0.51, df = 2 (P = 0.77); I² = 0%							
Test for overall effect: Z = 2.81 (P = 0.005)							
4.1.4 Liver dysfunction							
You 2012	26	50	20	55	8.0%	1.90 [0.87, 4.14]	
Zhang 2012	4	50	3	50	2.4%	1.36 [0.29, 6.43]	
Zhong 2011	1	14	8	14	6.5%	0.06 [0.01, 0.57]	
Subtotal (95% CI)		114		119	16.8%	1.11 [0.60, 2.06]	
Total events	31		31				
Heterogeneity: Chi² = 8.25, df = 2 (P = 0.02); I² = 76%							
Test for overall effect: Z = 0.34 (P = 0.73)							
4.1.5 No-infection fever							
Peng 2012	0	23	7	24	6.3%	0.05 [0.00, 0.93]	
Shi 2012	0	30	4	30	3.9%	0.10 [0.00, 1.88]	
Zhong 2008	0	44	4	22	5.1%	0.05 [0.00, 0.90]	
Zhong 2011	3	14	10	14	6.8%	0.11 [0.02, 0.61]	
Subtotal (95% CI)		111		90	22.1%	0.08 [0.02, 0.26]	
Total events	3		25				
Heterogeneity: Chi² = 0.39, df = 3 (P = 0.94); I² = 0%							
Test for overall effect: Z = 4.15 (P < 0.0001)							
Total (95% CI)		804		734	100.0%	1.33 [1.05, 1.70]	
Total events	340		301				
Heterogeneity: Chi² = 46.08, df = 22 (P = 0.002); I² = 52%							
Test for overall effect: Z = 2.33 (P = 0.02)							
Test for subgroup differences: Not applicable							

0.02   0.1   1   10   50
Favours CIK   Favours Non-CIK

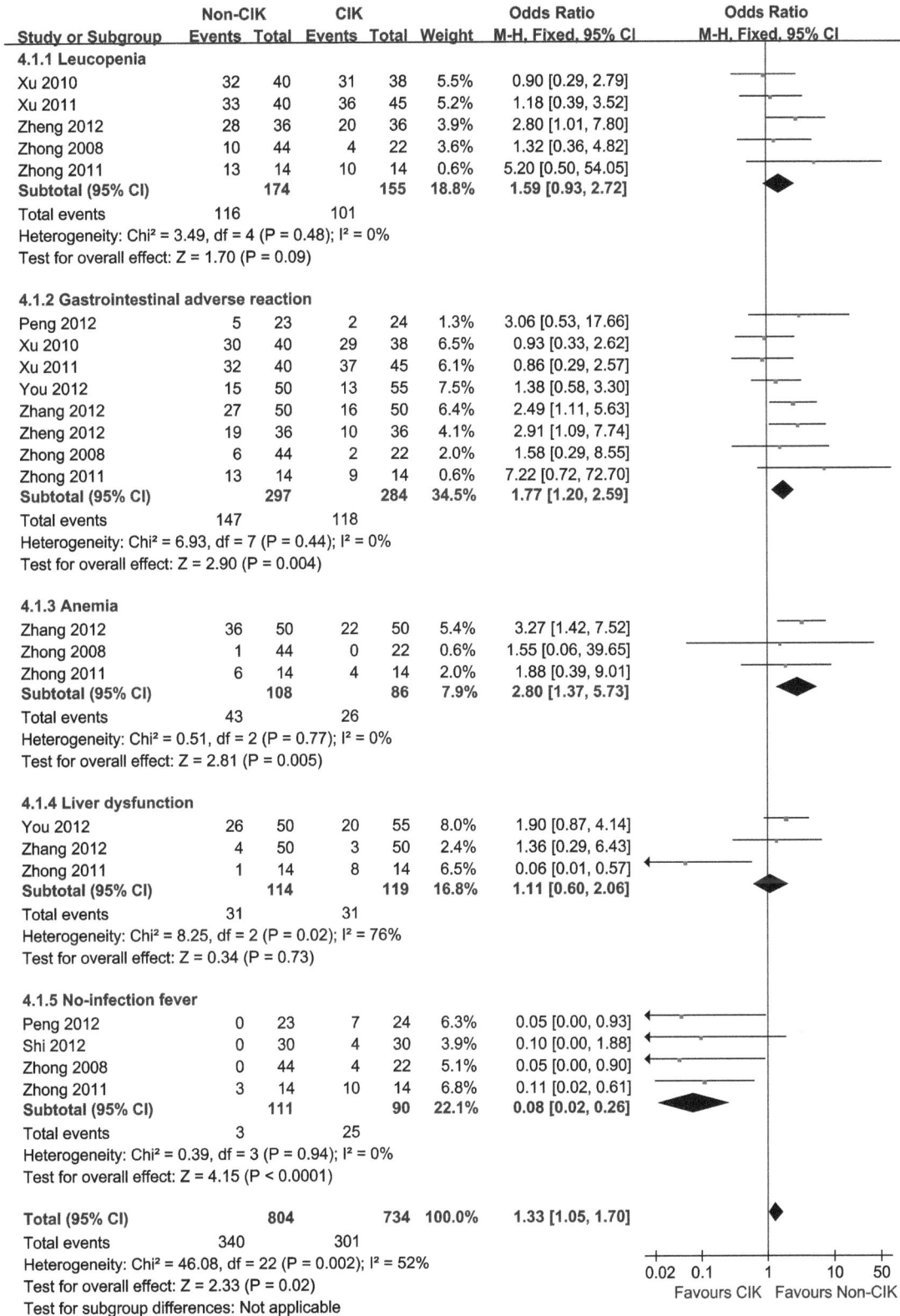

Figure 3. Forest plot comparing the toxicity and no treatment-related side effects between the CIK group and the non-CIK group.
Some serious adverse effects were observed significantly less frequently in the CIK group. Due to the lack of heterogeneity, the fixed-effect model was used.

main effector cells are eosinophils, basophils, and mast cells, as well as IgE B cells and IL-4/IL-5 CD4 T cells [27]. T regulatory cells express FoxP3 and produce TGF-β and $CD4^+CD25^+CD127^-$ T subgroups to suppress immune responses against Th1 and Th2. In addition, tumor cells also express high levels of $CD4^+CD25^+$ Treg cells, which help direct immunosuppressive cytokines to the tumor microenvironment [28], so the decrease of the Treg cell may be helpful to remove the immunosuppressive effect for NSCLC patients, and our results also demonstrated a lower number of Treg cells. Higher proportions of Treg and proliferating $CD8^+$ T cells were both associated with poor survival in malignancies lung cancer [41], suggesting that DC-CIK immunotherapy may play a role in enhancing the immune function of NSCLC patients.

Immunotherapy exerts its effect on the cellular immune response and requires time for immune cytokines to change the tumor burden or survival time. In our present study, we also evaluated T lymphocyte immune activity by Ag-NORs *in vivo* and the NSCLC tumor marker CEA. The significant increase in Ag-NORs ($p = 0.00001$) and the reduction in the CEA content ($p = 0.0008$) observed in the CIK group contributed to the prevention of short-term recurrence and improvement of clinical responses. We also analyzed clinical survival outcomes, clinical response rates, immunophenotypes and tumor markers, and we hypothesized that the CIK cells fight with tumor cells in several different ways, including direct cellular interactions (Fas/FasL pathway, granzyme B), the secretion of cytokines (IFN-γ, TNF-α, IL-2) and antibodies, and immune response regulations (T-lymphocyte variations) [29]. In all, our meta-analysis evaluated a variety of T-cell subgroups, and the differences in the cytokines used for immunotherapy, and we found that the results were consistent with the clinical therapeutic outcomes, such as the overall survival and clinical response.

In our analysis, CIK cell-based therapy yielded a disappointing result in non-infective fever ($P<0.0001$), and no other major side effect was observed. The pooled analysis showed that the adverse effects of gastrointestinal adverse reactions ($p = 0.004$) and anemia ($p = 0.005$) generated significant differences with fewer episodes in the CIK group. Thus, CIK cell immunotherapy with chemotherapy has proven to be a feasible and effective method for the treatment of NSCLC without severe side effects.

Limitation of the study

The 17 trials included in this meta-analysis were selected with an RCT to improve statistical reliability. To avoid bias in the identification and selection of trials, we minimized the possibility of overlooking published papers to the greatest extent. Although we selected using RCT as much as possible, there are some major criteria that did not receive a good grade under the Jadad scale, such as allocation concealment and intention-to-treat, meaning our study may have a moderate risk of bias. We also used a funnel plot to evaluate the publication bias. In our analysis, overall survival, clinical response rate, and side effects suffered low published bias; however, immunological assessment and T cell subgroups observed a high published bias. Therefore, there are some limitations to our study. First, CIK cell-based therapy is a greater concern for Chinese scholars; therefore, all 17 selected trials were from Asia, because there is a global lack of any multinational large-sample multicenter clinic research regarding CIK cell therapy for NSCLC. Second, some of the papers had to be excluded due to the lack of a control arm during the experimental design; however, some of the papers produced even better prognosis after the CIK treatment. Third, our analyzed data were selected from published papers rather than drawn first-hand

from patient records, potentially causing an overestimation of the analytical results. Therefore, only the enrollment of a larger sample could minimize this bias. However, various crucial issues for CIK cell-based immunotherapy need to be conquered before it can be approved as a standard treatment for NSCLC tumors due to several obstacles. First, the different dosage and treatment regimens of CIK cell transfusions may lead to different outcomes and immune responses. Second, although most of our selected papers focused on therapeutic outcomes based on chemotherapy RECIST criteria, due to the different tumor killing mechanisms, a novel immune-related response criterion (irRC) should also be used for the assessment of immunotherapy clinical activities [40]. Third, due to the poor immunogenicity of NSCLC, optimizing DC modifications combined with CIK cell infusion may contribute to more favorable clinical outcomes in NSCLC patients.

Taken together, the CIK-combined therapy for NSCLC presented a significantly prolonged overall survival, an improved clinical response rate, a strengthened immune system, and low rates of adverse side effects. The CIK therapy is more concerned with reducing the tumor burden stage than curing cancer. The CIK adoptive immune therapy showed potential regarding improved clinical outcomes, and there is increasing evidence that the CIK therapy treatment of NSCLC evokes specific humoral and cellular antitumor immune responses. However, the timing of the immunotherapy, dosage, regimens and efficient tumor antigens still require further research.

Conclusion

In total, 17 randomized controlled trials of NSCLC with 1172 patients were included in the present analysis. Combined CIK cell therapy for the treatment of NSCLC demonstrated significant superiority in terms of overall survival and objective response compared with the non-CIK group. The T-lymphocyte subgroups also seemed to favorably affect the immune system after chemotherapy. The data also indicated that CIK therapy relieves the side effects of chemotherapy without causing any additional major side effects aside from non-infective fever. This analysis supports a further larger-scale meta-analysis for the evaluation of the efficacy of CIK adoptive cell therapy for the treatment of NSCLC in the future.

Acknowledgments

This research work was supported by the National Natural Science Foundation of China (No. 31171427 and 30971651 to Zheng-Xu Wang), Beijing Municipal Science and Technology Project for Clinical Characteristics and Application Research of Capital (No. Z121107001012136 to Zheng-Xu Wang); the National Natural Science Foundation of China (No. 30700974 to Jun-Xia Cao) and the Postdoctoral Foundation of China (No. 20060400775 to Jun-Xia Cao).

Author Contributions

Conceived and designed the experiments: ZXW. Performed the experiments: MW JXC. Analyzed the data: MW JXC BLX XYZ J. Li J. Liu

HBW. Contributed reagents/materials/analysis tools: JHP YSL DL. Wrote the paper: MW JXC.

References

1. Parkin DM, Bray F, Ferlay J, Pisani P (2005) Global cancer statistics. CA Cancer J Clin 55: 74–108.
2. Chen WQ, Zheng RS, Zhang SW, Zhao P, Li GG, et al. (2013) Chinese cancer registration annual report: National cancer registration center of lung cancer. Chin J Cancer Res 25(1): 10–21.
3. Arango BA, Castrellon AB, Santos ES, Raez LE (2009) Second-line therapy for non-small-cell lung cancer. Clin Lung Cancer 10(2): 91–98.
4. National Institutes of Health (2012) Cancer of the Lung and Bronchus-SEER Stat Facts Sheet. http://seer.cancer.gov/statfacts/htm/lungb.html.
5. Jiang J, Liang X, Zhou X, Huang R, Chu Z, et al. (2013) Non-platinum doublets were as effective as platinum-based doublets for chemotherapy-naïve advanced non-small-cell lung cancer in the era of third-generation agents. J Cancer Res Clin Oncol 139(1): 25–38.
6. Wu C, Jiang J, Shi L, Xu N (2008) Prospective study of chemotherapy in combination with cytokine-induced killer cells in patients suffering from advanced non-small cell lung cancer. Anticancer Res 28(6B): 3997–4002.
7. Choi D, Kim TG, Sung YC (2012) The past, present, and future of adoptive T cell therapy. Immune Netw 12(4): 139–147.
8. Sangiolo D (2011) Cytokine induced killer cells as promising immunotherapy for solid tumors. J Cancer 2: 363–368.
9. Rutella S, Iudicone P, Bonanno G, Fioravanti D, Procoli A, et al. (2012) Adoptive immunotherapy with cytokine-induced killer cells generated with a new good manufacturing practice-grade protocol. Cytotherapy 14(7): 841–850.
10. Schmidt-Wolf IG, Finke S, Trojaneck B, Denkena A, Lefterova P, et al. (1999) Phase I clinical study applying autologous immunological effector cells transfected with the interleukin-2 gene in patients with metastatic renal cancer, colorectal cancer and lymphoma. Br J Cancer 81: 1009–1016.
11. Ma Y, Zhang Z, Tang L, Xu YC, Xie ZM, et al. (2012) Cytokine-induced killer cells in the treatment of patients with solid carcinomas: a systematic review and pooled analysis. Cytotherapy 14(4): 483–493.
12. Hontscha C, Borck Y, Zhou H, Messmer D, Schmidt-Wolf IG (2011) Clinical trials on CIK cells: first report of the international registry on CIK cells (IRCC). J Cancer Res Clin Oncol 137(2): 305–310.
13. Li XD, Xu B, Wu J, Ji M, Xu BH, et al. (2012) Review of Chinese clinical trials on CIK cell treatment for malignancies. Clin Transl Oncol 14(2): 102–108.
14. Jäkel CE, Hauser S, Rogenhofer S, Müller SC, Brossart P, et al. (2012) Clinical studies applying cytokine induced killer cells for the treatment of renal cell carcinoma. Clin Dev Immunol 2012: 473245.
15. Ma Y, Xu YC, Tang L, Zhang Z, Wang J, et al. (2011) Cytokine-induced killer (CIK) cell therapy for patients with hepatocellular carcinoma: efficacy and safety. Exp Hematol Oncol 1(1): 11.
16. Wang ZX, Cao JX, Liu ZP, Cui YX, Li CY, et al. (2014) Combination of chemotherapy and immunotherapy for colon cancer in China: A meta-analysis. World J Gastroenterol 20(4): 1095–1106.
17. Li H, Wang C, Yu J, Cao S, Wei F, et al. (2009) Dendritic cell-activated cytokine-induced killer cells enhance the anti-tumor effect of chemotherapy on non-small cell lung cancer in patients after surgery. Cytotherapy 11(8): 1076–1083.
18. Mo C, Gao J, Wang J, Huang Y, Wu X, et al. (2005) Clinical efficacy of DC-activated and cytokine-induced killer cells combined with chemotherapy in treatment of advanced lung cancer. Chinese J Cancer Biotherapy 17(4): 419–423. doi: 10. 3872/j. issn. 1007-385X. 2010. 04. 011.
19. Peng D, Li J, Yuan J, Liu Y, Yu W, et al. (2012) Efficacy and safety of autologous DC and CIK cells cominedPemetrexed in the treatment of elderly patients with non-small cell lung cancer. Chinese J Immunol 28(7): 648–652. doi: 10.3969/j.issn.1000-484X.2012. 07.017.
20. Sheng CH, Bao F, Xu S, Chang CY (2011) Clinical research on chemotherapy combined with dendritic cell-cytokine induced killer cells for non-small cell lung cancer. Journal of Practical Oncology 26(5): 503–506.
21. Shi SB, Ma TH, Li CH, Tang XY (2011) Effect of maintenance therapy with dendritic cells: cytokine-induced killer cells in patients with advanced non-small cell lung cancer. Tumori 98(3): 314–319.
22. Zhong R, Teng J, Han B, Zhong H (2011) Dendritic cells combining with cytokine-induced killer cells synergize chemotherapy in patients with late-stage non-small cell lung cancer. Cancer Immunol Immunother 60(10): 1497–1502.
23. Jadad AR, Moore RA, Carroll D, Jenkinson C, Reynolds DJ, et al. (1996) Assessing the quality of reports of randomized clinical trials: Is blinding necessary? Control Clin Trials 17: 1–12.
24. Shepherd FA, Douillard JY, Blumenschein GR Jr (2011) Immunotherapy for non-small cell lung cancer: novel approaches to improve patient outcome. J Thorac Oncol 6(10): 1763–1773.
25. Arens R, Schoenberger SP (2010) Plasticity in programming of effector and memory CD8 T-cell formation. Immunological Reviews 235: 190–205.
26. Mucida D, Cheroutre H (2010) The many face-lifts of CD4 T helper cells. Advances in Immunology 107: 139–152.
27. Neurath MF, Finotto S, Glimcher LH (2002) The role of Th1/Th2 polarization in mucosal immunity. Nature Medicine 8: 567–573.
28. Gallimore A, Godkin A (2008) Regulatory T cells and tumor immunity observations in mice and men. Immunology 123: 157–163.
29. Yu J, Zhang W, Jiang H, Li H, Cao S, et al. (2008) CD4+T cells in CIKs (CD4+ CIKs) reversed resistance to fas-mediated apoptosis through CD40/CD40L ligation rather than IFN-gamma stimulation. Cancer Biother Radio pharm 23(3): 342–354.
30. Li R, Wang C, Liu L, Du C, Cao S, et al. (2012) Autologous cytokine-induced killer cell immunotherapy in lung cancer: a phase II clinical study. Cancer Immunol Immunother 61(11): 2125–2133.
31. Xu Y, Xu D, Zhang N, Chen F, Liu J (2011) Observation of Chemotherapy Combined with Cytokine-induced Killer Cells and Dendritic Cells in Patients with the Advanced Non-Small Cell Lung Cancer. Prac J Cancer 25(2): 163–166.
32. Xu Y, Xu D, Zhang N, Chen F, Zhang G, et al. (2011) Effection of NP concurrent chemotherapy radiotherapy and sequential adoptive immunity cell for locally advanced non-small cell lung cancer. Chinese J Cancer Prev Treat 18(13): 1032–1035.
33. Yang L, Ren B, Li H, Yu J, Cao S, et al. (2013) Enhanced antitumor effects of DC-activated CIKs to chemotherapy treatment in a single cohort of advanced non-small-cell lung cancer patients. Cancer Immunol Immunother 62(1): 65–73.
34. You Z, Su X, Liu Y (2012) Observation on Clinical Efficacy of DC-CIK Biotherapy Auxiliary Interventional Chemotherapy on Central Non-Small-Cell Lung Carcinoma. Anti-tumor Phar 2(3): 193–196. doi: 10.3969/j.issn.2095-1264.2012.03.010.
35. Yuan J, Peng D, Li J (2011) Clinical effects of administering dendritic cells and cytokine induced killer cells combined with chemotherapy in the treatment of advanced non-small cell lung cancer. J Clin Pulmonary Med 16(12): 1910–1911.
36. Zhang J, Mao G, Han Y, Yang X, Feng H, et al. (2012) The clinical effects of DC-CIK cells combined with chemotherapy in the treatment of advanced NSCLC. Chin Ger J Clin Oncol 11(2): 67–71.
37. Zhong R, Han B, Zhong H, Gong L, Sha H, et al. (2008) Dendritic cells immunotherapy combined with chemotherapy inhibits postoperative recurrence and metastasis in stage IB of NSCLC after radical surgery. China Oncol 18(10): 760–764.
38. Zheng FC, Zhang XY, Feng HZ, Chen J, Sun Y, et al. (2012) Clinical Study of Stereotactic Conformal Body γ-knife Combined with Adoptive Immunotherapy (Dendritic Cell and Cytokine-induced Killer Cell) in the Treatment for Advanced Non-small Cell Lung Cancer. Journal of Chinese Oncology 18(11): 815–818.
39. Wang YY, Wang YS, Liu T, Yang K, Yang GQ, et al. (2013) Efficacy study of Cyber Knife stereotactic radio surgery combined with CIK cell immunotherapy for advanced refractory lung cancer. Exp Ther Med 5(2): 453–456.
40. Wolchok JD, Hoos A, O'DayS, Weber JS, Hamid O, et al. (2009) Guidelines for the evaluation of immune therapy activity in solid tumors: immune-related response criteria. Clin Cancer Res 15: 7412–7420.
41. McCoy MJ, Nowak AK, van der Most RG, Dick IM, Lake RA (2013) Peripheral CD8(+) T cell proliferation is prognostic for patients with advanced thoracic malignancies. Cancer Immunol Immunother 62(3): 529–539.

Permissions

The contributors of this book come from diverse backgrounds, making this book a truly international effort. This book will bring forth new frontiers with its revolutionizing research information and detailed analysis of the nascent developments around the world.

We would like to thank all the contributing authors for lending their expertise to make the book truly unique. They have played a crucial role in the development of this book. Without their invaluable contributions this book wouldn't have been possible. They have made vital efforts to compile up to date information on the varied aspects of this subject to make this book a valuable addition to the collection of many professionals and students.

This book was conceptualized with the vision of imparting up-to-date information and advanced data in this field. To ensure the same, a matchless editorial board was set up. Every individual on the board went through rigorous rounds of assessment to prove their worth. After which they invested a large part of their time researching and compiling the most relevant data for our readers.

The editorial board has been involved in producing this book since its inception. They have spent rigorous hours researching and exploring the diverse topics which have resulted in the successful publishing of this book. They have passed on their knowledge of decades through this book. To expedite this challenging task, the publisher supported the team at every step. A small team of assistant editors was also appointed to further simplify the editing procedure and attain best results for the readers.

Apart from the editorial board, the designing team has also invested a significant amount of their time in understanding the subject and creating the most relevant covers. They scrutinized every image to scout for the most suitable representation of the subject and create an appropriate cover for the book.

The publishing team has been an ardent support to the editorial, designing and production team. Their endless efforts to recruit the best for this project, has resulted in the accomplishment of this book. They are a veteran in the field of academics and their pool of knowledge is as vast as their experience in printing. Their expertise and guidance has proved useful at every step. Their uncompromising quality standards have made this book an exceptional effort. Their encouragement from time to time has been an inspiration for everyone.

The publisher and the editorial board hope that this book will prove to be a valuable piece of knowledge for researchers, students, practitioners and scholars across the globe.

List of Contributors

Zhengyu Ma
Department of Biomedical Research, Nemours/
A.I. duPont Hospital for Children, Wilmington,
Delaware, United States of America

David N. LeBard
Department of Chemistry, Yeshiva University, New
York, New York, United States of America

Sharon M. Loverde
Department of Chemistry, College of Staten Island,
City University of New York, Staten Island, New
York, United States of America

Kim A. Sharp
Department of Biochemistry and Biophysics,
University of Pennsylvania, Philadelphia,
Pennsylvania, United States of America

Michael L. Klein
Institute for Computational Molecular Science
and Department of Chemistry, Temple University,
Philadelphia, Pennsylvania, United States of
America

Dennis E. Discher
Department of Chemical and Biomolecular
Engineering, University of Pennsylvania,
Philadelphia, Pennsylvania, United States of
America

Terri H. Finkel
Department of Pediatrics, Nemours Children's
Hospital, Orlando, Florida, United States of America
Department of Biomedical Sciences, University
of Central Florida College of Medicine, Orlando,
Florida, United States of America

**Jadwiga Bienkowska, Norm Allaire, Alice Thai,
Jaya Goyal and Tatiana Plavina**
Translational Medicine, Biogen Idec, Cambridge,
Massachusetts, United States of America

**Ajay Nirula, Evan Beckman, Browning and Jeffrey
L.**
Immunobiology, Biogen Idec, Cambridge,
Massachusetts, United States of America

Megan Weaver, Charlotte Newman
Global Clinical Operations, Biogen Idec, Cambridge,
Massachusetts, United States of America

Michelle Petri
Johns Hopkins University School of Medicine,
Baltimore, Maryland, United States of America

**Isabel Cristina Can˜ eda-Guzmán, Norma Salaiza-
Suazo, Edith A. Fernández-Figueroa, Magdalena
Aguirre-García and Ingeborg Becker**
Unidad de Investigación en Medicina Experimental,
Facultad de Medicina, Universidad Nacional
Auto´noma de Mé xico, Hospital General de Mé
xico, México, D.F., México

Georgina Carrada-Figueroa
Universidad Autónoma Juárez de Tabasco,
Villahermosa, Tabasco, México

**Jill Seladi-Schulman, Patricia J. Campbell,
Suganthi Suppiah, John Steel and Anice C. Lowen**
Department of Microbiology and Immunology,
Emory University School of Medicine, Atlanta,
Georgia, United States of America

Karina Alves Toledo
Department of Biological Sciences, Universidade
Estadual Paulista – UNESP (FCL-Assis), Assis,
Brazil

**Marise Lopes Fermino, Camillo del Cistia
Andrade, Thalita Bachelli Riul, Renata Tomé
Alves, Vanessa Danielle Menjon Muller, Raquel
Rinaldi Russo, Victor Hugo Aquino and Marcelo
Dias-Baruffi**
Departmento de Análises Clínicas, Toxicoló gicas e
Bromatoló gicas,
Faculdade de Ciências Farmacêuticas de Ribeirão
Preto, Universidade de São Paulo, Ribeirão Preto,
Brazil

Sean R. Stowell and Richard D. Cummings
Emory University School of Medicine, Atlanta,
Georgia, United States of America

220   List of Contributors

Huawang Sun
Zhejiang Provincial Key Laboratory of Medical Genetics, School of Laboratory Medicine and Life Science, Wenzhou Medical University, Wenzhou, Zhejiang, China

Guo Li
College of Life Sciences, Zijingang Campus, Zhejiang University, Hangzhou, Zhejiang, China Institute of Aging Research, Hangzhou Normal University, Hangzhou, Zhejiang, China

Wenjuan Zhang, Jianxin Lu, Qi Zhou and Yena Yu
Zhejiang Provincial Key Laboratory of Medical Genetics, School of Laboratory Medicine and Life Science, Wenzhou Medical University, Wenzhou, Zhejiang, China

Ying Shi and Naiming Zhou
College of Life Sciences, Zijingang Campus, Zhejiang University, Hangzhou, Zhejiang, China

Stefan Offermanns
Department of Pharmacology, Max-Planck-Institute for Heart and Lung Research, Bad Nauheim, Germany

Mayumi Yoshimori and Honami Komatsu
Department of Hematology, Graduate School of Medical and Dental Sciences, Tokyo Medical and Dental University, Tokyo, Japan
Department of Laboratory Molecular Genetics of Hematology, Graduate School of Health Care Sciences, Tokyo Medical and Dental University, Tokyo, Japan

Ken-Ichi Imadome
Department of Infectious Diseases, National Research Institute for Child Health and Development, Tokyo, Japan

Ludan Wang, Tetsuya Fukuda, Osamu Miura and Ayako Arai
Department of Hematology, Graduate School of Medical and Dental Sciences, Tokyo Medical and Dental University, Tokyo, Japan

Yasunori Saitoh and Shoji Yamaoka
Department of Molecular Virology, Graduate School of Medical and Dental Sciences, Tokyo Medical and Dental University, Tokyo, Japan

Morito Kurata
Department of Comprehensive Pathology, Graduate School of Medical and Dental Sciences, Tokyo Medical and Dental University, Tokyo, Japan

Takatoshi Koyama
Department of Laboratory Molecular Genetics of Hematology, Graduate School of Health Care Sciences, Tokyo Medical and Dental University, Tokyo, Japan

Norio Shimizu
Department of Virology, Division of Medical Science, Medical Research Institute, Tokyo Medical and Dental University, Tokyo, Japan

Shigeyoshi Fujiwara
Department of Infectious Diseases, National Research Institute for Child Health and Development, Tokyo, Japan

Joanna Kern, Robert Drutel. , Silvia Leanhart, Marek Bogacz and Rafal Pacholczyk
Center for Biotechnology and Genomic Medicine, Georgia Regents University, Augusta, Georgia, United States of America

Johanna Raffetseder, Elsje Pienaar..a , Robert Blomgran, Daniel Eklund, Veronika Patcha Brodin, Henrik Andersson, Amanda Welin.b and Maria Lerm
Division of Microbiology and Molecular Medicine, Department of Clinical and Experimental Medicine, Faculty of Health Sciences, Linko¨ ping University, Linko¨ ping, SE-58185, Sweden

Marcio Fronza
Departamento de Análises Clínicas, Toxicoló gicas e Bromatoló gicas, Faculdade de Ciências Farmacêuticas de Ribeirão Preto, Universidade de São Paulo, Ribeirão Preto, São Paulo, Brazil
Departamento de Farmácia, Universidade de Vila Velha, Vila Velha, Espirito Santo, Brazil

Guilherme F. Caetano, Marcel N. Leite, Thiago A. M. Andrade and Marco A. C. Frade
Departamento de Clínica Mé dica, Divisão de Dermatologia, Faculdade de Medicina de Ribeirão Preto, Universidade de Sa˜o Paulo, Ribeirão Preto, São Paulo, Brazil

Claudia S. Bitencourt, Lú cia H. Faccioli and Francisco W. G. Paula-Silva
Departamento de Análises Clínicas, Toxicoló gicas e Bromatoló gicas, Faculdade de Ciências Farmacêuticas de Ribeira~o Preto, Universidade de São Paulo, Ribeirão Preto, São Paulo, Brazil

Irmgard Merfort
Department of Pharmaceutical Biology and Biotechnology, University of Freiburg, Freiburg, Germany

Baoping Zhang and Jizeng Wang
School of Civil Engineering and Mechanics, Lanzhou University, Lanzhou, 730000, PR China
Key Laboratory of Mechanics on Disaster and Environment in Western China, The Ministry of Education of China, Lanzhou University, 730000, PR China
Institute of Biomechanics and Medical Engineering, Lanzhou University, Lanzhou, 730000, PR China

Bin Liu
Institute of Biomechanics and Medical Engineering, Lanzhou University, Lanzhou, 730000, PR China
Department of Heavy Ion Radiation Medicine, Institute of Modern Physics, Chinese Academy of Sciences, Lanzhou 730000, PR China

Hong Zhang
Department of Heavy Ion Radiation Medicine, Institute of Modern Physics, Chinese Academy of Sciences, Lanzhou 730000, PR China

Mary M. Christopher
Department of Pathology, Immunology and Microbiology, University of California Davis, Davis, CA, 95616, United States of America

Michelle G. Hawkins
Department of Medicine and Epidemiology, University of California Davis, Davis, CA, 95616, United States of America

Andrew G. Burton
William R. Pritchard Veterinary Medical Teaching Hospital, University of California Davis, Davis, CA, 95616, United States of America

Ming-Qiang Zhang, Yang Jin, Jian-Bao Xin, Jian-Chu Zhang, Xian-Zhi Xiong, Long Chen and Gang Chen
Department of Respiratory and Critical Care Medicine, Key Laboratory of Pulmonary Diseases of Health Ministry, Union Hospital, Tongji Medical College, Huazhong University of Science and Technology, Wuhan, China

Yong Wan
Department of Respiratory and Critical Care Medicine WUHAN NO. 1 HOSPITAL, Wuhan, China

Flavio De Maio, Mariachiara Minerva, Ivana Palucci, Camassa, Michela Sali, Maurizio Sanguinetti, Giovanni Delogu and Raffaella Iantomasi
Institute of Microbiology, Universita' Cattolica del Sacro Cuore, Rome, Italy

Valentina Palmieri, Giuseppe Maulucci and Marco De Spirito
Institute of Physics, Universita' Cattolica del Sacro Cuore, Rome, Italy

Serena Wilber and t Bitter
Department of Medical Microbiology and Infection Control, VU University Medical Center, Amsterdam, Netherlands

Riccardo Manganelli and Saber Anoosheh
Department of Molecular Medicine, University of Padua, Padua, Italy

Kenji Sato
Department of Dermatology, Kochi Medical School, Kochi University, Nankoku, Japan
Pharmacology Department, Drug Research Center, Kaken Pharmaceutical Co., Ltd., Kyoto, Japan

Mikiro Takaishi and Shigetoshi Sano
Department of Dermatology, Kochi Medical School, Kochi University, Nankoku, Japan

Shota Tokuoka
Pharmacology Department, Drug Research Center, Kaken Pharmaceutical Co., Ltd., Kyoto, Japan

Conor Feehily, Aiden Finnerty and Conor P. O'Byrne
Bacterial Stress Response Group, Microbiology, School of Natural Sciences, College of Science, National University of Ireland, Galway, Galway, Ireland

Pat G. Casey, Colin Hill and Cormac G. M. Gahan
Alimentary Pharmabiotic Centre and School of Microbiology, University College Cork, Cork, Ireland

Kimon-Andreas G. Karatzas
Food Biosciences, University of Reading, Reading, United Kingdom

Min Wang, Yi-Shan Liu, Bei-Lei Xu, Duo Li, Xiao-Yan Zhang, Jun-Li Li, Jin-Long Liu, Hai-Bo Wang, Zheng-Xu Wang and Jun-Xia Cao
Biotherapy Center, General Hospital of Beijing Military Command, Beijing, China

Jian-Hong Pan
Department of Biostatistics, Peking University Clinical Research Institute, Peking University Health Science Center, Beijing, China

Index

www.ingramcontent.com/pod-product-compliance
Lightning Source LLC
Chambersburg PA
CBHW082059190326
41458CB00010B/3529